Coccidiosis in Livestock, Poultry, Companion Animals, and Humans

Praise for the Book

Coccidiosis in Livestock, Poultry, Companion Animals, and Humans is a long needed update and review for this group of clinically important protozoan parasites that infect a wide variety of hosts. It's been 25 years since the coccidia were thoroughly reviewed with updated information so it's timely and needed. The group of internationally recognized authors and subject matter experts have updated important aspects about Coccidiosis including detailed chapters on their biology, phylogeny, immunity, vaccination, modern molecular biology techniques, anticoccidial drugs, and new information on the coccidia of cattle. *Coccidiosis in Livestock, Poultry, Companion Animals, and Humans* will be a must have comprehensive resource for a wide range of global scientific disciplines for upper level undergraduate and graduate students, and researchers that include veterinary parasitologists, veterinarians, physicians, clinicians, and animal and poultry scientists.

Dr. Daniel E. Snyder
Veterinary Parasitology Consultant
Daniel E. Snyder, DVM, PhD Consulting, LLC

This book focuses on the genera *Eimeria, Cyclospora* and *Cystisospora*, which are apicomplexan parasites, known as conventional coccidia, and cause coccidiosis. Coccidiosis is one of the most important diseases of livestock, particularly poultry, but occurs also in many other farm and companion animals, as well as in humans. Coccidiosis has a huge economic impact, and represents a constant threat to the food supply. The extensive use of coccidiostats, especially against *Eimeria* in poultry, has led to widespread drug resistance, and this problem needs to be solved in the years to come, as there are many challenges ahead in order to ensure food security, but also food safety, for an ever-growing population on this planet. A plethora of studies on different aspects of coccidian biology, phylogeny, pathogenesis and treatment and prevention strategies have been carried out and published during the last 20–30 years, and it has become difficult to keep track and maintain an overview of the research developments in the field. Thus, this book summarizes in a concise and very structured manner the current knowledge on coccidiosis caused by conventional coccidia, and as such fills an important gap.

The driving force behind this book has been Dr. Jitender P. Dubey, which is clearly one of the most eminent parasitologists on this planet, and also known for his excellent books on *Toxoplasma, Cryptosporidium, Sarcocystis* and *Neospora*. Here, Dr. Dubey recruited scientists of high international reputation from all over the world to contribute chapters on the basic biology of coccidia, phylogeny, host immunity, vaccination, genomics, transcriptomics and proteomics, and on the current state of anti-coccidial drugs. These seven chapters provide an excellent and up-to-date overview on the covered subjects. The following chapters are dedicated to coccidiosis in the different major livestock species, including cattle, water buffaloes, pigs, sheep, goats, and most important, poultry. However, also other host species are covered, including camelids, rabbits, turkeys, ducks, horse and other equids, dogs, cats, and also humans. In these chapters the reader will encounter concise information on the different species of coccidia found in the different host species, the life cycle and morphological features, data on prevalence, on the pathogenesis, diagnosis, management and treatment options.

The book also contains stunning illustrations, showing the morphological, histological and structural features of the different coccidia, and how infections affect their hosts and cause disease. In addition, many tables are provided that summarize all this information in a concise and clear manner. Overall, I believe that this book represents an invaluable, highly useful resource and "must-have" for all interested in coccidian parasites, including students, biologists, veterinarians, parasitologists, government, academia and industry.

Dr. Andrew Hemphill
Institute of Parasitology
Department of Infectious Diseases and Pathobiology
Universität Bern
Switzerland

Coccidiosis in Livestock, Poultry, Companion Animals, and Humans

Edited by
J. P. Dubey

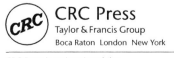

CRC Press
Taylor & Francis Group
Boca Raton London New York

CRC Press is an imprint of the
Taylor & Francis Group, an **informa** business

CRC Press
Taylor & Francis Group
6000 Broken Sound Parkway NW, Suite 300
Boca Raton, FL 33487-2742

First issued in paperback 2022

© 2020 by Taylor & Francis Group, LLC
CRC Press is an imprint of Taylor & Francis Group, an Informa business

No claim to original U.S. Government works

ISBN-13: 978-0-367-26592-2 (hbk)
ISBN-13: 978-1-03-233759-3 (pbk)
DOI: 10.1201/9780429294105

**Visit the Taylor & Francis Web site at
http://www.taylorandfrancis.com**

**and the CRC Press Web site at
http://www.crcpress.com**

*This book is dedicated to the memory of Drs. László P. Pellérdy (1907–1974),
Norman D. Levine (1912–1999), Datus M. Hammond (1911–1974),
Erich O. Scholtyseck (1918–1985), and Peter L. Long (1928–2005)
for their contributions to coccidiosis.*

Contents

Preface

Coccidiosis is one of the most important diseases of livestock, particularly poultry. Billions of dollars are spent on prevention worldwide to minimize coccidiosis in poultry. Traditionally, coccidiosis was considered an intestinal disease, caused by several distinct *Eimeria* species. The disease is so important and pervasive that until recently all poultry feed was medicated with anticoccidial drugs, mainly antibiotics. With the rapid development of drug resistance, and the increasing concern of feeding antibiotics to food animals and potential impact on public health, research has been directed to finding alternative methods of control of coccidiosis in poultry. Until 1970, coccidian parasites were considered host specific and confined to mainly the intestine. With the discovery of *Toxoplasma* as a coccidian of cats and infections in all warm-blooded hosts and subsequent discovery of *Sarcocystis*, and *Neospora* as coccidian parasites with generalized infections, research interest and activities in "conventional" coccidia, *Eimeria*, declined because of lack of funding and scientific researchers. There has been an explosion of research on non-*Eimeria* coccidians in the last 40 years. I have been involved in writing books on three subjects published by CRC Press: *Toxoplasma* (*Toxoplasmosis of Animals and Humans*, first edition, Dubey and Beattie, 1988; second edition, Dubey, 2010), *Sarcocystis* (*Sarcocystosis of Animals and Humans*, first edition, Dubey, Speer, and Fayer, 1989; second edition, Dubey, Calero-Bernal, Rosenthal, Speer, and Fayer, 2016), and *Neospora* (*Neosporosis in Animals*, Dubey, Hemphill, Calero-Bernal, and Schares, 2017). Additionally, I edited a multiauthored book on *Cryptosporidium* (*Cryptosporidiosis in Man and Animals*, Dubey, Speer, and Fayer, 1990).

All books on conventional coccidiosis were written more than 25 years ago (*The Coccidia*, Hammond and Long, University Park Press, 1973; *The Biology of Coccidia*, Long, Edward Arnold Press, 1982; *Coccidiosis of Man and Domestic Animals*, Long, CRC Press, 1990), and many of their authors are now deceased. Furthermore, in the last three books by Dr. Long, a lot of text was related to *Sarcocystis* and *Toxoplasma*. Thus, there is a need for a book dealing exclusively with conventional coccidia (*Eimeria, Cyclospora,* and *Cystoisospora*). Here, I enlisted scientists with international repute and specialized knowledge to write chapters on all major livestock species including cattle, pigs, sheep, and goats. Special emphasis is given to poultry coccidiosis because of economic impact. There are chapters on phylogeny, molecular biology, host-pathogen immunobiology and immunoprophylaxis, vaccines, genetics and genomics, biology, and chemotherapy. There is a special chapter on coccidiosis in chickens in China because most of the literature is in Chinese and often in local journals. There is also a chapter on intestinal coccidiosis in humans, including *Cyclospora*. We provide concise, authoritative, up-to-date information on coccidiosis, especially research in the last 28 years. Each host species chapter includes information on different species of coccidia, life cycle and biology, prevalence, epidemiology, pathogenesis, diagnosis, and treatment. All references are alphabetized by the first author and appear at the end of the book for the benefit of readers. Originals of each research papers were obtained to avoid mistakes in citations.

It is hoped that this book will be useful to biologists, veterinarians, parasitologists, and researchers from government, academia, and industry.

I would like to acknowledge those who made this possible; I cannot possibly list all of them. Christian Bauer from Germany and David Lindsay from the United States, and Camila Cezar, Fernando Murata, Meghan Sadler, and Oliver Kwok from my laboratory worked tirelessly to make this book possible.

J. P. Dubey

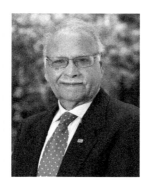

J. P. Dubey, MVSc, PhD, DSc, was born in India. He earned his veterinary degree in 1960 from Veterinary College, Mhow, India and masters in veterinary parasitology in 1963, from Veterinary College, Mathura, India. He earned a PhD in medical microbiology in 1966 from the University of Sheffield, England. Dr. Dubey received postdoctoral training from 1968 to 1973 with Dr. J.K. Frenkel, Department of Pathology and Oncology, University of Kansas Medical Center, Kansas City, Kansas. From 1973 to 1978, he was an associate professor of veterinary parasitology, Department of Pathobiology, Ohio State University, Columbus, Ohio, and professor of veterinary parasitology, Department of Veterinary Science, Montana State University, Bozeman, Montana, from 1978 to 1982. He is presently a senior scientist, Animal Parasitic Diseases Laboratory, Beltsville Agricultural Research Center, Agricultural Research Service, United States Department of Agriculture (USDA), Beltsville, Maryland.

Dr. Dubey has spent more than 55 years researching coccidian parasites, including *Eimeria*, *Toxoplasma*, *Neospora*, *Sarcocystis*, and related cyst-forming coccidian parasites of humans and animals. He has published over 1500 research papers in international journals. In 1985, he was chosen to be the first recipient of the Distinguished Veterinary Parasitologist Award by the American Association of Veterinary Parasitologists. Dr. Dubey is the recipient of the 1995 WAAVP Pfizer Award for outstanding contributions to research in veterinary parasitology. He also received the 2005 Eminent Parasitologists Award by the American Society of Parasitologists. The Thomson Institute for Scientific Information identified him as one of the world's most cited authors in plant and animal sciences for the last decade. In 2003, he was selected for the newly created Senior Science and Technology Service (SSTS) and is one of the few such scientists and executives within the USDA's Agricultural Research Service (USDA-ARS); selection for this position is by invitation only, on approval by the Secretary of Agriculture. In 2010, Dr. Dubey was elected to the U.S. National Academy of Sciences, Washington, DC, and inducted in the USDA-ARS Hall of Fame. In 2018, he was the first recipient of the William C. Campbell One-Health Award by the American Association of Veterinary Parasitologists. In the same year, he received the honorary Doctor of Science degree from McGill University, Montréal, Québec, Canada.

Contributors

G. Albanese
Departments of Population Health and Poultry Science
Poultry Diagnostic and Research Center
University of Georgia
Athens, Georgia

S. Almeria
Food and Environmental Microbiology
Office of Applied Research and Safety Assessment
Food and Drug Administration
Laurel, Maryland

B. Bangoura
Wyoming State Veterinary Laboratory
Department of Veterinary Sciences
University of Wyoming
Laramie, Wyoming

C. Bauer
Institute of Parasitology
Justus Liebig University Giessen
Giessen, Germany

D. Blake
Parasite Genetics, Pathobiology and Population Sciences
Royal Veterinary College
North Mymms
Hertfordshire, United Kingdom

R. Calero-Bernal
Department of Animal Health
Complutense University of Madrid
Madrid, Spain

C. K. Cerqueira-Cézar
Oak Ridge Institute for Science and Education (ORISE)
    Research Fellow
U.S. Department of Agriculture
Agricultural Research Service
Animal Parasitic Diseases Laboratory
Beltsville, Maryland

H. D. Chapman
Department of Poultry Science
University of Arkansas
Fayetteville, Arkansas

A. Chaudhury
Oak Ridge Institute for Science and Education (ORISE)
    Research Fellow at the Animal Biosciences and
    Biotechnology Laboratory
U.S. Department of Agriculture
Beltsville, Maryland

H. N. Cinar
U.S. Food and Drug Administration
Laurel, Maryland

A. Daugschies
Institute for Parasitology
Leipzig University
Leipzig, Germany

J. P. Dubey
U.S. Department of Agriculture
Agricultural Research Service
Animal Parasitic Diseases Laboratory
Beltsville, Maryland

U. Gadde
Huvepharma Inc.
Peachtree City, Georgia

M. C. Jenkins
U.S. Department of Agriculture
Agricultural Research Service
Animal Parasitic Diseases Laboratory
Beltsville, Maryland

A. Joachim
Institute of Parasitology, Department of Pathobiology
Veterinärmedizinische Universität Wien/Vetmeduni
    Vienna
Wien, Austria

B. Jordan
Departments of Population Health and
    Poultry Science
Poultry Diagnostic and Research Center
University of Georgia
Athens, Georgia

W. H. Kim
Oak Ridge Institute for Science and Education (ORISE)
    Research Fellow at the Animal Biosciences and
    Biotechnology Laboratory
U.S. Department of Agriculture
Agricultural Research Service
Beltsville, Maryland

O. C. H. Kwok
U.S. Department of Agriculture
Agricultural Research Service
Animal Parasitic Diseases Laboratory
Beltsville, Maryland

H. S. Lillehoj
Poultry Immunology, Genomics and Disease Resistance
Animal Biosciences and Biotechnology Laboratory
U.S. Department of Agriculture
Agricultural Research Service
Beltsville, Maryland

D. S. Lindsay
Department of Biomedical Science and Pathology
Virginia Maryland College of Veterinary Medicine
Center for One Health Research
Virginia Tech
Blacksburg, Virginia

X. Liu
College of Veterinary Medicine
China Agricultural University
Beijing, China

J. M. Molina
University of Las Palmas de G. C.
Faculty of Veterinary Medicine. Parasitology Unit
Las Palmas de Gran Canaria, Spain

F. H. A. Murata
Oak Ridge Institute for Science and Education (ORISE)
    Research Fellow
U.S. Department of Agriculture
Agricultural Research Service
Animal Parasitic Diseases Laboratory
Beltsville, Maryland

S. Noack
Molecular Discovery—Pharma R&D
Boehringer Ingelheim Vetmedica GmbH
Ingelheim am Rhein, Germany

M. Pakandl
Department of Research and Development
BIOPHARM, Research Institute of Biopharmacy and
    Veterinary Drugs
Prague. Czech Republic

T. Rathinam
Huvepharma Inc.
Peachtree City, Georgia

B. M. Rosenthal
U.S. Department of Agriculture
Agricultural Research Service
Animal Parasitic Diseases Laboratory
Beltsville, Maryland

A. Ruiz
Departmento de Patologia Animal
Produccion Animal, Bromatologia y Technologia de los
    Alimentos
University de Las Palmas de Gran Canaria
Las Palmas, Spain

R. K. Schuster
FTA Parasitology, FTA Tropical Veterinary Medicine
Central Veterinary Research Laboratory
Dubai, United Arab Emirates

P. M. Selzer
Molecular Discovery—Pharma R&D
Boehringer Ingelheim Vetmedica GmbH
Ingelheim am Rhein, Germany

A. Shrestha
Institute of Parasitology
Department of Pathobiology
Veterinärmedizinische Universität Wien/Vetmeduni
    Vienna
Wien, Austria

X. Suo
College of Veterinary Medicine
China Agricultural University
Beijing, China

L. Tensa
Departments of Population Health and Poultry Science
Poultry Diagnostic and Research Center
University of Georgia
Athens, Georgia

P. C. Thompson
U.S. Department of Agriculture
Agricultural Research Service
Animal Parasitic Diseases Laboratory
Beltsville, Maryland

F. Tomley
The Royal Veterinary College
North Mymms, Hatfield
Hertfordshire, United Kingdom

S. Wang
College of Veterinary Medicine
China Agricultural University
Beijing, China

CHAPTER 1

Biology of Intestinal Coccidia

J. P. Dubey, D. S. Lindsay, M. C. Jenkins, and C. Bauer

CONTENTS

1.1 INTRODUCTION AND BRIEF HISTORY

Coccidia have long been recognized as one of the most important groups of parasites that infect animals, especially domestic livestock. Most of the stages of the life cycle require a microscope for visualization, but some accumulations of stages cause gross lesions that can be observed in the intestinal tract. Coccidia were not discovered until the invention of the microscope by Leeuwenhoek, who probably saw coccidian life-cycle stages (now recognized as *Eimeria stiedai*) in the liver of a rabbit.[973–975] However, their economic importance was not realized until the early 1900s when outbreaks of bloody enteritis, caused by the coccidian *E. tenella*, were observed in the ceca of chickens.[228,232,1717] Despite improvements in modern animal husbandry practices, such as better management, hygiene, and sanitation, it is still almost impossible to raise livestock coccidia free.

Until the discovery of the two-host (polyxenous) life cycle of *Toxoplasma gondii* in 1970, conventional coccidia of the genus *Eimeria* were believed to have a simple oro-fecal one-host transmission life cycle with infections confined mostly to the intestines of the host. *T. gondii* is a tissue-dwelling coccidian that uses all warm-blooded animals, including humans, as intermediate hosts, but only felids can serve as the definitive host.[420] Since the discovery of the life cycle of *T. gondii*, a heteroxenous development has been demonstrated in several other coccidia as well. As stated in the preface, this book is concerned with those coccidia that have a direct life cycle completed in a single host,

Table 1.1   Different Genera Discussed in This Book

Genus	Sporocysts/ Oocyst	Sporozoites/per Sporocyst	Sporozoites/ Oocyst	Stieda Body	Tissue Cyst
Eimeria Schneider, 1875	4	2	8	Yes/no	No
Isospora Schneider, 1881	2	4	8	Yes	No
Cystoisospora Frenkel, 1977	2	4	8	No	Yes
Cyclospora Schneider, 1881	2	2	4	Yes	No
Wenyonella Hoare, 1933	4	4	16	Absent	No
Tyzzeria Allen, 1936	No	8 (free)	8	Present/absent	No

i.e., one-host parasites (homoxenous parasites). Only coccidia of domestic animals and humans are discussed in this book with minimal information on phylogeny of rodents, wildlife, fish, reptiles, and amphibians in Chapter 2. The taxonomy of these parasites is as follows:

Phylum: Apicomplexa; Levine, 1970
Class: Sporozoasida; Leuckart, 1879
Subclass: Coccidiasina; Leuckart, 1879
Order: Eimeriorina; Leger, 1911
Family: Eimeriidae Minchin, 1903

Definition: One-host parasites (homoxenous) with intracellular asexual and sexual development. Microgametes have two to three flagella, sporogony occurring outside the host.

The Family Eimeriidae and the genus *Eimeria* are named after Professor Theodor Eimer (1843–1898). Different genera of intestinal coccidia were initially distinguished based on the number of sporocysts within the oocyst and the number of sporozoites within each sporocyst (Table 1.1). Genera *Isospora* and *Cyclospora* were created by Professor Aimé Schneider (1844–1932), but their clinical importance was unknown until the 1970s. The genus *Wenyonella* was named after Charles Morley Wenyon (1878–1948), and the genus *Tyzzeria* was named after Ernest Edward Tyzzer (1875–1965); coccidians of both these genera parasitize only avians among the hosts discussed in this book. The genus *Cystoisospora* was created by Jacob Karl Frenkel (1921–2013) and is currently placed in Family Sarcocystidae; Poche, 1913.

Biologies of genera *Eimeria* and *Cystoisospora* are discussed in this chapter; genera *Tyzzeria* and *Isospora* are discussed in Chapter 18, and the genus *Cyclospora* is discussed in Chapter 22.

1.2 GENUS *EIMERIA* (SYN. *COCCIDIUM*)

1.2.1 Life Cycle of *Eimeria*

1.2.1.1 Oocyst

The **oocyst** is formed following sexual reproduction and is the result of fertilization of the macrogamont (female stage of the life cycle) by a microgamete (sperm) produced by a microgamont (male stage). It is the environmentally resistant stage of the life cycle that is excreted in feces. Initially, in freshly excreted feces, oocysts are unsporulated and not infectious (Figure 1.1A). Eimerian oocysts are from 10 to 108 μm long and vary in shape, size, and color depending on the species. Unsporulated oocysts contain a central mass (zygote, **sporont**) with a centrally located nucleus seen as a light area by light microscopy, and the sporont may occupy the whole oocyst, depending on the species (Figure 1.1A). The sporont is enclosed in a resilient oocyst wall, up to 11 μm thick, but in most species of *Eimeria* the wall is 1–3 μm thick. The oocyst wall has two to three layers and may be colorless, pale yellow, pinkish, or dark brown, with a smooth, pitted, or rough surface. In some species of *Eimeria*, the intracellular oocysts are enclosed in a thin layer (veil) that may be lost when oocysts are excreted in feces.[64]

The oocyst wall is permeable to gaseous exchange. Oocysts can remain viable and potentially infectious even after the removal of the outer layer by treatment with bleach (5%–6% sodium hypochlorite solution) (Figure 1.1C). At one pole, the oocyst wall may be thinned out (or partly absent); this area, if present, is called the **micropyle** (Figure 1.2)[1332] and may be covered by a dome-like structure, the micropylar cap. In some *Eimeria* species, caps are present at both poles.[1797] Small granules (polar granules) or hazy areas (hazy bodies) may be present between the sporont and the inner oocyst wall.

Oocyst maturation (sporulation) is an aerobic process that occurs in the environment. It depends on three factors, the presence of oxygen, temperatures between 10°C and 30°C, and humidity; sporulation is optimal between 22°C and 29°C. Meiosis (reduction division) occurs soon after excretion of unsporulated oocysts. In *E. tenella*, meiosis occurs within the first 8 hours of sporulation.[360] During early sporulation, the sporont shrinks and divides into four **sporoblasts**, each with a polar nucleus. After the mitotic division, from each sporoblast a **sporocyst** containing two sporozoites is formed (Figure 1.1C). Sporocysts may be circular, oval, piriform, or elongate and may contain a plug-like structure at one pole, the **Stieda body**. In some species of *Eimeria*, a substiedal body, below the Stieda body, may also be present (Figure 1.1C).[665] A residual mass, the oocyst residuum, is present in some *Eimeria* species, and its presence or absence in sporulated oocysts may be of taxonomic value.

Sporozoites are often banana shaped and contain a central vesicular nucleus, storage granules, and one or more

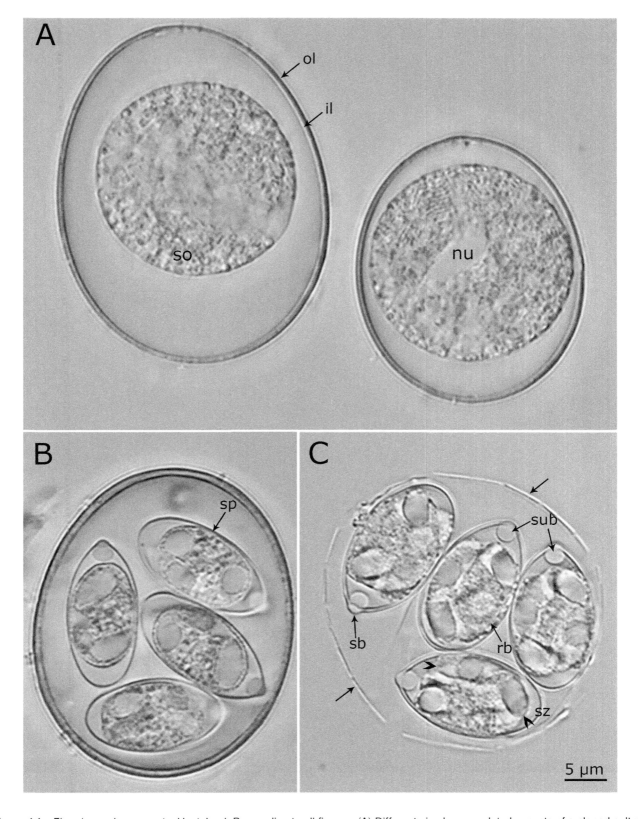

Figure 1.1 *Eimeria maxima* oocysts. Unstained. Bar applies to all figures. (A) Different-sized unsporulated oocysts of a cloned culture. The oocyst wall has two layers (ol, il), and a sporont (so) with a central nucleus (nu). (B) Sporulated oocysts with four sporocysts (st) (sp). (C) Partially flattened sporulated oocyst. The outer layer of wall has been removed by treatment with bleach (arrows). Note the Stieda (sb) and substida bodies (sub) at the narrow end of the sporocyst. Each sporocyst has two twisted sporozoites (sz) (opposing arrowheads) and a residual body (rb).

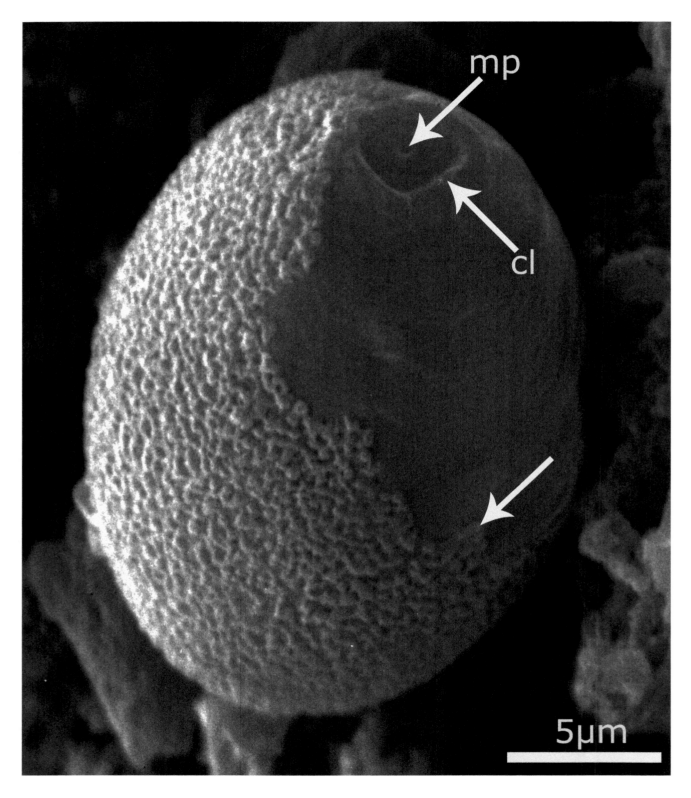

Figure 1.2   Scanning electron micrograph of *Eimeria stigmosa* oocyst. Note a micropyle (mp) surrounded by a collar (cl). The outer layer of the oocyst wall is corrugated and stripped (arrow) partly to expose the smooth inner layer. (Courtesy of Dr. Pecka, Z. Czech Republic.)[1322]

refractile bodies of varying sizes (Figure 1.1C). The refractile bodies are proteinaceous in nature, one to four in number, and may occupy two-thirds of the sporozoite[350,662]; they are thought to be linked to host cell invasion. Sporozoites of *Cystoisospora* do not have refractile bodies but have an inclusion called a crystalloid body in its place.

Oocysts can survive for months or years, depending on the species of *Eimeria* and environmental conditions. Anoxia, drought, and temperatures higher than 40°C are deleterious, and unsporulated oocysts are more susceptible to extremes of temperatures than when sporulated. Oocysts of ruminant coccidia can survive freezing temperatures and can over-winter on pastures. The survival of sporulated oocysts is dependent on stored energy reserves (polysaccharides) in their sporozoites. Sporulated oocysts are highly resistant to most commonly used disinfectants.[328]

1.2.1.2 Infection of the Host

Infection is acquired by ingesting sporulated oocysts present in contaminated food/litter, feces, or water. Sporozoites are released from oocysts inside the gut, and this process of excystation may differ depending on the host and the species of *Eimeria*.[1797] Sporozoites must first exit the sporocyst and then traverse the oocyst wall before they can be free to infect host intestinal cells. For example, in ruminants, passage through the rumen, exposure to carbon dioxide, and pH changes alter the oocyst wall increasing permeability to various molecules that induce excystation. In avian *Eimeria* species, passage through the gizzard can mechanically break the oocyst wall, thus facilitating release of the sporocysts. Exposure to bile salts and trypsin/chymotrypsin is considered key in excystation.[213] Bile salts stimulate motility of sporozoites, and their movement is noted before excystation occurs. During excystation, the Stieda and substiedal bodies are popped open or dissolved, thus allowing the escape of sporozoites. Excystation is completed in the small intestine. Not all oocysts excyst, and intact sporulated oocysts may be excreted in feces and retain their infectivity. Sporocysts of *Cystoisospora* do not contain Stieda bodies, and the excystation process is similar except the proteolytic enzymes act on sutures in plates in the sporocyst wall, and the sporocyst wall collapses along these plates to liberate sporozoites.

1.2.1.3 Asexual Development

Sporozoites are motile and migrate to the site of penetration/development by peristalsis or indirectly through host cells. They can rapidly enter enterocytes and remain inside them or leave to penetrate other cells.[65,263] Sporozoites of some species are carried to the lamina propria and to enterocytes of glands of Lieberkühn or to distant sites inside intraepithelial lymphocytes (IELs). As an example, *E. tenella* sporozoites are carried to ceca of chickens to continue their development; not all aspects of this transport are fully understood.

Once inside the enterocyte, sporozoites lose many of their organelles; this may take hours to several days dependent on the *Eimeria* species. In most *Eimeria* species, the sporozoite rounds up, to form a stage that has been called **trophozoite**.[264,265,974] We prefer the term **uninucleate zoite** because the trophozoites of *Eimeria* are nonmotile and contain a single nucleus to avoid confusion with the motile trophozoites of other protozoa that may contain two nuclei. In some *Eimeria* species (e.g., *E. auburnensis* of cattle,[265] *E. debliecki* of pigs,[1035] and *E. maxima* of chickens,[437] sporozoites retain their crescent shape and continue development and nuclear division—such organisms have been called **sporozoite-shaped schizonts**.[1423] They retain an intact apical complex, remain motile, and may escape from the original host cell and penetrate new cells. They can later transform into spheroidal schizonts and continue asexual development. In some *Eimeria* species (e.g., *Eimeria* species of rabbits), merozoites of the second generation can form multinucleated schizonts while retaining the crescent shape (see Chapter 14 on rabbits for more). The refractile body from the sporozoite can be carried through the divisional process and be present in merozoites.[584]

Intracellular sporozoites give rise to two or more organisms termed **merozoites**. Some *Eimeria* species can divide into two merozoites (Figures 1.3G and 1.4A), probably by endodyogeny (endo = inside, dyo = two, geny = progeny).[426] However, most *Eimeria* species divide by schizogony—a process in which the nucleus divides into four or more nuclei before merozoites are formed. The merozoites might be formed internally (endomerogony) or at the surface (ectomerogony)[659]; in most species of *Eimeria* of livestock, the division is by ectomerogony. Merozoites released from the schizonts may continue further cycles of multiplication; these have been designated as generations of schizonts. The concept of generations is based on time-limited occurrence of morphologically distinct schizonts and merozoites. For example, in *E. tenella*, there are three generations of schizonts.[974] Not all *Eimeria* species follow this sequence of development. As many as six generations of schizogony have been reported for *E. stiedai* of rabbits (see Chapter 14). The merozoites from different generations of schizogony may appear morphologically similar. We use the term **schizont** throughout the book, irrespective of the mode of division. Some authors use the term **merogony**, which is not specific to endodyogeny or schizogony.

In addition to asexual multiplication in enterocytes, some sporozoites might be transported to mesenteric lymph nodes and produce schizonts that can persist long after oocysts have been excreted in feces.[1044,1094]

The host cell and site of asexual development of schizonts may vary from an enterocyte to endothelial cell. The parasitized host cell nucleus can be indented and hypertrophied. Some species of *Eimeria* develop inside the host cell

Table 1.2 Unusual Aspects of *Eimeria* Species in Livestock and Poultry

Character	Species	Host	Remarks	Chapter
Largest oocysts	E. macusaniensis	Lama spp.	Up to 106 μm	13
	E. cameli	Camelus spp.	108 μm	12
	E. leuckarti	Equids	Up to 95 μm	19
Smallest oocyst	E. subspherica	Cattle	9–14 × 8–13 μm	7
Large schizonts	E. bovis	Cattle	Up to 435 μm	7
	E. zuernii	Cattle	Up to 338 μm	7
	E. auburnensis	Cattle	Up to 338 μm	7
	E. ninakohlyakimovae	Sheep	300 μm	9
	E. gilruthi	Sheep, goat	700 μm	10
Smallest schizonts	E. maxima	Chicken	5 μm	15
Large microgamonts	E. cameli	Camelus spp.	346 μm	12
	E. macusansiensis	Lama spp.	300 μm	13
	E. leuckarti	Equids	300 μm	19
Unusual location site	E. stiedai	Rabbit	Liver-bile duct	14
	E. alabamensis	Cattle	Host nucleus	7
	E. subspherica	Cattle	Host nucleus	7
	E. mulardi	Duck	Host nucleus	18
	E. gilruthi	Sheep, goat	Abomasum	9,10
	E. somateriae	Duck	Kidneys	18

nucleus, most notably *E. alabamensis* and *E. subspherica* of cattle (Table 1.2). Schizonts vary in size from 5 μm to being macroscopic and may contain hundreds of merozoites (Table 1.2; Figures 1.3 and 1.4).

1.2.1.4 Sexual Development

Merozoites released from the terminal schizogonic stage initiate the formation of male (micro) and female (macro) gamonts. In **microgamonts**, the nucleus divides several times and the nuclei move to the periphery of the cell, sometimes leaving a residual body (Figure 1.5). Two or three flagella are produced at the pole of the nucleus.

The **macrogamont** contains a single nucleus with a prominent nucleolus. With the growth of the macrogamont, the nucleus becomes surrounded by periodic acid Schiff (PAS)–positive granules, and eosinophilic forming bodies (wall-forming bodies [WFBs], also called plastic bodies) develop and migrate toward the periphery of the gamont (Figure 1.6). The WFB are of two types: WFB1 and WFB2.[1117] They vary in intensity of staining and size (Figure 1.6).

The microgamete swims to the macrogamont and fertilizes it. The secretion of WFB into membranes surrounding the developing macrogamont forms the oocyst wall (Figure 1.6). The oocyst wall has two to three layers. The unsporulated oocysts are liberated into the intestinal lumen and excreted in feces.

In Figure 1.7, the life cycle of *E. maxima* of chicken (*Gallus domesticus*) is depicted as an example. Asexual and sexual cycles of *E. maxima* take place in the small intestine but in different sites. First-generation schizonts are produced

in the glands of Lieberkühn, whereas the second and third generations of schizonts occur in villus enterocytes, and sexual stages are found in the lamina propria.

1.2.1.5 Extraintestinal Coccidia

Occasionally severe biliary and hepatic coccidiosis has been reported in cattle,[286] goats,[419] and dogs.[1053] These isolated cases are thought to be associated with unidentified species of intestinal coccidia. Presumably, merozoites or sporozoites from intestines are spilled over and colonize bile duct and gallbladder epithelium and induce severe inflammation to necrotic lesions. All stages from developing schizonts, gamonts, to unsporulated oocysts can be found in lesions (Figure 1.8).

The rare occurrence of these extraintestinal cases is different from the species of *Eimeria* that occur regularly in extraintestinal sites, such as *E. stiedai* in liver of rabbits or *E. truncata* in the kidney of geese.[974]

1.2.1.6 Description of *Eimeria* Species

Many criteria have been used to describe species of *Eimeria*, including morphology of oocysts, site of development, differences in endogenous stages, and molecular characteristics. The structure of sporulated oocysts has traditionally been used to describe new *Eimeria* species.[456] The size of oocysts can vary by more than 33%, and oocyst size can vary with infection dose (Figure 1.1A).[335] Color and oocyst wall surface might also vary in oocysts of a given species. For example, oocysts of *E. alabamensis* of cattle

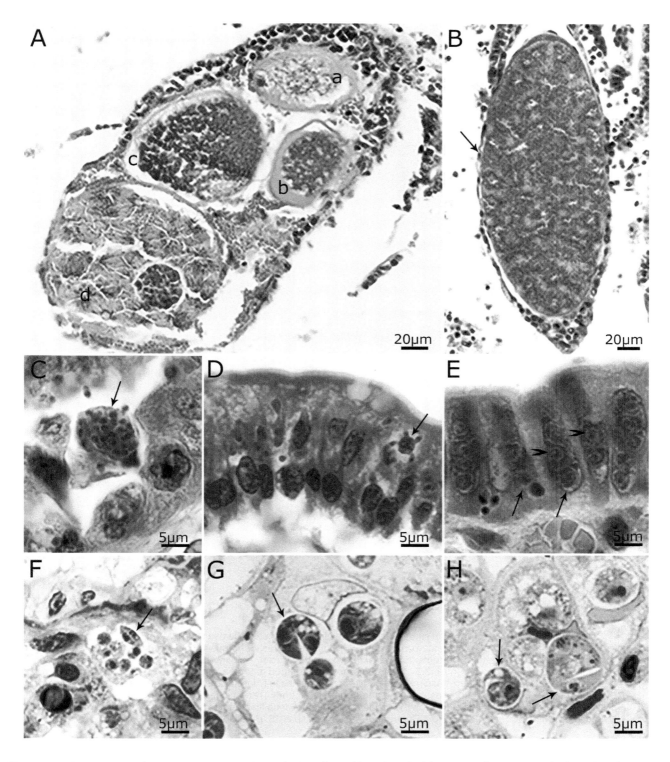

Figure 1.3 Development of *Eimeria* schizonts in histological sections of intestine. (A–E) Hematoxylin and eosin (HE) and (F–H) toluidine blue. (A) *E. bovis* of cattle. First generation in the lamina propria; a–d, in order of maturity. (B) *E. ellipsoidalis* of cattle. Mature first-generation schizont (arrow) in the lamina propria. (C) *E. bovis* of cattle. Mature second-generation schizont (arrow) in colon. Note small size, compared with first-generation schizonts in Figure 1.3A. (D) *E. maxima* of chickens. Second-/third-generation schizont with tiny merozoites around a large residual body (arrow). (E) *E. alabamensis* intranuclear schizonts (arrows). Arrowheads point to schizont nuclei. (F) *E. bareillyi* of water buffalo. Small group of parasites, one dividing into two merozoites (arrow). (G) *E. bareillyi* of water buffalo. Division of the parasite into two merozoites (arrow). (H) *E. bareillyi* of water buffalo. Merozoites splitting from the main groups (arrows).

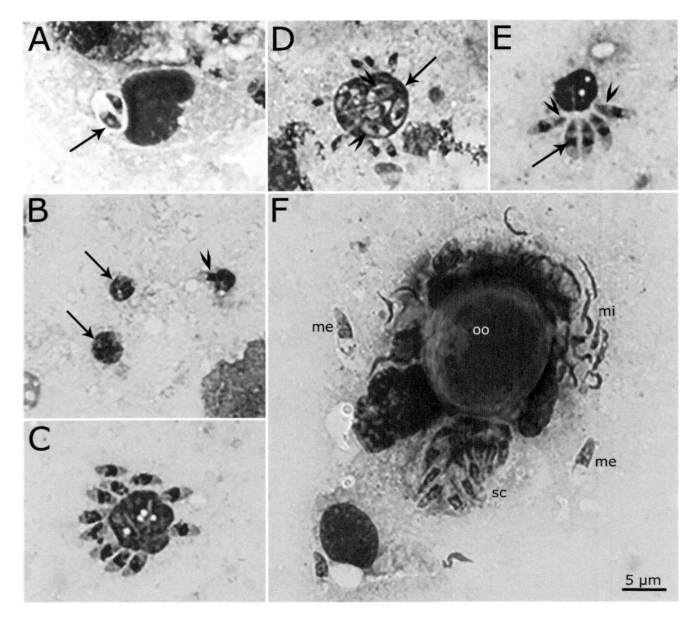

Figure 1.4   Development of *Eimeria* schizonts in smears of small intestines of chickens. Giemsa stain. (A–E) *E. maxima*, (F) *E. acervulina*. Bar applies to all figures. (A) Two merozoites (arrow) within one parasitophorous vacuole, apparently binary/endodyogeny division. (B) Three immature schizonts (arrows) with two or three nuclei. Arrowhead points to a merozoite arising at the two to three nucleated stage. (C) Small (3.5 μm long) merozoites arranged around a large undivided mass. (D) Small merozoites arising from a central undivided mass/residual body (arrow) that has fully formed merozoites. Arrowheads point to merozoites in the residual body. (E) Merozoites separating from a residual body. The apical end (arrowheads) of merozoite is stained distinctly from the central nucleus (arrow). (F) Note an oocyst (oo), long filamentous microgametes (mi), individual merozoites (me), and a schizont (sc). ([A–E] From Dubey, J.P., Jenkins, M.C. 2018. *Parasitology* 145, 1051–1058.)

may be piriform, elliptical, or spherical, and the crowding effect can affect the oocyst size.[1130] Some species are strictly site specific (e.g., *E. tenella* of chickens), whereas the site or region of intestine might change with progression of infection and dose. Molecular characteristics are helpful in taxonomy, especially in distinguishing *Eimeria* species from morphologically similar oocysts in different hosts.

1.3 GENUS *CYSTOISOSPORA*

Cystoisospora spp. oocysts have no micropyle and contain two sporocysts, each containing four sporozoites (Figure 1.9H). Additionally, sporocysts lack Stieda and substiedal bodies. The refractile body in sporozoites is crystalloidal in structure.

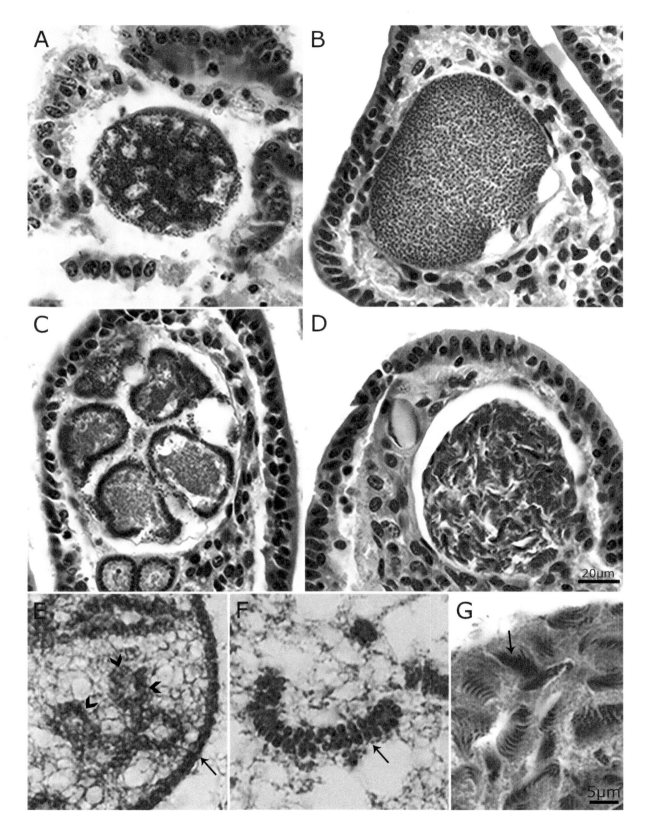

Figure 1.5 Development of microgamonts. (A–D) *Eimeria auburnensis* in the lamina propria of intestine of cattle. Note numerous nuclei. (E, F) *E. macusaniensis* in the lamina propria of llama. (E) Note arrangement of nuclei (arrows) in blastophores (circles, arrowheads). (F) Note a long chromatin strand with pairing of nuclei (arrow). (G) *E. auburnensis* microgametes arranged in whorls (arrow). Bar in (A–D) = 20 μm, bar in (E–G) = 5 μm.

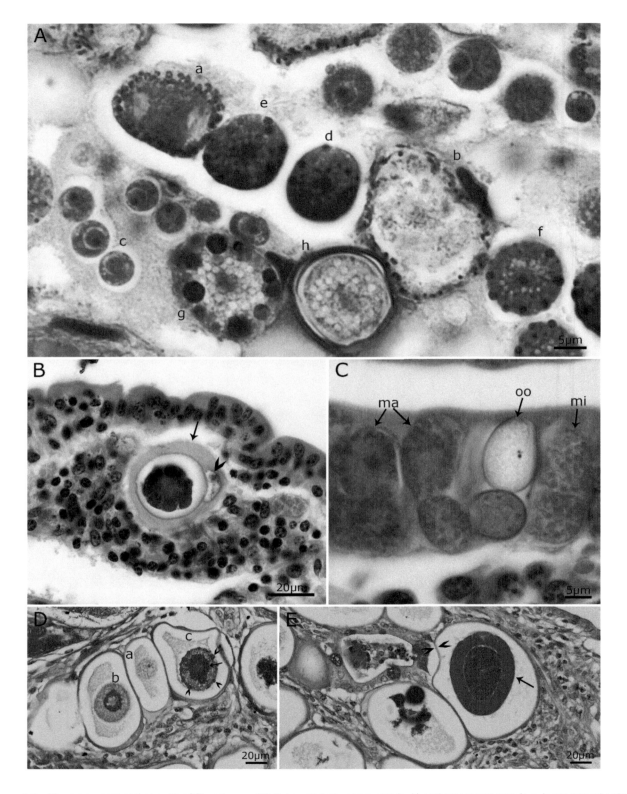

Figure 1.6   Macrogamonts and oocysts of *Eimeria* spp. (A) *E. bareillyi* microgamonts (a, b) and macrogamonts (c-g, in presumed order of development) and an oocyst (h). (B) Young macrogamont of *E. wyomingensis* in the lamina propria of intestine of cattle. Note thick parasitophorous vacuole (arrow) and hypertrophied indented host cell nucleus (arrowhead). (C). Intranuclear gamonts of *E. alabamensis* of cattle in surface epithelium. Note macrogamont (ma), microgamont (mi), and an oocyst (oo). (D) Three young macrogamonts of *E. macusaniensis* of intestine of llama (a) without WFB and PAS-positive granules, (b) with PAS-positive granules surrounding the nucleus, and (c) with PAS-positive granules (arrow) and WFB (arrowhead). (E) An oocyst (arrow) of *E. macusaniensis* in the lamina propria. Note the entire sporont is PAS positive. Also, note collapsed parasitopho-rous vacuolar membrane (arrowhead).

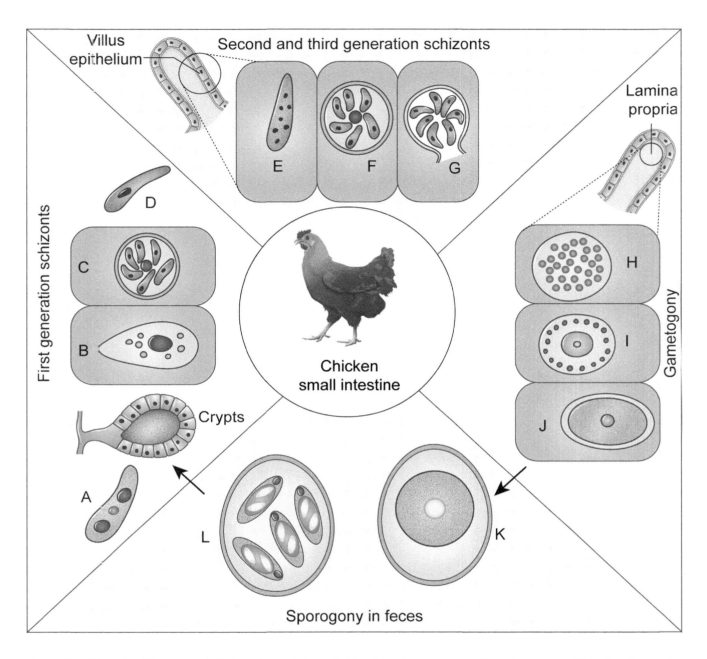

Figure 1.7 Life cycle of *E. maxima* of chickens. Asexual stages (schizonts) and gamonts occur throughout the small intestine. Sporozoites from first-generation schizonts in crypts, in glands of Lieberkühn (B, C). Merozoites (D) released from schizonts form a second (E–G) and possibly a third generation in villus epithelium. Microgamonts (H) macrogamonts (I) and oocysts (J) are found in the lamina propria. Unsporulated oocysts (K) are excreted in feces and sporulate in the environment. The host becomes infected by ingesting sporulated oocysts (L).

This book concerns only nine species of *Cystoisospora* (Table 1.3).

In general, the life cycle of *Cystoisospora* is comparable to *Eimeria* with minor differences in their asexual development (Figures 1.10 and 1.11). For example, *Cystoisospora* species sporozoites divide by endodyogeny during their initial development after entering host cells.[416] Merozoites can multiply for more than one cycle within the parasitophorous vacuole (PV); these are called "types" instead of generations

(Figure 1.10).[424,1438] The merozoites contain many amylopectin granules that stain bright red with PAS reaction.

Cystoisospora oocysts can sporulate rapidly (within 12 hours) (Figure 1.9). Omnivores and carnivores are definitive hosts for *Cystoisospora* species, and a variety of other hosts are paratenic hosts. In the paratenic host, *Cystoisospora* oocysts can excyst, and the sporozoites can invade extraintestinal tissues where they can encyst to form a monozoic tissue cyst (MZT)[1048] (Figures 1.11 and 1.12).

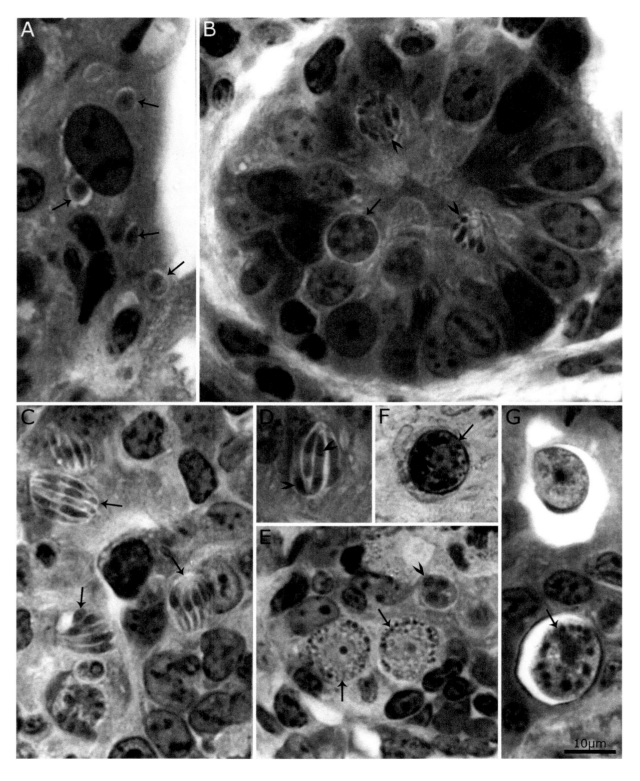

Figure 1.8   Endogenous stages of *Eimeria* sp. in the gallbladder of a goat. (A) Uninucleate zoites (arrows) in parasitophorous vacuoles in epithelial cells of the villous. HE stain. (B) Two immature schizonts (arrowheads) and a five-nucleate (arrow) schizont or microgamont. Iron hematoxylin stain (IH). (C) Mature schizonts (arrows). HE. (D) Schizont with six merozoites. Arrowheads point to the nucleus of the merozoite. Note, head (apical) to tail (nonconoidal end) of merozoites HE. (E) Two macrogamonts (arrows) each with a central nucleus, and a three-nucleate schizont (arrowhead). HE. (F) Partly formed oocyst (arrow) with a central nucleus and wall-forming bodies. Toluidine blue. (G) Two unsporulated oocysts with wrinkled walls. Wall-forming bodies are present in one oocyst (arrow) and absent in the other. IH. Bar applies to all figures. (From Dubey, J.P. 1986. *Proc. Helminthol. Soc. Wash.* 53, 277–281.)

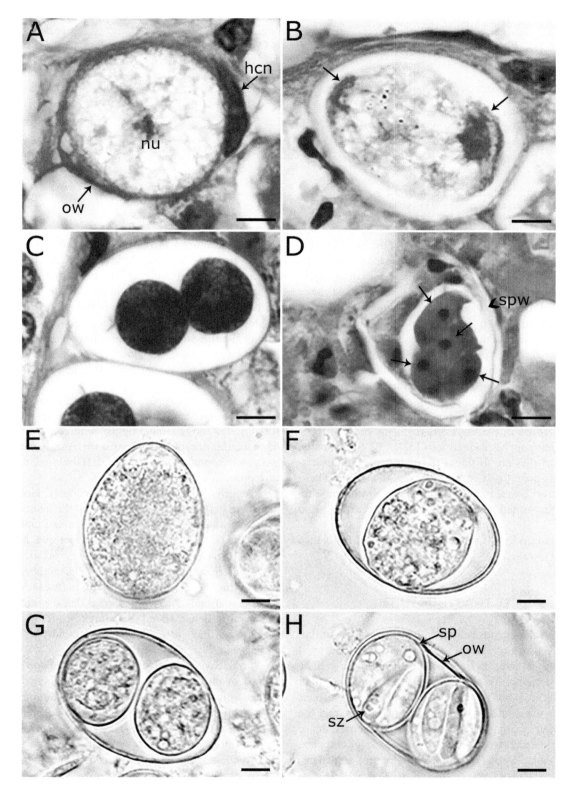

Figure 1.9 Sporulation of *Cystoisospora orlovi*. (A–D) Sporulation in colon of a camel. Histological section stained with HE. (E–H) Oocysts in feces. Bar = 5 μm and applies to all figures. (A) Intracellular unsporulated oocyst. Note host cell nucleus (hcn), oocyst wall (ow), and central nucleus (nu) of the sporont. (B) Sporulating oocyst with dense bodies (nuclei) at the poles (arrows). (C) Two sporoblasts. (D) Sporulated sporocyst with thin sporocyst wall (spw) showing four sporozoites (arrows). (E) Immature oocyst with sporont filling the interior of the oocyst. (F) Unsporulated oocyst with condensed sporont. (G) Oocyst with two sporoblasts. (H) Sporulated oocyst with thin oocyst wall (ow) with two sporocysts (sp), each with four sporozoites (sz).

Table 1.3 Summary of Important *Cystoisospora* Species

Name	Host	Location	Tissue Cyst	Paratenic Hosts	Pathogenicity	Chapter
C. suis	Pig	Small intestine	Unknown	Unknown	High	11
C. felis	Cat	Small intestine	Yes	Many	Low	21
C. rivolta	Cat	Small intestine	Yes	Yes	Low	21
C. canis	Dog	Small and large intestine	Yes	Yes	Moderate	20
C. ohioensis	Dog	Small intestine	Yes	Yes	Low	20
C. neorivolta	Dog	Small and large intestine	Unknown	Unknown	None	20
C. burrowsi	Dog	Small and large intestine	Yes	Unknown	None	20
C. orlovi	Camel	Large intestine	Unknown	Unknown	High	12
C. belli	Human	Small intestine	Yes	Unknown	Low[a]	22

[a] Can be severe in immunosuppressed patients.

The sporozoite can increase in size within the MZT. The MZT are formed in many organs, but most are seen in mesenteric lymph nodes. MZT persist in mice for the life of the mouse. The definitive host can acquire infection after ingestion of MZT.[560] Intestinal infections in definitive hosts after ingestion of MZT are identical to oocyst-induced infections but are a few hours faster.

The significance of the MZT and paratenic hosts in the life cycles of *Cystoisospora* is unknown. Perhaps it is an evolutionary link among coccidia with a direct fecal-oral transmission cycle (*Eimeria*) and coccidia with an obligatory two-host cycle (*Sarcocystis, Hammondia*). Although *C. suis* of pigs and *C. orlovi* of camel are included in the genus *Cystoisospora*, the MZT and paratenic hosts of these two species have not been identified (Table 1.3). Biologically, these two parasites are different from other coccidians discussed in this book (see Chapters 11, 12, 20, and 21). These parasites cause disease in nursing animals, and transmission is largely unexplained because their dams excrete few or no oocysts.

The sexual cycle of *Cystoisospora* (Figure 1.13) is also like that of *Eimeria*.

1.4 ULTRASTRUCTURE

Most coccidian parasites are ultrastructurally similar. Asexual stages (sporozoites and merozoites) contain various structures depicted in Figure 1.14B including a pellicle (outer plasma membrane and two inner membranes), refractile or crystalloid bodies, cytoskeletal elements (such as subpellicular microtubules, apical and polar rings, and the conoid), secretory organelles (rhoptries, micronemes, dense granules), a mitochondrion, a lipid body, a Golgi complex, ribosomes, endoplasmic reticula, a micropore, a nucleus, amylopectin granules, and an apicoplast. The pellicle consists of three membranes: a plasmalemma and two closely associated membranes that form an inner membrane complex (IMC). The IMC is formed from a patchwork of flattened vesicles. The inner membrane is discontinuous at the anterior tip above the polar rings, at the micropore, and at the basal complex posterior pore at the extreme posterior tip of the parasite (Figure 1.14A).[435] There are two apical and two polar rings (Figure 1.14B). The apical rings are located at the anterior tip of the parasite. Apical ring 1 encircles the top of the resting conoid. Polar ring 1 is an electron-dense thickening of the inner membrane complex at the anterior end of the parasite. Polar ring 2 anchors the subpellicular microtubules. The conoid is a truncated hollow cone and consists of tubulin structures wound like compressed springs. Twenty-two or more subpellicular microtubules originate from the inner polar ring and run longitudinally to about half or almost the entire length of the cell, dependent on the stage or species of the parasite. They are evenly spaced, and their distal ends are not capped. In addition, there are two 400 nm long intraconoidal tightly bound microtubules. The subpellicular microtubules form a rib cage and are arranged in a gentle counterclockwise spiral. Individual microtubules have prominent transverse striations.

Rhoptries are sac-like, homogenously electron-dense structures between the anterior tip and the nucleus and consist of an anterior narrow neck that extends into the interior of the conoid and a sac-like posterior end. Micronemes are electron-dense rod-like structures occurring mostly at the anterior end of the parasite. The number of micronemes is highly variable, and they are in flux moving toward the conoidal end. There are several dense granules, which are electron-dense round structures scattered throughout the parasite, but are predominantly found posterior to the nucleus end.

The nucleus consists of a nuclear envelope with pores, clumps of chromatin, and a nucleolus. There is one convoluted mitochondrion with tubular cristae and one enigmatic obligatory plastid organelle called the apicoplast (Figure 1.14A). The apicoplast is a membrane-bound, algae-derived obligatory endosymbiont structure that is no longer photosynthetic but has retained its own genome.[168]

Sporozoites and merozoites move by gliding, flexing, undulating, and rotating, and their motility is powered by the actin-myosin motor complex called **glideosome**, which is anchored to the IMC. The outermost IMC membrane is studded with myosin complexes, like a conveyor-belt system.

Functions of the conoid and the secretory components of rhoptries, micronemes, and dense granules are not fully

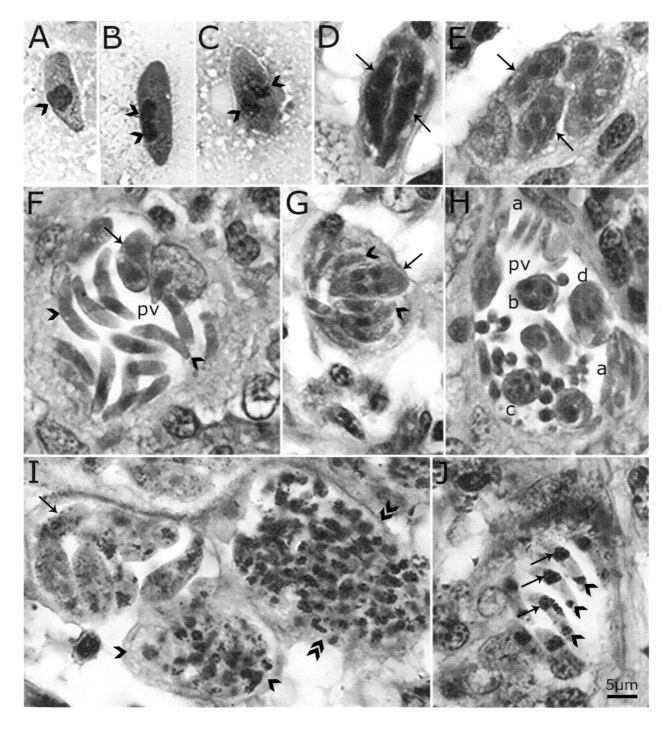

Figure 1.10 *Cystoisospora ohioensis* and *C. canis* asexual multiplication (A–C), *C. ohioensis*. Division of nuclei into two nuclei (arrowheads). Two daughter merozoites (arrowheads) are visible within one merozoite in (C). (D) Two elongated *C. canis* schizonts with multiple nuclei (arrowheads). (E) *C. canis* schizonts with multiple nuclei (arrows). (F) *C. canis*. A group of merozoites (arrows) in a parasitophorous vacuole (pv). Note one organism with two nuclei (arrow) and uninicleate merozoites (arrowheads). (G) *C. canis*. Schizont with mature merozoites (arrowheads) and one organism with four nuclei (arrow). (H) *C. canis*. Developing merozoites in a large pv. Note different shapes and sizes of merozoites including slender merozoites with single nucleus (a) multinucleate schizonts (b, c), and merozoites budding from a schizont (d). (I) *C. canis*. Three schizonts with varying degrees of periodic acid Schiff (PAS)–positive merozoites. Developing schizont containing multinucleated zoites (arrow), small schizont (arrowhead), and large schizont (double arrowheads). (J) *C. canis*. Schizont with mature merozoites. Note distribution of large (arrows) and small (arrowheads) PAS-positive granules. (A–C) Giemsa stain, smear; (D–H) HE stain; (I, J) PAS reaction counterstained with hematoxylin. Bar applies to all figures.

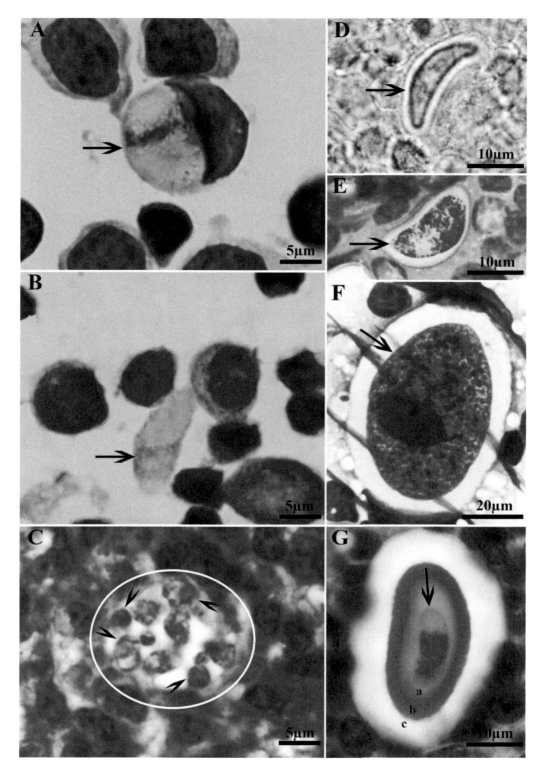

Figure 1.11 Extraintestinal stages of *Cystoisospora felis* in mesenteric lymph nodes of cats (A–C), and mice (D–G). All preparations are smears except (C) which is a histological section. (A) Zoite inside a lymphocyte (arrow). Giemsa. (B) Extracellular zoite (arrow). Giemsa. (C) Organisms (arrowheads) within a group (circle). Section stained with Giemsa stain. Organisms are stained lighter than the host cells, and sections had to be overstained to reveal the stages. (D) An unstained zoite (arrow). (E) A zoite (arrow) stained with periodic acid Schiff reaction counter-stained with hematoxylin (PASH). (F) A zoite (arrow) stained with Giemsa. (G) Monozoic tissue cyst. Arrow points to a sporozoite. Note bands of amylopectin stained red with PASH. The sporozoite is surrounded by lightly stained space (a), and intensely stained cyst wall (b), and a hollow space (c) surrounding the tissue cyst, perhaps an artifact of staining. (From Dubey, J. P. 2018. *Vet. Parasitol.* 263, 34–48.)

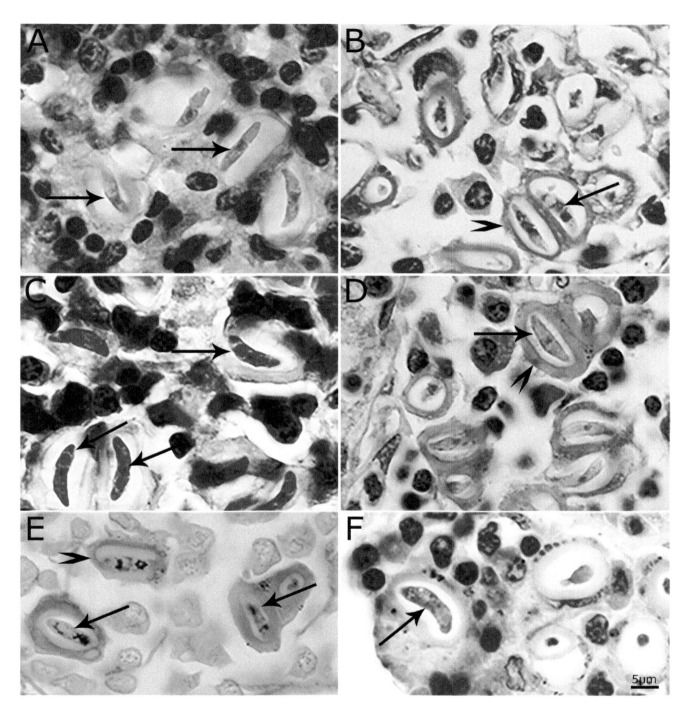

Figure 1.12 Monozoic tissue cysts of *Cystoisospora belli* in histological sections of mesenteric lymph node of a human AIDS patient after staining with different reagents/stains. Bar applies to all figures. Arrows point to sporozoites, and arrowheads point to cyst wall. Appropriate controls were used for each staining. (A) HE stain. The slide is overstained to reveal the light staining sporozoites. (B) Periodic acid Schiff (PAS). The cyst wall stains inconsistently with PAS. The sporozoites contain PAS-positive granules. (C) Trichrome stain. The sporozoites are stained brilliantly. (D) Immunohistochemical staining with 1:100 dilution of polyclonal antibodies to *Toxoplasma gondii*. Although *C. belli* does not react with anti-*T. gondii* antibodies, the digestion procedures reveal the parasite distinctive from host tissue. (E) Gomori's methamine silver stain is helpful in revealing the structure of the parasite. The cyst wall is negative, but the sporozoite has positive staining structures. (F) Toluidine blue stain. The tissue cyst is stained faintly.

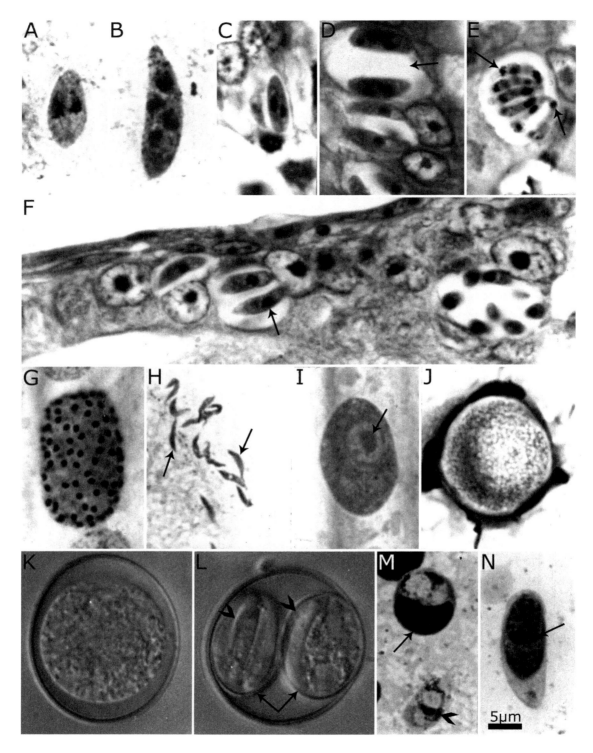

Figure 1.13 Life-cycle stages of *Cystoisospora rivolta* in cats and mice. (A, B, G–J, M, and N) Smears fixed in methanol and stained with Giemsa. (C,D,F) Sections stained with iron hematoxylin (IH). (E) Section stained with periodic acid Schiff reaction counterstained with hematoxylin (PASH). (K, L) Oocysts in fecal-float, unstained. (A) Division by endodyogeny. (B) A crescent-shaped schizont with four nuclei. (C) Division by endodyogeny. (D) Two multinucleated schizonts (arrow) in the same parasitophorous vacuole. (E) Merozoites with PAS-positive granules (arrows). (F) Schizonts and merozoites (arrow) of different sizes. (G) An immature microgamont with many nuclei. (H) Several mature microgametes (arrows). (I) Macrogamont with a large nucleus and prominent nucleolus (arrow). (J) An unsporulated intracellular oocyst. (K) Unsporulated oocyst containing a central sporont. (L) Sporulated oocyst containing two sporocysts (arrows) with sporozoites (arrowheads). (M) Extraintestinal zoites in the mesenteric lymph node of a cat. One zoite is in a monocyte (arrow), and another one is extracellular (arrowhead). (N) Extraintestinal tissue cyst containing a single zoite (arrow) in the mesenteric lymph node of a mouse. (From Dubey, J.P. 1979. *J. Protozool.* 26, 433–443.)

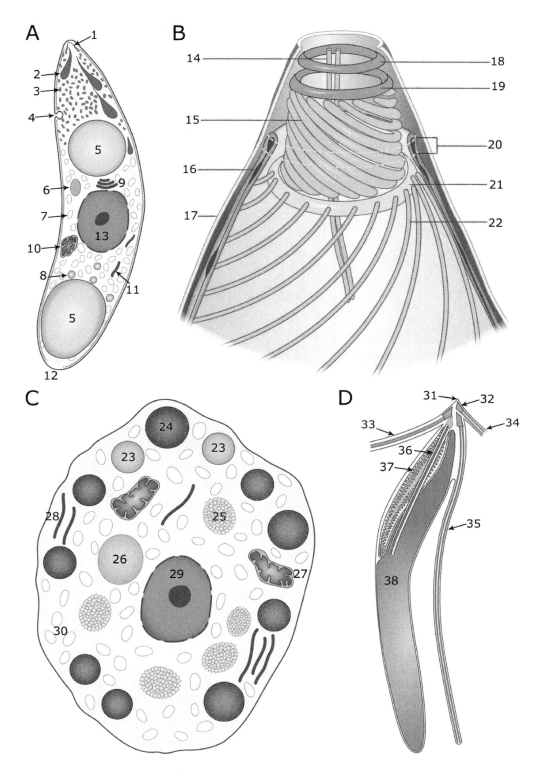

Figure 1.14 Coccidian stages. (A) Sporozoite. 1. Conoid. 2. Rhoptry. 3. Microneme. 4. Micropore. 5. Refractile body. 6. Apicoplast. 7. Amylopectin granules. 8. Dense granules. 9. Golgi body. 10. Mitochondrion. 11. Endoplasmic reticulin. 12. Posterior pore. 13. Nucleus. (B) Apical complex. 14. Internal microtubules. 15. Microtubules of conoid. 16. Inner membrane complex. 17. Plasmalemma. 18. Apical ring 1. 19. Apical ring 2. 20. Polar ring 1. 21. Polar ring 2. 22. Subpellicular tubules. (C) Macrogamont. 23. Veil-forming bodies. 24. Wall-forming bodies 1. 25. Wall-forming bodies 2. 26. Lipid body. 27. Mitochondrion. 28. Endoplasmic reticulum. 29. Nucleus. 30. Amylopectin granules. (D) Microgamete. 31. Perforatorium. 32. Basal body. 33. Flagellum 1. 34. Flagellum 2. 35. Flagellum 3. 36. Microtubule. 37. Mitochondrion. 38. Nucleus. ([A, C, D] Modified from Scholtyseck, E. 1973. Ultrastructure. In Hammond, D.M. and Long, P.L. [Ed.], *The Coccidia. Eimeria, Isospora, Toxoplasma, and Related Genera*. University Park Press. Baltimore, MD, 81–144; [B] from Dubey, J.P., et al. 2017. *Neosporosis in Animals*. CRC Press, Boca Raton, FL.)

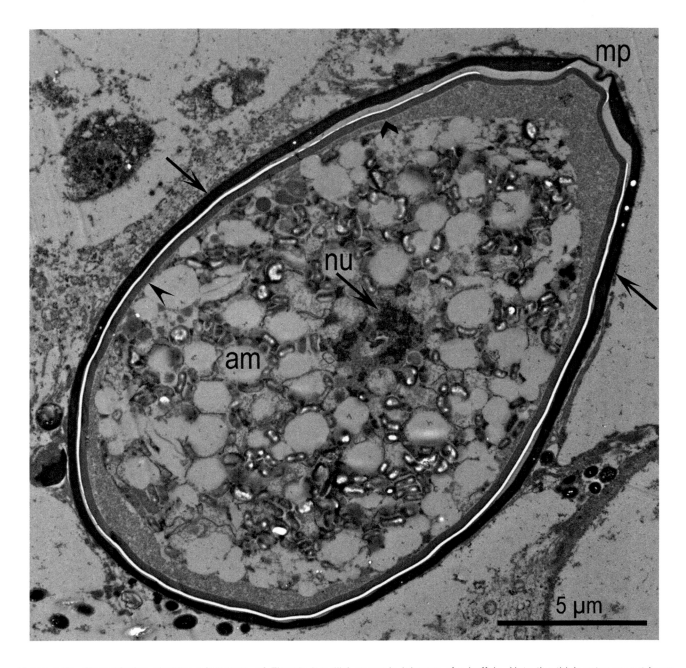

Figure 1.15 Transmission electron microscopy of *Eimeria bareillyi* oocyst in jejunum of a buffalo. Note the thick outer oocyst layer (arrows) and thinner inner oocyst layer (arrowheads). Note the sporont fills the interior of the oocyst. Note numerous amylopectin granules (am) and a central nucleus (nu). The oocyst is truncated at the micropylar end (mp) with thinning of the outer layer. (From Dubey, J.P. 2018. *Parasitology* 145, 1845–1852.)

known, but they were shown to be associated with host cell penetration and creating an intracellular environment suitable for parasite growth, development, and exit from the host cell. The conoid can rotate, tilt, extend, and retract as the parasite probes the host cell plasmalemma immediately before penetration. During host cell invasion, rhoptries and micronemes secrete their contents through the plasmalemma just above the conoid to the exterior. Sporozoites and merozoites can invade the host cell within seconds. Following invasion, sporozoites or merozoites are surrounded by the parasitophorous vacuolar membrane (PVM), evidently derived from the host cell plasmalemma. The PVM is not a homogenous structure of uniform thickness. Several molecules, secreted from dense granules and rhoptries, associate and modify the PVM, and a tubular membranous network (TMN) within the PV matrix is formed within hours following invasion. The TMN components are antigenically and structurally different from the PVM but are physically connected to it.

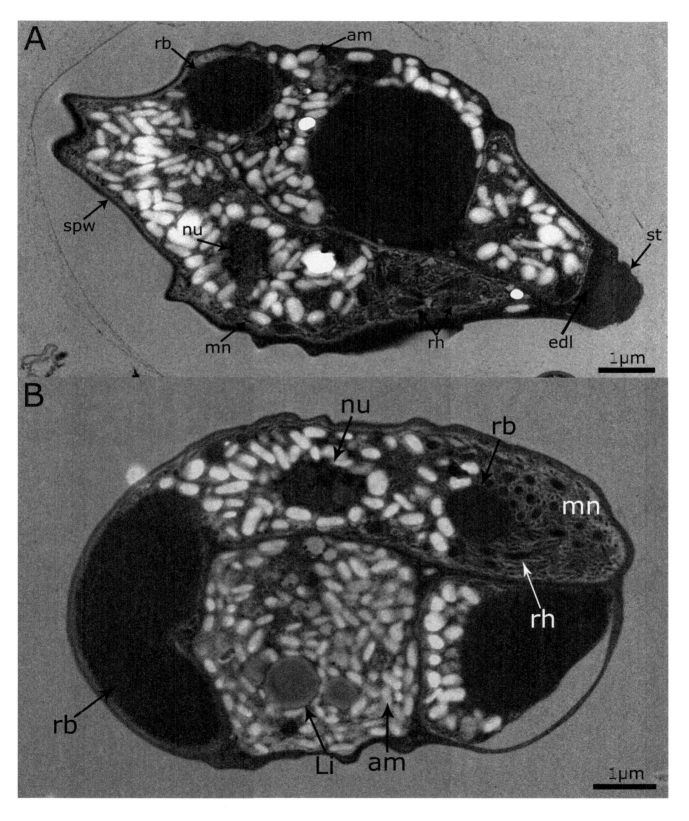

Figure 1.16 Transmission electron microscopy of sporocysts (A, B) of *Eimeria piriformis*. The sporocyst wall (spw) is crumpled in (A) but smooth in (B). Note a plug-like homogenous Stieda body (st), the electron dense layer (edl) immediately beneath the Stieda body, numerous amylopectin granules (am), two refractile bodies (rb), a small irregularly shaped nucleus (nu), rhopties (rh), lipid body (Li), and micronemes (mn). The sporozoites are twisted in sporocysts and are sectioned at different levels. (Courtesy of Dr. Michal Pakandl, Prague, Czech Republic.)

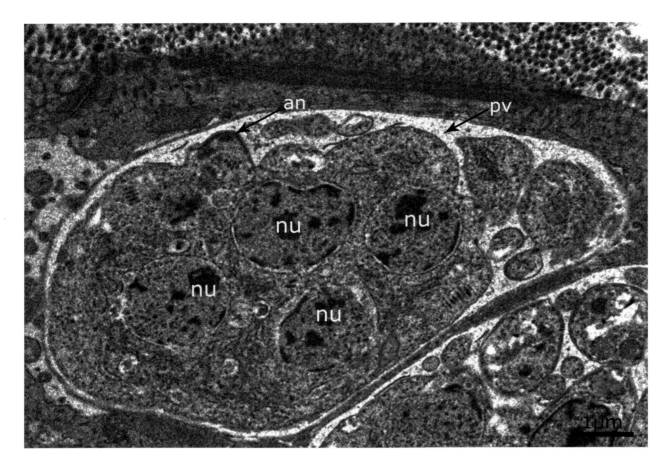

Figure 1.17 An immature schizont of *Eimeria meleagridis* of turkey in parasitophorous vacuole (pv). Note four nuclei (nu) and analagen (an) of the developing merozoite. (Coutresy of Dr. Michal Pakandl, Prague, Czech Republic.)

1.4.1 *Eimeria* Species

1.4.1.1 Oocysts, Sporocysts, Sporozoites

The wall of unsporulated oocysts of *Eimeria* species has one to three layers: the outer layer is often thick and electron dense, and the inner layer is thin and electron lucent (Figure 1.15). Unsporulated oocysts have a central nucleus and inner mass consisting of mainly amylopectin granules (Figure 1.15). With sporulation, the sporont shrinks and begins to divide to form sporocysts and sporozoites. *Eimeria* sporocysts have two sporozoites often arranged head to tail and suspended in a homogenous matrix. The sporocyst wall is smooth and has a Stieda body at the narrower end. The Stieda body consists of an upper homogenous portion and a lower portion that is more electron dense than the upper portion (Figure 1.16).[1312]

Eimeria sporozoites contain one to four refractile bodies and amylopectin granules.[1422] The refractile bodies are not membrane bound. They are located anterior and posterior to the nucleus (Figure 1.14A and 1.16). The amylopectin granules are often concentrated between the nucleus and the posterior refractile body. By light microscopy, they are

PAS-positive and appear as translucent or empty vacuoles by transmission electron microscopy (TEM). The position of the nucleus varies with species of *Eimeria*. Depending on the species of *Eimeria*, the nucleus may be pushed toward the conoidal end (e.g., in *E. bovis*), whereas it is located centrally in many other *Eimeria* species.[1422] The structure of the nucleus and the nucleolus can vary with species of *Eimeria*. For example, no nucleolus was found in *E. auburnensis* of cattle.[1422]

1.4.1.2 Schizonts and Merozoites

Sporozoites can enter host cells within 5 seconds.[263] During invasion, both the sporozoite and the host cell undergo changes. The sporozoite enters the host cell with the apical end and carries the host cell plasma membrane with it. This transformation from free living stage in the sporulated oocyst to intracellular phase is dependent on species of *Eimeria*. In most *Eimeria* species, sporozoites lose most of their organelles within 24 hours of entry in the host cell, but the process may be delayed for several days in some species. The earliest change is alteration in shape from crescentic to spheriodal. The inner layers of IMC are lost first followed

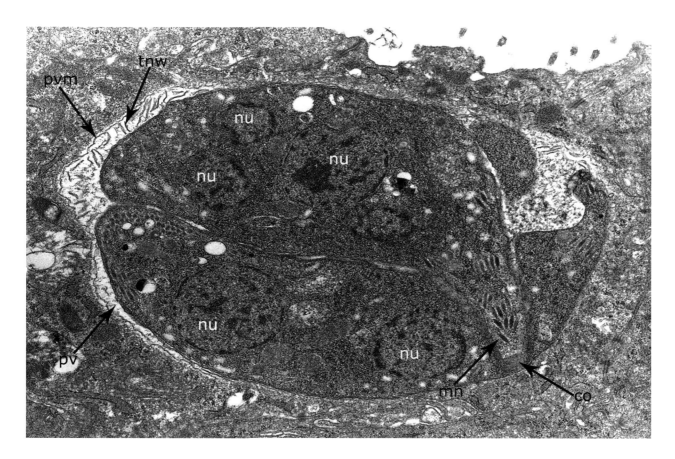

Figure 1.18 Transmission electron microscopy of schizonts of *Eimeria piriformis* in enterocyte of rabbit. Two schizonts are located within a parasitophorous vacuole (pv) that has a tubular network (tnw) connecting the parasite with parasitophorous vacuolar membrane (pvm). The schizonts are twisted and lying over each other. One schizont is cut longitudinally and has the conical conoid (co) and the round posterior non-conoidal end. Note few micronemes (mn) and multiple nuclei (nu). (Courtesy of Dr. Michal Pakandl, Prague, Czech Republic.)

by the loss of microtubules, conoid, micronemes, and rhoptries. The refractile body/bodies break up and are lost when the merozoites are formed. However, in a few *Eimeria* species, they are carried into first-generation merozoites or their progeny.

As stated earlier, coccidian parasites discussed in this book divide by endodyogeny or schizogony. In endodyogeny, the parent nucleus divides into two lobes that move into two apical complexes of daughter cells (progeny) that are formed at the narrow ends of the nuclear lobes. Eventually, the parent structures are consumed in the process of the formation of two daughter cells (progeny). Further progenies may be formed by simultaneous division of daughter cells; however, this type of division has not been demonstrated ultrastructurally for any *Eimeria* species. More commonly, the parent nucleus divides into four or more nuclei before merozoite formation (Figures 1.17 through 1.19). Merozoites may be formed internally as in *E. magna* of rabbits[320] or at the surface of the multinucleated schizont.[1549] The number of schizont generations is not genetically limited, and several *Eimeria* species from chickens and rabbits have been selected for precocious (fast) development by collecting the

oocysts from the first day of patency and repeatedly passing them in the host and collecting the first oocysts that are passed subsequently. This results in the shortening of the prepatent period, often lowering the pathogenicity, and this is caused by a loss of one or more schizont generations.[790] The precocious trait is stable and remains after the selection process has been stopped (see Chapter 14).

Ultrastructurally, merozoites are like sporozoites, except for a few minor differences such as the refractile bodies and amylopectin granules.[1549] Although most *Eimeria* merozoites do not have refractile bodies (Figure 1.19), there are exceptions. Also, merozoites usually have no or few amylopectin granules. As an example, two distinct morphological types of first-generation schizonts of *E. bovis* of cattle were described; the calves were euthanized 15 days postinoculation.[1601] Type I schizonts contained long (13 × 1.5 μm) merozoites, and type II schizonts had smaller (5.9 × 0.9 μm) merozoites. The schizonts had either short or long merozoites but not both. The long merozoites had numerous amylopectin granules and micronemes versus no amylopectin granules in the type II merozoites and few micronemes. These

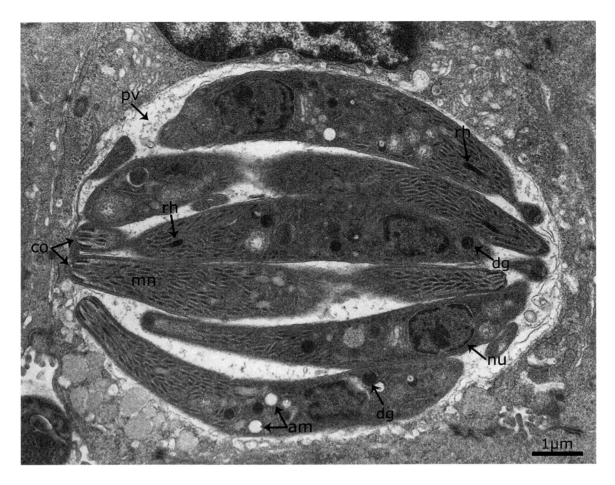

Figure 1.19 Transmission electron microscopy of a mature schizont of *Eimeria piriformis* of rabbit. Note slender merozoites with head-to-tail arrangement. Note few rhoptries (rh), dense granules (dg), and amylopectin granules (am), numerous micronemes (mn), a nucleus (nu) in the posterior half of the merozoite and conoid (co) anteriorly. The parasitophorous vacuole (pv) contains a tubular network. (Courtesy of Dr. Michal Pakandl, Prague, Czech Republic.)

observations made on *in vivo* schizonts were like those observed *in vitro* schizonts.[1601]

1.4.1.3 Microgamonts and Macrogamonts

After the last generation of schizogony, merozoites enter new host cells and form microgamonts (males) and macrogamonts (females). During microgametogenesis, the nucleus divides by mitosis into several nuclei that are usually vesicular. As the parasite enlarges, the nuclei move to the periphery and the nuclear chromatin is condensed. Two centrioles and a mitochondrion become associated with each nucleus.[1515] The centrioles give rise to flagella, the nucleus and the mitochondrion elongate, and the young spheriodal microgamete pinches off and is set free in the parasitophorous vacuole. The microgamete elongates and has two free flagella (Figure 1.20). A short third flagellum was seen in some species of *Eimeria*.[1515] One or more residual bodies are left after the microgamete formation (Figure 1.20). Microgametes can form at the surface leaving a single residual body (monocentric microgameteogenesis), or the surface can be increased

by folding and microgametes are produced on the compartments (blastophores) that leave more than one residual body (polycentric microgameteogenesis).

The earliest stage of macrogamont has a large central nucleus with a prominent nucleolus but very few other organelles other than endoplasmic reticulin. Amylopectin granules begin to accumulate, starting with the periphery of the nucleus (Figure 1.21). Other structures present in macrogamont are lipid bodies and mitochondrion. Three types of oocyst wall-forming bodies have been reported.[100,525,1117] Earliest to appear are veil-forming bodies (VFBs) that are scattered throughout the cytoplasm (Figure 1.14C). The WFBs are of two types: WFB1 and WFB2. The WFB1 are electron dense, and WFB2 are spongy (Figures 1.14C and 1.21). The oocyst wall is laid in patches (Figure 1.21), WFB1 forming the outer oocyst wall and WFB2 forming the inner oocyst wall. In some species of *Eimeria* (e.g., *E. maxima*), intracellular oocysts are surrounded by a thin transparent layer (veil) that is lost when oocysts are excreted in feces. The VFBs are linked to formation of the veil.[525] The WFBs disappear when the oocyst wall is formed.

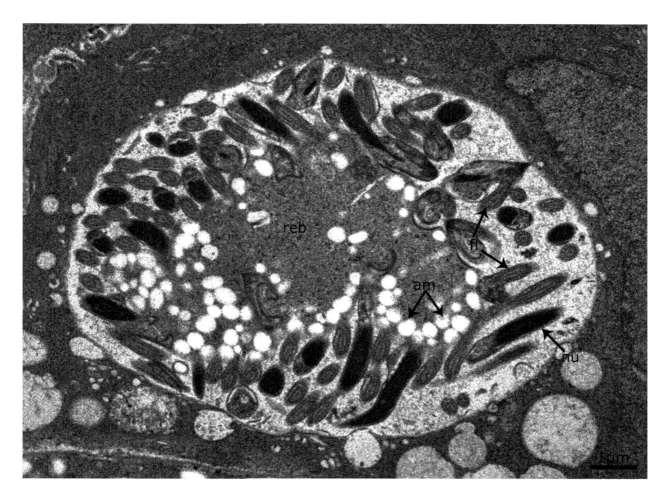

Figure 1.20 Transmission electron microscopy of mature microgamont of *Eimeria meleagridis*. Note a central residual body (reb), numerous amylopectin granules (am), microgametes with nucleus (nu), and flagella (fl). (Coutresy of Dr. Michal Pakandl, Prague, Czech Republic.)

1.4.2 *Cystoisospora*

The ultrastructure of *Cystoisospora* is essentially like *Eimeria* with the following differences:

1. The oocyst contains two sporocysts, each with four sporozoites. The sporocysts have four sutures through which sporozoites escape during excystation.[1357,1610]
2. Asexual multiplication occurs by endodyogeny or modified schizogony where the parasite can produce successive generation in the same host cell without rupture.[526]
3. *Cystoisospora* sporozoites contain a crystalloid body that is different than the refractile body of *Eimeria* (Figure 1.22). In some *Cystoisospora* species, sporozoites encyst in extraintestinal tissues and form MZT (Figure 1.22). The MZT cyst wall is up to 4 μm thick and consists of a homogenous material. The zoites in the MZT cysts usually have a crystalloid body.[441]
4. The gametogony of *Cystoisospora* is like that of *Eimeria* except that the WFBs are smaller than 2 μm in diameter.[527,528]

1.5 *IN VITRO* CULTIVATION

The species of coccidia discussed in this book are mostly site and species specific. Numerous attempts to successfully grow them *in vitro* from sporozoites to oocyst stages have been unsuccessful (Tables 1.4 and 1.5). Of all the species of coccidia in the present book, only *E. tenella* of chickens[385,389,392,1167,1624,1625] and *Cystoisospora suis* of pigs[1050,1821] have been reported to produce oocysts, starting with sporozoite inocula. The rodent coccidium *Eimeria nieschulzi* will also produce oocysts in fetal rat brain cell cultures if sporozoites are used as inoculum.[254] Additionally, if late-generation merozoites for the host intestines are used as inocula, *E. tenella* and *E. acervulina*[92,1228] from chickens, *E. meleagridis* of turkeys,[50] and *E. bovis* of cattle[1608] can complete their life cycles and produce oocysts. The studies by Doran[385] and McDougald and colleagues[1167] using *E. tenella* sporozoites of a precocious strain produced oocysts that sporulated and were infectious for chickens. Studies using third-generation merozoites of *E. meleagridis* from turkeys[50] and

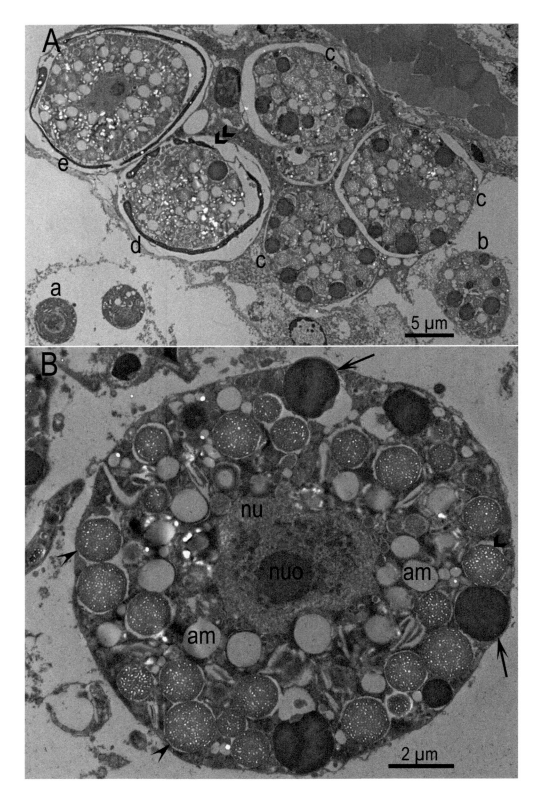

Figure 1.21 Transmission electron microscopy of macrogamonts and oocysts of *Eimeria bareillyi* in jejunum of a buffalo. (A) Gametogony and oocyst wall formation in presumed order of development (a–e). (a) Early macrogamont without wall forming bodies (WFB). (b,c) Developing macrogamonts with numerous WFB1, 2. (d) Oocyst wall formation in patches (double arrowheads) with one WFB and several WFB2. (e) Almost completed oocyst wall. (B) Higher magnification of a macrogamont. Note a centrally located nucleus (nu), nucleolus (nuo), amylopectin granules (am), electron-dense WFB1 (arrows), and electron lucent WFB2 (arrowheads). (From Dubey, J.P. 2018. *Parasitology* 145, 1845–1852.)

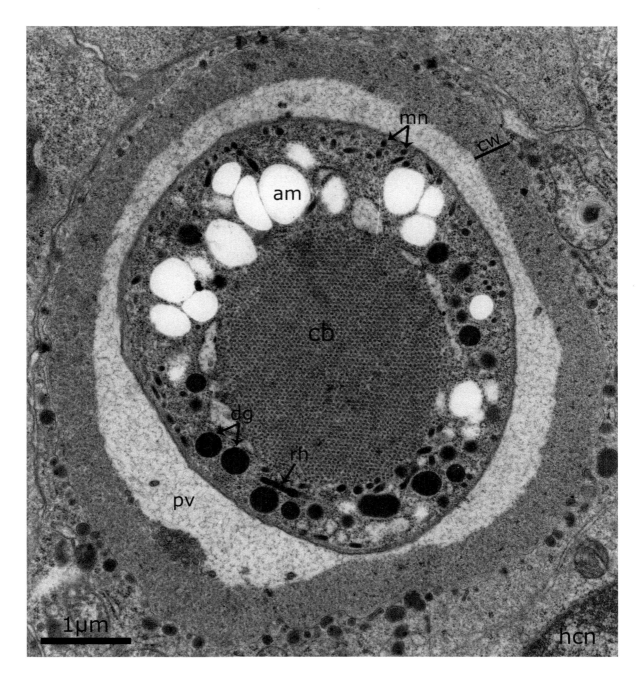

Figure 1.22   Transmission electron microscopy of tissue cyst of *Cystoisospora ohioensis* in mesenteric lymph node of a mouse. Note cross/ oblique section of sporozoite containing a large crystalloid body (cb), numerous amylopectin granules (am), a rhoptry (rh), several micronemes (mn), and dense granules (dg). The sporozoite is enclosed in a parasitophorous vacuole (pv) surrounded by a cyst wall (cw). Note host cell nucleus (hcn). (Modified from Dubey, J.P., Mehlhorn, H. 1978. *J. Parasitol.* 64, 689–695.)

E. magna from rabbits[1600] produced sporulated oocysts that were infectious for their natural hosts.

1.6 PATHOGENESIS AND LESIONS OF INTESTINAL COCCIDIOSIS

Pathogenicity of coccidia depends on many factors related to both the host and the coccidian species. The site of development, reproductive potential, type of cells parasitized, age of host, environmental conditions (weather), and the immune status of the host are important and can affect pathogenesis.[529,615,1077]

Most coccidia discussed in this book multiply in enterocytes, and lesions are caused by destruction of parasitized cells and mechanical alteration of adjacent tissue (Figures 1.23 through 1.27).

Infected cells as well as uninfected cells can undergo hypertrophy (increase in size) (Figure 1.28).[38,422,582,893] When

Table 1.4   Studies Describing Development of *Eimeria* and *Cystoisospora* from Domestic Animals in Cell Cultures

Host	Species	Stage Used	Development	Reference
Cattle	*E. alabamensis*	Sporozoites	SsM, T1 MS1, MZ1, T2	Sampson et al.[1481,1482]
Cattle	*E. auburnensis*	Sporozoites	SsM, T1, MS1, MZ1	Clark and Hammond[278]
Cattle	*E. bovis*	Sporozoites	T1, MS1, MZ1	Fayer and Hammond[520]
Cattle	*E. bovis*	MZ1	None	Hammond et al.[666]
Cattle	*E. bovis*	MZ1	MS2, MZ2, MaG, MiG, Oo	Speer and Hammond[1608]
Cattle	*E. bovis*	Sporozoites	Complete	Hermosilla et al.[705]
Cattle	*E. bovis*	MZ1	MS2, MZ2	Hermosilla et al.[708]
Cattle	*E. bovis*	Sporozoites	MS1, MZ1	López-Osorio et al.[1090]
Cattle	*E. canadensis*	Sporozoites	SsM T1, MS1, MZ1	Müller et al.[1212]
Cattle	*E. ellipsoidalis*	Sporozoites	T1 MS1, MZ1	Speer and Hammond[1604]
Cattle	*E. zuernii*	Sporozoites	MS1, MZ1	Speer et al.[1603]
Cattle	*E. zuernii*	Sporozoites	MS1, MZ1	López-Osorio et al.[1090]
Cattle	*E. zuernii*	MZ1 from culture	No growth	Speer et al.[1603]
Goats	*E. arloingi*	Sporozoites	MS1, MZ1	Silva et al.[1578]
Goats	*E. ninakohlyakimovae*	Sporozoites	MS1, MZ1	Ruiz et al.[1458]
Sheep	*E. crandallis*	Sporozoites	T1, MS1, MZ1	DeVos et al.[364]
Sheep	*E. ninakohlyakimovae*	Sporozoites	T1, MS1, MZ1	Kelley and Hammond[869,870,871]
Sheep	*E. ovinoidalis*	Sporozoites	MS1, MZ1	Carrau et al.[176]
Swine	*E. debliecki*	Sporozoites	SsM, MS1, MZ1, T2	Lindsay et al.[1035]
Swine	*C. suis*	Sporozoites	MS1, MZ1	Lindsay et al.[1041]
Swine	*C. suis*	Sporozoites	MS1, MZ1	Fayer et al.[519]
Swine	*C. suis*	Sporozoites	MS1, MZ1, MS2	Lindsay and Blagburn[1032]
Swine	*C. suis*	Sporozoites	Complete	Lindsay et al.[1050]
Swine	*C. suis*	Sporozoites	Complete	Worliczek et al.[1821]
Rabbit	*E. magna*	Sporozoites	SsM, MS1, MZ1, MMs1M, MS2, MZ2, E?	Speer and Hammond[1605]
Rabbit	*E. magna*	25-day merozoites from rabbits	MS3, MZ3, MiG, MaG, Oo	Speer and Hammond[1606]
Rabbit	*E. magna*	4.5- to 5-day merozoites (third generation) from rabbits	MS3, MZ3, MiG, MaG, AMaG	Speer and Hammond[1607]
Rabbit	*E. magna*	3- to 5.5-day Uni and multinuceate merozoites from rabbits	MS1, MZ1, MMs1M, MS2, MZ2, E?, MS3, MZ3, MiG, MaG, BiNHC	Speer et al.[1609]
Rabbit	*E. magna*	5.3- to 5.5-day merozoites (third generation) from rabbits	MiG	Speer and Danforth[1602]
Rabbit	*E. magna*	3-, 3.5-, 4-, 4.5-, 5-, 5.3-, and 5.5-day merozoites (first, second, third generation) from rabbits	3-day only MMs1M, MS2, MZ2, E?, MS3, MZ3 3.5 to 4 days mostly MS2, MZ2, E?, MS3, MZ3 few MaG, MiG, 4.5 days equal numbers MS2, MZ2, MS3, MZ3 and MaG, MiG 5 to 5.5 days mainly MiG, MaG, Oo, SOo SOo from culture infective *in vivo* Bile stimulates motility of microgametes	Speer[1600]

Abbreviations: AMag, Motile amoeboid movement in macrogamonts; BiNHC, binucleate host cells induced by stages (cytochalasins B-like?); Complete, asexual and sexual stages with oocysts; E?, development suggestive of endodyogeny; MaG, macrogamonts; MiG, microgamonts; MMs1M, multinucleate merozoite-shaped first-generation merozoites; MS1, first-generation schizonts; MS2, second-generation schizonts; MZ1, first-generation merozoites; MZ2, second-generation merozoites; Oo, oocyst; SOo, sporulated oocyst; SsM, sporozoite-shaped schizonts; T1, first-generation trophozoites; T2, second-generation trophozoites.

the numbers of cells increase markedly, it is hyperplasia; for example, bile duct epithelial cells infected with *E. stiedai* of rabbits undergo marked hyperplasia. Formation of grossly visible polyps due to accumulation of oocysts and gamonts in ovine and caprine coccidiosis is a good example of extreme hyperplasia (Figure 1.28). The mesenteric lymph nodes in animals affected with intestinal coccidia are often enlarged, perhaps reacting to antigens absorbed through the damaged epithelium.

Edema, congestion of blood and lymph vessels, hemorrhage, desquamation, and necrosis of the epithelium and submucosa can lead to diarrhea, dysentery, and even death. Blood can be rapidly expelled from the anus at distances of up to 2 meters from calves with *E. zuernii* or *E. bovis* infections. The straining to defecate (tenesmus) can cause rectal prolapse in calves with coccidiosis.

Concurrent infections with enteric helminths, other protozoa, bacteria, viruses, and environmental conditions may

Table 1.5 Development of *Eimeria* Species from Chickens, Turkeys, and Bobwhite Quail in Cell Culture

Species	Stage Used	Development	Reference
E. tenella	Sporozoites from oocysts	MS1, MZ1,	Patton[1330]
E. tenella	MZ2 from chickens	MaG, MiG, Oo	Bedrnik[92]
E. tenella	Sporozoites from oocysts	MS1, MZ1	Matsuoka et al.[1153]
E. tenella	Sporozoites from oocysts	AllAS, MaG, MiG	Strout and Cuellette[1624]
E. tenella	Sporozoites from oocysts	Complete, SOo	Doran[385]
E. tenella	Sporozoites from oocysts of a precocious strain	MS1, MZ1, MaG, MiG, Oo, SOo	McDougald and Jeffers[1167]
E. tenella	Sporozoites from oocysts	Complete	Strout and Cuellette[1625]
E. tenella	Sporozoites from oocysts	Complete	Doran[386,387]
E. tenella	Sporozoites from oocysts	AllAS, MaG, MiG	Klimes et al.[300]
E. tenella	Sporozoites from oocysts	Complete, MnMaG	Doran and Augustine[392]
E. tenella	Sporozoites from oocysts	Complete	Doran and Augustine[393]
E. tenella	Sporozoites from oocysts	Complete	Doran and Augustine[395]
E. tenella	MZ1, MZ2 from cultures	NS	Doran[390]
E. acervulina	Sporozoites from oocysts	NS	Doran and Vetterling[397]
E. acervulina	Sporozoites from oocysts	T1, iMS1	Strout et al.[1326]
E. acervulina	MZ4 from chickens	AllAS, Mag, MiG, Oo	Naciri-Bontemps[1228]
E. acervulina	Sporozoites from oocysts	AllAS	Naciri-Bontemps[1228]
E. brunetti	Sporozoites from oocysts	MS1, MZ1, MS2, MZ2	Shibalova[1557]
E. brunetti	Sporozoites from oocysts	MS1, MZ1, T2, MS2, MZ2	Ryley and Wilson[1474]
E. dispersa turkey isolate	Sporozoites from oocysts	?AS	Doran and Augustine[394]
E. maxima	Sporozoites from oocysts	NS	Doran[388]
E. mivati	Sporozoites from oocysts	NS	Doran[388]
E. necatrix	Sporozoites from oocysts	MS1, MZ1	Doran and Vetterling[397]
E. necatrix	Sporozoites from oocysts	MS1, MZ1, MS2, MZ2	Doran[388]
E. praecox	Sporozoites from oocysts	NS	Doran[388]
E. adenoeides	Sporozoites from oocysts	MS1, MZ1	Doran[384]
E. gallopavonis	Sporozoites from oocysts	NS	Doran and Vetterling[397]
E. gallopavonis	Sporozoites from oocysts	?AS, MaG	Doran and Augustine[394]
E. meleagrimitis	Sporozoites from oocysts	MS1, MZ1	Doran and Vetterling[397]
E. meleagrimitis	Sporozoites from oocysts	?AS	Doran and Vetterling[397]
E. meleagrimitis	Sporozoites from oocysts	AllAS	Augustine and Doran[50]
E. meleagrimitis	Sporozoites from turkey intestine	AllAS, MaG	Augustine and Doran[50]
E. meleagrimitis	MZ1 from turkey intestine	T2, MS2, MZ2, T3	Augustine and Doran[50]
E. meleagrimitis	MZ2 from turkey intestine	MS3, MZ3, MaG, MiG, Oo	Augustine and Doran[50]
E. meleagrimitis	MZ3 from turkey intestine	MS2, MZ2, MS3, MZ3, MaG, MiG, Oo SOo	Augustine and Doran[50]
E. dispersa from bobwhite quail	Sporozoites from bobwhite quail oocysts	MS1, MZ1, MS2, MZ2	Fisher et al.[535]

Note: Oocysts from culture were viable and sporulated. They were infectious for normal host by oral inoculation.
Abbreviations: AllAS, All asexual generations; ?AS, undetermined number of asexual generations; Complete, asexual and sexual stages with oocysts; iMS1, immature first-generation schizonts; MaG, macrogamonts; MiG, microgamonts and microgametes; MnMa, multinucleate macrogamonts; MS1, first-generation schizonts; MS2, second-generation schizonts; MS3, third-generation schizonts; MS4, fourth-generation schizonts; MZ1, first-generation merozoites; MZ2, second-generation merozoites; MZ3, third-generation merozoites; MZ4, fourth-generation merozoites; NS, no development observed; Oo, unsporulated oocysts; SOo, sporulated oocyst; T1, first-generation trophozoites; T2, second-generation trophozoites; T3, third-generation trophozoites.

adversely interact with coccidian infections. Thus, enterotoxaemia due to *Clostridium perfringens* is a common consequence of some eimerian infections, such as *E. macusaniensis* of South American camelids and *E. maxima* of chickens. Cold and dry weather, transport stress, crowding, and poor nutrition can all contribute to the development of coccidiosis in ruminants.

1.7 DIAGNOSIS

The detection of oocysts in feces, detection of lesions in appropriate locations, and identification of endogenous stages at necropsy can all aid in obtaining a definitive diagnosis. There are excellent papers on the techniques that can be employed.[336,459,974]

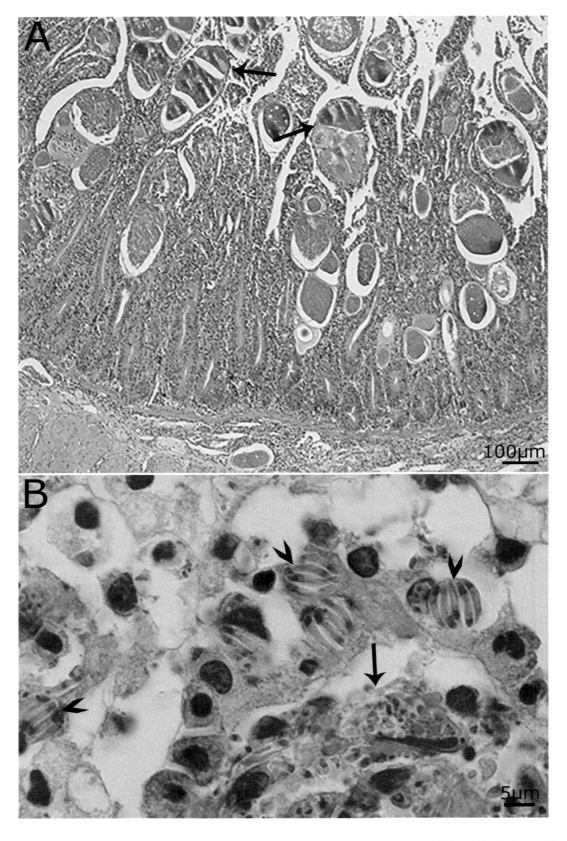

Figure 1.23 Pathogenesis of coccidiosis. HE stain. (A) Numerous large, first-generation schizonts of *Eimeria bovis* (arrows) in an experimentally infected calf but no inflammation. (B) Small schizonts of *E. bareillyi* (arrowheads) causing necrosis of crypts and plugging (arrow) of their lumen in small intestine of a 3-week-old buffalo calf.

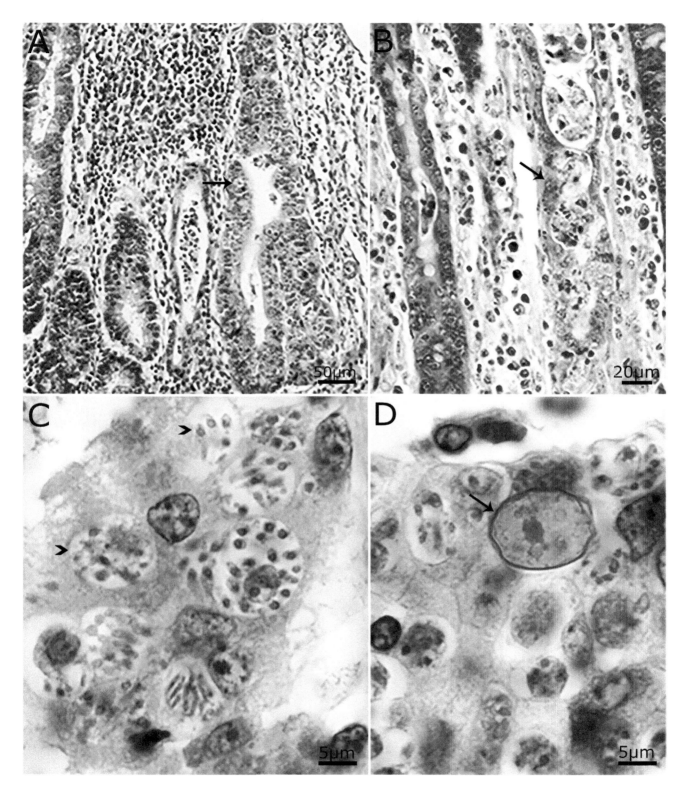

Figure 1.24 Lesions associated with *Eimeria zuernii* in colon of a naturally infected cattle. HE stain. (A) The crypts are heavily infected with *E. zuernii*. The lamina propria is infiltrated with leukocytes, primarily mononuclear cells (arrow). (B) Necrosis of the lamina propria (arrow). (C) Numerous second-generation schizonts (arrowheads); some of them are very small. (D) An unsporulated oocyst (arrow).

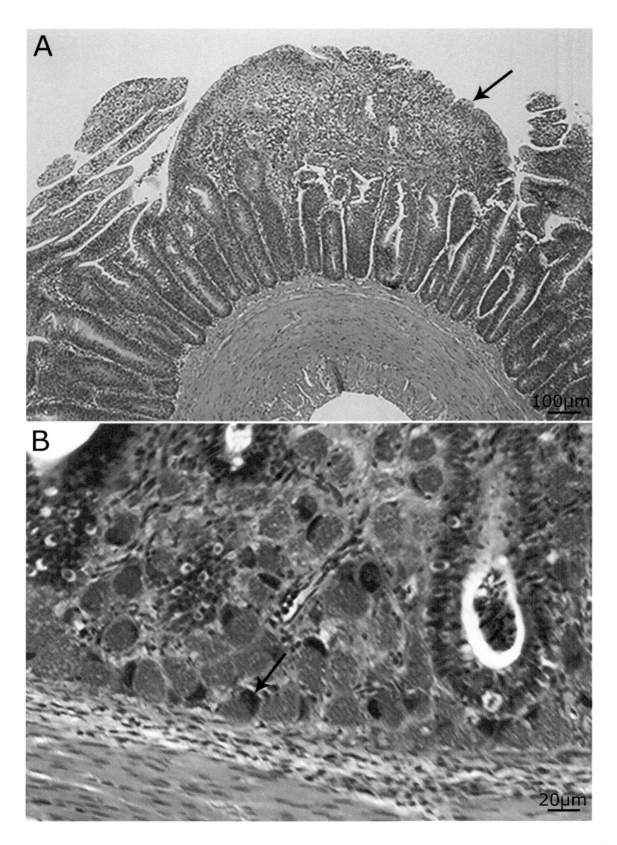

Figure 1.25 Lesions of coccidiosis. (A) Fusion of villi (arrow) in the small intestine in chicken caused by *Eimeria maxima*, HE stain. (B) Second-generation schizonts (arrow) in cecum of chicken experimentally infected with *E. tenella*. HE stain.

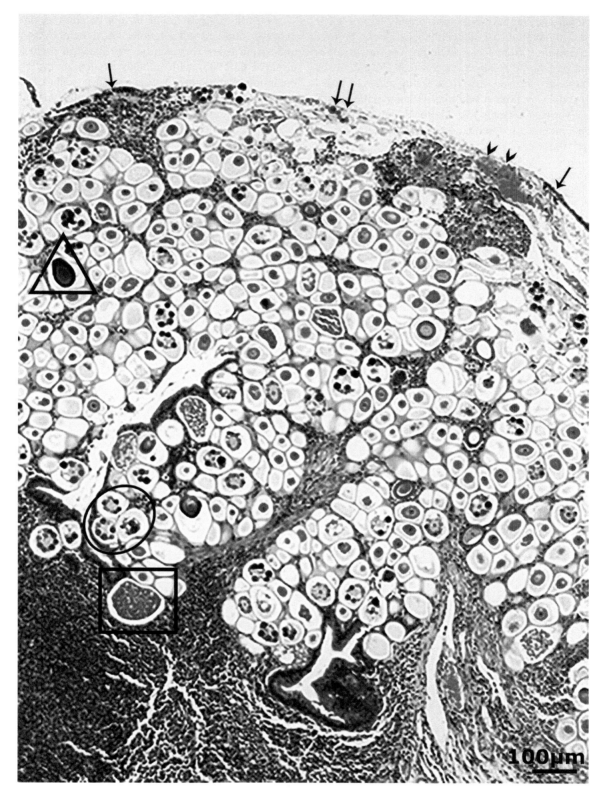

Figure 1.26 Severe infection in jejunum of an alpaca associated with *Eimeria macusaniensis*. Biopsy specimen from the case reported by Johnson et al.[829] HE stain. Double arrows point to loss of surface mucosal villous structures. Arrows point to remnants of intact surface epithelium. The mucosa is replaced with numerous macrogamonts (circle), few microgamonts (rectangle), and rare oocysts (triangle). Note severe inflammation within the underlying submucosa. (Courtesy of Dr. Gerald E. Duhamel, Cornell University, Ithaca, New York.)

Coccidian oocysts have a specific gravity (sg) of 1.1 or higher. Several solutions of higher than 1.1 sg can be used for their separation from feces, including saturated salt or sugar solutions. Some *Eimeria* species (e.g., *E. macusaniensis* of camelids) are very large (~100 um) and very heavy (sg > 1.3) and do not float in solutions with a specific gravity of 1.3 or lower (see Chapter 13). Sedimentation techniques, commonly employed for trematode eggs, are useful for the detection of these heavy oocysts.

Overall, sugar solution is less deleterious on oocysts than the saturated salt solutions. Once the oocysts are separated from feces, they can be sporulated at room temperature (22°C–25°C) with enough oxygen in the container. Potassium dichromate (2.5%) or sulfuric acid (2%) solutions can be used to inhibit microbial growth. After sporulation, oocysts can be stored at 4°C for up to 1 year; thereafter, the infectivity declines. Some species of *Eimeria* and *Cystoisospora* autofluoresce under ultraviolet light.[329]

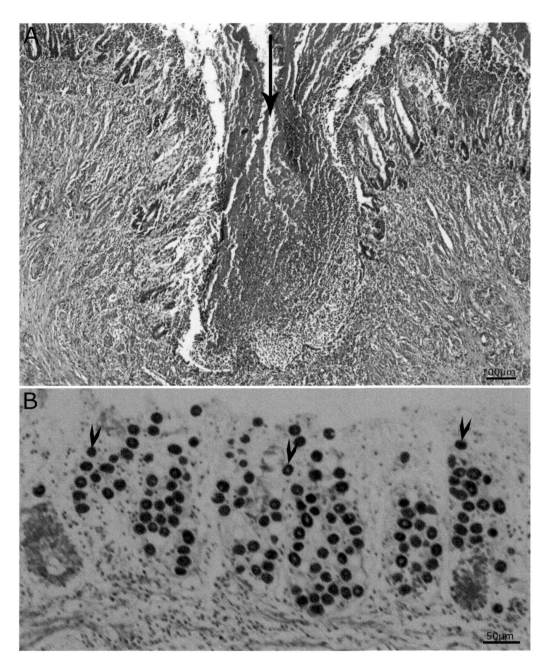

Figure 1.27 *Cystoisospora orlovi* colitis in a naturally infected nursing camel calf. Hemorrhage in colonic mucosa. (A) Denudation and exudation of intestinal contents in lumen (arrow), HE stain. (B) Masses of female gamonts (arrowheads). Periodic acid Schiff reaction counterstained with hematoxylin. (Specimen courtesy of Joerg Kinne, Central Veterinary Laboratory, Dubai, UAE.)

Polymerase chain reaction (PCR) and variations of PCR can be used as an aid for diagnosis and are most commonly employed in detection of *Eimeria* in chickens. Several PCR-based methods have been described (for review see Chapman et al.[232]) that typically use high copy number DNA targets, such as genes coding for ribosomal RNA (18S, ITS1 and ITS2) or the mitochondrial DNA (Cox1, Cox3, or CytB). Detection may entail analytical techniques such as gel electrophoresis of PCR amplicons or real-time PCR analysis, thus requiring special equipment and facilities. The relative difficulty in isolating large amounts of *Eimeria* DNA from oocysts and the presence of substances that are inhibitory of PCR requires the use of internal standards to control for false-negative reactions. These and other factors

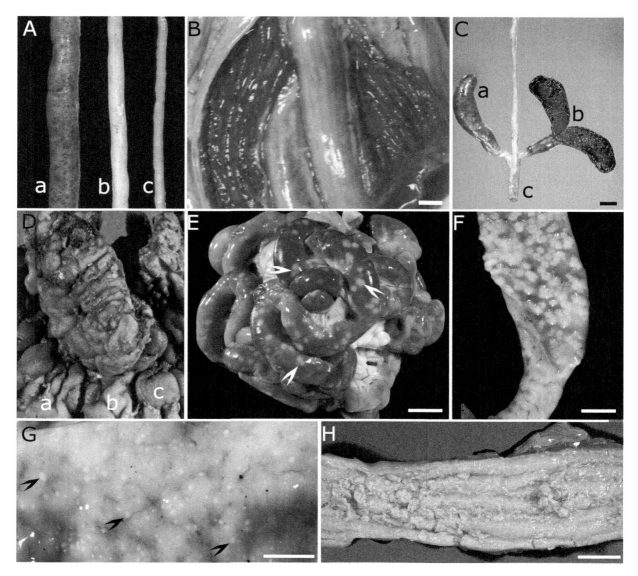

Figure 1.28 Gross lesions of intestinal coccidiosis. Unstained. (A) Serosal view of unopened small intestine of chickens. (a) *Eimeria necatrix* infection with hemorrhage and edema. (b) *E. acervulina* infection with moderate edema and distention. (c) Uninfected. (B) Hemorrhage in the colon of a camel calf naturally infected with *Cystoisospora orlovi*. (C) Necrosis and hemorrhage in experimental *E. tenella* infection. Intact (a) and opened (b) ceca, and terminal ileum (c). (D) Proliferative enteritis in the ileum of an alpaca. Note, fusion and proliferation of villi (a, b, c). (E, F) Severe *Eimeria* spp. infection in the large intestine of goats. Note congestion and yellowish-white plaques that are visible even through serosa (arrowheads). (G) Macroscopic schizonts (arrowheads) in abomasum of a naturally infected sheep. (H) Pseudomembranous enteritis in a pig due to *C. suis* infection. Note cracks in mucosa and adherent desquamated tissue. Bars = 1 cm in (B, C, E, F, H) and 0.5 cm in (G). ([A] From Gardiner C.H. et al. 1988. *An Atlas of Protozoan Parasites in Animal Tissues*. Agriculture handbook number 651. U.S. Department of Agriculture [USDA], Agricultural Research Service [ARS], Washington, DC; [B] From Kinne, J. et al. 2002. *J. Parasitol.* 88, 548–552; [C] From Gardiner, C.H. et al. 1988. *An Atlas of Protozoan Parasites in Animal Tissues*. Agriculture handbook number 651. USDA, ARS, Washington, DC; [D] Courtesy of Robert Bildfell, Oregon State University and from Dubey, J.P. 2018. *Parasitol. Res.* 117, 1999–2013; [E,F] Courtesy of Dr. Kim Newkirk, University of Tennessee; [G] From Ammar, S.I. et al. 2019. *J. Vet. Diagn. Invest.* 31, 128–132 and Courtesy of Dr. Linden Craig, University of Tennessee.)

have limited the widespread application of PCR for *Eimeria* oocyst detection to specially equipped laboratories.

Necropsy examination is often necessary to determine the etiology of a disease. Some coccidian species are identifiable by gross examination with a high certainty; as an example, *E. tenella* produces characteristic lesions in ceca of chickens (Figure 1.27B). Endogenous stages can be identified by making smears of lesions on glass slides (Figure 1.4). Sometimes the demonstration of characteristic oocysts in smears will confirm a diagnosis. In some cases, the smears can be fixed in methyl alcohol and examined after staining with Giemsa (Figure 1.4). For intestines fixed and processed for histological examination, endogenous stages can be visualized by conventionally used HE staining methods. The PAS reaction is useful in differentiating endogenous stages, as macrogamonts are PAS-positive, whereas microgamonts are usually PAS-negative. Schizonts and merozoites of some coccidia (e.g., *Cystoisospora* species of cats and dogs) are often PAS-positive (Figure 1.10).

1.8 CONTROL

Coccidian oocysts are environmentally resistant and can survive for months under harsh conditions. They are also resistant to most disinfectants available when used at recommended concentrations.[328] Some chemicals can be effective but are at concentrations that are also harmful to humans and livestock so they are not used. Desiccation and steam (>70°C) can kill oocysts.[521,1324] Metam sodium was effective in preventing sporulation of chicken *Eimeria* in poultry litter.[532] In general, oocysts of coccidian parasites are environmentally resistant.

Prevention and control of coccidiosis are discussed with each host chapter. Chemotherapy of coccidiosis is discussed in Chapter 6.

REFERENCES

38, 50, 64, 65, 92, 100, 168, 176, 213, 228, 232, 254, 263–265, 278, 286, 320, 328, 329, 335, 336, 350, 360, 364, 384–390, 392–395, 397, 416, 419, 420, 422, 424, 426, 435, 437, 441, 456, 459, 519–521, 525–529, 532, 535, 560, 582, 584, 615, 659, 662, 665, 666, 705, 708, 790, 829, 869, 870, 871, 893, 900, 973–975, 1032, 1035, 1041, 1044, 1048, 1050, 1053, 1077, 1090, 1094, 1117, 1130, 1153, 1167, 1212, 1228, 1312, 1322, 1324, 1330, 1332, 1357, 1422, 1423, 1458, 1474, 1481, 1482, 1515, 1549, 1557, 1578, 1600–1610, 1624–1626, 1717, 1797, 1821

CHAPTER 2

Phylogeny of Coccidian Parasites

P. C. Thompson and B. M. Rosenthal

CONTENTS

2.1 INTRODUCTION

Hundreds of *Eimeria* species have been described. Our purpose here is to review what is known regarding their diversity and the extent, timing, and drivers of their speciation, referring to the best available estimates of their phylogenetic history.

As described in Chapter 1, coccidian parasites belong to the phylum Apicomplexa,[977] a group of eukaryotes in the kingdom Alveolata. This phylum was originally described to accommodate many organisms that did not group clearly into other groups of protists, with limited understanding as to the evolutionary relationships among its members. Subsequent evaluations have defined characteristics demonstrating their common descent.[9] These single-celled organisms share the conoid, an apical organelle that facilitates entry into host cells. They infect virtually all metazoan hosts and are ubiquitous. As recently as 25 years ago, most phylogenetic analyses were restricted to morphological characters to estimate their relationships. Since then, a revolution in molecular markers has helped to clarify evolutionary relationships among the constituents, but some controversy remains concerning the divisions among subgroups within the phylum.

Coccidians fall within Class Sporozoea Leuckart 1879 and are the largest Subclass within the apicomplexans, containing around 2300 named species. They are further classified within the Order Eucoccidiida, which has two suborders:

Adeleorina Leger 1911 and Eimeriorina Leger 1911. Various authors have included haemosporids and piroplasms as belonging to the coccidians, but consensus places only the adeleorinids and eimeriorinids into this group. The adeleorinids consist of monoxenous parasites of invertebrates, and will not be discussed further here. Members of the suborder Eimeriorina have both monoxenous and heteroxenous life cycles, parasitizing all vertebrate types, including fish, reptiles, birds, and mammals.

In a major reorganization of coccidians in the 1970s,[977] the Eimeriorina suborder was subdivided into two groups based on the presence or absence of Stieda bodies; those lacking Stieda bodies were placed within the Sarcocystidae, and those with Stieda bodies were situated within the Eimeriidae.[1723] Later it was shown that this bifurcation also divided those with heteroxenous life cycles from those with homoxenous life cycles, but the presence of a Stieda body did not suffice as a basis to establish monophyly.

Other physical or phenotypic characters have been proposed for reconstructing evolutionary relationships among the Eimeriorina but suffer from the difficulty in comparably preserving such characters in fixed samples and the need for specialized skills to properly prepare specimens for light or electronic microscopic examination and properly interpreting the results.

Since the 1990s, researchers have increasingly incorporated molecular phylogenetics to investigate divisions within the Eimeriorina, inferring descent relationships by reconstructing the history of changes in homologous DNA sequences. Subdivision of the two sister families has been confirmed by analyzing a variety of loci and most recently by comparing complete genomic sequences.[177,1260,1404] Molecular phylogenetics has further enabled fine-scale examination of the evolution within families and genera.

2.2 LIMITS OF MORPHOLOGY OR PHENOTYPE IN DIAGNOSING RELATED PARASITE TAXA

Among related species of *Eimeria,* the distribution of morphological and phenotypic characteristics does not always respect deeper phylogenetic relationships; this suggests that they are capable of evolving more rapidly than needed in order to use them to trace deeper historical patterns. This point is illustrated by one clade consisting of 11 parasite species exclusive to rabbits.[931] Two sister clades within this parasite assemblage have been recognized based on variation in 18S rDNA; the members of only one of these clades possess an oocyst residuum, the presence of which is presumed to represent an ancestral condition. Other morphological and phenotypic characters do not consistently differ among these two clades: no specific lineage is especially pathogenic. (Indeed, the two most pathogenic lineages, *E. intestinalis* and *E. flavescens,* appear only distantly related.)

Instead of seeking those characters capable of consistently resolving interrelationships among a given subset of organisms, it would be preferable to employ attributes varying in a wide range of organisms whose states can be definitively and reproducibly described by those lacking intimate knowledge of each lineage. These principles underly the growth and reliance on molecular phylogenetics as a basis to understand the evolutionary history of these parasites.

2.3 MOLECULAR MARKERS USED IN PHYLOGENETICS

Most extant molecular phylogenetic studies of these organisms have relied exclusively on variation in the ribosomal DNA small subunit 18S locus. It has been the workhorse of phylogenetic studies, because structural constraints define highly conserved regions of the molecule that are interspersed by more variable regions that record changes capable of diagnosing groups of taxa sharing especially close common ancestry. This ubiquitous locus typically occurs repetitively in the nuclear DNA but evolves in a concerted fashion. For most species, only a single sequence has been documented; researchers should, however, be cautioned that variation among paralogous copies has occasionally been described and may be more common than is generally appreciated. Such variation might confuse estimates of relationships, especially among the most closely related of taxa.

Within the family Eimeriidae, at least 17 genera and more than 1500 species have been named. To date, hundreds of 18S sequences, representing about 200 putative species, have been deposited to public databases. Given the likelihood that tens of thousands of undiscovered *Eimeria* species exist, the available data should be understood as but a small sample of the actual diversification history; moreover, the bias in sampling effort (toward parasites of humans and livestock of value to us) may distort our impression of parasite diversity and of the forces responsible for their diversification and success. Our understanding will undoubtedly change as more sequence data are considered.

The genera best represented in the literature are those of known medical or economic importance assigned to the genera *Eimeria, Goussia, Caryospora, Lankesterella, Atoxoplasma, Isospora,* and *Cyclospora.* Recent molecular studies have shown that the subdivisions are not clear among genera and may merit future revision.

By far, the 18S locus provides the best available means to estimate genealogical relationships because, for many parasite taxa, only 18S has thus far been characterized. Notwithstanding other advantages of this locus, overreliance on any single gene precludes independent tests of phylogenetic relationships, may bias inferences, and may preclude resolution of recent distinctions among closely related taxa.

Recently, certain other genetic loci have been explored for their diagnostic and phylogenetic potential, most notably the large subunit ribosomal DNA (28S),[1453] the mitochondrial cytochrome oxidase I (COI) gene,[1145,1189,1266,1756] and the apicoplast RNA polymerase subunit β (*rpoB*) gene.[1266] The species characterized at any of these loci number only in the tens.

Recent advances in sequencing technology have, however, afforded the research community complete draft genomes of some species of *Eimeria,*[699,1404] providing a wealth of loci yet to be explored as candidates for diagnosing taxa and reconstructing their evolutionary relationships.

2.4 HOW WE KNOW WHAT WE KNOW, AND THE EXTENT OF WHAT REMAINS UNEXPLORED

Fewer than 10% of the 1500 named species of *Eimeria* are represented in any published phylogeny. More inclusive phylogenies should provide more meaningful and more stable estimates of evolutionary relationships but may very likely complicate our view of intrageneric relationships. Parasite clades that now appear restricted to certain, closely related hosts may be found to share a close relationship to others, parasitizing unrelated hosts. There are at least two distinct lineages of *Eimeria* that infect rodents, only one of which derives from an ancestor that also gave rise to parasites in bats, suggesting a history of host switching between bats and rodents.[11] There is also experimental evidence that although most *Eimeria* are host specific, some can infect hosts belonging to different families.[1757]

2.5 ORIGINS OF *EIMERIA*

The earliest branching eimeriid lineages contain numerous species that infect sharks and other kinds of fish, assigned to the genus *Goussia* (which itself is composed of at least four significantly differentiated subclades) (Figure 2.1).[821,1200,1453,1829] An examination of 18S sequences from fish parasites found that piscine *Eimeria* (and those in the genus *Calyptospora*) branched off very early in the history of *Eimeria*. For those species examined, *Eimeria*

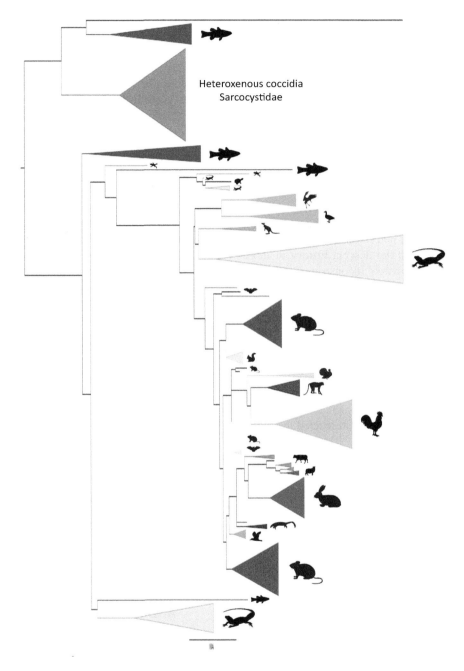

Figure 2.1 Diversification history of eimeriid parasites of various vertebrate host types, as reconstructed from phylogenetic trees reconstructed under the criterion of maximum likelihood. Triangles reflect natural groups of parasites of particular host groups. The breadth of each triangle is proportional to the number of such taxa that have been characterized to date. While the existence of each colored grouping enjoys strong statistical support, the precise placement of some of them (including the group parasitizing marsupials and the group parasitizing primates) are more equivocal and deserve additional analysis with more sequence data. Broadly speaking, Eimeriid parasites appear to have origins as parasites of fish. Among parasites in terrestrial vertebrates, early branching lineages parasitize amphibian, reptilian, and certain avian hosts. Distinct lineages are evident among parasites of placental and nonplacental mammals. The complete history of this ubiquitous parasite group awaits far more comprehensive sampling but is enough to show that certain host groups (e.g., rodents) have been successfully colonized by more than one, independent Eimeriid parasite lineage.

infecting fish were found in a strongly supported clade at the base of the *Eimeria* tree with consistently large genetic distances among isolates (indicating extensive time since diverging from one another). The basal evolutionary position of these parasites of aquatic vertebrates indicates that the Eimeriidae evolved very early in the history of life, parasitizing progenitors of land animals. This finding was confirmed by a smaller sample of sequences from the large subunit 28S rDNA. Eimeriids remain sister to Sarcocystidae with a well-supported clade of fish *Eimeria* at the base of the Eimeriidae.

Thereafter, this group was likely carried onto land with their diversifying hosts and now parasitizes every major group of terrestrial vertebrates. In support of this evolutionary hypothesis, *Eimeria arnyi* (from a snake) and *Eimeria ranae* (from frogs) appear to be derived from lineages that commenced their independent evolution prior to the origins of parasites of avian and mammalian hosts.[820] Incongruously, *Eimeria* now parasitizing marsupial hosts appear to have diversified before the diversification of parasite groups infecting birds and placental mammals, conflicting with what we know about the descent history of those host groups. Resolving this apparent inconsistency might be achieved by systematically characterizing *Eimeria* in early branching hosts from each major vertebrate lineage.

The present view of *Eimeria* in birds and mammals, based on analyses of nuclear 18S and mitochondrial COI loci, suggests a more complicated, and possibly intertwined, history.[1266] As previously stated, the earliest-branching lineage known in mammals is restricted to marsupials and (to available sampling) now appears most closely related to certain species of *Eimeria* infecting snakes and frogs. The earliest lineage *Eimeria* known in birds, restricted to cranes, branches off in this portion of the tree. This same lineage then gave rise to parasites of bats and rodents. Later, a clade of parasites specific to passerine birds split from one specific to other bats and rodents. Eventually, this line led to a well-supported division between parasites in pigs, ungulates, and rabbits, each diversifying within a phylogenetically limited host range. The most-derived (most recently diversified) species define parasites ascribed to *Cyclospora* and to the galliform avian *Eimeria* associated with agriculture.

Robust phylogenetic trees based on 18S sequences have been described for those *Eimeria* imposing significant losses to poultry production[79,1189] and provide some insight into evolutionary mechanisms engendering diversity among species of *Eimeria*. The branching of the various species correlates with variation in certain morphological and phenotypic characteristics; for example, species of similar size are closely related and probably diversified through sympatric speciation, evolving from a common lineage to infect specific areas of the chicken intestinal tract.

Several recent publications have sought to use multiple loci or even whole genomes to test conclusions based on the analysis of variation in 18S, alone.[1266] Mitochondrial markers

were used in addition to 18S sequences to explore evolutionary relationships among *Eimeria* species that infect chickens. The additional locus confirmed previous observations of monophyly among these species and established that *E. tenella* and *E. necatrix* form a sister clade to the other major chicken pathogens. They later extended their investigation of Eimeriidae to include genes from the nucleus (18S), mitochondria (COI, 16S, and 23S), and plastid genomes (rpoB) as a proof of principle for using a genome-level sequence to investigate phylogenetics of a wide range of coccidia, including both Sarcocystidae and Eimeriidae. Concatenated alignments of these genes resulted in well-supported Bayesian trees resembling those that had previously been reconstructed from variation in 18S alone. Fundamental observations from this study include the following: Eimeriidae are monophyletic with respect to the Sarcocystidae; the genera *Lankesterella*, *Isosopora*, *Atoxoplasma*, and *Cyclospora* fall within the clade encompassing all eimeriids; and the 18S locus is best for distinguishing among genera, whereas COI sequences are suitable for distinguishing among congeneric species. Not explicitly stated in this paper but evident in the phylogenetic trees is that host association is not a definitive factor in locating any species within the tree; for example, multiple avian and mammalian lineages are evident. Nevertheless, the available evidence (based on admittedly spotty sampling) appears to substantiate parasite lineages that have evolved with, and are restricted to, primates, rabbits, and galliform birds.

Taken altogether, it is evident that *Eimeria* evolved for a prolonged period in aquatic vertebrates prior to commencing a complex history of diversification in terrestrial vertebrates. There is ample evidence from clades containing both bird and mammal eimeriids that these parasites have at least occasionally switched among vertebrate host types. Further diversity has been elaborated within groups restricted to a given host type, as is exemplified by the parasites of chickens. Further sampling will be needed to reveal the important evolutionary connections between different groups of hosts, which in turn may provide insight into past ecological ties among vertebrate species.

2.6 LESSONS LEARNED FROM THE MOST-STUDIED PARASITES OF LIVESTOCK, AND POSSIBLE CONSEQUENCES OF SUCH INVESTIGATOR BIAS

Current information, for example, substantiates a belief that *Eimeria* in domesticated goats and sheep form a natural group subsumed within the broader *Eimeria* tree and closely related to the *Eimeria* in cattle.[881,1266] Understanding the origins of this parasite group, and any role human activity has played in this group's diversification and spread, requires broader examination of bovid and other wild host groups. Only with the benefit of considerably broader sampling will we know if the parasites now abundant in bovid livestock originated in wild bovids, whether extant wild bovids serve as reservoirs for infection in managed herds, and whether parasites in our bovid livestock derive from more than one introduction from exogenous sources. Should a "bovid" parasite one day be found in a bird or a reptile (or should evolutionarily close species pairs be identified in such disparate host types), our present notions of host specificity would require reassessment.

2.7 HOW MUCH MORE HAS YET TO BE DISCOVERED?

Theory and observations demonstrate benefits to sexual parasites adapting to the conditions typical of a given definitive host, and the risks a parasite might face in reproducing in "the wrong place" with "the wrong mates." Total fidelity of a parasite to a given host would result in (at least) as many parasite species as host species. Moreover, the most-studied systems (e.g., poultry parasites) indicate that any given host may simultaneously or sequentially harbor numerous parasite taxa, each perhaps specialized on a distinct transmission strategy, physical substrate, and suite of immunological markers and signals.

Experimental data show that certain parasites fail to establish or reproduce even in exogenous hosts closely related to their host of origin.[723,1724,1757] We frankly do not know how generally this principle holds, lacking empirical data one way or the other. Nonetheless, intuition and experience strongly argue that many more species of *Eimeria* await discovery and description. Humility demands we should proceed cautiously in inferring the history and relationships among organisms we have not yet even encountered.

Molecular systematics has reaffirmed certain foundational premises derived from microscopy and has necessitated revision of certain other prior conclusions. Nonetheless, vast untapped stores of information await definition. By subjecting a broader range of heritable information to systematic comparison from a broader array of taxa, genomics and metagenomics will enrich our understanding of the diversity, history, and best classification of *Eimeria* species. Having traced their distant origins in the seas to their establishment on land, and having discerned their ancient subdivision into the major and ubiquitous groups, we are now positioned to examine the nuances of what makes each unique, and how their specific attributes influence their actual and potential impact on us and the animals in our care.

REFERENCES

9, 11, 79, 177, 699, 723, 820, 821, 881, 931, 977, 1145, 1189, 1200, 1260, 1266, 1404, 1453, 1723, 1724, 1756, 1757, 1829

CHAPTER 3

Host Immunity in Coccidiosis

H. S. Lillehoj, W. H. Kim, and A. Chaudhury

CONTENTS

3.1 INTRODUCTION

Avian coccidiosis is one of the most widespread infectious diseases of livestock and poultry and poses a significant economic threat to animal husbandry.[1565] Prophylactic medication that has been successful in reducing coccidiosis and dramatically increased the efficiency of commercial livestock and poultry production over the last 50 years is no longer applicable due to governmental regulatory changes to meet the rising consumers' demand for antibiotic-free meat. Therefore, new strategies for coccidiosis prevention and treatment are needed for sustainable commercial meat production in the antibiotic-free era. The etiology of coccidiosis is complex and may differ among different animal species. However, in general, it involves many host- and parasite-associated factors, including genetics, diet, environment, and management. While more than 1700 species of *Eimeria* have been described, only seven are known to infect chickens: *E. acervulina, E. tenella, E. maxima, E. brunetti, E. mitis, E. necatrix,* and *E. praecox*. All seven species are distributed worldwide, with *E. acervulina, E. tenella,* and *E. maxima* being the most common (see Chapters 15 and 16).

Eimeria parasites are obligate intracellular pathogens that primarily infect the intestinal tract with various levels of damage to the gut epithelium, decreased nutrient absorption, inefficient feed utilization, and impaired growth rate, which, in severe cases, may lead to mortality. The increased incidence of coccidiosis and escalating restriction on antibiotic growth promoters in livestock and poultry production worldwide indicate that there is a timely need to understand host-pathogen immunobiology in coccidiosis to facilitate the development of effective novel control strategies. However, the current limited understanding of host immune systems and parasite biology and antigenicity complicates the development of effective anticoccidial prevention and treatment strategies in livestock and poultry.

Mammalian and avian immune systems are complex and possess both innate and adaptive immune responses as well as humoral and cell-mediated components.[1010,1014,1016,1017] Coccidial parasites are intracellular pathogens that develop in the gut, even though infection engenders a systemic response to produce humoral antibodies and a cell-mediated immune response. The innate immune system in mammals and poultry comprises cells and their secreted products that defend the host against infection in a nonspecific manner. Host pattern recognition receptors (PRRs) constitute a critical component of innate immunity, and they recognize conserved components of pathogens, the pathogen-associated molecular patterns (PAMPs). Protozoan PAMPs are potent stimulators of innate immune responses, although their cognate PRRs are not well defined, compared with those that recognize bacterial and viral PAMPs.[586] Antigen-specific, adaptive immunity is mediated by T cells expressing T-cell receptors (TCRs), B cells expressing surface immunoglobulins, and their secreted antibodies, cytokines, and chemokines. In the intestine, gut-associated lymphoid tissue (GALT) mediates adaptive immunity through three interrelated processes: antigen processing and presentation, production of intestinal antibodies, and activation of cell-mediated immunity. In immune hosts, parasites that enter the gut are prevented from further development, suggesting that acquired, cell-mediated immunological memory resulting from initial pathogen exposure inhibits natural progression of parasite development.[1014,1707,1870]

The immunobiology of avian coccidiosis involves a complex interplay between the various life stages of *Eimeria* parasites and host intestinal epithelial and immune cells. Adaptive immunity is highly specific and regulates antigen-specific immune responses to prevent colonization and growth of the pathogen inside the host. In mammals and poultry, two major lymphocyte types, B cells (producing surface immunoglobulins) and T cells (TCRs), are the major components of adaptive immune responses. Although B-cell depletion studies have revealed that antibodies do not play a specific role in anticoccidian protective immunity, other studies have emphasized the importance of passively transferred humoral immunity to *Eimeria* infection in chickens and other animals.

One of the most immediate and significant outcomes of coccidiosis is devastating destruction of the intestinal mucosa because of parasite infection, and replication and development of following life-cycle stages within the intestinal epithelia. This pathological effect, and the associated retardation of chicken growth, has been the major impetus for development of anticoccidial control strategies. Synthetic coccidiostatic drugs have played a major role in mitigating the negative consequences of *Eimeria* infection in commercial animal production. It is also clear, however, that alternatives to antibiotic chemotherapy are becoming an increasing priority for modern livestock and poultry production to maintain commercial profitability, reduce the emergence of drug-resistant parasites, and ensure consumer confidence in providing safe, consumable foods. A major challenge for developing new disease prevention and control strategies against coccidiosis is determining the nature of protective host immune responses, virulence factors associated with parasite pathogenesis, and the best mode of vaccine delivery to induce protective immunity against all variants of *Eimeria* parasites. At present, there is a limited number of immunological reagents in poultry to identify various effector components of cell-mediated immunity, which represents a major effector arm of host immunity against coccidiosis. Thus, there has been limited progress in our understanding of host immunity against many pathogens including *Eimeria* parasites.

In this chapter, we review various aspects of the host immune response against coccidiosis in different animal species with a primary focus on chicken coccidiosis and identify the major components that are involved in immunity to *Eimeria* spp. A better understanding of host-parasite immunobiology will facilitate the development of prevention and treatment strategies against coccidiosis in the era of antibiotic-free animal production.

3.2 IMMUNITY IN CHICKENS

3.2.1 Innate Immunity in Chickens

Eimeria parasites induce robust innate immune responses in chickens that are indicated by increased numbers of macrophages and monocytes, and increased secretion of soluble effector molecules such as nitric oxide (NO), cytokines, and chemokines.[1182] In avian coccidiosis, innate immune response to *Eimeria* is initiated upon initial exposure to sporozoites, which then expands in complexity involving many different components of the local immune system as coccidia undergo life-cycle changes. Host adaptive immunity follows after innate immunity becomes stronger with each subsequent exposure to oocysts.[1379] As the first line of defense, innate immunity protects the host against invading pathogens. The host innate immune system comprises cells and their secreted products that protect the host against the microbial infection in a nonspecific manner. These include physical barriers such as intestinal mucosa, phagocytic immune cells such as macrophages and leukocytes, and cytokines and chemokines. Innate immunity is initiated upon initial recognition of conserved PAMPs by PRRs on and within the hemopoietic or epithelial cells. Toll-like receptors (TLRs) and nucleotide-binding oligomerization domain-like receptor (NOD)-like receptors (NLRs) are transmembrane PRR proteins that recognize specific PAMPs, usually a conserved entity from the pathogens.[157,920] PAMPs are diverse molecules such as proteins, lipids, carbohydrates, and nucleic acids that are derived from bacteria, viruses, fungi, and protozoa.[586,920] Some of the well-known PAMPs include viral nucleic acids, lipopeptides, bacterial lipopolysaccharides (LPSs), glycolipids, and CpG DNA. In mammals, TLRs were the first-described PPRs,[968,1170] and several TLR homologs are now well defined in chickens.[157,1642,1692] Although cognate PPRs are not well defined for protozoan PAMPs, they induce potent innate immune responses.

In chickens, 10 TLRs have been identified so far: TLR1LA, TLR1LB, TLR2A, TLR2B, TLR3, TLR4, TLR5, TLR7, TLR15, and TLR21.[157,1692] Out of these, six chicken TLRs (TLR2A, TLR2B, TLR3, TLR4, TLR5, and TLR7) have orthologs in mammals and fish. Phylogenetic analyses have revealed that TLR21 is only shared by fish, and the remaining three TLRs (TLR1LA, TLR1LB, and TLR15) are unique to chickens. The role of TLRs in innate immunity against coccidiosis is yet to be established, although the expression of TLR3, TLR4, and TLR15 is upregulated in chickens following infection with *E. praecox*. Chickens that are infected with *E. tenella* have increased levels of TLR1LA, TLR4, TLR5, TLR7, and TLR21 as early as 3 hours postinoculation (HPI) in 1-day-old chickens and at 12 HPI in 3-week-old chickens, with TLR5, TLR1LA, and TLR21 remaining highly expressed at 72 HPI.[1881] Similarly, *in vitro* stimulation of heterophils and monocyte-derived macrophages with *E. tenella* live sporozoites induces high expression of TLR4, TLR5, and TLR adaptor protein, MyD88 as early as 2 hours.[1916] Expression of these innate molecules is significantly higher in macrophages stimulated with heat-killed than in live sporozoites, suggesting that application of heat-killed sporozoites induces a robust innate immune response against avian coccidiosis when used as a vaccine.[1916] However, the relevance of these observations on host protective immune response in coccidiosis needs to be validated using specific TLR gene knock-out models *in vivo*.

Currently, not many TLR agonists expressed by *Eimeria* spp. have been recognized. One well-known *Eimeria* PAMP is profilin, which is a 19-kD protein that was originally isolated as a recombinant protein from *E. acervulina* merozoites[1014,1182] and expressed in all developmental stages of their life cycle. This conserved protein is believed to serve as a major TLR ligand and stimulated IFN-γ production.[533,1014] Immunization with profilin protein confers significant protection against experimental coccidiosis in chickens.[779–783,883,964,1014] Despite its functional role in chicken splenic cell proliferation and interferon (IFN)-γ production, a cognate TLR receptor for *Eimeria* profilin has not yet been identified in avian species. In mammals, toxofilin, a protein from *Toxoplasma gondii*, is homologous with profilin. Toxofilin is a TLR11 ligand and induces a potent interleukin (IL)-12 response in mouse dendritic cells (DCs).[1855] It is debatable whether profilin induces innate immune responses via a MyD88-dependent pathway or TIR-domain-containing adapter-inducing IFN-β(TRIF)-dependent pathway. Nevertheless, the importance of *Eimeria*-profilin in inducing innate immunity against coccidiosis is inevitable. Besides its role in anticoccidial immunity, profilin also has antiviral and anticancer properties in mammals.[608,848,849,1452] In addition, profilin serves as a potent adjuvant in mammalian models such as *T. gondii* infection. Profilin, as an adjuvant, increases protective immunity against *T. gondii* in experimentally infected mice. The role of profilin in innate immunity against avian coccidiosis, and its use as an adjuvant in human as well as veterinary medicine, warrants further investigation. Some of the other mammalian TLR agonists such as CpG DNA (TLR9) activate chicken macrophages and offer increased protection against avian coccidiosis. The adjuvant effect of CpG DNA on *Eimeria* protein vaccines protects chickens from experimental coccidiosis induced by *E. acervulina* and *E. tenella*. However, chickens do not express TLR9 or any other equivalent TLR; therefore, it is unclear how CpG DNA activates chicken macrophages and induces innate immunity to avian coccidiosis. Similarly, heat shock protein (HSP) 70 from *E. tenella* can induce anticoccidial immunity in chickens. HSP70 is a well-known ligand for TLR2 and TLR4. In chickens, it is yet to be defined.

Other than TLRs, cells involved in innate immune responses to *Eimeria* at different phases are natural killer (NK) cells, DCs, epithelial cells, heterophils, and macrophages. In particular, NK cells play a major role in inducing innate immunity during *Eimeria* infection.[888,889,1008,1014] The high-throughput sequencing of the intestinal cDNA library of *Eimeria*-infected chickens has identified a novel anticoccidial peptide secreted by NK cells homologous to mammalian NK-lysin.[732,888] NK-lysin transcripts are significantly increased in response to *Eimeria* infection. Avian macrophages are also involved and play a major role in innate immunity against coccidiosis. In response to *Eimeria* sporozoites, avian macrophages produce a large amount of NO, which is the first major innate response against coccidiosis. In general, a TLR4 ligand, LPS from gram-negative bacteria, induces a strong NO response in macrophages with a well-known mechanism, thus inducing the first innate response of the host to the bacterial infection. Avian macrophages respond to coccidian sporozoites in a similar way, although the mechanism is yet to be discovered.[1015] Additionally, macrophage migration inhibitory factor (MIF) plays a crucial role in mediating innate immunity in coccidiosis.[1644] MIF is produced by macrophages, monocytes, T cells, and nonlymphoid cells, and is highly conserved in vertebrates as well as invertebrates.[169] Mammalian MIF induces expression of inflammatory markers such as IL-1β, IL-6, IL-8, IFN-γ, and tumor necrosis factor (TNF)-α.[1740] In avian coccidiosis too, *Eimeria*-infected chickens induce high levels of the chicken MIF gene transcript in the gut.[780] When stimulated with recombinant MIF protein, chicken macrophages produce increased levels of IL-6, IL-17, and TNF superfamily member (TNFSF) 15. Additionally, intestinal DCs initiate strong protective innate immunity against avian coccidiosis.[355,356] Immunization with DC-derived exosomes protects against *Eimeria* infection in chickens, with a robust innate immune response.[358] More recently, involvement of exosomes derived from chicken antigen-presenting cells infected with *Eimeria* showed promising results in protecting chickens from coccidial parasites.[359] However, it is not practical to produce such exosomes on a large scale; therefore, serum exosomes from *Eimeria*-infected chickens are isolated and used for protective immunity against avian coccidiosis.

Besides NK cells and macrophages, B and T lymphocytes are also engaged in producing strong innate immune responses after primary infection with *Eimeria* in chickens.[1870] Based on early investigations, B- and T-cell-mediated innate immunity plays an important role in anticoccidial immunity in mammalian and avian species.[1018,1446,1445,1761] After primary infection in bursectomized chickens, high numbers of oocysts are produced but do not induce clinical coccidiosis after secondary infection due to the protective innate immunity acquired after the primary infection.[1182] In particular, higher numbers of CD8[+] cytotoxic T cells (CTLs) are induced after primary coccidial infection, thus indicating the key role of T cells in mediating innate anticoccidial immunity.[153,154,1007,1011,1182] Additionally, CD4[+] and CD8[+] T cells offer resistance to primary coccidial infection.[1447,1454] With the use of avian lymphocyte-specific immune reagents, flow cytometry of intraepithelial lymphocytes (IELs) in naïve as well as *Eimeria*-infected chickens showed the relevance of T cells in mediating anticoccidial innate immune responses.[1009–1011] The increased T-cell populations in primary infection produce elevated levels of proinflammatory cytokine IFN-γ. IFN-γ has an immunoregulatory as well as antiparasitic effect by mainly inhibiting parasite development.[266,1012,1013,1451] It is a major cytokine that has anticoccidial effects by inhibiting the invasion or development of *Eimeria*.[1012] The significant role of IFN-γ in anti-*Eimeria* immunity has been studied extensively. It is now clear that lymphocytes from birds exposed to primary *Eimeria* infection produce large amounts of IFN-γ.[153] It is proposed that, at the site of infection, T-cell priming occurs, resulting in production of IFN-γ at the infection site, thus regulating anticoccidial immunity.[155,1009,1869] *In situ* hybridization has shown that, following *Eimeria* challenge, IFN-γ is produced by the cells (predominantly T cells) at the site of infection (cecum) and by splenocytes.[1455]

As stated earlier, the innate immune response in avian coccidiosis is characterized by secretion of several cytokines and chemokines produced by innate cells. Besides IFN-γ, a wide variety of cytokines such as IL-1, IL-2, IL-4–IL-6, IL-8, IL-10, IL-12, IL-13, and IL-15–IL-18, TNF-α, LPS-induced TNF-α factor (LITAF), TNFSF15, transforming growth factor (TGF)-β1–TGF-β4, and granulocyte-macrophage colony-stimulating factor (GM-CSF) is produced in response to primary infection with several species of *Eimeria* in chickens.[52,352,571,733,734,776,807,855,909,1017,1183–1185,1319,1456,1510,1511,1596,1867,1887] Primary infection with *E. maxima*, *E. acervulina*, and *E. tenella* induces a robust cytokine response as opposed to the subdued response after secondary infection.[733,735] After primary infection with these three species, IELs show increased expression of cytokines such as IFN-γ, IL-2, IL-4–IL-6, IL10, IL-12, IL-13, and IL-15–IL-18 as early as 2 or 6 days postinfection.[733,735] The secondary infection with the same species, however, shows subdued expression of these cytokines, indicative of T-cell involvement in primarily regulating anticoccidial innate immunity in chickens. Several immunodominant antigens such as proteases and sporozoite antigens from *E. tenella*, *E. acervulina*, and *E. maxima* have been identified by immunoproteomics analysis.[937,1062] These molecules can cause profuse inflammatory and cellular innate immune responses that contribute to the pathogenesis and severity of coccidial infection.[937,1062]

The role of host genetics in influencing susceptibility to coccidiosis demonstrates that non-MHC molecules may have a major influence on disease susceptibility, although chickens with certain MHC types have higher susceptibility

to *Eimeria* infection.[882,1009] Among the two parental broiler breeder lines, A and B, A is resistant to bacterial and coccidial infections, and this is attributed to stronger innate immune responses observed in line A than in line B.[1655] Recently, two genetically B-complex disparate Fayoumi chicken lines, M5.1 and M15.2, showed differential innate and adaptive responses and thus different resistance patterns to *E. tenella* infection.[963] Similarly, immunological variation among the different strains of the same *Eimeria* species is also observed in chickens.[843,1250] These intraspecific variations are due to *Eimeria* oocyst morphology, pathogenicity, and drug sensitivity.[232,789]

Overall, innate immunity to avian coccidiosis is still being explored, and more information on this will elucidate the role of innate immunity against avian coccidiosis. Most of the literature on innate immunity to avian coccidiosis is based on the observation of expression of gene transcripts or transcriptomic analysis of the gut. Thus, as for their mammalian counterparts, more efforts directed toward identifying anticoccidial innate immune mechanisms in chickens are required. Also, this knowledge will aid in identifying possible innate immune-derived molecules for their potential application against avian coccidiosis.

3.2.2 Adaptive Immunity in Chickens

Adaptive immunity is antigen-specific resistance to infections and is required for complete pathogen clearance in most cases. The mechanism of adaptive immunity to coccidiosis in chickens is less elucidated than that of innate immunity. Earlier studies have shown that immunity to reinfection with a homologous *Eimeria* spp. involves acquired immunity in coccidiosis in chickens.[1449] Treatment of chickens with immunosuppressive drugs such as cyclosporine A or dexamethasone abolishes protective immunity with reduced T-cell proliferation and cytokine production, suggesting that T-cell-dependent cell-mediated immune response is responsible for protection against coccidiosis.[1007,1446] Cell-mediated immune response comprises many different cell types, including cytotoxic T cells and various cytokines.[887,1016] Given the importance of cell-mediated immune response in protective immunity to coccidiosis, *E. tenella*–specific T-cell proliferation in response to sporozoites, merozoites, or soluble antigen has been reported.[1006] Regarding the subset of T cells required for the development of active immunity in chickens, both CD4[+] and CD8[+] T cells are recruited to the site of *Eimeria* infection. Initially, CD8[+] γδ T cells were implicated in the inhibition of the parasite,[1016] but later data indicated that the CD4[+] αβ T cells are also important in protective immunity against *Eimeria* because they represent the subpopulation of cells that remain elevated during secondary infection, and this elevation correlates with protective immunity.[882] The differential role of T-cell subsets such as CD4[+] and CD8[+] T cells has also been described.[1446,1454] *In vivo* depletion of CD8[+] or αβ-TCR[+]

cells by administration of respective monoclonal antibodies in chickens shows significantly more oocysts in feces compared to either untreated control or CD4-depleted chickens following secondary infection with either *E. tenella* or *E. acervulina*.[1707] The proportion of CD8+ T cells is increased in the intestines and peripheral blood of chickens infected with *E. tenella*.[154,1011] Furthermore, CD8+ T cells have been shown to produce IFN-γ upon *Eimeria* sporozoite antigen stimulation, and *E. acervulina* sporozoites are primarily found inside these cells.[153,1706] It is suggested that these cells are responsible for protective immunity to coccidiosis regarding sporozoite transport and cytokine expression. In *E. maxima* infection, both CD4+ and CD8+ T cells are seen in the small intestine, with a higher proportion of CD8+ T cells. Although CD8+ T cells are believed to be the primary subset of T cells involved in protective cell-mediated immunity against coccidiosis, other studies have shown enhanced CD4+ T cells in the local immune response to coccidiosis. When two strains of chickens displaying differential protective immunity to coccidiosis were compared, duodenal CD4+ T cells increased after primary and secondary *E. acervulina* infection in resistant SC (B2B2) as compared to susceptible TK (B15B21) chickens.[266] The underlying mechanism mediated by CD4 cells may include cytokine secretion.[294,1742] In the cecal tonsil, increased interferon (IFN)-γ transcript is observed in *E. tenella*–infected SC chickens, and selective depletion of CD4+ but not CD8+ T cells reduces expression of IFN-γ, suggesting that CD4+ T cells are also involved in the production of cytokines in coccidiosis.[1870] With an enhanced understanding of subsets of CD4+ cells with mammalian studies, it became clear that several studies have focused on the role of other subsets of T cells such as Th17 and regulatory T (Treg) cells in coccidiosis. Chicken IL-17, isolated from *Eimeria*-infected IELs, has a proinflammatory role in coccidiosis.[1183] The exact role of Th17 cells in chickens is poorly understood due to the lack of immunological reagents to study the complex network of the IL-17 cytokine pathway in chickens. Following infection by *E. acervulina* or *E. maxima*, IL-17 mRNA levels are increased in IELs compared to uninfected controls.[732] In *E. tenella* infection, IL-17 expression in IELs is downregulated, except in the later stage of infection.[734] Similarly, it was reported that chicken IL-17 expression is downregulated in inflamed intestinal tissue following *E. tenella* infection, and treatment with IL-17 or IL-17F induces expression of proinflammatory cytokines in chicken fibroblasts.[886] These results suggest that IL-17 is induced during chicken coccidiosis in the gut dependent on the species of *Eimeria*. Th17 response can play protective and pathological roles in protozoan infections. The cloning of IL-17 receptor A (IL-17RA), which binds IL-17A and IL-17F in chickens, has revealed that *Eimeria* infection downregulates expression of IL-17RA, and modulation of this receptor facilitates the host to reduce intestinal pathogenesis amplified by IL-17/IL-17RA signaling.[885] Recent evidence seems

to support a role for Th17 cytokines in host immunopathology in coccidiosis in chickens. Treatment with IL-17-neutralizing antibody in *E. tenella* infection induces lower neutrophil recruitment, inflammatory cytokine expression, and parasite burden in the intestinal tract, resulting in enhanced body weight gain, reduced oocyst production in feces, and intestinal lesions.[1882] IL-17 is also involved in the initiation and migratory response of epithelial cells during intracellular development, and maturation of parasites, contributing to pathogenesis in the intestinal tract. Following *E. tenella* infection, chickens treated with IL-17 neutralizing antibodies have a reduced number of second-generation schizonts and cecal lesions.[357] In contrast to other T cells, Treg cells are a subset of T cells expressing both CD4 and CD25 and are involved in immunosuppression. In chickens, the ortholog of mammalian forkhead box (Fox) P3 has yet to be identified, although there is a report of an avian foxp3 gene.[362,1534] Thus, CD4+CD25+ T cells in chickens have been characterized as Treg cells showing suppression of activated immune cells.[1539] These cells produce high amounts of IL-10, transforming growth factor (TGF)-β, cytotoxic T-lymphocyte-associated antigen-4, and lymphocyte-activation gene-3, as in mammals.[1531] IL-10 showed 29-fold higher expression in CD4+CD25+ cells compared to CD4+CD25− cells, and its immunosuppression in chickens has been extensively studied.[1539] In coccidiosis, IL-10 is considered to play an important role in evasion of the host immune response. One possible mechanism to explain its role in coccidiosis is that coccidial parasites have evolved to stimulate Treg cells to express IL-10, and it helps parasites to facilitate invasion and survival in chickens through suppression of the IFN-γ-related Th1 response that is critical for protective immunity against coccidial parasites. Two inbred lines of chickens that differ in their resistance or susceptibility to *Eimeria* infection have revealed that expression of IL-10 is the major difference between the two lines. Expression of IL-10 is induced in chickens susceptible to *Eimeria* infection among the genes related to different Th lineages, such as IFN-γ for Th1, IL-4 for Th2, and IL-10 and TGF-β for Treg cells, while IL-10 is suppressed in the age-matched resistant line.[1456] *Eimeria*-infected chickens treated with IL-10 antibody show improved growth rate compared to those with control antibody, but IL-10 antibody has no effect on fecal oocyst production.[43,1484] A study reported that supplementation of vitamin D induces IL-10 expression as well as Treg cells and decreases production losses associated with coccidial infection.[1208] These results indicate that regulation of the protective immune response to *Eimeria* infection by Treg cells is important, and IL-10 plays a role in pathogenesis in chicken coccidiosis. Recently, it has been reported that oral treatment of aryl hydrocarbon receptor ligand modulated the ratio of Treg/Th17 cells in *Eimeria*-infected chickens. Dietary indole, 3,3′-diindolylmethane increased the proportion of Treg cells in cecal tonsil, while Th17 cells are decreased and the elevated the ratio of

Treg/Th17 cells in coccidiosis was related to reducing the level of local inflammatory response and facilitating the repairing process of an inflamed intestine.[890]

Although the minimum role of serum antibodies for protective immunity against coccidiosis came from studies in B-cell-[1445] and T-cell-suppressed[1007] chickens, several studies have reported that protection against coccidiosis in young animals is provided via transfer of antibodies from hens to young chickens. Unlike mammals, this occurs via egg yolk and includes maternal IgY (equivalent to IgG in mammals) in chickens. Transfer of antibodies has been shown to protect chickens from *E. tenella* or *E. acervulina* infection.[1440,1450] Maternally transferred antibodies also show partial protection against heterologous infection, possibly via cross-recognition of conserved epitopes in different *Eimeria* spp.[1593] Sera obtained at 2 weeks after *E. maxima* infection can transfer protection to naïve chickens. Some of the chickens are protected almost completely against infection.[1440,1442] It has been demonstrated that the protection conferred by transferred sera is correlated with levels of *Eimeria*-specific IgG.[1767] Based on these findings, there have been many efforts to protect against coccidiosis using *Eimeria*-specific antigens obtained from various sources such as egg yolk, or genetically engineered bacteria or yeast.[135,1542] The possibility of using pathogen-specific egg yolk antibodies as an antibiotic alternative in avian coccidiosis needs further exploration.[572]

3.3 IMMUNITY AGAINST COCCIDIA IN OTHER SPECIES

Besides coccidiosis in chicken, only limited information is available on immune response to coccidia in other species including cattle, sheep, pigs, dogs, and cats. Generally, coccidia can infect animals of all ages and usually cause no clinical signs as immunity is quickly acquired and maintained by continuous exposure to reinfection. Young animals exposed for the first time are often more susceptible to severe infection and clinical disease. Following recovery from coccidiosis, animals are immune to reinfection with the same species.

3.3.1 Turkeys

Although not much information is available in terms of immune response to coccidia in species other than avian species, immunity to coccidiosis in several other animals has been documented. Of relevance, coccidiosis in turkeys is well established, and there is some information available on immunity. There are seven well-known *Eimeria* species in turkeys that cause coccidiosis (Chapter 17). Turkeys display age resistance to coccidial infection that is not related to previous exposure. This resistance to coccidiosis in turkeys has been reported as innate immunity against

the parasite.[279,1785] The age resistance phenomenon is well established in turkeys; however, the mechanisms involved have not yet been explained, and there are some conflicting reports available.[229] Age resistance among turkeys could be due to previous exposure to the parasite and thus involvement of acquired immunity.[225] This notion is supported by the observation that when turkeys are raised in isolators designed to exclude any possibility of extraneous infection, they are susceptible to *Eimeria meleagrimitis* at 10 weeks of age.[1083] This further indicated that turkeys are more susceptible to infection as they age, with the contingency of providing a coccidia-free environment.

As stated earlier, not much information is available on humoral or cellular immune responses to *Eimeria* infection in turkeys. Although antibodies against metabolic products or the inner contents of merozoites of *E. meleagrimitis* are present in turkey serum, the protective role against infection remains unclear.[49] As an innate immune response to primary infection with *E. adenoeides*, changes in peripheral blood leukocytes and macrophage function have been studied.[229] It was observed in that study that circulating lymphocytes were decreased after 4 days of infection and migrated from the blood to the site of infection, characterized by mucosal infiltration. As a protective response to the infection, lymphocytes and heterophils were elevated at 11 days post-inoculation (DPI). However, no differential phagocytic activity of macrophages was observed after infection. Also, the NO production, which is commonly observed in *Eimeria*-infected chickens, was not observed in turkeys after coccidial infection. These findings strongly suggested that components of innate immunity were activated in response to primary infection with *E. adenoeides*. Also, immunity to coccidiosis in turkey is species specific as no cross-protection is observed among the species, as demonstrated by findings such as immunization with one species does not protect against challenge with another. This species specificity among turkey *Eimeria* spp. is used extensively to accurately identify the species based on their antigen-specific immune responses.[1083,1085]

More recently, cell-mediated immune mechanisms occurring in turkeys after oral infection with *E. adenoeides* have been reported, with increased leukocyte infiltration at the site of infection (cecal tissues). This response was characterized by high numbers of CD4+ and CD8+ cells in the ceca at 9 and 11 DPI in infected poults compared with uninfected controls.[569] Also, chemokine CXCL2 was significantly increased at 4 and 7 DPI, and IL-10 and IFN-γ, and IL-1β and IL-13, at 4 and 7 DPI, respectively. In *E. adenoeides*–infected turkey poults, leukocyte infiltration occurred as early as 6 DPI and continued to be higher at 10, 12, 16, and 18 DPI, with increased CD4+ and CD8+ lymphocyte infiltration in the ceca at 12, 16, and 18 DPI. Similarly, coccidial infection in turkeys induced high expression of cytokines such as IFN-γ, IL-1β, IL-2, IL-10, IL-12β, IL-13, and IL-18 from 12 to 16 DPI.[571]

3.3.2 Ruminants

In cattle, primary infection with *Eimeria* protects animals from subsequent clinical disease due to reexposure to oocysts.[333,1654] However, it depends on the number of oocysts to which the animal is exposed, as infection with a low to moderate number of oocysts does not induce adaptive immunity in cattle.[287,333] There is little evidence of passive transfer of antimerozoite antibodies such as IgG1, IgG2, and IgM to calves from their dams.[534] Immunoglobulins such as IgM, IgA, and IgG2 are directly correlated with oocyst excretion. IgG2 secretion is the major humoral type 2 immune response to *Eimeria* infection. Like chicken coccidiosis, IFN-γ is secreted by NK cells and promotes IgG2 synthesis in response to infection. Antibody response to coccidia only reflects exposure to the infection and mainly depends on the level of infection and thus may not confer protection.[534] Cellular immunity plays an integral role in protection against infection.[534,538,736] It is believed that CD4+ T cells and other lymphoid cells are passively transferred to the calf via colostrum.[510,534] Upon hormone treatment of calves, CD2+, CD4+, and CD8+ lymphocytes and mononuclear cells are increased, and this ultimately reduces the severity of coccidiosis. This notion is supported by the fact that hormonal treatment promotes T-cell responsiveness that protects the calves from coccidial infection as compared to the untreated calves.[692] CD2+, CD4+, and CD8+ phenotypes are proportionally increased during *E. bovis* infection. Lymphocytes from *E. bovis*–infected calves show a proliferative response when stimulated with antigen, thus concluding that in coccidial infection in cattle, there is prolonged reactivity of the T-cell population.[705,755] This T-cell activation may not be able to interrupt the parasite life cycle in primary infection, but it interferes with the level and duration of oocyst excretion and has a protective role in subsequent infections in cattle.[706] CD4+ T cells reflect Th1 response to coccidial infection in cattle, characterized by IFN-γ-driven NO release, and thus clearance of the primary infection.[706] Like chickens and mice, involvement of γδ cells in bovine coccidiosis is also suggested, although there is no clear evidence to support this. Other than IFN-γ, IL-4 and TNF-α are associated with the coccidial infection in cattle. IL-4 expression is elevated, whereas TNF-α expression is reduced during infection.[706,755] A periparturient rise in oocyst excretion is also observed in cattle, possibly due to calving-related stress and immunosuppression.[510] Although immunization is a preventive measure, vaccination with virulent oocysts of *E. alabamensis* has been reported to provide partial protection against infection.[1654] There are reports of vaccinating calves with oocysts of either one or mixed *Eimeria* spp., but no significant protection has been observed.[287,333] Herd-specific immunization using radiated oocysts does not offer any protection either.[333] Therefore, vaccination is not an alternative to treatment of bovine coccidiosis at

present.[1686] Additionally, cattle remain exposed to infection throughout their lives, and immune responses do not necessarily guarantee protective immunity.

However, recent research in this area has provided some insightful findings regarding the immune response to *Eimeria* infection. More detailed analysis of T-cell subpopulations after primary and secondary *E. bovis* infection has revealed that CD4+, CD8+, and γδTCR+ cells are increased at the site of infection, especially after primary infection. This indicates that these cell types are involved in protection against coccidial infection.[1641] Similarly, bovine umbilical vein endothelial cells express *E. bovis*–specific antigens.[55] Neutrophil extracellular trap (NET) formation by polymorphonuclear neutrophils reduces the coccidial infection rate by increasing expression of TNF-α, inducible NO synthase (iNOS), and cytokines such as IL-6, IL-8, IL-10, and IL-12, and are now considered to be an early innate immune mechanism in bovine coccidiosis.[96,97] It is now apparent that *E. bovis* NET formation is dependent on CD11b, extracellular signal-regulated kinase 1/2, p38 mitogen-activated protein kinase, and store-operated calcium entry.[1222] These findings have potential for vaccine development to prevent bovine coccidiosis.

Along with *E. bovis*, other coccidian parasites such as *Neospora caninum* and *Toxoplasma gondii* have a significant role in immunomodulation in coccidiosis. *Eimeria* sporozoites and tachyzoites of *N. caninum* and *T. gondii* invade and replicate in endothelial cells.[1679] However, the immunomodulation is distinct between *Eimeria* sporozoites and tachyzoites of the other two pathogens. *T. gondii and N. caninum* tachyzoites induce profound upregulation of the CXC chemokines GRO-α, IL-8, and IFN-γ-inducible protein (IP)-10, CC chemokines monocyte chemoattractant protein (MCP)-1 and RANTES, and GM-CSF, cyclo-oxygenase (COX)-2, and iNOS, as early as 2 HPI.[1679] In contrast, *E. bovis* sporozoites moderately upregulated IL-8 and IP-10, CC chemokines MCP-1 and RANTES, and GM-CSF, but failed to induce transcription of CXC chemokine genes and COX-2. This difference may indicate a specific invasion strategy of *E. bovis* sporozoites to persist in the host cell for a long time. Nevertheless, host cell infection with these coccidian parasites induces profound proinflammatory and immunomodulatory responses, thus exhibiting innate immune reactions and further indicating the transition to adaptive immunity.[1679]

Coccidiosis in small ruminants such as sheep and goats affects mostly young animals in the field and is also species specific, such that lambs immune to one species of *Eimeria* are susceptible to others.[880] The susceptibility of lambs to coccidiosis increases with age until about 4 weeks. Young lambs are relatively resistant to infection with a mixture of pathogenic species of coccidia. Lambs inoculated at 4–6 weeks of age develop severe diarrhea, whereas the same inoculum given at 1 day of age causes no clinical disease.[618] With regard to maternal immunity in sheep, IgG1 is a predominant isotype transmitted in sheep with colostrum, and it has a half-life of 11–13 days. Maternal antibodies can be detected until 40 days after birth and can protect the animals against *Eimeria* infection. Afterward, the level of maternal antibodies is reduced, and the animal becomes susceptible to disease.[379,1401] Experimental infection with *E. ovinoidalis* and *E. faurei* in sheep demonstrates a significant increase in specific antibodies during both primary and challenge infections.[1244] Even though levels of immunoglobulin do not correlate with *E. ninakohlyakimovae* oocyst counting in feces of goat kids, *Eimeria*-infected kids show increased serum IgG and IgM, and increased IgA in ileal mucus.[1144] Resistance to *Eimeria* infection is thymus dependent and is largely mediated by T-cell-promoted intracellular killing directed mainly against asexual stages such as sporozoites or merozoites.

3.3.3 Rabbits

Although rabbits are an intermediate host for several coccidia belonging to *Toxoplasma, Cryptosporidium,* and *Besnoitia, Eimeria* coccidiosis is well studied in terms of immune responses in rabbits. In rabbits, GALT, including the appendix, sacculus rotundus, Peyer's patches (PP), intestinal epithelial lymphocytes, and lamina propria leukocytes, plays a significant role in maintaining immunity.[1300] The GALT components are the specific site of the endogenous development of *E. coecicola* in rabbits. In response to *E. intestinalis* infection, the percentage of CD4+ lymphocytes in the intestinal lamina propria and CD8+ lymphocytes in mesenteric lymph nodes (MLNs) is increased at 14 DPI with CD8+ lymphocytes in MLNs remaining high up to 21 DPI.[1409] MLN cells from infected rabbits proliferate when stimulated with parasite antigen with some antigen-specific humoral response (IgG). Protection against infection is more attributed to an effective mucosal immune response after primary infection followed by increasing systemic responses after subsequent infections. *E. intestinalis*, which is highly immunogenic, infection is characterized by increased CD8+ cells in the ileal epithelium.[1309] Cellular immune responses to *E. intestinalis* are age dependent in rabbits and occur at 15 days of age onward, when a significant increase in T-cell populations is observed.[1310] Thus, the immune system of rabbits reacts to the infection after 25 days of age, and vaccination at this age appears to be a suitable approach. Compared to chicken and mice, fewer studies have investigated the immune response of rabbits to coccidiosis, and the reduced numbers of sporozoites in GALT, oocyst shedding postinfection, and weight gain are related to immune responses to infection.[1300,1311]

3.3.4 Horses

E. leuckarti is the only species that infects horses, donkeys, and zebra.[430] Immunity to *E. leuckarti* can be acquired through reinfection. Experimental infection with *E. leuckarti* oocysts indicates that the number of oocysts excreted after challenge is significantly lower than after primary infection, suggesting partial immunity.

REFERENCES

43, 49, 52, 55, 96, 97, 135, 153–155, 157, 169, 225, 229, 232, 266, 279, 287, 294, 333, 352, 355–359, 362, 379, 430, 510, 533, 534, 538, 569, 571, 572, 586, 608, 618, 692, 706, 732–736, 755, 776, 779–783, 789, 807, 843, 848, 849, 855, 880, 882, 883, 885–890, 909, 920, 937, 963, 964, 968, 1006–1018, 1062, 1083, 1085, 1144, 1170, 1182–1185, 1208, 1222, 1244, 1250, 1300, 1309–1311, 1319, 1379, 1401, 1409, 1440, 1442, 1445–1447, 1449–1452, 1454–1456, 1484, 1510, 1511, 1531, 1534, 1539, 1542, 1565, 1593, 1596, 1641, 1642, 1644, 1654, 1655, 1679, 1686, 1692, 1706, 1707, 1740, 1742, 1761, 1767, 1785, 1855, 1867, 1869, 1870, 1881, 1882, 1887, 1916

CHAPTER 4

Vaccination

M. C. Jenkins

CONTENTS

4.1 INTRODUCTION

Several factors have contributed to the increased use of live *Eimeria* oocyst vaccines to control coccidiosis in broiler and layer chickens. Between 2010 and 2016, worldwide broiler production has increased by 17% to approximately 23 billion broilers (PoultryTrends.com). In the same time period, the number of eggs produced has increased 12.5% to 1350 billion eggs (PoultryTrends.com). This is because the relative cost of raising broilers and egg-layers is low compared to other food animal commodities which is due in part to greater efficiency of feed conversion in commercial breeds of chicken (~1.6–1.8 kg feed/kg body weight). Also, egg production can, depending on whether the eggs are for consumption (table eggs) or serve as a source of chicks for broiler replacement, exceed 250 eggs/year. The short life span of broilers (5–8 weeks depending on market) and the rapid growth rate that in 1950 required 10 weeks to produce a 1.4 kg broiler now requires only 5 weeks to produce the same size broiler has led to intensive poultry production. Depending on its size, a typical broiler house will contain up to 35,000 chickens, and four to six houses on a single farm are common. Improvements in nutrition and health and increased efficiencies within vertically integrated poultry companies have also contributed to the rapid growth of the industry. Typically, broilers are raised near one another at a stocking density of ~0.075 m²/chick during growout, which is ideal for rapid transmission of infectious agents between chickens in a poultry house.

Eimeria oocysts are well adapted to withstand a wide range of temperatures, humidities, and ammonia levels that are typically found during growout in a poultry house. The oocysts rapidly undergo sporulation after being excreted in the feces of infected chickens. Outbreaks of coccidiosis and associated diseases, such as necrotic enteritis (NE), result from nonimmune chicks ingesting fully sporulated *Eimeria* oocysts in litter. Physical and enzymatic activity in the intestinal tract acting on oocysts and sporocysts causes the release of sporozoites that invade *Eimeria* species-specific regions of the gut. For instance, although the regions overlap to some extent, *E. acervulina* is found predominantly in the duodenum, *E. maxima* in the jejunem and ileum, and *E. tenella* in the cecum. Asexual (schizongony) and sexual (gametogeny) development within intestinal cells lining the gut leads to poor nutrient uptake resulting in reduced egg production (layers), lower weight gain, and poorer feed conversion efficiencies (broilers).

Early control of avian coccidiosis relied on medication of feed with synthetic chemicals, such as nicarbazin, zoalene, and decoquinate followed by clopidol, robenidine, diclazuril, and halofuginone (for review see Greif et al.[624]). However, resistance to all chemicals developed rapidly in

Eimeria, which prompted the development of ionophore drugs such as lasalocid, monensin, narasin, maduramicin, and semduramicin. The advantage of ionophores is that, unlike synthetic chemicals, they allow for some *Eimeria* development (thus the term **leaky**), which may stimulate immune-mediated resistance to subsequent *Eimeria* infection. Another advantage of ionophores is that they have activity against gram-positive bacteria, which may account for their growth-promoting effects. However, drug resistance in *Eimeria* to ionophores has been observed by several authors leading to alternative strategies for prophylaxis (for review see Peek and Landman[1336]). One way that poultry companies have extended the life of anticoccidial drugs (ACDs) is to use shuttle programs, whereby a synthetic chemical may be used in the starter feed followed by an ionophore in the grower feed. Another approach to reduce the number of drug-resistant *Eimeria* in a poultry house is to rotate the use of ACDs with live *Eimeria* oocysts vaccines, which are composed of drug-sensitive strains of *Eimeria*. The basis for this approach and a review of the literature related to live *Eimeria* oocyst vaccines are given later. Although there has been and continues to be considerable effort on developing subunit or recombinant *Eimeria* vaccines, this review covers only live virulent or attenuated *Eimeria* vaccines. The reader is alerted to several excellent reviews specifically on recombinant vaccines and generally on vaccination against coccidiosis.[244,1160,1566, 1567,1695,1804,1805]

4.2 BASIS FOR DEVELOPMENT OF LIVE *EIMERIA* OOCYST VACCINES

Although the first commercial coccidiosis vaccine was released in the early 1950s, research in the 1920s gave insight into the possibility of using *Eimeria* oocysts to elicit immune protection in chickens against *Eimeria* challenge infection. As early as 1925, it was found that a single oral dose of *Eimeria* residing in the ceca could induce a protective immune response to coccidiosis.[90] In the 1930s to early 1950s, pioneer researchers found that oral inoculation of chickens with low numbers of *E. acervulina*, *E. maxima*, or *E. tenella* oocysts elicited strong immunity against challenge infection.[371,372,465,835] Depending on *Eimeria* species, a single infection provoked at least partial resistance to homologous challenge.[1449] Complete immunity often requires repeat inoculations of low doses of oocysts, often called **trickle infection**.[694–697,846,847] This boosting effect of repeated exposure to oocysts is supported by the observation that chickens grown in contact with litter develop stronger immunity to *Eimeria* infection than those housed in wire cages.[234,235] The term **cycling** is often used to describe ongoing *Eimeria* oocyst infections that arise by chickens pecking in litter and ingesting oocysts therein.

In the early days of coccidiosis research, it was thought that young chicks (<3 days old) could not be immunized by infecting them with *Eimeria* oocysts. Indeed, research in the 1960s and 1970s showed that chicks 1–3 days old produced fewer oocysts than older chicks.[396,1081,1439] This is probably due to multiple factors, including less-developed gizzard to release sporocysts from oocysts to fewer intestinal cells for sporozoites to invade, all influenced by the well-established crowding effect.[1803] However, the evidence for immunity developing in newly hatched chicks that protects them against challenge at 3–4 weeks is overwhelming (see Williams[1804,1805]) and is the basis for spray vaccination of chicks with *Eimeria* oocysts at the hatchery. The excretion of *Eimeria* oocysts by chicks that had been inoculated *in ovo* with oocysts, sporocysts, or sporozoites at 18 days' incubation lends further support for early immunization.

Although strong immunity can be elicited by repeatedly dosing chicks with low numbers of *Eimeria* oocysts, the immune response appears to be extremely species-specific (for review see Rose[1443]). For instance, infecting naïve chickens with *E. maxima* oocysts does not protect them against subsequent challenge with *E. acervulina* oocysts. There are a few reports showing some cross-immunity between *E. tenella* and *E. necatrix*[1438] in that heterologous challenge gave rise to lower numbers of oocysts shed compared to oocyst shedding in nonimmune animals. However, the general rule is that immunity to *Eimeria* is species-specific, and this is the reason that all commercial coccidiosis vaccines are composed of multiple *Eimeria* species.

4.3 *EIMERIA* DEVELOPMENTAL STAGES THAT INDUCE AND ARE TARGETED BY PROTECTIVE IMMUNITY

The primary and secondary immune responses to *Eimeria* are unique because the former may have little impact on the parasite completing its life cycle,[1585] while acquired immunity is completely effective against challenge infection. This is because *Eimeria* have a tightly controlled patent period involving timed events such as sporozoite invasion, three to four rounds of schizogony, gamete formation, and fusion followed by oocyst excretion. Those extracellular forms (i.e., sporozoites, merozoites, microgametes) are present in the lumen for a short time before invading another epithelial cell, and thus may escape natural killer (NK) cell lysis or macrophage ingestion. While there is little doubt that a primary oocyst infection provokes a strong protective immune response against secondary *Eimeria* challenge, which developmental stages induce and are targeted by the avian immune system remain controversial. Work in the mid-1980s showed that arresting the *in vivo* development of *E. tenella* sporozoites with decoquinate did not allow for development of protective immunity against subsequent *E. tenella* challenge.[794] However, our studies in the mid-1990s on the effects of γ-irradiation on *E. acervulina*, *E. maxima*, and *E. tenella* showed that protective immunity could be elicited with irradiated oocysts in the absence of any detectable merogonic development.[799,800,801,806] Staining of intestinal tissue with monoclonal antibodies specific for different developmental stages revealed that sporozoite invasion arising from optimally irradiated oocysts was unaffected, but schizont development was negligible. Also, oocysts were not detected in feces of chickens inoculated with irradiated *E. acervulina*, *E. maxima*, or *E. tenella* oocysts. It is possible that sufficient schizogonous development and oocyst excretion transpired from irradiated oocysts and were below the detection limit of the histological and oocyst counting methods. Arguing against sporozoites playing a major role in eliciting immunity is the finding by others that protective immunity induced by irradiated *Eimeria* was only observed when oocyst development took place (i.e., oocysts shedding).[24] Earlier studies using drugs to inhibit schizogony indicated that second-generation schizonts were critical to immunity.[739,740,872] Supporting this was the research by Johnson and colleagues[830] who found that an attenuated *E. tenella* strain (WisF-96), which is missing the second and third schizont generations, was unable to protect against nonattenuated *E. tenella* (Wis). Working with *E. maxima*, Rose and Hesketh[1444] found that the second schizont generation is probably most important for eliciting protective immunity.

It also is unclear which *Eimeria* developmental stage is targeted by the protective immune response. Work by Horton–Smith and colleagues in the mid-1960s found that immunity was directed at the sporozoite-infected (trophozoite) host cell with lower numbers of intracellular parasites seen at 24–48 hours, few at 72 hours, and none at 120 hours postchallenge.[742] This observation was confirmed by others who found that the number of intracellular stages in immune chickens after *E. tenella* oocyst challenge was appreciably less compared to nonimmune chickens.[951] Further, in immune chickens, the number of invading *E. tenella* sporozoites is slightly lower than in *E. tenella*–infected naïve birds, but the main effect appears to be inhibition of transport of sporozoites by intraepithelial lymphocytes (IELs) from the surface epithelium to crypt enterocytes.[1448] Nevertheless, the target of immunity may depend on *Eimeria* species. For instance, another study found that sporozoite invasion in *E. tenella*- or *E. adenoides*-immune animals after homologous challenge was about 50% of that in nonimmune animals.[48] However, sporozoite numbers postchallenge were not decreased and in some instances, increased in upper intestinal species, such as *E. acervulina* and *E. meleagrimitis*.[48] Currently, it seems that for *E. tenella*, and possibly other *Eimeria* species, resistance to challenge infection involves immune recognition of sporozoite-infected host cells and/or developing second-generation schizonts during a primary infection. After resistance is established, both extracellular sporozoites and developing sporozoites (trophozoites) inside epithelial cells of the gut are the targets of the acquired immune response, which appears to involve both CD4+ and CD8+ T cells and associated cytokines, such as IFNγ (for review see Chapman et al.[232]). These findings may reflect the existence of common and unique antigens expressed by different *Eimeria* developmental stages.[1161]

4.4 VIRULENT VACCINES

Although research in the 1920s–1940s showed that inoculation of chickens with *Eimeria* oocysts could elicit a protective response against coccidiosis,[90,371,372,835] the first commercial *Eimeria* vaccine was not released until the mid-1950s[461,462,465] (for an excellent review see Williams[1805]). This first product, named "DM Cecal Coccidiosis Vaccine," was composed of a single *Eimeria* species, *E. tenella*, owing to the perceived importance of this protozoan at that time. Improvements to the original vaccine arose and were sold by different companies and contained additional *Eimeria* species depending on geographical region among other considerations. These include "Coxine," "Nobicox," and finally "Coccivac." The latter name has remained and contains a mixture of low doses of *E. acervulina*, *E. maxima*, *E. tenella*, and *E. mivati*, although recent work puts in doubt the existence of *E. mivati*, which may in fact be *E. mitis*.[1758] Coccivac has been delivered to chicks in a variety of ways, including in drinking water, in feed, intraocular, and by spraying on chicks in the hatchery (see Section 4.9). In the late 1990s, Lee and his coworkers reported on a product called "Immucox" that contained *E. acervulina*, *E. tenella*, and two strains of *E. maxima*.[321,324] Immucox was delivered to chicks by suspending the oocysts in gelatin slabs and placing the slabs in the chick transport boxes to allow chicks to ingest vaccine during transport from the hatchery to the poultry farm. Other vaccines include Inovocox that contained *E. acervulina*, *E. maxima*, *E. mitis*, and *E. tenella* and was designed for *in ovo* injection of embryonated eggs at 18 days' incubation. NobilisCoxA™ was a vaccine containing ionophore-resistant *Eimeria* that can be used in conjunction with ionophore drugs so that immunity can develop in conjunction with ACD in feed to prevent coccidiosis outbreaks due to wild-type strains in litter. Several authors expressed concern about intentionally releasing drug-resistant *Eimeria* strains into poultry facilities, which is no longer an issue because the product is no longer available. "Advent" is another vaccine based on a mixture of low doses of *E. acervulina*, *E. maxima*, and *E. tenella* that, per the manufacturer, has known viability because of testing using a Viacyst assay. One of the problems associated with production of live *Eimeria* oocyst vaccines is that the time from collection and sporulation of oocysts to U.S. Food and Drug Administration (FDA) approval of a batch can be lengthy due to the requirement for efficacy testing. Viability testing of live oocyst vaccines is important before a product is used to ensure that *Eimeria* oocysts contained therein can initiate an infection and thereby elicit a protective immune response.

Several studies have confirmed that *Eimeria* oocyst vaccines are effective in protecting chicks against coccidiosis.[650,955,1366,1652] As pointed out earlier, there were initial concerns about the capacity of young chicks to be immunized against coccidiosis via oral inoculation with *Eimeria* oocysts. These concerns have been alleviated by several studies. For instance, Shiotani and his colleagues[1559] showed that over 80% of *E. tenella* and 97% of *E. maxima* oocysts given to 4-week-old chickens had excysted and presumably initiated an infection. A few years later, it was found that in 2-day-old chicks, over 90% of inoculated *E. tenella* oocysts had excysted and possibly infected epithelial tissue.[1799] Moreover, successful *in ovo* inoculation of *Eimeria* oocysts followed by shedding of oocysts by vaccinated hatchlings suggests that uptake can occur very early and patent infection occurs.[1786,1788]

However, several issues have been noted with live *Eimeria* oocyst vaccine use including lower average daily gain and poorer feed conversion efficiencies (higher FCR)[1323] as well as increased incidence of NE. This is probably not unexpected because without uniform vaccination and complete immunity in every chick, there will be lower growth and greater susceptibility to NE in chicks that either ingested too much or too little vaccine. In spite of these negative effects, several authors have found that by 35–42 days, compensatory gain takes place in oocyst-vaccinated chickens that achieve body weights equivalent to ACD-treated controls.[319,321,1137,1323] The addition of bacitracin methylene disalicylate (BMD) in feed to control *Clostridium* and other bacteria does not appear to compromise the effectiveness of live *Eimeria* vaccines in eliciting immunity.[237] The addition of BMD along with *Eimeria* vaccination serves to hinder NE incidence. At present, the most deleterious side effect of *Eimeria* oocyst vaccination is the occasional blips in mortality observed at 2.5–4.5 weeks of age, which is due to *Clostridium perfringens* invading intestinal tissue that has been first damaged by developing *Eimeria* parasites.

Several variables affect the efficacy of live *Eimeria* oocyst vaccines. First is the uniformity and efficiency of vaccination. In our studies, as high as 50% of newly hatched chicks given oocysts by spray vaccination received an insufficient amount of vaccine as indicated by shedding of *Eimeria* oocysts.[803] Immunity in battery cage studies indicated that the level of resistance elicited by spray vaccination was significantly lower than by oral gavage or ingestion of gelatin beads containing an equivalent number of oocysts. This effect could be overcome by growing vaccinated chicks in contact with litter, which probably reflects an exposure to *Eimeria* oocysts present in the litter.[804] In fact, several authors have shown a cohort effect of housing vaccinated and nonvaccinated chicks together in the same floor pen.[531,1734] As mentioned earlier, "cycling" of *Eimeria* oocysts serves to boost immunity, but this depends on oocysts being fully sporulated and viable. Variables such as temperature, moisture content, and oxygen levels affect the

sporulation rate. In the 1950s, optimal conditions for sporulation in litter were described—temperatures between 25°C and 28°C and moisture content ~30%.[463,464] Drier litter, because it allowed higher levels of oxygen, was found to be better than wet litter in promoting *E. maxima* sporulation.[1763] In *E. acervulina*, 60% sporulation was achieved within 1 day of being excreted into litter, with 100% sporulation achieved by 3 days.[609] This is like another study that found that over 95% of *E. acervulina* oocysts had sporulated by 5 days in litter.[1801] However, by 3 weeks about 70% of these oocysts appeared damaged and were becoming nonviable.[1801] Due to inefficient and nonuniform vaccination methods and the presence of viable *Eimeria* oocysts carried over from the previous batch of chickens, there is probably a continuum of oocysts excretion during normal growout that ensures viable oocysts are present for a long time. With 100% vaccine uptake, one would expect that oocyst numbers in litter would peak at about 3 weeks of age by the first and second rounds of oocyst development.[805] In the field, the dynamics of *Eimeria* oocyst levels in litter are much more complex due to incomplete vaccination, varying levels of drug sensitivity (in an ACD program) in the resident *Eimeria* population, and litter quality.[805]

Despite these drawbacks, which may be overcome with improvements in vaccine delivery, live *Eimeria* oocyst vaccines offer a viable way to control avian coccidiosis by allowing immunity to check outbreaks. The advantage of live *Eimeria* oocyst vaccines is that because they are composed of drug-sensitive strains of the parasite, they can and have been used in rotation with ACD to replace the drug-resistant strains present in litter. The concept that drug-sensitive *Eimeria* strains would interbreed with or outcompete drug-resistant ones in a poultry house was put forth in the 1970s.[792] This approach serves to extend the useful life of synthetic chemicals and ionophores by using immunity rather than drug treatment to control coccidiosis infection.

4.5 ATTENUATED VACCINES

One of the drawbacks to coccidiosis vaccines based on live virulent *Eimeria* is that overall performance is depressed because chicks may ingest high numbers of oocysts that are randomly distributed in litter during growout. To reduce the pathogenicity of *E. tenella* without affecting its immunogenicity, an attenuated strain of this parasite was generated by collecting oocysts shed from *E. tenella*–infected chickens starting at 125 hours postinoculation (HPI). Peak excretion of *E. tenella* oocysts normally occurs around 144 hours. By selecting earlier in each subsequent infection, researchers could generate a "precocious" strain of *E. tenella* that completed its life cycle in 96 hours, thus the term *E. tenella* WisF-96. Comparing the attenuated strain (WisF-96) to the parent strain (WisC), it was observed that defective second-generation schizonts, reduced pathogenicity, attributed to an increase in developmental rate.[1167] A pioneering study reported that the second- and third-generation schizont stages of *E. tenella* WisF-96 were missing, and gametogeny proceeded directly from first-generation schizonts.[1167] In his original work, Jeffers[790] showed that the precocious trait was stable for at least 25 generations, and subsequently showed that it had a genetic basis because it could be used to generate recombinants with a nonattenuated strain of *E. tenella*.[791]

Since Jeffers' report, a number of groups have produced precocious lines of *Eimeria* (for review see Williams[1804,1805]) so that by 1990 a vaccine called Paracox® was released that contained attenuated strains of *Eimeria* species infectious for chickens. Currently, there are at least three products: Paracox-5 that is composed of precocious *E. acervulina*, *E. mitis*, *E. tenella*, and two strains of *E. maxima*; Paracox-8 that contains the Paracox-5 strains plus *E. brunetti*, *E. necatrix*, and *E. praecox*; and HatchPak Cocci III which contains *E. acervulina*, *E. maxima*, and *E. tenella*. Paracox-5 and HatchPak Cocci II are designed generally for broilers, while Paracox-8 is for broiler breeders. In the early 1970s, an attenuated *E. tenella* strain was produced by serial passaging of this parasite in chick embryos.[1075,1079] The loss of pathogenicity was due to the inability of attenuated *E. tenella* to produce large schizonts.[1076] However, attenuation appeared to be reversible by two passages in chickens. This reversion depended on how many times the parasite was passaged in embryos, with 42 cycles allowing reversion but 62 cycles not allowing reversion.[1075,1079] Embryo-passaged *E. tenella* is the source of this parasite for the Livacox vaccine line that also contains one to three additional strains of *E. acervulina*, *E. brunetti*, and *E. maxima* that have been selected using the procedure initiated by Jeffers and optimized by others (see Williams[1805]).

The advantage of live oocyst vaccines based on precocious strains of *Eimeria* is that strong immunity is elicited without the occasional negative impact on performance often observed with vaccines based on virulent *Eimeria* strains. A single dose of Paracox in broiler breeders can confer strong immunity against *E. necatrix* infection.[1809] While the acquisition of sterile immunity (absence of oocyst excretion after challenge) was only possible with boosting, a single Paracox-5 immunization was sufficient to prevent clinical coccidiosis. Similar findings have been made with Paracox and Livacox immunization in protecting against experimental *E. acervulina*, *E. brunetti*, *E. maxima*, or *E. tenella* infection[831,1561,1806] as well as improving performance in field operations.[1804,1805] The disadvantage of attenuated coccidiosis vaccines is that they are considerably more expensive to produce than vaccines based on virulent *Eimeria*.[239] This is primarily due to the lower fecundity of precocious *Eimeria* strains that, depending on the strain, produce 85%–97% fewer oocysts compared to nonattenuated *Eimeria*. As such, precocious *Eimeria* vaccines are used on a limited basis except in regions where regulations disallow the use of vaccines containing virulent *Eimeria* oocysts.

4.6 USING VACCINES IN CONJUNCTION WITH ANTICOCCIDIAL DRUGS

In the early years of applying *Eimeria* oocyst vaccines, it was standard practice to administer subeffective drugs, such as amprolium, at 10 days' posthatch to suppress vaccine reactions.[1804] Subsequent work showed that immunity could develop in oocyst-vaccinated chicks given feed containing ionophores.[465,1634] With the release of highly effective synthetic chemicals, the administration of live oocyst vaccines in conjunction with ionophores lost favor as a means of controlling coccidiosis. However, resistance of *Eimeria* to synthetic anticoccidial chemicals arose rapidly, especially with repeated use, which prompted research on immunity to *Eimeria* during ionophore control programs. A study found that monensin-treated chickens developed strong immunity against *Eimeria* infections as measured by clinical signs.[214] An interesting phenomenon that was borne out in subsequent work is that broilers given feed containing salinomycin during growout were immune to *Eimeria* oocyst challenge possibly because parasite development and oocyst cycling at some level had taken place.[218] These findings were corroborated by others[1086] who found that monensin at 40–50 ppm allowed for development of immunity to all seven *Eimeria* species infecting chickens. A general trend is that immunity develops more slowly the longer medication is applied and more rapidly in used litter compared to new litter.[225,226,243] An interesting approach is to vaccinate chicks and then place them in poultry houses containing medicated feed.[57] A similar approach was suggested by Seeger[1528] to vaccinate at the hatchery and then provide ionophore drugs 24–48 hours later. If applied in a judicious way, synthetic chemicals can also be used to control coccidiosis in young chicks and then be withdrawn, allowing for immunity to develop by virtue of chicks ingesting *Eimeria* oocysts in litter. This is exemplified in another study that revealed that chicks grown on starter feed containing nicarbazin, halofuginone, or robenidine not only showed better performance later in growout, but also became immune to challenge.[238] Shuttle programs involving medication of starter feed with nicarbazin (days 0–21) followed by salinomycin in grower feed (days 21–44) allowed for immunity as judged by protection against depressed weight gain associated with *E. acervulina*, *E. maxima*, or *E. tenella* challenge,[218] but not oocyst output.

Taken together, these findings suggest that ionophores are not completely effective in preventing parasite replication. Ionophores are active against *Eimeria* extracellular stages (i.e., sporozoites, merozoites); thus, there is a race between the parasite invading new host cells or being impeded from invasion by the drug. If sufficient numbers of *Eimeria* developmental stages escape the inhibitory effects of an ionophore or are inherently resistant, then immunity may develop. Synthetic chemicals are more effective in blocking parasite development due to their mode of action. Thus, immune-mediated resistance to challenge generally does not develop until these drugs are withdrawn. Shuttle programs incorporating a synthetic chemical in the starter feed followed by an ionophore in the grower feed may be the best solution to protecting chicks against coccidiosis early in life while allowing immunity to develop during later stages of growout. It is likely that there is a continuum in the infection dynamics in each poultry house with the interplay of drug resistance and levels of *Eimeria* oocysts in litter at any one time that results in either coccidiosis and NE or resistance to both. As one would predict, the percentage of healthy and diseased chickens in a house depends on the combination of all these factors and litter condition.

4.7 USING LIVE *EIMERIA* OOCYST VACCINES TO REDUCE DRUG RESISTANCE IN *EIMERIA* POPULATION

The repeated use of anticoccidial drugs, particularly synthetic chemicals, eventually leads to *Eimeria* drug resistance (for review, see Chapman[219,224] and Chapman and Jeffers[239]). Drug resistance appears to be a stable trait in *Eimeria* and under genetic control because the genotype can be transferred to drug-sensitive strains *in vivo*.[216,789,791,1563] Of concern is that the drug-resistant phenotype is not lost even in the absence of drug treatment and that cross-resistance to a broad class of ionophores is possible.[217,219] This phenomenon was the basis for the development of a live *Eimeria* oocyst vaccine (Nobilis Cox ATM) that contains ionophore-resistant strains of *E. acervulina, E. maxima,* and *E. tenella.* The rationale behind this product is that immunity can be elicited in chicks at an early age while simultaneously preventing infection with drug-sensitive strains present in litter.

Poultry growers have addressed the lack of drug sensitivity in several ways. One approach is to use a "shuttle" program, whereby two different drugs are employed at different times during growout, such as a synthetic chemical in the starter feed and an ionophore in the grower feed. A second approach, termed *rotation* is to switch drugs between different sets of chickens such as a synthetic chemical in flock *n* and an ionophore in flock *n* + 1. Several authors have found that sensitivity of *Eimeria* in a poultry house to anticoccidial drugs is greater in operations that utilize live *Eimeria* oocyst vaccines. For instance, monensin sensitivity was greater in farms that had switched to an anticoccidial vaccine from ionophores,[221] and diclazuril sensitivity was restored on farms after just two growout cycles of using Coccivac B.[1138] Others have observed the same phenomenon with sensitivity to monensin and diclazuril on farms using Paracox-5.[1335] Similarly, Jenkins and his colleagues[798] found that salinomycin sensitivity was greater in *Eimeria* isolated from vaccine-utilizing farms than those recovered from farms using ionophores. The concept of rotating drugs and vaccines during the year so that drug-sensitive strains in the vaccine would replace drug-resistant strains present in litter

was proposed by Jeffers in the 1970s. While genetic recombination between drug-sensitive and drug-resistant *Eimeria* strains has been demonstrated, this mechanism is thought to play a minor role in increasing the relative number of sensitive *Eimeria* in a population. Likely, introduction of vaccine-derived oocysts into a poultry house in which anticoccidial drugs are not being used just serves to displace the drug-resistant parasites already present. The drug-resistant strains may be 2–3 months older than the newly excreted vaccine derived oocysts and thus may not be as fecund as the recently shed vaccine-originating oocysts. Chapman and his colleagues have suggested a yearly schedule for rotating between anticoccidial drugs and live oocyst vaccines to extend the useful life of the former.[236,239]

4.8 GENETIC DIVERSITY IMPACTING EFFICACY OF VACCINATION

The species specificity of the immune response to avian *Eimeria* has been known for a long time.[1441,1443] Although there have been a few reports of infection with one *Eimeria* species conferring partial resistance to another, solid immunity against even the most sensitive parameter, oocyst excretion, is generally only seen in homologous challenge. This indicates that antigen(s) involved in protective immunity are unique to each *Eimeria* species, or at least there are important differences in the host immune response to each of the seven *Eimeria* infecting chickens. With *E. acervulina* and particularly *E. maxima*, infra-immunological variation has been described by several authors.[843,1078,1082,1132,1250] The most thoroughly studied is immunological variation in *E. maxima*. Long[1078] found that infection with *E. maxima* Houghton does not completely protect against challenge with *E. maxima* Weybridge, findings later confirmed by Norton and Hein.[1250] Long and Millard[1082] observed that inoculating chicks with a mixture of four different *E. maxima,* including the Houghton and Weybridge strains, elicited protective immunity against seven different field isolates of *E. maxima*. This work forms the basis for including two different *E. maxima* strains in several commercial coccidiosis vaccines (e.g., Paracox, Immucox). Cross-protection or lack thereof between *E. maxima* Houghton and Weybridge is more complicated than originally thought because immunizing dose and genetic background of the host may influence the level of immunity.[133,1586] In other species that have been tested, such as *E. tenella* and *E. mitis*, no infra-immunological variation has been found.[536,845]

What is the reason that immunological variation in *Eimeria* is not as common as observed in other apicomplexans, such as *Plasmodium,* the causative agent of malaria? It has been suggested that because *Eimeria* are homoxenous, parasite development from sporozoite invasion to oocyst formation is so rapid, and the short life span (e.g., 5–8 weeks in broiler chickens) and an ample supply of naïve hosts to infect, there is little need for the parasite to evade immunity.[135] Most authors believe that innate immunity has little effect on *Eimeria* completing its life cycle in a primary infection.[276,1585] One reason is that extracellular parasites (i.e., sporozoites, merozoites, microgametes) exist outside the cell for a relatively short period of time and therefore would not be quickly attacked by NK cells or macrophages. In fact, IELs are known to transport sporozoites from the epithelial villi to crypts, possibly reflecting a way that *Eimeria* avoids destruction by harnessing immune cells for transport. Both common and unique antigens are expressed by different developmental stages,[1161] but the parasite may complete its entire life cycle in 4–6 days before acquired immunity has a chance to establish. This does not explain why solid immunity as judged by oocyst development and excretion can be achieved by *Eimeria* infection that with *E. maxima* requires only a single dose of 20 oocysts, and is boosted with multiple low doses of oocysts. One possible explanation is that immunity is directed at functional proteins such as AMA-1 or IMP-1 whose role in metabolism, host cell invasion, or parasite replication is more critical to *Eimeria* than immune evasion.[135] This would explain the lack of genetic diversity in these immunogenic proteins.[135] However, it remains unknown why *Eimeria* has not evolved in a way similar to *Plasmodium* that during secondary infection directs the immune response to variable regions of surface proteins that may have little functional role in the parasite (for review, see Kirkman and Deitsch[896]). In *P. falciparum*, for instance, micro- and macrogamete fusion and zygote formation occur in a second host (mosquito), with asexual development occurring in the intermediate host (humans). There may be more opportunity for genetic recombination in *Plasmodium* compared to *Eimeria*, the latter restricted to a single host, while in malaria the definitive host (mosquito) may ingest multiple parasite genotypes in a single or multiple blood meals. It is possible that selection is at the population level, and because there are sufficient numbers of susceptible hosts to infect, the emergence of *Eimeria* capable of varying epitope expression to avoid immunity is minimal. Another possibility is that the relative number of immune variants is extremely low compared to wild type that are continually being shed over the course of growout. It is interesting, however, that immunological variation is observed in the most immunogenic species—namely, *E. maxima*.

4.9 DELIVERY OF LIVE VACCINES

Almost all research showing that immunization with *Eimeria* oocysts can confer protection against homologous challenge has been done by inoculating one chick at a time. Taking this approach from theory into practice requires a practical, cost-effective administration method that can be used to vaccinate over 23 billion broiler chickens and 5.5 billion layers produced worldwide each year. A number of delivery methods have been tried, including spraying on feed, adding to drinking water with or without a thickening agent (for review, see Williams[1804,1805]), or incorporating oocysts into an edible gel[324] or in gelatin beads.[803,804,1251] Using a Bioinjector II equipped with an immunizer attachment for injecting Marek's disease virus (MDV) vaccine, an intraocular route of oocyst vaccine delivery showed promise. Inoculation through the eye worked because oocysts passed through the lacrimal duct into the nasal cavity, eventually reaching the intestinal tract via the oropharynx.[222,236,1804] This technique fell out of favor with the widespread delivery of MDV into embryonated eggs. A technique that showed great promise was *in ovo* injection of a coccidiosis vaccine into 18-day-old eggs.[370] A number of authors showed that chicks hatching from eggs injected at 18- to 19-day incubation with *Eimeria* sporozoites, sporocysts, or oocysts excreted oocysts within 1 week after hatch.[376,969,1364,1786,1787,1788] *In ovo* vaccination was not detrimental to hatchability but also elicited a protective immune response later in life.[376,969,1364,1787,1788] For reasons unknown, *in ovo* delivery of *Eimeria* oocysts vaccines is no longer being employed.

Currently, spray vaccination of an aqueous or gel solution containing a mixture of *Eimeria* spp. oocysts onto newly hatched chicks is the preferred method of administration. In one study, Albanese and her coworkers[21] found no difference in the number of oocysts excreted from and immunity developing in chicks given vaccine by aqueous or gel spray. In theory, each newly hatched chick ingests a low-dose mixture of *Eimeria* oocysts, generally *E. acervulina*, *E. maxima*, and *E. tenella*, by preening themselves or other chicks in a shipping box. Once placed in a poultry house, immunity initiated by the primary vaccination is boosted by the ingestion of *Eimeria* oocysts present in litter. Edgar[466] recognized the importance of uniformity in live oocyst vaccination. Achieving uniform protection in young chicks is important because high numbers of viable oocysts are present in litter during growout.[685,798,805,1087,1613] In practice, it is likely that only a small percentage of chicks are getting the desired dose at the hatchery, while others are ingesting too many or not enough oocysts.[236,1804] Those ingesting too few or no oocysts are fully susceptible to *Eimeria* challenge infection once placed in the poultry house. Those ingesting too many oocysts could be the source of high numbers of *Eimeria* oocysts in litter that can cause outbreaks of coccidiosis and NE during growout. Thus, more effort is needed to develop practical, cost-efficient ways of delivering live *Eimeria* oocyst vaccines to newly hatched chicks.

4.10 CONCLUSIONS

Avian coccidiosis is regularly listed by poultry veterinarians as the most important poultry disease affecting performance of broilers and egg-layers. Worldwide, this parasitic disease costs poultry growers and companies over

$1 billion in losses due to unrealized weight gain, poor feed conversion efficiency, and the cost of anticoccidial controls, be it drugs or live *Eimeria* oocyst vaccines. Increased mortalities in broilers between 2.5 and 3.5 weeks of age are most often due to necrotic enteritis associated with acute coccidiosis infection. Like *Eimeria* oocysts, *Cl. perfringens* spores are capable of resisting inactivation in litter and are prevalent throughout growout. *Eimeria* vaccines are attractive because they can be used in rotation throughout the year in place of ionophores and synthetic chemicals, and thereby stem the inevitable anticoccidial drug resistance that occurs when these compounds are continually used. The major obstacle in the use of live *Eimeria* vaccines is how to ensure each chick ingests a minimum dose of oocysts so that subsequent exposure to *Eimeria* oocysts in litter has a boosting effect rather than causing outright enteric disease. Improving vaccine delivery, reducing the carryover of viable *Eimeria* oocysts during downtime (2–3 weeks) in a poultry house, and gaining an understanding of how genetic diversity affects vaccine design are just three of the many research areas ripe for investigation.

REFERENCES

21, 24, 48, 57, 90, 133, 135, 214, 216, 217, 218, 219, 221, 222, 224, 225, 226, 232, 234–239, 243, 244, 276, 319, 321, 324, 370–372, 376, 396, 461–466, 531, 536, 609, 624, 650, 685, 694–697, 739, 740, 742, 789–792, 794, 798–801, 803–806, 830, 831, 835, 843, 845–847, 872, 896, 951, 955, 969, 1075, 1076, 1078, 1079, 1081, 1082, 1086, 1087, 1132, 1137, 1138, 1160, 1161, 1167, 1250, 1251, 1323, 1335, 1336, 1364, 1366, 1438, 1439, 1441, 1443, 1444, 1448, 1449, 1528, 1559, 1561, 1563, 1566, 1567, 1585, 1586, 1613, 1634, 1652, 1695, 1734, 1758, 1763, 1786, 1787, 1788, 1799, 1801, 1803–1806, 1809

CHAPTER 5

Genomics, Transcriptomics, and Proteomics of the *Eimeria* Species

D. Blake and F. Tomley

CONTENTS

5.1 INTRODUCTION

Understanding of the molecular composition, structure, and functional interactions of cellular biomolecules including DNA, RNA, and proteins has advanced considerably for *Eimeria* in the last decade. Access to technologies such as next-generation sequencing and high-throughput proteomics, facilitated by reduced costs and template requirements, has been key. Here, we discuss progress toward understanding the genomes, transcriptomes, and proteomes of eimerian parasites. Details of cell biology and specific protein actions and interactions have been reviewed elsewhere.[232,305]

5.2 *EIMERIA* GENOMES

Eimeria contain distinct nuclear, apicoplast, and mitochondrial genomes. The nuclear genome occurs as a single haploid copy per cell throughout much of the eimerian life cycle except for the fertilized zygote and unsporulated oocyst, which are diploid.[292,1764] The oocyst undergoes meiosis within the first 8 hours of sporulation to generate four haploid sporoblasts.[360] Sporoblasts mature into sporocysts within which a single mitotic division leads to the production of daughter sporozoites.[1249,1468] In common with many other apicomplexans including *T. gondii* and the *Plasmodium* species, the *Eimeria* species studied to date possess haploid karyotypes with more than 12 chromosomes, as

defined by pulsed-field gel electrophoresis or genome optical mapping.[134,1404,1560] Confirmation that *E. tenella* possesses 14 chromosomes came from electron microscopic observation of synaptonemal karyotypes in oocyst spreads.[361] Individual chromosomes vary in size; for *E. tenella* the smallest is ~1 Mbp and the largest ~7 Mbp.[1560] The smallest *E. tenella* chromosome, termed chromosome 1, was the first to be fully sequenced and assembled.[1052] This revealed a striking organizational structure, featuring distinct chromosomal regions rich in simple sequence repeats including the trinucleotide CAG/CTG (and other closely related trinucleotides) and the heptanucleotide AAACCCT/AGGGTTT, interspersed with regions that are largely devoid of repeats (termed *repeat-rich* and *repeat-poor*, respectively). Comparison of repeat-rich and repeat-poor regions revealed no clear association with gene function or density, although gene length and intron number were higher in the repeat-rich regions where transposon-like sequences were also more common.[1052] A first draft genome assembly for *E. maxima* comprised 42.5 Mbp from the Houghton strain in 22,256 contigs; this high level of fragmentation was most likely due to repeat-rich regions scattered throughout the genome.[130] More comprehensive datasets became available in 2014 with genome assemblies for all seven *Eimeria* species that infect chickens.[1404] Six of these sequences derive from Houghton reference strain parasites, the exception being the Weybridge strain for *E. maxima*. Notable features included evidence that the repeat-rich/repeat-poor segmental structure of eimerian chromosomes is conserved across all species that infect the chicken. A genome assembly for the mouse-infecting species *Eimeria falciformis* showed a similar distribution of trinucleotide and heptanucleotide repeats resulting in segmented chromosomal structures like those of the chicken-infecting species, indicating a conserved evolutionary background.[699] Finally, a draft genome assembly was generated recently for the rat-infecting species *Eimeria nieschulzi*, as part of a study exploring gametocyte and oocyst wall proteins.[1796]

Comparing *Eimeria* genome assemblies reveals considerable variation in predicted genome size, ranging from 45.8 to 72.2 and 43.7 to 62.9 Mbp for *Eimeria* that infect chickens and rodents, respectively (Table 5.1). Some of the difference is likely due to the variable quality of assemblies; however, optical mapping supports the estimates for *E. acervulina*, *E. maxima*, *E. necatrix*, and *E. tenella*.[1404] Currently, the *E. tenella* genome assembly is the best curated for those species that infect chickens, termed "tier 1" since it included bacterial artificial chromosome (BAC) and fosmid end sequences and was enhanced by directed manual improvements for targeted regions. The *E. acervulina*, *E. maxima*, and *E. necatrix* genome assemblies are termed "tier 2," benefitting from automatic postassembly improvements, while those for *E. brunetti*, *E. mitis*, and *E. praecox* are drafts or "tier 3."[1404] Detection of core eukaryotic genes annotated in the *T. gondii* genome assembly suggest that tier 1 and 2 *Eimeria* genomes are 93%–99% complete, although each assembly remains highly fragmented. Tier 1 and 2 genome assemblies have between 3415 and 4664 scaffolds, which is 10-fold higher than for the *T. gondii* assembly.[1404] The tier 3 assemblies remain less refined, with between 5317 and 15,978 scaffolds. It is likely that the high repeat content of the genomes has hindered effective assembly at many locations because of the short sequence reads produced by the Illumina next-generation sequencing technology employed. The future inclusion of longer sequence reads should improve each of the genome sequence assemblies. All genome sequence assemblies are

publically available through sequence repositories such as GenBank, the European Nucleotide Archive (ENA) and the DNA Data Bank of Japan (DDBJ). Assemblies for all seven *Eimeria* species that infect chickens, and *E. falciformis*, can also be accessed through the web resource ToxoDB (http://toxodb.org/) where comparative analyses with other coccidian parasites is facilitated.

Comparison of *Eimeria* genome sequence assemblies again emphasizes the occurrence of dispersed regions rich in repetitive sequences, with considerable conservation of repeat boundaries between species. Building on the findings from *E. tenella* chromosome 1, the repeat-rich regions are more precisely defined as areas with a repeat density greater than 5%.[1404] Of particular note is that transcribed and translated repetitive regions code for homopolymeric amino acid repeats (HAARs), which are found in *Eimeria* species at a greater frequency than recorded in any other organism to date. HAARs in *Eimeria* proteins, resulting from translation of five or more triplet simple tandem repeats (STRs), most commonly encode alanine or glutamine, and to a lesser extent serine. For *E. tenella*, 57% of gene models are predicted to contain HAARs, with supporting evidence of transcription and translation.[1404] Consideration of gene ontogeny does not reveal links between HAARs and any functional protein class, although occurrence is lower in genes that code for proteins associated with host-parasite interactions such as surface antigens, microneme proteins, and rhoptry kinases. Other nucleotide repeats detected within *Eimeria* genomes include a series of fragmented retrotransposon-like elements. These were first seen in the *E. tenella* chromosome-1 assembly and are related to chromovirus long-terminal repeat (LTR) retrotransposons.[1052,1404] A high level of disruption suggests that these retrotransposons are unlikely to have been functional for many generations.

Complete mitochondrial genomes are published for a range of *Eimeria* species. For chickens, sequences are available for multiple isolates from all seven of the recognized

Table 5.1 Summary of Published Genome Assemblies for *Eimeria* Species

Host	Species	Strain	Assembly Size (Mbp)	Gene Count (total)	Reference
Gallus gallus	*E. acervulina*	Houghton (H)[a]	45.83	7,037	Reid et al.[1404]
	E. brunetti	Houghton (H)[a]	66.89	8,893	Reid et al.[1404]
	E. maxima	Weybridge (Wey)[a]	45.98	6,249	Reid et al.[1404]
		Houghton (H)	42.52	na	Blake et al.[130]
	E. mitis	Houghton (H)[a]	72.24	10,254	Reid et al.[1404]
	E. necatrix	Houghton (H)[a]	55.01	8,864	Reid et al.[1404]
	E. praecox	Houghton (H)[a]	60.08	7,894	Reid et al.[1404]
	E. tenella	Houghton (H)[a]	51.86	8,634	Reid et al.[1404]
		Nippon-2 (Nt2)		na	Reid et al.[1404], Blake et al.[132]
		Wisconsin (Wis)		na	Reid et al.[1404], Blake et al.[132]
Mus musculus	*E. falciformis*	Bayer Haberkorn 1970[a]	43.67	6,037	Heitlinger et al.[699]
Rattus norvegicus	*E. nieschulzi*	Landers	62.95	na	Wiedmer et al.[1796]

Abbreviation: na, not provided.
[a] Assembly and gene count figures downloaded from ToxoDB (https://toxodb.org/toxo/), accessed September 21, 2018.

Eimeria species as well as the cryptic operational taxonomic units currently referred to as OTUs X, Y, and Z.[1028,1057,1205,1268] Sequences are also available from several *Eimeria* that infect turkeys[1267] and rabbits.[1058,1697] The mitochondrial genome sequences from *Eimeria* are highly conserved and contain ~6200 bp DNA with a concatemeric topology,[716] ranging from 6148 to 6214 bp for those which infect chickens, 6165–6238 bp for turkeys, and 6168–6261 bp for rabbits. Sequences are also available for some species that infect cattle (*E. zuernii*) and rodents (*E. falciformis*).[1205] The mitochondrial genome sequences are biased in nucleotide content toward adenine and thymine (A+T), presenting more than 60% A+T. All of the mitochondrial genomes include the protein-coding genes cytochrome c oxidase subunit I (COI), cytochrome c oxidase subunit III (COIII), and cytochrome b (CytB), as well as ribosomal large and small subunit rRNA sequences.[1267]

In addition to nuclear and mitochondrial genomes, apicomplexan parasites contain a vestigial plastid of algal origin referred to as the apicoplast, which houses an ~35 Kb circular genome.[1619] The complete apicoplast genome is sequenced for *E. tenella*,[168] revealing a high A+T bias as described for the mitochondrial genomes. The gene organization within the *E. tenella* apicoplast is comparable to *T. gondii*, although sequence similarity is low. Analysis of each *Eimeria* genome sequence assembly reveals contigs representing apicoplastid genomes, and shows that many ancestral plastid genes are now located within the nuclear genomes.[1404]

A fourth type of genome has been described within many *Eimeria* isolates, representing one or more double-stranded RNA viruses.[961,1412] Several report multiple RNA species typically associated with segmented RNA viruses, for example, in *E. necatrix*,[486,960,961] *E. nieschulzi*,[1426,1532] *E. acervulina*,[961] *E. brunetti*,[961] and *E. tenella*.[670] However, amplification and sequencing of putative whole viral genomes from *E. brunetti* (Laboratory of Arthur Gruber, Accession number AF356189.1), *E. tenella*,[1823] and *E. stiedae*[1832] suggests these are nonsegmented dsRNA viruses, belonging to the Family Totiviridae, within the genus *Victorivirus*, and are distinct from other viruses reported to infect protozoa. For all three of these species, viral RNA sequencing has generated assemblies of ~6000 bp, and it is proposed that *Eimeriavirus* be considered a new subgenus.[1823] The genome assemblies include open reading frames coding for putative capsid and RNA-dependent RNA polymerase (RdRp) proteins, although sequence similarity is relatively low (≤51% amino acid similarity). The consequences of viral infection for *Eimeria* species is unclear, with no evidence of significantly harmful or beneficial effects.

5.3 *CYCLOSPORA CAYETANENSIS*

The coccidian *Cyclospora* species are morphologically distinct from *Eimeria*; for example, including two sporocysts in each sporulated oocyst instead of four.[1285] Nonetheless,

phylogenetic comparison of loci including the mitochondrial and apicoplast genomes consistently place parasites such as *C. cayetanensis* among the eimerians.[1666] Genome sequencing *C. cayetanensis* has produced an assembly of 51.9 Mbp across 2297 supercontigs.[1068] Analysis of the assembly has shown conservation of the eimerian repeat-rich/repeat-poor segmental structure within the *C. cayetanensis* genome, including shared STR and LTR sequences and suggesting a common evolutionary history.

5.4 *EIMERIA* TRANSCRIPTOMES

The first systematic studies of *Eimeria* gene transcription relied on sequencing and analysis of expressed sequence tag (EST) libraries, with data published for *E. acervulina*, *E. brunetti*, *E. maxima*, and *E. tenella*.[1,901,1188a,1239,1524,1770] Included within the dataset are ESTs produced using the open reading frame expressed sequence tag (ORESTES) approach, increasing sequence representation across the transcriptome and reducing 3′ bias.[1253] Transcriptomic data were used to identify coding and untranslated region (UTR) sequences with relevance to *Eimeria* taxonomy, host-parasite interactions and vaccine development. A small number of full-length cDNA sequences were produced using an oligo-capping method.[37] Analysis of EST, ORESTES, and full-length cDNA sequences confirmed the widespread occurrence of the triplet STRs within *Eimeria* transcriptomes. Average full-length cDNA and UTR sequences were longer in *E. tenella* than *T. gondii* or *C. parvum*, reflecting the higher repetitive content. Analysis of sequences at transcriptional start sites of several *E. tenella* genes indicates that these contain an initiator element (Inr core promoter) but lack a classical TATA box.[1353] Consensus sequence of translational initiation sites found A to be dominant at positions −3, −2, and −1, with G most common at position +4. At position ~4, C and G were both found to be common, suggesting a Kozak sequence of (G/C)AAAAUGG for *E. tenella* with high similarity to *T. gondii*.[37]

EST and ORESTES sequences were combined with sequences from other closely related coccidians, such as *T. gondii*, and used to annotate *E. tenella* chromosome 1.[1052] Subsequently, RNA sequencing using next-generation sequencing technologies (RNAseq) provided considerably more information, with replicate datasets from unsporulated and sporulated oocysts, sporozoites, and second-generation merozoites used in the *E. tenella* genome annotation.[1404] The resulting gene models were then used to predict orthologous genes for the other *Eimeria* species. Total gene numbers predicted for each genome ranged from 6249 to 10,254 for *Eimeria* species that infect chickens (*E. maxima* and *E. mitis*, respectively), and 6037 for *E. falciformis* (Table 5.1). A clear distinction can be made between gene numbers in *Eimeria* species considered to cause hemorrhagic rather than malabsorptive disease, although the use of *E. tenella* as the reference may have introduced some bias. Except for *E. mitis*, genomes of all hemorrhagic-type species are predicted to encode more than 8000 genes, while the malabsorptive species encode fewer than 8000.[1404] The outlier, *E. mitis*, is currently represented by a tier-3 genome assembly. Further sequencing and assembly improvement might resolve the apparent conflict. It is not known whether the apparent difference in gene number is causally related to pathogenicity.

At the time of publication, ~70% of gene models developed for *E. tenella* were hypothetical, with no function assigned to the encoded proteins. Of interest is the identification of novel *Eimeria*-specific gene families.[1404] Two of these, *Eimeria*-specific families 1 and 2 (*esf1* and *esf2*), code for 18–50 or 2–23 putative novel proteins per species, respectively. The function of these ESF proteins is currently unknown, but *esf* genes have relatively high K_a/K_s ratios, indicative of diversifying selection and suggesting that they are likely to be involved in interaction with the host. Other multigene families are known to encode variable *Eimeria* surface antigens (SAGs): single-domain, membrane-bound proteins attached to the surface of invasive zoites by glycophosphatidylinositol anchors.[1659] Each species of *Eimeria* possesses tandem arrays of *sag* genes that are differentially expressed during the endogenous development cycle. For species that infect chickens, the *sag* genes cluster into three, phylogenetically distinct subfamilies, all with low but significant homology to the cysteine-rich secretory protein superfamily (CAP).[594,1404] *SagA* genes are present in all chicken-infecting *Eimeria* species; however, *sagB* genes are found only in *E. tenella* and *E. necatrix*, while *sagC* genes are expanded in the other five species. The mouse-infecting species *E. falciformis* possesses related *sag* genes with a single gene grouping phylogenetically into the *sagA* family and the others forming an independent *sag* gene clade that is not present in the chicken-infecting species.[699]

The precise function of *Eimeria* SAGs is not known; however, their surface location, high variability, and regulation of expression between invasive zoite stages suggests they are important in the interaction of parasites with host cells, as is the case for GPI-linked surface antigens in *T. gondii*.[691,851] For *E. tenella,* it has been shown that SAGs of the *sagA* gene family bind epithelial cells in culture.[1404] As all eight *Eimeria* species examined to date (seven from the chicken, one from the mouse) contain at least one *sagA* gene (varying from 1 to 145 genes), it seems likely that SAGs of the *sagA* subfamily play a conserved role across all the species, possibly related to host cell binding. However, investigation of the *in vitro* effect that 10 different recombinant *E. tenella* SAGs had on chicken macrophages suggests that some (but not all) members of the *sagA* subfamily can induce pro-inflammatory responses, indicating that there is divergence in their specific interactions with host cells.[267] In contrast, SAGs of the *sagB* subfamily did not bind epithelial cells[1404] or induce pro-inflammatory responses.[267] The much more restricted species distribution of the non-*sagA* subfamilies of SAGs

and the fact that all species examined do possess a non-*sagA* subfamily suggests that these more divergent clades of SAGs fulfill more specific functions, possibly related to host and site specificity of invasion. Interestingly, the genome of *C. cayetensis* contains four putative *Eimeria*-type surface antigens that are distantly related to the *sagA* gene family, but only one of these is predicted to have both a signal peptide and GPI-anchor. This suggests that the coccidian that is phylogenetically most closely related to *Eimeria* species, and which infects humans, may use a different class of surface antigens in its initial interaction with host cells.[1068]

RNAseq offers semiquantitative measurement of transcription, permitting the construction of stage-specific expression profiles. Several endogenous eimerian life-cycle stages have not yet been analyzed, primarily because protocols to obtain sufficient quantities of pure intracellular stages are not yet available. A notable exception is the sexual stages (gametocytes) of *E. tenella*. Protocols established initially for the purification of *E. maxima* gametocytes were used to purify *E. tenella* gametocytes (micro- and macrogametocytes) as template for RNAseq.[1765,1768] While the proportion of contaminating host transcripts was higher than reported for RNAseq from extracellular life-cycle stages, sufficient parasite sequences were produced to explore the biology of eimerian sexual stages.[1765] Transcription profiles for genes associated with macro- and microgametocytes were obtained, and gametocyte-specific proteins were defined. For example, transcription of two macrogametocyte-specific proteins with unknown functions was recorded, together with a microgametocyte gamete fusion protein, EtHAP2. A similar study published more recently for *E. necatrix* produced comparable results,[1637] including upregulation of genes that code for oocyst wall proteins and a series of subtilisin-like proteases. These results provide an important resource for other coccidian parasites such as *T. gondii* and *Neospora caninum* for which culture and recovery of sexual stages in the respective definitive hosts (cats and dogs) are very challenging.

The *Eimeria* genome assemblies have enabled comparative transcriptomic studies exploring variation among parasite life-cycle stages, among strains or lines of parasites, and examination of changes in host-parasite gene expression during infection. Comparing a given parasite's life-cycle stages consistently identifies complex, stage-specific transcription profiles for unsporulated and sporulated oocysts, sporozoites, several different merozoite stages, and gametocytes.[746,1404,1636,1765] Transcriptome sequencing of parasites selected for abbreviated prepatent periods (termed *precocious* and used in live-attenuated anticoccidial vaccines[1561]) identifies numerous differentially expressed genes (DEGs) that are up- or downregulated compared to the parental ("wild-type") strain. Thus, sporozoite transcriptomes of the attenuated Nt-P110 and parental Nt lines of *E. tenella* (with a difference of 30 hours between prepatent periods) showed attenuation to coincide with significant reductions in transcripts related to carbohydrate metabolism and cell attachment, and increases in transcripts associated with cell proliferation.[1149] Transcriptomes of merozoites, sporulated and unsporulated oocysts from the attenuated *E. maxima* BJ-PL-98 line and the parental Beijing strain, with prepatent periods of 98 and 130 hours, respectively, similarly showed high numbers of DEGs.[746] It is important to note that 22 passages through chickens were required to generate the precocious BJ-PL-98 line and that some quantitative variation in transcript abundance would be expected to have occurred through genetic drift. The development of next-generation sequencing technologies has also permitted detailed comparative characterization of interacting host and pathogen transcriptomes. The most detailed study published to date used the mouse (*Mus musculus*) system with *E. falciformis*. The authors demonstrated significant changes in the host transcriptome following exposure to a pathogenic parasite dose.[471] Immune mediators such as transforming growth factor beta (TGF-β), epidermal growth factor (EGF), tumor necrosis factor (TNF), and interleukins (IL)-1 and IL-6 were all differentially transcribed in the presence or absence of parasite infection. While the parasite transcriptome demonstrated significant variation between life-cycle stages, there was no significant effect of host infection history on sporozoite transcriptomes. The study went on to compare immunocompromised (*Rag1-/-* knockout mice, lacking in mature B and T cells) and competent host lines, again detecting significant differences in host, but not parasite, transcriptomes. The authors speculated that the lack of variation in parasite transcriptomes, irrespective of host immunocompetence or exposure history, indicated a lack of plasticity that might limit their potential to switch between hosts, in part explaining the high host specificity of many *Eimeria* species. It has also been suggested that the short eimerian life cycle, coupled with stage-specific expression of many proteins relevant to host interaction and invasion, might limit selection by the host immune response and avoid a major driver for transcriptome plasticity.[135]

5.5 *EIMERIA* PROTEOMES

Proteomic studies of *Eimeria* species can be divided into three broad categories: those that focus on specific parasite compartments or organelles, those that compare different life-cycle stages, and those that assess host-parasite interactions. For *E. tenella*, several papers describe the proteinaceous contents of microneme, refractile body, and rhoptry organelles.[156,350,1258] A critical phase for each of these studies was the development and validation of protocols for the disruption of whole sporozoites and enrichment of the target subcellular organelles. Outputs from each study have been used to confirm and annotate gene models predicted from genomic/transcriptomic datasets and provide information on the location and/or timing of expression of

target proteins. Several proteins identified in these studies have also been examined as recombinant proteins for subunit vaccine development. Proteomic analysis of *E. tenella* micronemes (MICs) confirmed the relatively low complexity of these organelles and identified several new candidate MIC proteins.[156] Work on the refractile body highlighted the abundance of a small number of known proteins including the aspartyl proteinase eimepsin and a previously studied refractile body protein, SO7, both of which are present in multiple isoforms.[350] Analysis of the *E. tenella* rhoptry proteome revealed a larger rhoptry neck protein (RON) repertoire than had hitherto been described for related coccidians such as *T. gondii* and *N. caninum* with distinct stage-specific expression profiles for many, leading the authors to speculate that the molecular components of host cell invasion vary among life-cycle stages.[1258] It also revealed that the sporozoite stage expressed only two secreted rhoptry kinases out of what is now known to be a total repertoire of 28 *ropk* genes.[1661]

Whole cell proteomics has been used to define the protein content of individual life-cycle stages such as *E. tenella* sporozoites[349] and second-generation merozoites,[1063] and to compare protein repertoires of multiple life-cycle stages.[937] The latter study was comprehensive, identifying 1868 proteins and adding to the subcellular organelle datasets by building associations for paralogous proteins including the identification of multiple apical membrane antigens and members of different RON families. Assessing protein abundance by functional category illustrated the key roles for each life-cycle stage, consistently highlighting the importance of glycolysis and gluconeogenesis in parasite metabolism with varied rankings in abundance of surface, transcription, protein synthesis, and cell transport pathways according to parasite stage. Comparison of stage-specific proteomes from parasites with distinct selectable phenotypes, such as drug resistance/susceptibility, has been used to explore the consequences and underpinning molecular mechanisms of anticoccidial effects. For example, Shen and colleagues compared proteomes from second-generation *E. tenella* merozoites of diclazuril resistant and susceptible lines, identifying 13 differentially expressed proteins.[1551]

5.6 MOLECULAR STUDIES OF GENETIC DIVERSITY

As previously described, *Eimeria* genomes are relatively complex, comprising 42–72 Mbp DNA organized in more than 12 chromosomes. Despite such complexity, genetic diversity has until recently been assessed using just two loci; the nuclear rRNA locus (including the 18S rRNA gene and internal transcribed spacer [ITS] regions 1 and 2) and the mitochondrial cytochrome oxidase subunit I (COI) coding sequence. While such approaches can provide effective discrimination of species, low levels of sequence diversity and the presence of polymorphic duplicates, even within individual parasite genomes, limit their use for assessment of variation between strains.[275,1758] Low-throughput strategies, such as multilocus sequence typing (MLST), random amplification of polymorphic DNA-polymerase chain reaction (RAPD-PCR), and amplified fragment length polymorphism (AFLP) have been developed as alternatives to sample additional regions of the genome (reviewed elsewhere),[91] although uptake of these techniques has been limited. Recently, access to multiple genome sequence assemblies for species such as *E. tenella* has facilitated the identification of molecular genetic markers including single nucleotide polymorphisms (SNPs) and insertions/deletions (indels). Using a panel of 55 SNPs in a genome-wide haplotyping study, it was found that population structure varies for *E. tenella* in different geographical regions of the world. *E. tenella* samples collected from chicken farms in North Africa and northern India showed relatively low levels of haplotype diversity, in direct contrast to samples from sub-Saharan Africa and southern India where whole genome haplotype diversity was very high.[132] Network analysis illustrated the widespread occurrence of a small number of genetically distinct haplotypes in North Africa and northern India, contrasting with numerous diverse, often unique, haplotypes in Nigeria and southern India. Subsequent analyses using a closely related SNP-based polymerase chain reaction-restriction fragment length polymorphism (PCR-RFLP) panel indicated

distinct but tightly restricted genetic diversity in the United Kingdom and Ireland.[1342] Comparative analysis of genetic diversity at the *ama1* and *imp1* loci, both of which code for anticoccidial vaccine candidates,[131,1327] revealed considerably lower levels of polymorphism with little or no evidence of balancing selection.[132,924] The absence of notable coding sequence polymorphism suggested that, at least for AMA1 and IMP1 in *E. tenella*, functional constraints may preclude the development of variants capable of evading immunity. The relevance of such findings is unclear but may prove of value to ongoing attempts to develop subunit vaccines for *Eimeria*. Limited antigenic diversity for vaccine candidates supports the feasibility of developing subunit vaccines that are appropriate for use in field populations around the world. Sampling additional *E. tenella* populations and extending studies to other species are likely to be informative, as will expanding the density of genetic markers.

REFERENCES

1, 37, 91, 130, 131, 132, 134, 135, 156, 168, 232, 267, 275, 292, 305, 349, 350, 360, 361, 471, 486, 594, 670, 691, 699, 716, 746, 851, 901, 924, 937, 960, 961, 1019, 1028, 1052, 1057, 1058, 1063, 1068, 1149, 1188a, 1205, 1239, 1249, 1253, 1258, 1267, 1268, 1285, 1327, 1342, 1353, 1404, 1412, 1426, 1468, 1524, 1532, 1551, 1560, 1561, 1636, 1637, 1659, 1661, 1666, 1697, 1758, 1764, 1765, 1768, 1770, 1796, 1823, 1832

CHAPTER 6

Anticoccidial Drugs of Livestock and Poultry Industries

S. Noack, H. D. Chapman, and P. M. Selzer

CONTENTS

6.1 INTRODUCTION

In this chapter, we aim to give an overview of the efficacy and mode of action of the current compounds used to control coccidiosis in poultry and livestock and provide a brief outlook of research needs for the future. This chapter complements previous reviews of this subject.[223,1243,1336]

6.2 DRUG CATEGORIES

Anticoccidial drugs belong to one of two categories as follows.[28,223]

6.2.1 Polyether Antibiotics or Ionophores

Polyether antibiotics or ionophores are produced by the fermentation of *Streptomyces* spp. or *Actinomadura* spp. These drugs disrupt ion gradients across the cell membrane of the parasite:

a. Monovalent ionophores (monensin, narasin, salinomycin)
b. Monovalent glycosidic ionophores (maduramicin, semduramicin)
c. Divalent ionophore (lasalocid)

6.2.2 Synthetic Compounds

Synthetic compounds, popularly known as "chemicals," are produced by chemical synthesis, often with a specific mode of action:

a. Inhibition of parasite mitochondrial respiration (decoquinate, clopidol)
b. Inhibition of the folic acid pathway (sulfonamides)
c. Competitive inhibition of thiamine uptake (amprolium)
d. Unknown mode of action (e.g., diclazuril, halofuginone, nicarbazin, robenidine)

Combination products, consisting of either a synthetic compound and ionophore (e.g. nicarbazin/narasin-Maxiban, Elanco) or two synthetic compounds (clopidol/methyl benzoquate-Lerbek, Impextraco NV), are also available. Arsenical drugs such as roxarsone, that has some anticoccidial efficacy, arsanilic acid, carbarsone, and combinations thereof have been discontinued in many countries since 2015, based on scientific reports that indicated organic arsenic could transform into inorganic, highly toxic arsenic.[1227,1852]

6.3 CONTROL OF COCCIDIOSIS IN POULTRY

Satisfactory control of coccidiosis in poultry requires strict attention to hygiene and sanitation, and biosecurity measures that limit human access to poultry facilities.[231] Adequate ventilation and leak-free watering systems are important to reduce excessive moisture because wet litter aids sporulation of the infective stage of the life cycle (the oocyst). Nevertheless, despite such measures, eradication has not proved possible, and the parasites persist in poultry flocks.[233] Preventative strategies may employ pharmaceutical ingredients in medicated food or drinking water, or immunization involving the use of live attenuated or nonattenuated vaccines.[901] By these means, it is estimated that most broiler chickens produced worldwide receive treatment with drugs or are vaccinated.[236] Prophylaxis is preferred as most of the damage occurs before clinical signs become apparent and because drugs cannot completely prevent infection.

The concept of coccidiosis prevention in chickens by inclusion of drugs in the feed (prophylaxis) was first described in 1948 and involved the use of sulfaquinoxaline, the first feed additive for poultry (reviewed by Chapman[230]).[629] In the years that followed, many other drugs were introduced, and until the introduction of ionophores in the 1970s, chemoprophylactic control of coccidiosis was based on the use of such synthetic anticoccidials.[1472] No new chemicals have been introduced for decades, and resistance has been documented for all the drugs approved for use in chickens,[223] although the onset of resistance can be slowed by using rotation programs with different chemicals and/or ionophores.[241] Nevertheless, resistance to the available chemicals and ionophores has become widespread.[1336] Drugs with novel molecular modes of action, and hence unprecedented targets, will be necessary if control of coccidiosis by chemotherapy is to be achievable in the future.[892,1526] Very little effort to discover new drugs has been undertaken or, at least, published in recent years, but this may change with the advent of genomics technology.[232] Examples of the successful application of novel drug discovery could be shown for other protozoa that are relevant for the animal health industry, for example, for the pig parasite *Cystoisospora suis*.[1572]

6.3.1 Ionophores

For many years, ionophores have been the principal choice to control coccidiosis because resistance to them develops slowly and because they do not completely suppress parasite development, thus allowing the development of immunity in the host after first exposure.[225,226,241] They are characterized by multiple tetrahydrofuran rings that are connected in the form of spiroketal moieties[1418] and are effective against the asexual and sexual life-cycle stages of coccidia, disturbing the normal transport of ions across surface membranes of sporozoites or early trophozoites.[51,1587–1590] Ionophores are only used in livestock and are not employed for any purpose in human medicine. They are not active against most foodborne bacteria of poultry, for example, *Escherichia coli*, *Salmonella* spp., and *Campylobacter* spp., and are not, therefore, included in the World Health Organization (WHO) list of medically important antimicrobials.[1667,1795] Their use is not an issue for public health.

These drugs have a rather narrow safety margin,[399] and most are incompatible with several therapeutic antibiotics. Among those are tiamulin,[1720,773] chloramphenicol, erythromycin, oleandromycin,[158,1350,1721] and certain sulfonamides, leading to intoxication manifested by severe temporary clinical signs.[399,1520] In addition, ionophores are incompatible with some antioxidants.[399,932,933,1336,1721]

Monovalent ionophores can form lipid-soluble complexes with sodium and potassium cations, whereas divalent ionophores can bind calcium and magnesium cations only. Polyether ionophores arrest the development of sporozoites by increasing the concentration of intracellular Na^+ ions. In addition, they increase the activity of $Na^+/K^+/ATPase$[1784] and affect merozoites by causing the cell membrane to burst.[1174] Toxic effects in horse, cattle, dogs, cats, rats, and avian species are thought to be mediated by disrupting ion gradients of cell membranes, leading to mitochondrial damage and thus depletion of cellular energy. Well-known toxic effects are cardiac toxicity and muscle degeneration and neuropathy, the latter being manifested by myelin degeneration and ataxia.[231,862]

6.3.1.1 Monovalent Ionophores

6.3.1.1.1 Monensin

In 1967, the structure of monensic acid (Figure 6.1E), a fermentation product of *Streptomyces cinnamonensis,* was first described, and the compound was reported to have a broad-spectrum effect against *Eimeria.*[14] It forms lipid-soluble complexes with sodium and potassium cations, leading to increased permeability of the membrane for these ions. Monensin can transport sodium ions through membranes in both electrogenic and electroneutral manners.[1199] Horses are particularly susceptible to monensin poisoning.[1154] Accidental deadly poisoning of horses with monensin has been published.[116,125,383]

6.3.1.1.2 Salinomycin

Salinomycin (Figure 6.1A) was isolated from *Streptomyces albus.* It exhibits not only activity against *Eimeria* of poultry but also against gram-positive bacteria including mycobacteria and some filamentous fungi.[1193] Salinomycin is an ionophore with strict selectivity for alkali ions and a strong preference for potassium, interfering with transmembrane potassium potential and promoting the efflux of K^+ ions from mitochondria and cytoplasm. Recently, it has been shown to kill human cancer stem cells and to inhibit breast cancer growth and metastasis in mice.[1235] Salinomycin is the least toxic of all the ionophores.[1265]

6.3.1.1.3 Narasin

Narasin (Figure 6.1B) is a polyether antibiotic obtained from *Streptomyces aureofaciens.*[795] It is a derivative of salinomycin having an additional methyl group, therefore, alternatively called (4S)-4-methyl salinomycin. When combining different ionophores with nicarbazin, Challey and Jeffers[209] found that combinations of nicarbazin and narasin had synergistic activity. A combination product containing both active pharmaceutical ingredients (API) in a 1:1 ratio was developed (Maxiban). Very high levels of narasin caused death in sows, leg muscle weakness in turkeys, and cardiopulmonary clinical signs in 15% of the rabbits from Brazilian rabbit farms.[1265]

6.3.1.2 Monovalent Glycosidic Ionophores

6.3.1.2.1 Maduramicin

The ionophores maduramicin (also called Yumamycin; Figure 6.1C) was first isolated from the bacterium *Actinomadura yumaensis.*[1054] It is a large heterocyclic compound with a series of electronegative crown ethers able to bind monovalent or divalent metal ions[1127] and is widely used for commercial broiler production. Maduramicin is the most toxic of all the ionophores for nontarget animals[1265] and humans.[1541] It might cause severe cardiovascular defects,[1568] as it inhibits proliferation and induces apoptosis in myoblasts.[256]

6.3.1.2.2 Semduramicin

Semduramicin (Figure 6.1D) can be isolated from *Actinomadura roserufa.*[1715] It is a highly effective drug against *Eimeria* and is well tolerated by chickens.[1072,1417]

6.3.1.3 Divalent Ionophores

6.3.1.3.1 Lasalocid

Compound X-537A (later named lasalocid A; Figure 6.1F) was isolated from *Streptomyces lasaliensis.*[107] It was shown to have anticoccidial activity in chickens[1192] and to increase weight gain and feed conversion.[1405]

Except for salinomycin, lasalocid is the one with lowest toxicity.[1265] Nevertheless, dogs appear to be more sensitive to lasalocid intoxication than other species, and accidental poisoning of dogs by lasalocid has been reported.[506,1529]

6.3.2 Synthetic Compounds

Based on chemical structure, synthetic drugs include the quinolones, pyridones, alkaloids, guanidines, thiamine analogues, and triazine derivatives (Figure 6.2). The mode of action of some synthetic anticoccidials has been described,[1774,1775] but for others their mode of action needs to be investigated (e.g., diclazuril, halofuginone, nicarbazin, robenidine). Such information and its relevance to the inhibition of specific developmental stages of the life

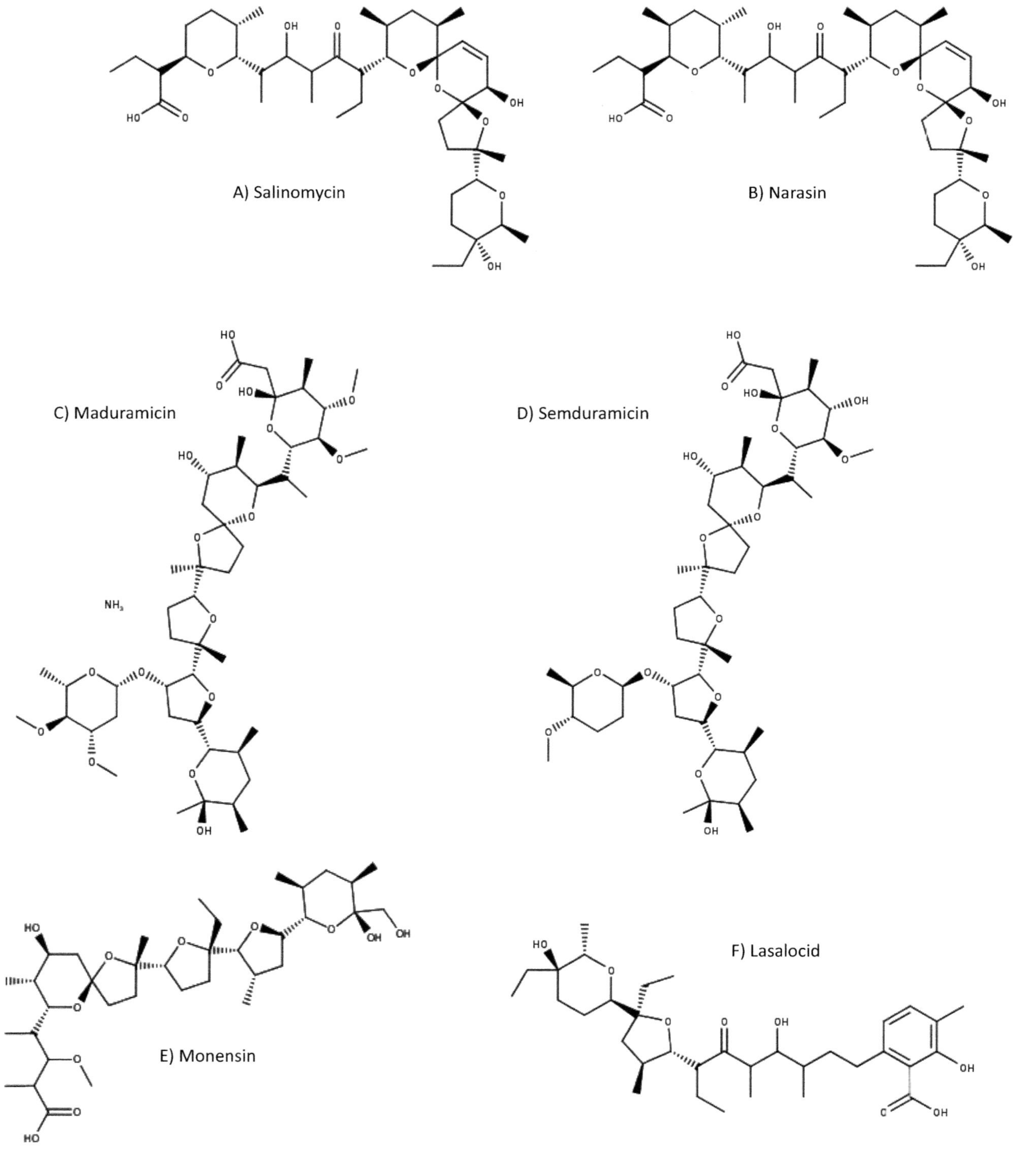

Figure 6.1 Ionophores used as anticoccidials. While salinomycin, narasin, maduramicin, semduramicin, and monensin (A–E) belong to the monovalent ionophores, lasalocid (F) is a divalent ionophore.

cycle of the parasites are important in understanding toxicity and adverse effects of synthetic anticoccidials, and to obtain optimal control by correct timing of prophylaxis. Structures of synthetic anticoccidials are shown in Figure 6.2.

6.3.2.1 Inhibition of Parasite Mitochondrial Respiration

One of the main targets for anticoccidial drugs is the respiratory chain, which is different from vertebrates as *E. tenella* oocysts predominantly use succinate or malate plus pyruvate

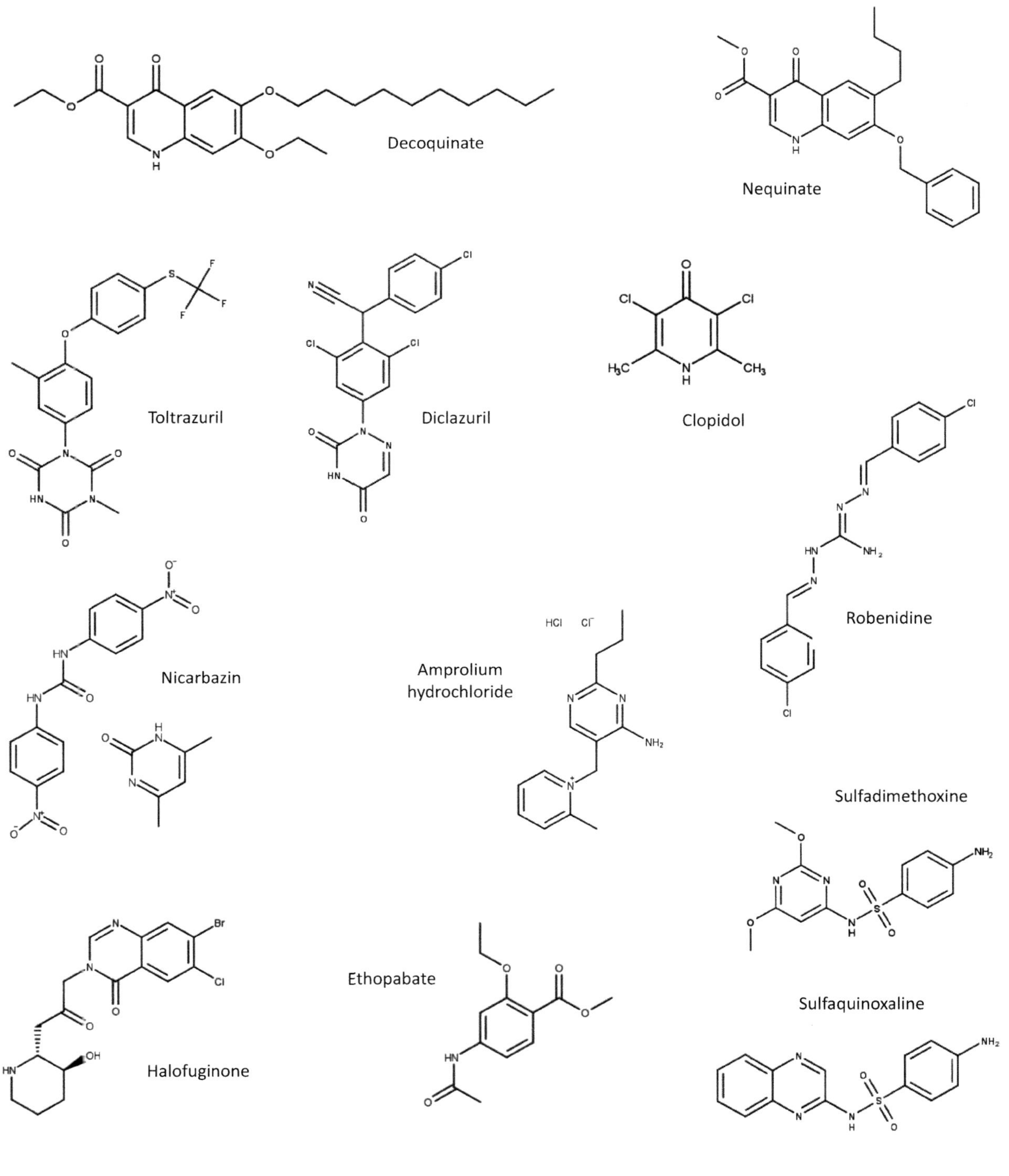

Figure 6.2 Synthetic anticoccidial active pharmaceutical ingredients.

to consume oxygen.[1774] As the respiratory chain of protozoa is relatively insensitive to rotenone and amytal, it can be assumed that NADH dehydrogenase is less important than succinate dehydrogenase.[674] Clopidol and quinolones inhibit mitochondrial energy production during the early stages of *Eimeria* development but act on different stages of the coccidia.[564,854]

6.3.2.1.1 Quinolones (Decoquinate, Nequinate [Methyl Benzoquate])

Quinolones were first discovered in 1962 and since then have undergone numerous modifications to their nucleus to improve spectrum as well as pharmacokinetics.[576] They arrest or kill sporozoites or early trophozoites, but even though they cover a broad spectrum, they are not able to fully control coccidiosis. Quinolone coccidiostats inhibit the respiration by blocking electron transport in the parasite mitochondrion reversibly, probably acting at a site near cytochrome b.[1772,1773]

Methyl benzoquate, an alkoxy-quinolone ester, acts synergistically with clopidol, a pyridone derivative, to prevent *Eimeria* infections in chicken.[1471] Decoquinate (6-ethyl-[decycloxy]-7-ethoxy-4-hydroxy-3-quinolinecarboxylate) was introduced in 1967.[1807] It also shows synergistic effects when combined with clopidol in low concentrations, inhibiting the electron transport more effectively than the sum of their individual actions.[564,1772,1800] Thus, both APIs are often used in combination products with clopidol. Nevertheless, quinolones and their combination with clopidol are used less frequently today because of the relatively rapid development of resistance.[223,867]

6.3.2.1.2 Clopidol

Clopidol, also known as meticlorpindol or clopindol, is a pyridinol with broad coccidiostatic activity against early development of *Eimeria* spp. by inhibiting mitochondrial energy production in sporozoites and trophozoites.[858] A synergistic effect between meticlorpindol and 4-hydroxyquinolones has been described.[209,793] To achieve complete control, combination products with quinolones are marketed.

6.3.2.1.3 Toltrazuril

Toltrazuril interacts with the mitochondrial pyrimidine biosynthesis linked to the respiratory chain; thus, it presumably inhibits mitochondrial dihydroorotate dehydrogenase.[674,828] In addition, toltrazuril might affect the apicoplast.[653]

Toltrazuril is one of the triazines that acts on intracellular stages of the life cycle that are undergoing schizogony and gamogony,[652] especially affecting mitochondria and the endoplasmic reticulum.[1173] Respiratory chain enzymes like succinate-cytochrome C reductase, NADH oxidase, and fumarate reductase as well as enzymes involved in pyrimidine synthesis are inhibited by toltrazuril. However, if one considers the high concentrations needed for inhibition of the latter enzymes, it is questionable whether this mechanism would translate into an anticoccidial effect.[674] In addition, nuclear division in schizonts and microgamonts as well as the wall-forming bodies in macrogamonts are disturbed.[1173]

6.3.2.2 Inhibition of the Folic Acid Pathway

The folic acid antagonists include sulfonamides, 2,4-diaminopyrimidines, and ethopabate, which are structural analogs of folic acid or of para-aminobenzoic acid (PABA), a precursor of folic acid. They interfere with the synthesis of folic acid by competing with PABA, thereby inhibiting folate synthetase and thus preventing cellular

replication.[952] Diaveridine and ormetoprim are active against the protozoan enzyme dihydrofolate reductase.[1038] As coccidia rapidly synthesize nucleic acids, they have high requirements of folic acid, in contrast to their hosts, which can utilize folic acid from feed and thus have no need for PABA.[1871]

6.3.2.2.1 Sulfonamides

Sulfonamides (sulfadimethoxine, sulfaquinoxaline) inhibit dihydropteroate synthetase.[1158] They have broad-spectrum activity against gram-negative and gram-positive bacteria as well as protozoa. Accidental human consumption of sulfonamide-contaminated products can cause central nervous system effects, gastrointestinal disturbances, and hypersensitivity reactions.[952] Sulfonamides act on developing schizonts and on sexual stages.

Sulfonamides are only used rarely in U.S. broiler production because of the high potential for residues. On rare occasions only, a combination of sulfadimethoxine and ormetoprim is used in a "prestarter feed" for birds under 16 weeks of age to prevent mortality from coccidiosis and bacterial infections with a 5-day meat withdrawal period.[1722] In Europe, sulfonamides are not approved for prevention of coccidiosis in poultry.

6.3.2.2.2 Ethopabate

Ethopabate is an antagonist of folic acid or of its precursor, PABA, thus inhibiting the synthesis of nucleic acid and limiting the production of new cells.[854] It is most active against *E. maxima* and *E. brunetti*.[1336] As it lacks activity against *E. tenella* cecal stages, it is often used in combination products together with amprolium.

6.3.2.3 Competitive Inhibition of Thiamine Uptake

6.3.2.3.1 Amprolium

Amprolium hydrochloride (1-[(4-amino-2-propyl-5-pyrimidinyl) methyl]-2-methylpyridinium chloride monohydrochloride) is an analog to thiamine (vitamin B1) but lacks the hydroxyethyl functionality that thiamine possesses and thus is not phosphorylated to a pyrophosphate analog.[862] It inhibits the uptake of thiamine by second-generation schizonts of *E. tenella* and prevents formation of thiamine pyrophosphate, which is required for many essential metabolic reactions, for example, as cofactor of several decarboxylase enzymes involved in cofactor synthesis.[778]

As amprolium is only poorly active against some *Eimeria* spp., it is largely used in combination products or mixtures with the folic acid antagonists ethopabate or sulfaquinoxaline to extend its spectrum of activity. The primary use of amprolium today is for water treatment during clinical outbreaks. Amprolium is the only active pharmaceutical ingredient approved for prevention and treatment in laying chicken. It has a large safety window (at least 5:1 when used at the recommended level in feed [125 ppm]).[1469]

6.3.2.4 Other Modes of Action

6.3.2.4.1 Nicarbazin

Nicarbazin is an equal molar complex of 4,4'-dinitrocarbanalide and 2-hydroxy-4,6-dimethylpyrimidine.[220] It was the first anticoccidial drug with true broad-spectrum activity and has been in common use since 1955.[854] The 4,4'-dinitrocarbanilide components of nicarbazin inhibit transglutaminase activity, whereas the 2-hydroxy-4,6-dimethylpyrimidine portion increases transglutaminase activity. In addition, nicarbazin increases lipoprotein lipase activity and acts as a calcium ionophore.[1866] Nicarbazin and narasin show synergistic activity,[208] and a combination product of these drugs was developed. Nicarbazin has only a small safety window. As it disrupts the ion and water equilibrium, medicated birds are at increased risk of heat stress under hot and humid weather conditions.[874] In addition, it is highly toxic to layers, symptoms include bleaching of brown-shelled eggs, mottling of yolks, reduced hatchability, and decreased egg production.[838]

6.3.2.4.2 Diclazuril

Like toltrazuril, diclazuril belongs to the chemical class of triazines, developed together with clazuril by Janssen Pharmaceuticals.[1113] Diclazuril is a nucleoside analog thought to be involved in nucleic acid synthesis, possibly affecting later phases of coccidia differentiation.[1737] It has been shown to affect parasite wall synthesis resulting in the formation of an abnormally thickened, incomplete oocyst wall and zygote necrosis in both *E. brunetti* and *E. maxima*.[1738] In addition, diclazuril has been shown to cause disruption of the transmembrane potential of mitochondria and to induce ultrastructural changes in merozoites.[1908] Nevertheless, it is not clear if this is the true mode of action or is just a consequence of cell death. Diclazuril was shown to downregulate mRNA expression of the serine/threonine protein phosphatase type 5 (PP5) significantly by 51.4% in *E. tenella*.[1910] PP5s of many eukaryotic organisms have important regulatory functions in the cell cycle[375,1030] and are associated with the apoptosis signal-regulated kinase 1 (ASK1).[929]

6.3.2.5 Unknown Modes of Action

6.3.2.5.1 Halofuginone

Halofuginone hydrobromide is a quinazolinone derivative related to the antimalarial drug febrifuginone. It was originally extracted from leaves and roots of the traditional Chinese herbal *Cichroa febrifuga* plant, which is used traditionally in Chinese medicine to treat malaria.[1358] It is effective against asexual stages of most species of *Eimeria*, delaying development.[1875]

6.3.2.5.2 Robenidine

Robenidine (1-3-*bis* [p-chlorobenzylideneamino]-guanidine hydrochloride) is a synthetic derivative of guanidine introduced in 1972,[873] which does not affect initial intracellular development of coccidian but prevents maturation of schizonts. Its mechanism of action is presumed to interfere with energy metabolism by the inhibition of respiratory chain phosphorylation and ATPases, and to inhibit oxidative phosphorylation.[858,1814]

6.3.3 Markets and Market Products

About 59 billion broilers, 5.8 billion layers, and 1.4 trillion eggs are produced each year worldwide. The global anticoccidial poultry market as estimated by the animal health industry is approximately US$1 billion (Boehringer Ingelheim internal analysis, 2016). Academic estimates calculate that the global loss due to coccidiosis in poultry is more than US$3 billion.[1566,1802] Specifying a value of the market and the cost of coccidiosis in poultry is not an easy task (and may be impossible) because small errors in such calculations can cause huge differences, and there are many different estimates and continuously changing factors involved (e.g., currencies, inflation, energy cost).[1802] Nevertheless, it is reasonable to speculate how much of these costs can be exploited commercially. If only half of the estimates are calculated, it would still be in the range of US$0.5 billion and therefore deserving of further research. To illustrate distinctions in differently regulated markets, we focus in the next sections on marketed products in Europe, the United States, and Australia (Figure 6.3A, B).

6.3.3.1 European Union

In the European Union (EU), chemicals are rarely used apart from the synthetic/ionophore combination product Maxiban. In contrast, in the United States, synthetic anticoccidials are often employed in rotational programs with ionophores. Nevertheless, they represent a minor part of the

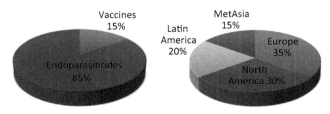

A) Percentage of market shares for vaccines and endoparasiticides

B) Split by geographic region

Figure 6.3 The global anticoccidial poultry market. (A) Endoparasiticides make up 85% of the total global anticoccidial poultry market. (B) The North American and European poultry markets are currently the most relevant ones. (From Noack, S. et al., 2019. *Parasitol. Res.* 118, 2009–2026.)

Table 6.1   Anticoccidial Products and Active Pharmaceutical Ingredients (APIs) Approved in Europe for Use in Poultry

Anticoccidial API	Trade Name	Company
Decoquinate	Deccox	Alpharma BVBA; Zoetis SA
Diclazuril	Clinacox	Eli Lilly and Company Ltd; Janssen Pharmaceutica NV
	Coxiril	Huvepharma NV
Halofuginone	Stenorol	Huvepharma NV
Lasalocid A	Avatec	Alpharma BVBA; Zoetis SA
Maduramicin	Cygro	Alpharma BVBA; Zoetis SA
Monensin	Coxidin	Huvepharma NV
	Elancoban	Eli Lilly and Company Ltd
Narasin	Monteban	Eli Lilly and Company Ltd
Narasin + Nicarbazin	Maxiban	Eli Lilly and Company Ltd
Nicarbazin	Koffogran (Nicarb)	Phibro Animal Health SA
Robenidine	Robenz (Cycostst)	Alpharma BVBA; Zoetis SA
Salinomycin	Huvesal, Sacox	Huvepharma EOOD; Huvepharma NV
	Salinomax	Alpharma BVBA
Semduramicin	Aviax 5%	Phibro Animal Health SA
Toltrazuril	Baycox	Bayer AH

Source: Data retrieved from the European Food Safety Authority (http://www.efsa.europa.eu/), Department for Environment, Food and Rural Affairs (https://www.vmd.defra.gov.uk/ProductInformationDatabase).

coccidiosis control program. Ionophores are most widely used in the EU, also due to their antibiotic affects in the intestine, for example, against dysbacteriosis caused by Clostridia. The ionophores salinomycin, narasin, monensin, lasalocid, maduramicin, and semduramicin and the chemical anticoccidial drugs robenidine, decoquinate, halofuginone, nicarbazin, and diclazuril are licensed in the EU as zootechnical feed additives under regulation 1831/2003/EC in species where coccidiosis is systematic for biological and zootechnical reasons, which is the case for poultry and rabbits (Table 6.1). Systematic means that in these hosts, diagnosis of coccidiosis is not required; therefore, no prescription is necessary. By contrast, in species where coccidiosis is not systematic, anticoccidials are registered as veterinary medicines (e.g., for cattle; regulated in the EU by Directive 2001/82/EC). In the United Kingdom, more than 40% of all antimicrobials sold for use in food and nonfood animals are employed for the control of coccidia (277 tons of active ingredient in 2011; mostly for control of *Eimeria*), with ionophores representing more than 70% of these.[1744]

6.3.3.2 United States

Rotation programs including ionophores and synthetic anticoccidials are the standard in intensive broiler production in the United States. These programs sometimes are also combined with vaccination. In contrast to the EU,[182] the use of antibacterials for growth promotion is allowed in the United States. However, with the Guidance for Industry (GFI) 209 of the U.S. Food and Drug Administration (FDA), 2012 and GFI 213 (FDA, 2013), the FDA has enhanced control of use of medically important antibacterials, eliminating the use of them for growth promotion. In addition, in 2017, the United States restricted the use of medically important antibiotics in feed to Veterinary Feed Directives (VFDs) that require veterinary oversight. The use of a VFD drug in feed is permitted only under the professional supervision of a licensed veterinarian (https://www.fda.gov/animalveterinary/developmentapprovalprocess/ucm455416.htm), while administration in drinking water still requires prescription. This restriction led to the withdrawal of some old anticoccidials, as for all, new VFD registrations were required, especially for combination products. Table 6.2 summarizes the products approved for use in the United States.

6.3.3.3 Australia

All agricultural and veterinary chemical products sold in Australia must be registered by the Australian Pesticides and Veterinary Medicines Authority (APVMA). The "Guideline for the evaluation of the efficacy and safety of coccidiostats" (https://apvma.gov.au/node/427) must be followed. Registered products are summarized in Table 6.3.

6.4 CONTROL OF COCCIDIOSIS IN RUMINANTS AND SWINE

There are several anticoccidial drugs available for treatment and prevention of coccidiosis in ruminants, both from the class of synthetic drugs (e.g., sulfonamides, amprolium, decoquinate, the triazines diclazuril and toltrazuril) and

Table 6.2 Anticoccidial Products and Active Pharmaceutical Ingredients (APIs) Approved by the U.S. Food and Drug Administrations for Use in Poultry

Anticoccidial API	First Approved	Trade Names	Company	Combination Products Available With
Amprolium	1960	Amprol; Corid; Amprolium-P	Huvepharma EOOD	Bacitracin, Bambermycins, Virginiamycin
		AmproMed P	Cross Vetpharm Group Ltd.	
		Cocciprol	Phibro Animal Health Corp.	
Clopidol	1968	Coyden 25	Huvepharma EOOD	Bacitracin, Bambermycins, Chlortetracycline
Decoquinate	1970	Deccox	Zoetis Inc.	Bacitracin, Chlortetracycline, Lincomycin
Diclazuril	1999	Clinacox	Huvepharma EOOD	Bacitracin, Bambermycins, Virginiamycin
Halofuginone	1987	Stenorol	Huvepharma EOOD	Bacitracin, Bambermycins
Lasalocid	1976	Avatec	Zoetis Inc.	Bacitracin, Bambermycins, Virginiamycin
Maduramicin	1989	Cygro	Zoetis Inc.	—
Monensin	1971	Coban 90 Coban 60	Elanco US Inc.	Avilamycin, Bacitracin, Bambermycins, Chlortetracycline, Lincomycin, Ractopamine, Oxytetracycline, Virginiamycin, Tilmicosin
Narasin	1988	Monteban 45	Elanco US Inc.	Avilamycin, Bacitracin, Bambermycins
Nicarbazin	1955	Nicarb 25%	Phibro Animal Health Corp.	Bacitracin, Bambermycins
		Nicarbazin; Carbigran 25	Elanco US Inc.	
		Nicarmix 25	Planalquimica Industrial Ltda.	
Robenidine	1972	Robenz	Zoetis Inc.	Bacitracin, Chlortetracycline, Lincomycin, Oxytetracycline
Salinomycin	1983	Bio-Cox Type A Medicated Article Sacox 60	Huvepharma EOOD	Avilamycin, Bacitracin, Bambermycins, Chlortetracycline, Lincomycin, Oxytetracycline, Virginiamycin
Semduramicin	1995	Aviax	Phibro Animal Health Corp.	Bacitracin, Virginiamycin
Sulfachloropyrazine		ESB 3	Zoetis Inc.	—
Sulfamethazine	1945	SMZ-Med 454	Cross Vetpharm Group Ltd.	—
		Sulmet Soluble Powder	Huvepharma EOOD	
Sulfadimethoxine		ALBON; AGRIBON	Zoetis Inc.	—
		SDM Sulfadimethoxine Concentrated Solution 12.5%	Cronus Pharma LLC	
		Sulfadimethoxine Soluble Powder	Phibro Animal Health Corp.	
		Sulfamed-G	Cross Vetpharm Group Ltd.	
		Sulfasol Soluble Powder; Sulforal	Med-Pharmex, Inc.	
		DI-METHOX; Sulfadimethoxine 12.5% Oral Solution; Sulmet Drinking Water Solution, 12.5%	Huvepharma EOOD	
Sulfaquinoxaline	1948	20% Sulfaquinoxaline Sodium Solution; 25% S.Q. Soluble; S.Q. 40%; Sul-Q-Nox Sulquin 6-50 Concentrate	Huvepharma EOOD Zoetis Inc.	—
Zoalene	1960	Zoalene 90 Medicated Coccidiostat Zoamix Type A Medicated Article	Zoetis Inc.	Bacitracin, Bambermycins, Lincomycin
Amprolium + Ethopabate	1997	Amprol Plus	Huvepharma EOOD	Bacitracin, Bambermycins, Chlortetracycline
		Amprol Hi-E		
		Amprol Plus 3-Nitro		
Narasin + Nicarbazin	1989	Maxiban 72	Elanco US Inc.	Avilamycin, Bacitracin, Bambermycins
Ormetoprim + Sulfadimethoxine	1970	Rofenaid 40	Zoetis Inc.	—
Sulfamethazine + Sulfaquinoxaline	2006	PoultrySulfa	Huvepharma EOOD	Sulfamerazine

Source: Data retrieved from U.S. Food and Drug Administration (https://www.fda.gov/AnimalVeterinary/default.htm).

Table 6.3   Anticoccidial Products and Active Pharmaceutical Ingredients (APIs) Approved in Australia for Use in Poultry

Anticoccidial API	First Approved	Trade Names	Company
3,5-Dinitro-O-toluamide	1994	Dot	Dox-Al Australia PTY Ltd.
		Dot premix	Bec Feed Solutions PTY Ltd.
		Doteco	International Animal Health Products PTY Ltd.
		Nutridot	Nutriment Health PTY Ltd.
		Phibrodot	Phibro Animal Health PTY Ltd.
Amprolium	1996	Amprolium	Parafarm PTY Ltd.
Decoquinate	2016	Deccox	Zoetis Australia PTY Ltd.
Lasalocid	2001	Avatec	Zoetis Australia PTY Ltd.
Maduramicin	1997	CyGro	Zoetis Australia PTY Ltd.
		Maduradox	Dox-Al Australia PTY Ltd.
Monensin	1994	CCD Monensin, Rumensin	Elanco Australasia PTY Ltd.
		Coxidin	Huvepharma EOOD
		Doxaban	Dox-Al Italia S.P.A.
		Monendox	Dox-Al Australia PTY Ltd.
		Moneco	International Animal Health Products PTY Ltd.
		Neove Monensin	Nutriment Health PTY Ltd.
		Phibromonensin	Phibro Animal Health PTY Ltd.
Narasin	1984	Elanco Narasin, Monteban	Elanco Australasia PTY Ltd.
Nicarbazin	1996	Carbidox	Dox-Al Australia PTY Ltd.
		Cycarb	Zoetis Australia PTY Ltd.
		Elanco Nicarbazin, Carbigran	Elanco Australasia PTY Ltd.
		Keymix	International Animal Health Products PTY Ltd.
		Nutrinicarb	Nutriment Health PTY Ltd.
		Phicarb	Phibro Animal Health PTY Ltd.
Robenidine	2003	Cycostat	Zoetis Australia PTY Ltd.
		Nutrirob	Nutriment Health PTY Ltd.
Salinomycin	1996	Bio-Cox, Sacox	Huvepharma EOOD
		CCD Salinomycin	CCD Animal Health PTY Ltd.
		Coxistac	Phibro Animal Health PTY Ltd.
		Neove	Nutriment Health PTY Ltd.
		Sadox, Salindox	Dox-Al Australia PTY Ltd.
		Doxalino	Dox-Al Italia S.P.A
		Saleco	International Animal Health Products PTY Ltd.
Semduramicin	1998	Aviax	Phibro Animal Health PTY Ltd.
Sulfaquinoxaline	1983	Inca Sulpha-Quin	Inca (Flight) Co PTY Ltd.
Toltrazuril	1993	Baycox, Toltracox Poultry	Bayer Australia Ltd. (Animal Health)
		Coxi-Stop	Abbey Laboratories PTY Ltd.
Diaveridine + Sulfaquinoxaline	1990	Keymix Solquin	International Animal Health Products PTY Ltd.
Amprolium + Ethopabate	1989	Keymix Keystat	International Animal Health Products PTY Ltd.
Maduramicin + Nicarbazin	2005	Gromax	Zoetis Australia PTY Ltd.
Methyl benzoquate + Clopidol	1993	Lerbek	Feedworks PTY Ltd.

Source: Data retrieved from Australian Pesticides and Veterinary Medicines Authority (https://apvma.gov.au).

ionophores (monensin, lasalocid). These drugs are used either therapeutically for the treatment of young animals showing signs of infection (e.g., amprolium, sulfonamides; triazines) or for prevention by inclusion in the feed (e.g., decoquinate, monensin, lasalocid). As most of the damage to the intestine is already present before diagnosis of coccidiosis occurs, therapy is mostly not sufficient to cure but rather useful to hinder further spread of disease. Therapy should be combined with palliative application of electrolytes, glucose, and antidiarrheals to help to maintain hemostasis.[333]

Only three APIs are currently used for treatment of porcine coccidiosis: narasin, salinomycin, and toltrazuril. Resistance against toltrazuril has been observed not only for *Eimeria* isolates from chicken[1615] and ovine *Eimeria* field isolates[1264] but also in a field isolate of *Cystoisospora suis*, the usual cause of coccidiosis in very young pigs.[1570]

6.4.1 Ionophores

The divalent ionophore lasalocid has been shown to decrease oocyst production in naturally infected lambs and cattle and in a few instances improve performance and reduce clinical signs of disease when included in the feed.[548,737] The efficacy of the monovalent ionophore monensin, employed as a preventive drug by incorporation in the feed of livestock, is well documented.[108,541,620,965,1162]

6.4.2 Amprolium

Amprolium has been used for many years for the control of coccidiosis in sheep and cattle. The drug is principally used for the treatment of animals showing clinical signs of disease but may be employed for prevention by inclusion in the feed. It is available as an oral solution, soluble powder, or pelleted feed additive. The drug was shown to reduce oocyst production in lambs when given as an in-feed medication, and an outbreak of clinical coccidiosis was successfully controlled by single drenching followed by medication.[1662] Amprolium was effective for the control of coccidiosis in feedlot lambs[59] and in cattle.[1246]

6.4.3 Decoquinate

This drug is used for the prevention of coccidiosis in young ruminants by incorporation in the feed. Its efficacy has been demonstrated in sheep, goats, and cattle.[542,545,1186]

6.4.4 Triazines

Numerous studies have shown that diclazuril and toltrazuril, when administered orally to young cattle, lambs, or pigs prior to the onset of clinical signs (referred to as metaphylactic treatment), decreases oocyst production in natural and artificial infections with *Eimeria* species[142,326,496,1215,1217,1220] or *Cystoisospora suis*.[401,917,1219] In some cases, improvements in performance have been demonstrated.[1460,1507]

6.4.5 Sulfonamides

Various sulfonamides, such as sulfaquinoxaline and sulfaguanidine, have been used for many years for the treatment of livestock showing clinical signs of coccidiosis.[667] As appetite is depressed in infected animals, then inclusion in the drinking water is preferable for treatment.[1573]

6.5 REGISTERED ACTIVE PHARMACEUTICAL INGREDIENTS IN DIFFERENT MARKETS

6.5.1 European Union

In the EU, only a few anticoccidial APIs are registered for use in ruminants and/or pigs (mostly piglets): decoquinate, diclazuril, lasalocid, monensin, and toltrazuril (European Medicines Agency, https:// www.EMA.Europa.eu).

6.5.2 United States

In the United States, anticoccidials for use in ruminants and pigs are mainly used in combinations as feed additives, combined with antibacterials and growth promotors. Registered APIs are as follows:

Amprolium	Clopidol	Decoquinate	Dexamethasone
Diclazuril	Ethopabate	Halofuginone	Lasalocid
Maduramicin	Monensin	Narasin	Nicarbazin
Ormetoprim	Robenidine	Salinomycin	Semduramicin
Sulfachloropyrazine	Sulfadimethoxine	Sulfamerazine	Sulfamethazine
Sulfaquinoxaline	Tylosin	Zoalene	

Source: U.S. Food and Drug Administration (https://www.fda.gov/AnimalVeterinary/default.htm).

6.5.3 Australia

In Australia, only lasalocid, monensin, narasin, salinomycin, and toltrazuril are registered anticoccidials for treatment of ruminants and/or pigs (Australian Pesticides and Veterinary Medicines Authority, https://apvma.gov.au).

6.6 RESISTANCE AND RESEARCH FOR NEW ANTICOCCIDIALS

Development of resistance is a threat for all drugs that are used extensively for a prolonged time. A consequence of this is documented resistance for all drugs in intensive poultry production (Table 6.4).[223] In a survey conducted in the United States from 1995 to 1999, it was found that anticoccidials were universally used by 99% of commercial broiler operations.[227]

The polyether ionophores became the drug of choice in 1972 and remain the most extensively used drugs as of today. While the development of resistance to ionophores is rather slow, probably due to their unique mode of action, resistance development in synthetic drugs that have a specific mode of action seems to appear more rapidly, involving genetic mechanisms. Sometimes resistance was reported shortly after marketing a new drug an example being arprinocid (Figure 6.4).[215] Another example is the quinolone buquinolate (Figure 6.4) that was "commercially dead" within 6 months of its introduction due to the sudden appearance of

Table 6.4   Summary of Reported Resistance to Anticoccidials in Field Strains of *Eimeria*

Drug	Year of Introduction	Country Where Resistance was First Described	Year Resistance was First Described	Species[a]
Sulfaquinoxaline	1948	United States	1954	*Et*
Nitrofurazone	1948	United States	1955	Not given
Nicarbazin	1955	Britain	1964	*Et*
Dinitolmide	1960	Britain	1964	*Et, En*
Amprolium	1960	Britain	1964	*Eb*
Clopidol	1966	Britain	1969	*Ea, Em, Et*
Buquinolate	1967	United States	1968	Not given
Methyl benzoquate	1967	Britain	1970	*Et*
Decoquinate	1967	Britain	1970	*Et*
Monensin	1971	United States	1974	*Em*
Robenidine	1972	United States	1974	*Em*
Halofuginone	1975	France	1986	*Ea, Et*
Lasalocid	1976	United States	1977	*Ea*
Arprinocid	1980	Britain	1982	*Et*
Salinomycin	1983	United States	1984	Various
Diclazuril	1990	Brazil	1994	*Ea, Em, Et*
Toltrazuril	1986	Netherlands	1993	Not given

Source: Adapted from Chapman, H.D., 1997. *Avian Pathol.* 26, 221–244.
[a]   Species: *Ea, E. acervulina*; *Eb, E. brunetti*; *Em, E. maxima*; *En, E. necatrix*; *Et, E. tenella*.

drug resistance. Development of resistance against buquino-late was found to take place after a single experimental passage of *Eimeria*.[212] By comparison, drug resistance against toltrazuril did not occur in at least five successive drug exposures in field studies.[274]

A study on 10 *Eimeria* field isolates from northern Germany detected resistance in 9 out of the 10 isolates of *Eimeria*, with 7 out of the 10 having developed multiple resistance.[1615] Similar results have been shown in isolates from broiler farms in the United Kingdom[219] and the Netherlands,[1335] showing the enormous threat of development of broad resistance against all classes of anticoccidial drugs. As drug sensitivity in a population of coccidia can be altered by the introduction of drug-sensitive coccidia, for example, through the use of coccidiosis vaccines, or by the use of drug-sensitive laboratory-maintained lines or other

reservoirs,[63,792,1168] these measures have to be combined in an attempt to control coccidiosis. Restoration of sensitivity to drugs following the use of vaccines comprising drug-sensitive strains of *Eimeria* has been demonstrated for the ionophores, monensin and salinomycin, and the synthetic drug diclazuril.[221,239,240,798,1138,1335] Partial restoration of sensitivity to diclazuril and monensin was also observed following use of attenuated vaccine.[1335] Therefore, a yearly rotation program has been proposed in which use of ionophores is alternated in successive flocks with vaccination.[241]

The development of resistance led to increasing efforts for the identification of new, resistance-breaking drugs. One recent example is nitromezuril, a new triazine anticoccidial. It shows only limited cross-resistance with diclazuril or toltrazuril,[522] but these results must be further evaluated before this drug might finally enter the market.

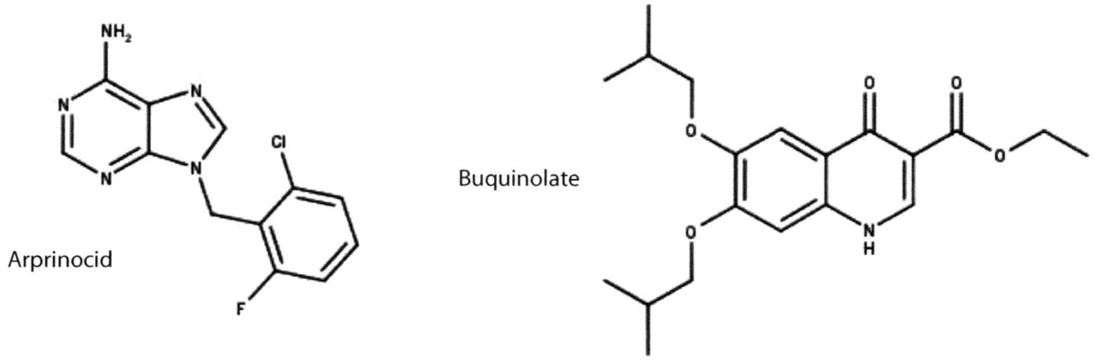

Arprinocid

Buquinolate

Figure 6.4   Chemical structures of arprinocid and buquinolate.

6.7 CONCLUSION

In light of the continuously expanding livestock industry and its growing significance for global food production, control of coccidiosis, perhaps the most widespread and intractable disease of poultry and other livestock, is of great importance. However, relatively little drug discovery effort has been made on *Eimeria* infections of domestic livestock.[493 1125,1213,1638] In view of advances in biotechnology, modern approaches toward the discovery of novel resistance-breaking drug candidates may be anticipated. Genomic analysis of all seven *Eimeria* species that cause coccidiosis in poultry has been accomplished,[1404] and this may allow the identification and validation of species-specific protein targets. Novel drug discovery rationales including high-throughput screening, structural biology, and the elucidation of the mode of action of active compounds can be envisioned. Combining target-based approaches with parasite *in vitro* and *in vivo* testing and medicinal chemistry generates a comprehensive view on the genotype-to-phenotype-to-compound correlation, which could allow for the design of novel drug candidates. Unfortunately, resistance develops rapidly following the introduction of drugs in the field. The current approach to delay the onset of resistance is to employ rotation programs combined with good husbandry, chemoprophylaxis, and/or live parasite vaccination.[135] However, for the control of coccidiosis in the future, both novel cost-effective preventative chemotherapy and subunit or recombinant vaccines are desperately needed.

REFERENCES

14, 28, 51, 59, 63, 107, 108, 116, 125, 135, 142, 158, 182, 209, 212, 215, 219–221, 223, 225–227, 230–233, 236, 239–241, 274, 326, 333, 375, 383, 399, 401, 493, 496, 506, 522, 541, 542, 545, 548, 564, 576, 620, 629, 652, 653, 667, 674, 737, 773, 778, 792, 793, 795, 798, 828, 838, 854, 862, 867, 868, 873, 874, 892, 901, 917, 929, 932, 933, 952, 965, 1030, 1038, 1054, 1072, 1113, 1125, 1127, 1138, 1154, 1158, 1162, 1168, 1173, 1174, 1186, 1192, 1193, 1199, 1213, 1215, 1217, 1219, 1220, 1227, 1235, 1243, 1246, 1256, 1264, 1265, 1335, 1336, 1350, 1358, 1404, 1405, 1417, 1418, 1460, 1469, 1471, 1472, 1507, 1520, 1526, 1529, 1541, 1562, 1568, 1570, 1572, 1573, 1587–1590, 1615, 1638, 1662, 1667, 1715, 1720–1722, 1737, 1738, 1744, 1772–1775, 1784, 1795, 1800, 1802, 1807, 1814, 1852, 1866, 1871, 1875, 1908, 1910

CHAPTER 7

Coccidiosis in Cattle

B. Bangoura and A. Daugschies

CONTENTS

7.1 INTRODUCTION

Coccidiosis is an economically important disease of cattle worldwide. Cattle coccidia belong to the genus *Eimeria*. Historically, bloody diarrhea associated with coccidiosis has been known for more than 100 years, but life cycles of bovine *Eimeria* were not known until the 1950s. The present chapter is focused on coccidiosis in cattle (*Bos taurus*, *Bos* spp.).

7.2 MORPHOLOGY AND LIFE CYCLE

Currently, 12 *Eimeria* species are considered valid[333] (see Tables 7.1 and 7.2). The status of eight or more species is uncertain.[972]

Like other *Eimeria* species, oocysts are excreted in feces. Their morphology is highly distinct for most bovine *Eimeria* spp. and can be used for species identification (see Figure 7.1).

The endogenous development of bovine *Eimeria* follows the general life cycle of *Eimeria* spp. that takes place, mostly within enterocytes. It involves one or two (rarely three) asexual generations, followed by sexual replication. Until now, the number and localization of schizonts have been described for some, but not all, *Eimeria* species of cattle. The available data on the endogenous developmental stages are summarized in Tables 7.3 and 7.4. *E. bovis* and *E. zuernii* are the two most important species in cattle followed by *E. alabamensis*. The other described *Eimeria* species are considered non-pathogenic.

Table 7.1　Oocyst Morphology of Cattle *Eimeria* Species

Character	E. bovis (Züblin, 1908) Fiebiger, 1912	E. zuernii (Rivolta, 1878) Martin, 1909	E. alabamensis Christensen, 1941	E. ellipsoidalis Becker and Frye, 1929	E. subspherica Christensen, 1941	E. auburnensis Christensen and Porter, 1939
			Oocyst			
Shape	Pear shaped to ovoid	Subspherical to spherical	Pear shaped to ovoid	Ellipsoidal to slightly ovoid	Spherical to subspherical	Elongate ovoid
Size range	23–34 × 17–23	15–22 × 13–18	13–24 × 11–16	12–32 × 10–29	11–14 × 10–13	32–38 × 19–21
Size mean	28 × 20	18 × 16	19 × 13	23.1 × 16.1	12.7 × 11.8	34 × 20
Wall thickness	1.7	0.7	0.6–0.7	0.8 (thinner at one pole)	0.5–0.6	1.0–1.8
Wall appearance	Smooth, colorless to yellow-brown	Smooth, colorless	Smooth or granulated, colorless to pale yellow-brown	Smooth, colorless	Smooth, colorless to pale yellowish	Smooth, colorless or yellowish, rarely mamillated
Micropyle	+ (3.5–5.6, mean 4.3)	–	+	– (slightly thinner wall at one pole)	–	+ (4.4–8.2, mean 6.2)
Micropylar cap	–	–	–	–	–	–
			Sporocysts			
Shape	Elongate-ovoid	Elongate-ovoid	Elongate, one end bullet-like	Elongate-ovoid	Elongate-ovoid	Elongate-ovoid
Size range	13–19 × 6–8	9–11 × 5–6	11–16 × 4–5	11–16 × 5–6	7–10 × 3–4	16–18 × 6–8
Size mean	14.9 × 6.6	10.1 × 5.5	12 × 5	13 × 5	7.8 × 3.5	16.8 × 6.9
Stieda body	+ (flat)	+ (tiny)	+ (tiny)	Flat or missing	+ (small)	+ (small)
Special features of sporulated oocysts	No oocyst residuum	No oocyst residuum	No oocyst residuum, but polar granule	No oocyst residuum	No oocyst residuum	No oocyst residuum, but polar granule
Sporulation time (d)	2–3	2–10	4–8	2–3	4–9	2–3
References	Floriao et al.[544], Levine and Ivens[978]	Floriao et al.[544], Levine and Ivens[978]	Davis et al.[341], Levine and Ivens[978]	Gräfner and Weichelt[613], Levine and Ivens[978]	Levine and Ivens[978], Oda and Nishida[1261]	Floriao et al.[544], Davis and Bowman[339], Levine and Ivens[978]

All measurements are in micrometers.

Table 7.2 Oocyst Morphology of Cattle *Eimeria* Species

Character	E. cylindrica Wilson, 1931	E. pellita Supperer, 1952	E. bukidnonensis Tubangui, 1931	E. brasiliensis Torres and Ramos, 1939	E. canadensis Bruce, 1921	E. wyomingensis Huizinga and Winger, 1942
Oocyst						
Shape	Cylindrical	Ovoid	Pyriform	Ellipsoidal	Slightly ovoid or ellipsoidal	Pyriform
Size range	20–24 × 15–17	32–42 × 22–27	43–51 × 30–35	31–40 × 22–30	28–38 × 22–26	36–44 × 26–30
Size mean	23 × 16	38.2 × 24.2	47.4 × 33.0	35.7 × 25.6	35 × 24	39.9 × 28.3
Wall thickness	0.7 (one pole) – 1.2 (sides)	1.8	3.5	1 (pole) –1.8 (sides)	1.8	2.5
Wall appearance	Smooth, colorless	Heavily pitted, velvety, dark yellow to brown	Rough surface; appears striated	Smooth, brownish yellow	Smooth, rarely rough; colorless to yellow	Rough surface; few striations
Micropyle (width)	–	+ (5–7, mean 6)	+ (3.5)	+ (overlaid by polar cap)	+ (3.0–8.1, mean 5.9)	+ (3.5)
Polar cap	–	–	–	12 × 1.5–2.0	–	–
Sporocysts						
Shape	Elongate-ellipsoidal, one end truncate	Elongate-ellipsoidal	Elongate-ellipsoidal	Elongate-ellipsoidal	Elongate-ellipsoidal	Elongate-ellipsoidal
Size range	13–16 × 5–6	17–20 × 7–9	18–21 × 9–11	16–22 × 7–10	19–22 × 8–9	17–20 × 8–10
Size mean	13.9×5.5	18.5×8.3	19.6×9.8	19.2×9.2	21.0×8.2	18.7×8.6
Stieda body	–	+ (small, flattened)	+	–	+	+
Special features of sporulated oocysts	No oocyst residuum, but shattered polar granules	No oocyst residuum, but shattered granules	No oocyst residuum	No oocyst residuum	No oocyst residuum	No oocyst residuum
Sporulation time (days)	2–3	10–12	5–27	5–7	3–5	3–7
References	Floriao et al.[544], Levine and Ivens[978]	Ernst and Todd[504]	Courtney et al.[304], Lee[957]	Lee and Armour[958], Marquardt[1128], Ernst et al.[503]	Floriao et al.[544], Levine and Ivens[978]	Courtney et al.[304], Lee and Armour[959]

All measurements are in micrometers.

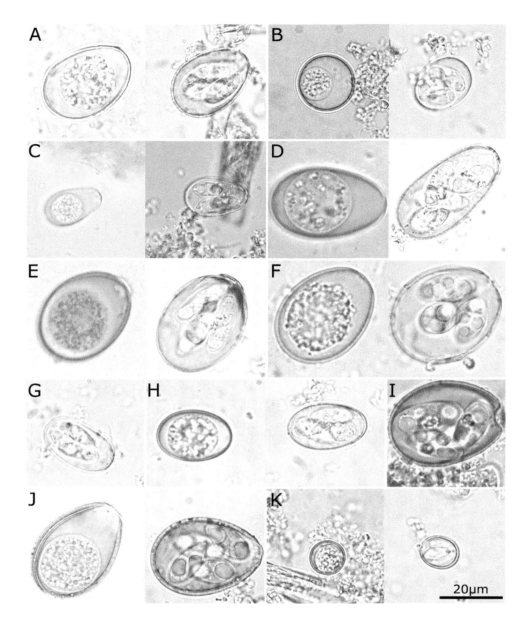

Figure 7.1 Oocyst morphology of different bovine *Eimeria* spp. (A–F,H,I,K): unsporulated (left) and sporulated (right) oocysts of (A) *E. bovis*, (B) *E. zuernii*, (C) *E. alabamensis*, (D) *E. auburnensis*, (E) *E. brasiliensis*, (F) *E. canadensis*, (H) *E. ellipsoidalis*, (J) *E. pellita*, (K) *E. subspherica*. (G,I) Sporulated oocysts of (G) *E. cylindrica*, (I) *E. wyomingensis*. Scale bar refers to all pictures. Light-microscopy, native, 1000× (except for unsporulated *E. auburnensis* and unsporulated *E. brasiliensis*: 400×). Note differences in size, wall thickness and color, shape, and presence of micropyle/polar cap.

7.2.1 *Eimeria bovis*

First-generation schizonts occur in the cytoplasm of enterocytes of the gut mucosa as well as endothelial cells of the central lacteals in the posterior part of the small intestines, mainly caudal jejunum and ileum[562,661,1719] (Figure 1.3, Chapter 1). The schizonts in the central lacteals of the villi may be visible by the naked eye since their diameter can reach more than 435 µm; they can contain up to 120,000 merozoites per schizont, at this stage also referred to as

macroschizont,[661,658] and are observed up to 20 days postinoculation (DPI). Invaded enterocytes may be deformed and syncytia may be formed in the lower ileum leading to a cogwheel pattern of epithelial cells in histological sections.[562] In addition, first-generation schizonts have been observed in the mesenteric lymph nodes of experimentally infected cattle, but their clinical and biological significance are unknown.[1044] The second-generation schizogony and gametogony take place in the epithelium of mainly cecum and colon. These stages invade undifferentiated stem cells of the crypts.[660,614]

Table 7.3 Endogenous Development of Cattle *Eimeria* Species—Morphology and Biological Features

Character	E. bovis	E. zuernii	E. alabamensis	E. ellipsoidalis	E. subspherica	E. auburnensis
Mature Schizont I						
Size	281 × 303 (207–435 × 134–267)	122 × 167 (115–225 × 78–202)	8.4 × 7.4 (7.0–11.9 × 5.6–9.8)	10.6 × 9.4 (9–16 × 7.5–15)	nd	178.3 × 114.2 (133.6–337.9 × 95.2 × 171.9)
Merozoite size	13.2 × 1.5 (9.8–14.5 × 1.3–1.8)	11.2 × 1.7	(7–9 × 1.4–2.1)	10.4 × 2 (8–12 × 1.5–2.5)	nd	12.7 × 2.2 (10.4–13.8 × 1.7–2.9)
Number of merozoites	120,000	500–1000[a]	16–32	24–36	nd	Several thousands
Localization	Endothelial cells in lacteals of villi posterior half of small intestine	Lamina propria of lower jejunum and ileum	Intranuclear in epithelial cells of lowest one-third of the small intestine	Small intestine	Intranuclear, rarely in cytoplasm, in epithelial villus cells of the jejunum	Epithelial cells in crypts of jejunum and ileum
Mature Schizont II/III						
Size	8.9 × 10 (7.2–11.4 × 7.2–11.4)	14 × 13.5 (13–18 × 13–18)	12.4 × 9.4 (8.4–17.5 × 4.9–14.0)	nd	nd	8.5 × 6 (6–12 × 5–9)
Merozoite size	5.9 × 0.9 (4.8–6.7 × 0.7–1.1)	6.5 × 1.5 (5.5–7 × 1–2)	4.2 × 1.4	nd	nd	8 × 1.5 (7–9 × 1–2)
Number of merozoites	30–36	Mean 32	16–32	nd	nd	7 (4–11)
Localization	Cecum, colon epithelial cells	Epithelial cells of colon and cecum	Intranuclear in epithelial cells of small intestine, mainly ileum	Ileum and lower duodenum	nd	Epithelial cells in crypts of jejunum and ileum
Mature Gamonts						
Macrogamont size	nd	11.2 × 13.4 (8.4–14 × 10.5–14.7)	9.1 × 12.0 (7–19.6 × 7–11.9)	nd	nd	Mean 17.9
Localization	Epithelial cells of intestinal glands in cecum and colon	Epithelial cells of intestinal glands in colon and cecum	Intranuclear in epithelial cells of lower small intestine, expansion to cecum and upper colon in heavy infections	nd	Intranuclear in epithelial villus cells of the jejunum	Subepithelial in lamina propria of villi in lower three-fourths of the small intestine
Prepatent period (days)	21–23	15–22	6–11	8–13	7–9 (–18)	18–20
Patent period (days)	6–10	2–8	1–13	12	4–15	2–7
Pathogenicity	+++	+++	++	+	– to +	– to +
References	Daugschies et al.[327], Speer[1601], Hammond et al.[661], Hammond et al.[660]	Bangoura and Daugschie[68], Stockdale[1617], Davis and Bowman[338]	Davis et al.[341]	Speer and Hammond[1604]	Ernst and Courtney[500], Enemark et al.[491], Koreeda et al.[908]	Enemark et al.[491], Hammond et al.[664], Chobotar et al.[265], Levine[974]

Abbreviation: nd, not described, sporulation time strongly dependent on environmental temperature.

All measurements are in micrometers.

[a] *In vitro* observations.

Table 7.4 Endogenous Development of Cattle *Eimeria* Species—Morphology and Biological Features

	E. cylindrica	*E. pellita*	*E. bukidnonensis*	*E. brasiliensis*	*E. canadensis*	*E. wyomingensis*
Mature Schizont I						
Size	nd	nd	nd		93 × 67.5 (72–125 × 37–106)[a]	nd
Merozoite size	nd	nd	9–13 long		10.5 × 1.5 (9–12 × 1–2)[a]	nd
Number of merozoites	nd	nd	nd		nd	nd
localization	nd	nd	Small intestine		nd	nd
Mature Schizont II/III						
Size	nd	nd	nd			nd
Merozoite size			nd			nd
Number of merozoites			nd			nd
Localization			nd			nd
Mature Gamonts						
Macrogamont size	nd	nd	nd			25 × 20 (19–30 × 16–27)
Localization	nd	nd	Beneath epithelium in lamina propria of the ileum			Lamina propria of villi in lower 5 m of small intestine
Prepatent period (days)	11–20	nd	16–18			13–15
Patent period (days)	nd	nd	2–12			1–7
Pathogenicity	+		+			– to +
References	Enemark et al.[491]	–	Courtney et al.[304], Davis and Bowman[340]	Ernst et al.[503]	Müller et al.[1212]	Courtney et al.[304], Ernst and Benz[498], Lindsay et al.[1046]

a = average, nd = no data. All measurements are in micrometers.

7.2.2 *Eimeria zuernii*

First-generation schizonts are found as early as 10 DPI and up to 21 DPI in the ileum.[1618] These stages may be macroscopic,[1090,1603] though this finding is inconsistently described *in vivo*.[338,1617] Smaller second-generation schizonts as well as sexual stages including oocysts are observed from 16 to at least 22 DPI in the cytoplasm of epithelial cells in colon and cecum[1617] (Figure 1.24, Chapter 1). The gametogony takes place in epithelial cells of proximal colon and cecum mainly between days 18 and 21 post-inoculation (PI).[1221,1618]

7.2.3 *Eimeria alabamensis*

The endogenous development of *E. alabamensis* is much shorter than in *E. bovis* and *E. zuernii* (see Table 7.2). Another important difference compared to the other two pathogens is that the development of *E. alabamensis* takes place within the host cell nucleus of epithelial cells instead of the cytoplasm (Figure 1.6, Chapter 1) Small, immature schizonts are observed as early as 2 DPI in the lower third of the small intestines.[341] Schizonts are visible up to about 8 DPI. The gametogony starts on 4 DPI, reaching high numbers of macro- and microgamonts around 8 DPI. Oocysts are formed quickly. They are visible from 6 DPI onward and concentrate in the ileum with up to five oocysts per host cell nucleus.[341]

7.3 EPIDEMIOLOGY

Cattle *Eimeria* species are widespread worldwide, irrespective of their names often referring to geographical areas. Bovine coccidiosis is diagnosed frequently not in individual animals but as a herd health issue.[293,540,1293] Calves start excreting pathogenic *Eimeria* oocysts typically a few weeks after grouping and rehousing in the barn or turnout on pasture.[714] Due to a comparatively long endogenous development phase of about 15–22 days in *E. bovis* and *E. zuernii*, it may take several weeks from initial exposure to *Eimeria* until the infection spreads widely within the animal group. Often a small proportion of the animal group is initially infected in a low-contaminated environment by few oocysts, leading to a considerable oocyst excretion by these individuals. This is the basis for infection of more animals in the group—i.e., coccidiosis builds up as a herd disease over several infection cycles. Frequently, all susceptible animals become infected over time, meaning that on-farm prevalences reach up to 100% for the naïve exposed population.[1140]

Studies indicate that water hygiene management, climate, and bedding are important factors influencing the risk of severe coccidiosis for indoor-reared calves.[70,611,612,1190] Considering different husbandry types, there is a high variation in prevalence. Cattle housed at a high animal density, for example, feedlot cattle, are prone to higher infection intensities and extensities compared with cattle grazing on pasture.

This is caused by a higher environmental contamination and increased infection pressure by overcrowding. In Illinois, prevalences of 82% were observed for bovine *Eimeria* spp. in calves, with 32% and 17% for *E. bovis* and *E. zuernii*, respectively.[1657] In Brazil, the prevalence of *Eimeria* spp. in calves was 51%, with 30% for *E. bovis* and 22% for *E. zuernii*.[174] In India, a study comparing calves, heifers, and adult cattle found the highest *Eimeria* prevalence in heifers (45%), followed by calves (33%) and adults (21%). Similar results were obtained by Tomczuk and colleagues[1699] in Poland. Thus, in general, all ages could be affected by *Eimeria* infections, though clinically relevant infections are by far more common in younger, naïve animals.

Regarding the occurrence of different *Eimeria* spp., bovine coccidiosis in indoor settings is commonly caused by *E. bovis* and *E. zuernii*. However, on pasture, all three pathogenic cattle *Eimeria* spp. including *E. alabamensis* are seen regularly. Accordingly, *E. zuernii* and *E. bovis* are regarded as ubiquitous pathogens.[333,540]

The eradication of *Eimeria* spp. from a contaminated site is extremely challenging because of the high reproduction potential of these protozoa combined with a high tenacity of the oocysts in the environment.[1129,1152] Hence, notwithstanding implementation of hygienic measures like cleaning and disinfection, subsequent production cycles in the same environment will often suffer from coccidiosis problems because pathogen removal is incomplete, and every infected animal contributes to further environmental contamination for the next animal group. Generally, the main reservoir for *Eimeria* is the young animal population passing the parasite from one production cycle to the next. This is supported by negative age-oocyst excretion data.[948] High oocyst production because of lacking immunity renders calves epidemiologically much more important than the parental population that may excrete only low oocyst numbers in most cases. A peri-parturient rise of oocyst output in pregnant cows was observed[510] but is generally not considered epidemiologically relevant given the generally low *Eimeria* oocyst numbers excreted with the feces of adult animals.

7.4 PATHOGENESIS

The typical lesions are caused by parasite multiplication and the host's inflammatory reaction. Thus, the damage is partially induced directly by intracellular parasite replication, leading to intestinal cell destruction, and partially related to the host's immune response.

The role of the immune reaction in the pathogenesis is not yet clarified. It is known that innate and adaptive cellular immunity play a major role in the immunological reaction to bovine *Eimeria* and in the immunoprotection against challenge infections,[899,1678] as in a variety of coccidia infections in different hosts. It is complemented by a humoral response.[841] However, immunopathology and the impact of

self-destruction caused by immune attack to the pathogen in bovines have not yet been investigated in detail. The extent of the induced immune response appears to be linked to the pathogenicity of the respective *Eimeria* sp. Interestingly, *E. bovis* induces a strong humoral response-related IL-4 expression in the early prepatent period, concurrent with a delayed cellular immune response and thus a higher replication potential for the parasite. In the less pathogenic *E. alabamensis*, this mechanism of immune evasion seems to be less pronounced. Additionally, in *E. bovis* and *E. alabamensis*, apoptosis is described to be inhibited *in vitro* by activation of the NFκB pathway, securing the parasite survival in the host cell. A stronger inhibition is seen in the more pathogenic *E. bovis*.[23] Inflammation markers in blood serum, like haptoglobin and serum amyloid A, are increased in calves severely affected by *E. zuernii* coccidiosis, underlining the importance of the inflammatory response in clinical disease.[945]

Irrespective of the pathogenicity of the various *Eimeria* species, lesions are aggravated in coinfections with other bacterial or viral pathogens. On commercial farms, *Eimeria* spp. are usually pathogens among others. Experimental studies corroborated that *Eimeria* infections in cattle interact especially with pathogenic clostridia, which leads to a more severe enteritis.[895,1221]

7.5 LESIONS

Intestinal lesions are observed in infections with pathogenic *Eimeria* spp. Though nonpathogenic *Eimeria* also destroy intestinal epithelial cells during their replication, the impact on gut integrity is not relevant.

7.5.1 *Eimeria bovis*

Starting at 19 DPI, the ileum is inflamed and features blunt, shortened villi with ulcerated tips. First-generation schizonts can induce profound tissue destruction due to subepithelial parasite development mainly in the ileum.[562] Second schizogony and gametogony lead to extensive epithelial destruction and a long regeneration period. Around day 16 PI, hemorrhagic and fibrinoid typhlitis and colitis develop in consequence of late schizogony and gametogony. The mucosa and submucosa of colon and cecum appear edematous. Starting on 19 DPI, lesion severity increases, and necrotizing diphtheritic typhlitis and colitis are seen. Colon and cecum are edematous down to the muscular layers, and show congestion and ulceration (see Figure 7.2), resulting in a visible thickening of colon and cecal walls. On the mucosal surface of these regions, often fibrin strands and fibrinous pseudomembranes are visible. Microscopically, the epithelium is eroded and lost comprehensively, especially in the cecum, and the denuded lamina propria is infiltrated with leukocytes (see Figure 7.3) and covered by fibrin strands. The large intestinal edema and hemorrhages persist

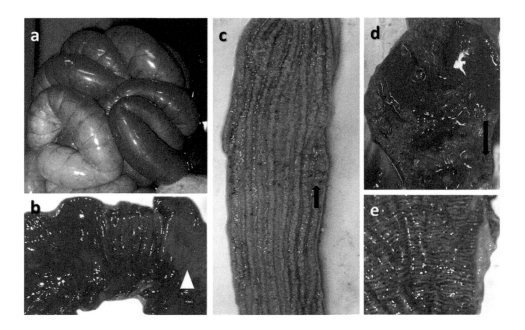

Figure 7.2 *Eimeria bovis* infection-induced enteritis. (a,b) hemorrhagic colitis of proximal colon with reddening and extensive loss of superficial mucosa (arrowhead); (c) diphtheric colitis of distal colon with multiple erosions and ulcerations (arrow); (d) diphtheric typhlitis colon with multiple erosions and ulcerations (arrow); (e) hemorrhagic proctitis with reddening and "tiger-stripe" pattern. Significant wall edema observed in large intestine (cecum, distal colon, rectum [c–e]).

at least until 26 DPI. Crypt hyperplasia and reepithelization are visible starting day 20 PI in colon and cecum.[1719] The intestinal lesions mainly occur during late schizogony and gametogony, with most damage related to the presence of sexual stages.[562]

7.5.2 *Eimeria zuernii*

Gross lesions become visible starting at day 18 PI. Initially, most affected are cecum and proximal colon. There, an extensive loss of the superficial epithelium occurs, while fibrinous casts may be present.[1618] The remaining mucosa

features petechiae, sometimes forming a "tiger-stripe" pattern[1617] (see Figure 7.2) most common but not restricted to *E. zuernii*. The underlying submucosa and deeper layers of the gut wall are edematous and visibly thickened around 20 DPI.[1618] Only mild histopathological changes associated with first-generation schizonts are observed in the posterior 3 m of the small intestine, mainly ileum. Likewise, the second-generation schizonts cause little damage compared to the sexual stages. The gametogony induces pronounced lesions in proximal colon and cecum most visible days 18 through 21 PI.[1221,1618] In these locations, increasing significant epithelial losses are observed during this period. A diphtheric

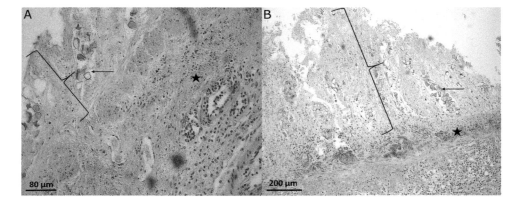

Figure 7.3 Histopathological changes associated with (A) colitis (400× magnification) and (B) typhlitis (100× magnification) due to *E. bovis* infection. Extensive loss of epithelium and mucosal villous structure (brackets), presence of intraepithelial parasitic stages in (mainly oocysts, arrows) and detritus on mucosa. Mononuclear inflammatory cell infiltration (stars). Hematoxylin and eosin stain.

membrane is built on the luminal surface, containing large amounts of blood. These superficial changes of the mucosa are accompanied by comprehensive edema of the submucosa and muscular layer of cecum and colon as well as mononuclear inflammatory infiltration of the submucosa. The intestinal contents are bright or dark red because of severe hemorrhages. Starting around day 22 PI, the lesions heal and are sequentially resolved until day 32 PI.[1618] In less severe *E. zuernii* infections, moderate lesions are seen, which are widely repaired within 1 or 2 weeks after the onset of oocyst excretion.[1221]

7.5.3 *Eimeria alabamensis*

The pathology of *E. alabamensis* infections strongly depends on the dose. In general, much higher doses are required to induce significant pathological changes and clinical disease than in the other two pathogenic species. In high-dose infections, enteritis with hyperemia is observed in the posterior half of the small intestines. Comprehensive epithelial destruction with concomitant leukocytic infiltration and villi destruction occur.[341]

7.6 CLINICAL DISEASE

The observed presence of pathogenic *Eimeria* spp. on a farm does not necessarily have to correlate with the observation of clinical outbreaks. In many instances, natural trickle infections take place (i.e., repeated uptake of low oocyst doses) and induce protective immunity as well as endemic stability. Susceptibility to clinical coccidiosis, that is, diarrheic disease of varying severity (see Figure 7.4), depends on several factors such as the *Eimeria* sp. involved,

its replication potential, the induced tissue inflammation in interaction with the host's immune response, as well as additional factors like stress, inadequate feeding, and concurrent infections with other pathogens.

Mostly, clinical disease is observed in young animals, which is owed to a naïve immune status and not to age-specific resistance in older animals.[333] Based on the parasite's life cycle, coccidiosis is a self-limiting disease, though clinical signs may persist longer than oocyst excretion until the intestinal damage has been repaired.

Susceptible cattle typically are infected with several *Eimeria* spp., which may often include two or three pathogenic species,[499] which entails a pronounced pathology and clinical disease.[1623]

Clinical signs are dominated by diarrhea due to mucosal destruction and by related pathological metabolic changes. These include dehydration and reduced weight gain and result in increased treatment costs and economic losses. Clinical signs are most pronounced in young, naïve calves that undergo primary infections with pathogenic *Eimeria* species.

The adverse health effects are prolonged, and bovine *Eimeria* infections are considered to have a lasting impact on animal performance[946] in terms of retarded growth and fertility. *Eimeria* infections facilitate secondary bacterial infections.[895] Importantly, due to the high contagiosity and high tenacity of oocysts in the environment, bovine coccidiosis is rather a herd disease than a problem of single individuals. It gains greatest relevance in husbandries defined by high animal density and intensive production. Clinical coccidiosis causes obvious direct losses; however, the clinical disease only accounts for a limited proportion of lost revenues. Especially, subclinical infections inflict significant economic damages that are difficult to quantify.[946]

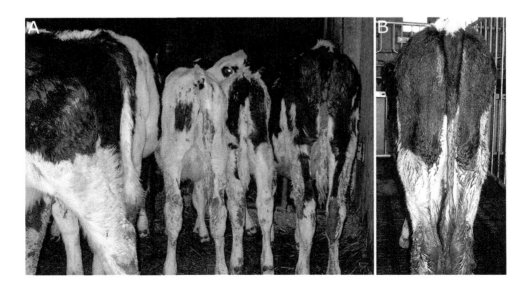

Figure 7.4 Clinical signs of bovine coccidiosis due to pathogenic *Eimeria* spp. in a group of young animals include (A) profuse catarrhal to (B) hemorrhagic diarrhea.

7.6.1 *Eimeria bovis* and *Eimeria zuernii*

In clinically relevant infections, severe diarrhea occurs toward the end of the prepatent period,[68,1619] that is, about 2–3 weeks after infection (see Table 7.2 for prepatent and patent periods). The diarrhea quality varies from mucous to watery and hemorrhagic (see Figures 7.4 and 7.5). Often lots of fibrin and tissue strands are excreted (see Figure 7.5).[1619,327] Affected calves develop inappetence and a sudden and marked weight depression that may entail a long-term performance decrease. Fever may occur[692] but not in all cases. Moribund calves may be hypothermic. Related to the occurrence of severe diarrhea, the electrolyte and acid-base balances are impacted, and acidosis may occur,[67] while a catabolic metabolism is inflicted.[69] Mortality varies greatly depending on infection pressure, immune competence, and other abiotic and biotic factors. It may be as high as 20%.[552]

7.6.1.1 Neurological Signs Associated with Coccidiosis

Besides the directly plausible diarrhea-related health issues, a rare phenomenon called "bovine nervous coccidiosis" is described in both *E. bovis* and *E. zuernii* infections.[850] Affected calves show epileptic-type seizures with opisthotonus and nystagmus. In Northern America, a temporal clustering in winter is reported.[1382] Feedlot calves seem to be most susceptible to this syndrome and generally, a low percentage of the animals with clinical coccidiosis seems affected. However, once the signs of neurological coccidiosis develop, the mortality is high, up to 75%.[1410] The actual underlying mechanism remains unclear, though *Eimeria* infection–related neurotoxin production, electrolyte imbalances, or vitamin A deficiency were discussed as causes.[774,1410] The syndrome is difficult to diagnose exactly because there are no specific gross lesions in the central nervous system related to the observed clinical signs.[1410]

7.6.1.2 Winter Coccidiosis

In the Northern hemisphere, especially in Canada and the Northwestern part of the United States, clinical coccidiosis is often observed in 6- to 12-month-old calves during fall and winter seasons.[1241] The resulting enteric disease, affecting 20%–50% of animals in a herd, is caused by *E. bovis* and/or *E. zuernii* and entails significant economic losses. Studies from the mid-twentieth century indicated that the mortality in young cattle suffering from winter coccidiosis may reach 10%–15% without treatment.[549] The severity of clinical winter coccidiosis is not based on particularly high infection doses but is assumed to be triggered by a higher susceptibility to diseases during cold weather conditions.[1241] Interestingly, infections with pathogenic *E. bovis* and *E. zuernii* are both found to be significantly more prevalent in first-year cattle during fall and winter compared to spring and summer,[537] contributing to the high morbidity and mortality seen during winter coccidiosis. Though the impact of winter coccidiosis seems to be highest in North America, an increased probability for bovine coccidiosis to occur during winter has been observed in Northern Europe as well.[947]

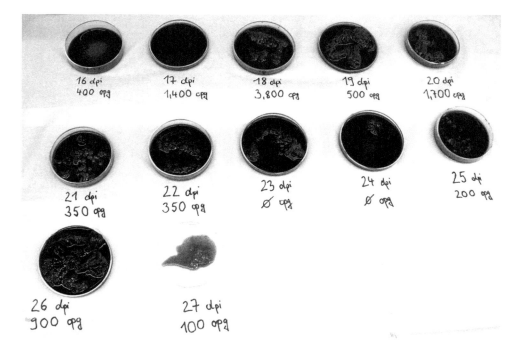

Figure 7.5   Fecal quality over time in an animal with clinically relevant *E. bovis* infection (DPI, days after infection) along with oocyst excretion (opg, oocysts per gram of feces). Note watery quality, blood contents, and fibrinous casts on days 18–26.

7.6.2 *Eimeria alabamensis*

The extent of clinical disease is clearly dose dependent. Low-level infections often remain subclinical, whereas massive infections of at least 10 million oocysts may lead to severe watery diarrhea and reduced weight gain, while mortality is generally low.[736] As in *E. bovis* and *E. zuernii*, the calves' performance can be reduced for a prolonged period. Interestingly, immunity after primary infection is low in *E. alabamensis*, and reinfections result in significant oocyst excretion and subclinical or clinical coccidiosis.[337]

7.6.3 Coccidiosis in Water Buffaloes and Bison

In general, there are no bison-specific *Eimeria* spp. described. It is widely assumed that bison share *Eimeria* spp. with cattle.[512,1348,1367,1368,1470] There is no published information on clinical coccidiosis in bison. Coccidiosis in water buffaloes is described in Chapter 8.

7.7 DIAGNOSIS

Generally, the fecal flotation method is used to detect excreted *Eimeria* oocysts. In groups of exposed calves, examination of a collective sample is an option to determine the general presence of *Eimeria* spp. on a farm. If oocysts are present, species differentiation is necessary to allow the identification of pathogenic and/or apathogenic species so the treatment demand can be evaluated. Bovine *Eimeria* spp. can be differentiated by microscopic oocyst morphology analysis (see Tables 7.1 and 7.2, Figure 7.1). Enumeration of oocysts is helpful in individual fecal samples of diseased animals to determine the severity of infection. Furthermore, oocyst counts are mandatory if a herd health status is to be monitored over several successive calving cycles to assess the efficacy of applied prevention measures. It allows for evaluation of management, hygienic measures, and drug efficacy. Therefore, counting methods using Flotac chambers or McMaster slides are established in many diagnostic laboratories.

Species diagnosis can also be achieved by polymerase chain reaction.[864] Currently, diagnosis is based on the ITS-1 region of ribosomal RNA genes. Sequences are described for six bovine *Eimeria* spp., including the three pathogenic species *E. bovis*, *E. zuernii*, and *E. alabamensis*.

Serologic detection has been established for *E. bovis*.[510] An enzyme-linked immunosorbent assay (ELISA) to detect IgG is described though the diagnostic value is more on a herd level than on an individual level. Positive IgG may reflect the late stage of endogenous development of the parasite or previous parasite replication (postpatency). Thus, for individual pro- or metaphylaxis, serologic analysis is not suitable.

7.8 CONTROL

Prevention greatly relies on herd management and reduction of the infection pressure by cleaning and disinfection measures. Additionally, individual preventive drug treatment is often applied. Successful prevention also comprises measures to reduce clinical disease susceptibility for infected animals, for example, by stress reduction. Since *Eimeria* generally induce protective immunity, vaccination might be a potentially optimal means to control bovine coccidiosis. However, respective data are lacking, and no respective products are available, yet.

7.8.1 Management

Naïve calves that are susceptible to infection (i.e., for *E. alabamensis*, all young calves) should be kept in a clean environment and separate from shedders. Considering the short sporulation time of environmental oocysts, an all-in–all-out management system with regular bedding change and hygienic procedures is advantageous wherever possible, especially on dairy farms and in feedlots. Mechanical transmission of oocysts between groups of animals is a risk of infection. To minimize the transmission risk between herds or animal groups within a herd, equipment should not be moved without disinfection, and clothing should be changed by caretakers and veterinarians. The youngest calves should be fed and looked after first before attending older animals to avoid direct transmission from potential oocyst excretion to susceptible calves. Stress or concomitant infections often contribute to the disease process. Accordingly, husbandry conditions should be optimized. This includes climate, nutrition, group size, and prevention of crowding, as well as general animal health prophylaxis by hygiene, vaccination against common pathogens, and regular screening of the calves' health. Little is known regarding the impact of selective cattle breeding on susceptibility toward coccidiosis though individual studies indicate a certain potential to breed partially resistant cattle.[1326] Administration of colostrum is advantageous mainly in terms of prevention of concomitant infections. However, a targeted effect on coccidiosis is not seen.[534]

7.8.2 Cleaning and Disinfection

Removal and inactivation of oocysts from the environment is of major importance to prevent coccidiosis. Physical measures like ultraviolet (UV) light application and heat are suitable disinfection measures for confined environments where the building and technical structures allow for their application. Targeted chemical disinfection of *Eimeria* oocysts is limited and mostly less effective than physical measures. Chemical disinfection aiming at effective inactivation of *Eimeria* oocysts is widely restricted to hazardous substances like chlorocresols,[328,1538] which in many countries are not available due to their ecotoxicity. Formaldehyde did not effectively inactivate sporulated bovine *Eimeria* spp. oocysts.[137] In addition, even if chemical disinfection with a highly effective disinfectant is applied properly (application on clean and dry surfaces only), surface properties like cracks or porosity or low temperature may reduce disinfection efficacy. For bovines on pasture, disinfection options are even more limited. However, simple cleaning of water troughs more often than once per month can reduce subclinical cattle coccidiosis markedly by lowering the infection pressure.[1190] Physical treatment is effective in *Eimeria* oocyst disinfection. However, the only practically feasible treatment is natural UV light on pasture, which is highly efficient in oocyst inactivation.

7.8.3 Feed Additives

Anticoccidial feed additives are potent drugs applied as a long-term treatment, mostly for several weeks, while animals are under the (highest) risk of infection. They are used mainly in feedlot cattle but also in other calf-raising facilities to prevent both clinical and subclinical coccidiosis. This form of prophylaxis and metaphylaxis (i.e., application before and during infection) is widespread in many countries, however, not approved in others, for example, in the European Union. Typically used feed additives can have a coccidiostatic or coccidiocidal activity. The mode of action varies by drug class. Anticoccidial drugs are discussed in Chapter 6.

In contrast to chicken *Eimeria*, no drug resistances in cattle *Eimeria* have been reported in the field so far. In general, a risk of drug resistance development can be assumed since drug resistance is promoted by continuous and low-dose use of an anticoccidial compound.

7.8.4 Individual Treatment

In animal groups with diseased calves, treatment of the whole group of young animals is applied due to animal welfare and economic reasons. Another benefit of early implementation of group treatments (i.e., during prepatency) is the reduction of the infection pressure by suppressing oocyst excretion and thus environmental contamination. The treatment time point is highly important. It should be applied as early metaphylaxis at best or latest when the first animals start excreting oocyst in the respective group.[492,496] Therapeutic treatment, that is, during patency, is less advantageous but necessary in case of clinical disease. Once lesions develop, treatment will be of limited benefit in terms of sustained health and reduction of oocyst excretion; however, the duration of disease and oocyst excretion may be shortened if therapy is provided immediately. The major challenge in scheduling metaphylactic treatment is the determination of the optimal time point. During prepatency, there is no way to obtain an *in vivo* diagnosis on the current state of infection. It cannot be determined which animals are infected or which endogenous parasitic phase is present. Thus, herd monitoring over several calving cycles (seasons) is needed to schedule group treatment accurately. A rule of thumb is to treat animals during late asexual replication. Thus, depending on the *Eimeria* spp. present in the respective host group, it should be approximately 14 days after exposure of the animal group to a contaminated environment for *E. bovis* and *E. zuernii*. Exposure normally starts with stabling, beginning of the grazing period, or similar moving events.

Anticoccidial drugs used for treatment in a defined number of single animals at risk are the triazines toltrazuril and diclazuril (see Chapter 6). They must be administered only once if the time point is well chosen—that is, in the prepatent period for most animals of the treated group.[326,1220,1719] Triazines are approved for control of bovine coccidiosis in certain countries only (e.g., EU). As an alternative, sulfonamides are widely used for coccidiosis treatment, mainly therapeutically. However, the anticoccidial benefit is limited due to the long administration period potentially overlapping with the natural end of patency.

REFERENCES

23, 67, 68, 69, 70, 137, 174, 265, 293, 304, 326–328, 333, 337–341, 491, 492, 496, 498–500, 503, 504, 510, 512, 534, 537, 540, 544, 549, 552, 562, 611–614, 658, 660, 661, 664, 692, 714, 736, 774, 841, 850, 864, 895, 899, 908, 945–948, 957, 958, 959, 972, 974, 975, 978, 1044, 1046, 1090, 1128, 1129, 1140, 1152, 1190, 1212, 1220, 1221, 1241, 1261, 1293, 1326, 1348, 1367, 1368, 1382, 1410, 1470, 1538, 1601, 1603, 1604, 1617–1619, 1623, 1657, 1678, 1699, 1719

Coccidiosis in Water Buffaloes (*Bubalus bubalis*)

J. P. Dubey

CONTENTS

8.1 INTRODUCTION AND HISTORY

The water buffalo (*Bubalus bubalis,* referred hereafter as buffalo) is important to the economy of several countries in Asia and South America, and there are also isolated herds in Europe. Historically, clinical coccidiosis in buffalo was first reported in India,[128] but the species of coccidia was not identified. There is considerable confusion concerning the species of *Eimeria* in buffaloes. Much of the confusion is because most of the species were originally described from cattle and assumed to be the same in buffaloes. Recently, I reviewed in detail history, taxonomy, and biology of coccidia and coccidiosis in buffaloes.[423] Here, essential information concerning the biology of bubaline coccidiosis is summarized. Among the genera of coccidia discussed in this book, only *Eimeria* species are known to parasitize buffaloes.

8.2 SPECIES OF *EIMERIA* IN BUFFALO

Eleven or more *Eimeria* species, originally described from cattle, have been reported in buffalo (Table 8.1).[423] Additionally, *E. illinoisensis* was reported from Iran,[58] *E. pellita* (regarded as synonym of *E. bukidnonsis* by some authors) from Italy,[306] and *E. gokaki* (regarded as synonym of *E. brasiliensis*) from Brazil.[1691] Two species, *E. bareillyi*

and *E. ankarensis,* were originally described from buffalo,[595,1504] and they are not transmissible to cattle (Table 8.2).[423] Information from these two species is summarized first.

8.2.1 *Eimeria bareillyi* Gill, Chhabra, and Lall, 1963

It was first found in buffalo from a farm in Bareilly, Uttar Pradesh, India, and hence so named.[595] Since then it has also been reported from Brazil, Italy, the Netherlands, Egypt, and Turkey (Table 8.3, indicated in bold).[423] *E. bareillyi* was not transmissible to cattle.[1491] Three cattle and three buffaloes were inoculated orally with 100,000 *E. bareillyi* oocysts and necropsied 7, 14, and 21 days postinoculation (DPI).[1491] Neither parasitic stages nor oocysts were detected in cattle fed oocysts. All three buffaloes fed oocysts became infected.[1491]

8.2.1.1 Morphology and Life Cycle

The following description of its oocysts is a summary of description by different authors.[120,449,595,1390,1691] Its oocysts are morphologically distinctive. Unsporulated oocysts are yellowish to brown in color, often pyriform, and sometimes with asymmetrical sides (Figure 8.1).[423] The narrower (anterior) end is truncated/flattened, 5–6 μm wide. Unsporulated oocysts are 23–35 × 15–25 μm, with a length-to-width ratio of about 1.4. The sporont is about 16 μm in diameter and

Table 8.1 Morphology of Oocysts of *Eimeria* Species Common to Cattle and Buffalo

Eimeria Species	Oocyst Size[a]	Oocyst Shape	Sporocyst Size	Sporozoite Size	Distinctive Character
E. alabamensis	21 × 14 (17–24 × 12–16)	Pyriform, subellipsoidal	10.4 × 5.2 (10–11 × 5–6)	9 × 2.6	Pyriform, small
E. auburnensis	38 × 24 (31–34 × 20–27)	Ovoid, ellipsoidal	19 × 8 (17–21 × 8–9)	15–18 × 4	
E. bovis	28 × 21 (23–43 × 15–26)	Ovoid	16 × 6.6 (15–17 × 6–7)	13 × 3	
E. brasiliensis	39 × 27 (31–44 × 20–29)	Ovoidal, ellipsoidal	20 × 8.4 (17–21 × 8–9)	16 × 4.7	Micropylar cap present
E. bukidnonensis	42 × 31 (38–46 × 25–35)	Pyriform, spotted	17 × 9 (15–19 × 8–11)	13.3 × 5.3	Pyriform, large, spotted wall
E. canadensis	31 × 22 (25–37 × 18–28)	Ellipsoidal	16 × 7.5 (13–17 × 6.6–8.0)	14 × 3	
E. cylindrica	26 × 14 (20–34 × 12–17)	Subcylindrical	10.4 × 5.2 (9–13 × 4–6)	7.6 × 2.1	Cylindrical shape
E. ellipsoidalis	20 × 14 (15–26 × 12–16)	Ellipsoidal	12.2 × 5.4 (10–13 × 5–6)	11 × 2.6	
E. subspherica	11 × 10 (9–13 × 8–12)				Smallest size
E. wyomingensis	41 × 28 (37–44 × 26–31)	Egg shaped	22 × 8.6 (21–24 × 8–9)	20 × 4	Egg shape, rough wall
E. zuernii	17 × 16 (14–22 × 13–19)	Subspherical	9.9 × 6.0 (8.0–10.5 × 5–7)	9 × 3	Subspherical, small sporozoites

Source: From Dubey, J.P. 2018. *Vet. Parasitol.* 256, 50–57.
[a] All measurements are in micrometers (μm).

occupies the posterior and middle portion of the oocyst. A mass of few granules is present at the anterior tip. The micropyle is 2–6 μm wide. Micropylar cap, oocyst residuum, and polar granules are absent. Sporocysts are elongate-ovoid, 12–19 × 6–8 μm with pointed and broader ends. The Stieda body is indistinct 2.1 × 0.4 μm. Sporozoites are 10–12 × 4 μm. Sporulation time at 22°C–29°C is 3–4 days.

In experimentally infected buffaloes, endogenous development occurred in jejunum and ileum.[1491–1493,1543,1546] Schizonts occurred in enterocytes in crypts of Lieberkühn and in villi of small intestine 5–14 DPI; they were 11.5–20.7 μm and contained 24–36 slender 10–15 μm long merozoites. Gamonts were detected 14–15 DPI. Macrogamonts were 12.5–23.3 × 11.1–16.7 μm, and microgamonts were 15–30 × 10–23 μm. Oocysts in sections were 21.0–31.7 × 15–20 μm. The prepatent period was 12–15 days.

8.2.1.2 Pathogenicity and Clinical Coccidiosis

E. bareillyi was pathogenic in experimentally infected buffaloes.[1491–1493,1543,1546]

Clinical coccidiosis has been reported in 3-week-old to 4-month-old buffaloes from India,[1544,1545,1547] Brazil,[84,86,345] and the Netherlands.[449] In India, *E. bareillyi*-associated illness was diagnosed in 18- to 45-day-old buffaloes born in winter months at a dairy in Prabhani, Maharashtra.[1544,1545,1547] Fifteen 18- to 45-day-old buffaloes developed yellowish mucoid diarrhea 1–2 days before discharge of *E. bareillyi* oocysts. Some animals were moribund 4–7 days after the onset of illness. Whether other enteric pathogens were involved in those reports is not clear. However, in a well-managed buffalo farm in Limburg, the Netherlands, 9 of 22 calves

Table 8.2 Attempted Experimental Transmission of *Eimeria* Species from Buffalo to Cattle

Eimeria species	Dose	Fed to	Testing	Success	Remarks	Country (Reference)
E. ankarensis, and others[a]	50–3500	Three 1-week-old cattle	Fecal	Only E. ankarensis not transmitted[a]	No clinical signs	Turkey (Sayin[1504])
E. bareillyi	100,000	1-month-old cattle (three) and buffaloes (three)	Necropsy 7, 14, 21 days postinoculation	Cattle not infected, all three buffaloes infected; prepatent period 14–15 days	Endogenous stages in buffaloes, not cattle	India (Sanyal et al.[1491]; Sanyal and Ruprah[1490])
E. ellipsoidalis	100,000	1-month-old cattle (three) and buffaloes (three)		Yes; longer prepatent periods in homologous infected calves	Soft feces in cattle and diarrhea in buffaloes; endogenous stages in buffaloes and cattle	
E. zuernii	50,000	1-month-old cattle (three) and buffaloes (three)		Yes	Hemorrhagic enteritis in cattle and in buffaloes	
E. bovis + E. zuernii	30,000	1.5- to 4-month-old buffaloes	Fecal	Yes; diarrhea	No clinical signs	Egypt (Ghanem et al.[588])

Source: From Dubey, J.P. 2018. *Vet. Parasitol.* 256, 50–57.
[a] Cattle fed 3500 E. zuernii, 1500 E. ellipsoidalis, 1000 E. bovis, 500 E. auburnensis excreted oocysts with prepatent periods of 13, 10, 18, 21 days, respectively. No oocysts were excreted after feeding 50 E. bareillyi oocysts.

Table 8.3 Prevalence of *Eimeria* Species in Water Buffaloes Worldwide

Country/Region	Age Range	Number Tested	Number Positive (%)	Number of *Eimeria* spp.	*Eimeria* Species and Remarks	Reference
Bangladesh						
Different regions	NS	480	11 (2.3)	1	*E. zur*	Islam et al.[772]
Kurigram	6 m–>5 yr	236	8 (3.39)	NS	NS	Mamun et al.[1120]
Brazil						
Pará	2–48 wk	825	104 (12.2)	4	*E. aub*, *E. elp*, *E. sub*, *E. zur*	Láu[949]
São Paulo	15 d–12 mo	1920	699 (36.4)	8	*E. aub* 1.5%, *E. bov* 8.3%, *E. buk* 0.3%, *E. can* 3.1%, *E. cyl* 4.4%, *E. elp* 4.7%, *E. sub* 4%, *E. zur* 10%	Rebouças et al.[1399]
São Paulo	Newborn	24	24 (100)	NS	NS. Two calves infected in the second wk of life, 58% at the third wk and 100% at the sixth wk	Barbosa et al.[72]
São Paulo	Different	720	313 (43.6)	10	*E. alb* 0.4%, *E. bov* 21.1%, *E. brs* 0.8%, *E. buk* 1.4%, *E. can* 4.4%, *E. cyl* 3.5%, *E. elp* 5.3%, *E. sub* 9.4%, *E. wym* 0.8%, *E. zur* 9.7%	Rebouças et al.[1400]
São Paulo	3–45 d	106	106 (100)	NS	NS	Ribeiro et al.[1415]
Minas Gerais	Newborn	48	48 (100)	4	9 d: *E. bov* 100%; 20–25 d: *E. bov* 80%, *E. elp* 7%, *E. sub* 10%, *E. zur* 3%; Two calves were found infected at 2 days of age, whereas all calves were found infected after 7 days of age	Bastianetto et al.[85]
Minas Gerais	Newborn	109	NS	5	13–16 d: **E. bar 77%**, *E. bov* 33%; 15–18 d: **E. bar 33%**, *E. bov* 16%, *E. aub* 10%, *E. sub* 41%; 20–23 d: **E. bar 34%**, *E. bov* 12%, *E. cyl* 2%, *E. sub* 41%	Bastianetto et al.[86]
Mato Grosso do Sul	>1 yr	36	Not clearly stated	5	*E. aub*–like 19%, *E. elp* 19%, *E. cyl*–like 22%, *E. sub*–like 7.5%, *E. zur* 11%; Calves started oocyst excreting 6–29 days of age; feces tested from the first day of birth; of 18 calves tested, 6%–17% infected 22–156 days old and 28%–78% at 157–367 days old	de Noronha et al.[346]
Rio de Janeiro	Calves and adults	33	3 (9)	1	**E. bar**	Ramirez et al.[1390]
Rio de Janeiro	Young calves	121	80 (66.1)	11	*E. alb*, *E. ank* 8.2%, *E. aub*, **E. bar 3.3%**, *E. bov*, *E. brs*, *E. cyl*, *E. elp*, *E. gok* 2.4%, *E. sub*, *E. zur* 51.8%	Teixeira Filho et al.[1691]
Egypt						
Assiut	6 mo	500	60 (12)	NS	NS	Tawfik[1681]
Beni Suef	Calves	812	99 (12)	5	*E. bov* 33.3%, *E. cyl* 23.3%, *E. elp* 20%, *E. sub* 10%, *E. zur* 13.3%; prevalence was 12.4% at the first mo of age and 14.4% at 5–6 mo old	El-Sherif et al.[479]
Lower Egypt	1 wk–12 mo	191	124 (64.9)	NS	NS. 92.1% prevalence was revealed using the coproantigen ELISA	Ahmed and Hassan[17]
Giza	Different	485	4 (0.8)	NS	NS	Hashem[679]
Menoufiya	Calves	79	17 (21.5)	NS	NS. Calves had diarrhea; infection was 17.9% (7/39) in suckling calves and 25% (10/40) in weaned calves	Ramadan et al.[1388]
El-Minia	Calves	480	91 (18.9)	NS	NS. 40.8 (20/49) in suckling calves >2 mo old, 33.3% (14/42) in weaned calves >6 mo old	El-Ashram et al.[475]
Dakahlia	Different	175	49 (28)	10	*E. alb* 0.6%, *E. aub*–like 0.6%, *E. aub* 2.3%, **E. bar 5.7%**, *E. bov* 10.8%, *E. can* 1.1%, *E. cyl* 4%, *E. elp* 2.3%, *E. sub* 2.8%, *E. zur* 9.7%	El-Alfy et al.[474]
Greece						
Serres	NS	110	44 (40)	NS	NS	Founta et al.[551]

(Continued)

Table 8.3 (*Continued*)   Prevalence of *Eimeria* Species in Water Buffaloes Worldwide

Country/Region	Age Range	Number Tested	Number Positive (%)	Number of *Eimeria* spp.	*Eimeria* Species and Remarks	Reference
India						
Uttar Pradesh	<1 yr	305	230 (75.4)	12	*E. alb* 2.9%, *E. aub* 29.8, **E. bar 5.2%,** *E. bov* 31.3%, *E. brs* 2.2%, *E. buk* 4.5%, *E. can* 8.4%, *E. cyl* 8.8%, *E. elp* 16.7%, *E. sub* 16.3%, *E. wym* 4.2%, *E. zur* 16.3%	Bhatia et al.[120]
Punjab	<6 mo	1582	683 (54.5)	NS	NS	Jyoti et al.[853]
Thiruvannamalai	<1 yr>1 yr	50	2 (16)	NS	NS	Aruna et al.[44]
Punjab	NS	956	338 (35.4)	10	*E. alb, E. aub, E. bov, E. brs, E. can, E. cyl, E. elp, E. ill, E. sub, E. zur*	Gupta et al.[647]
Haryana	Calves	427	247 (57.8)	11	*E. alb* 12.9%, *E. aub* 7.2%, **E. bar 38.4%,** *E. bov* 34.8%, *E. can* 19.3%, *E. cyl* 8.1%, *E. elp* 9.3%, *E. pel* 4.4%, *E. sub* 29.9%, *E. wym* 6.1%, *E. zur* 31.9%. 63.1% prevalence in calves 0–3 mo and 43.4% in calves 4–6 mo	Nain et al.[1230]
Assam	Different	1258	57 (4.5)	NS	NS	Das et al.[323]
Indonesia						
Different	Different	340	102 (30)	NS	NS	Nurhidayah et al.[1255]
Iran						
Tabriz	NS	NS	NS	8	*E. aub* 5%, *E. bovis* 10%, *E. pellita* 10%, *E. buk* 20%, *E. can* 5%, *E. cyl* 10%, *E. ill* 5%, *E. zur* 35%. 50.6% infection in adults and 49.4% in calves	Yakhchali and Zareei[1841]
Khuzestan	≤6 mo	108	108 (100)	11	*E. alb* 14.8%, *E. aub* 18.5%, *E. bov* 76.8%, *E. pel* 11.1%, *E. brs* 19.4%, *E. buk* 2.7%, *E. can* 62.9%, *E. elp* 26.8%, *E. ill* 5.5%, *E. sub* 25.9%, *E. zur* 47.2%	Bahrami and Alborzi[58]
Urmia	<9 mo	317	112 (35.3)	8	*E. aub* 0.6%, **E. bar 2.5%,** *E. bov* 15.1%, *E. buk* 2.2%, *E. cyl* 0.9%, *E. elp* 7.3%, *E. ovo* 1.3%, *E. zur* 23.3%	Tavassoli et al.[1680]
Iraq						
Bablyon	Different	200	32 (16)	NS	NS	Obayes et al.[1259]
Diwanyiah	NS	85	24 (38)	2	*E. brs, E. zur*	Karawan et al.[861]
Italy						
Southern Italy	1 mo	13 herds	NS	3	*E. aub, E. bov, E. zur*	Galiero and Consalvo[577]
Caserta	Different	1620	408 (25.1)	7	*E. aub, E. bar, E. bov, E. elp, E. pel, E. sub, E. zur* 50.3% of 540 calves, 16.5% of 632 yearlings and 8% of 548 adults were infected. *E. zur* was the prevalent followed by **E. bar**	Guarino et al.[632]
Southern Italy	<4 mo	42	42 (100)	7	*E. aub,* **E. bar 100%,** *E. bov, E. elp, E. pel, E. sub, E. zur* 4 calves infected with *E. bareillyi* at the 5th day of age	Fusco et al.[567]
Malaysia						
NS	Calves	20	20 (100%)	3	*E. bov, E. cyl, E. sub.* All calves had mixed infection with 3 spp.	Sani and Chandrawathani[1489]
Pakistan						
Faisalabad	Different	500	73 (14.6)	4	*E. bov* 19.1%, *E. cyl* 24%, *E. elp* 12%, *E. zur* 45% The prevalence was 29.1% in diarrheic animals and 13.8 in healthy ones	Hayat et al.[689]
Hyderabad	Calves	1000	66 (6.6)	1	*E. bov*	Mirani et al.[1187]
Toba Tek Singh	3–10 yr	585	290 (49.6)	6	*E. alb, E. bov, E. can, E. cyl, E. elp, E. zur*	Khan et al.[875]
Faisalabad	1–8 yr	162	7 (4.3)	NS	NS	Hussain et al.[756]
Lahore	6 mo or more	250	157 (58.8)	6	*E. alb* 15.6%, *E. bov* 52.3%, *E. can* 31.2%, *E. cyl* 11.5%, *E. elp* 23.1%, *E. zur* 46.9%	Jahanzaib et al.[775]
Philippine						
Laguna and Cavite	<1 yr - >5 yr	200	33 (16.5)	4	*E. alb* 14%, *E. bov* 32%, *E. elp* 18%, *E. zur* 36% Prevalence in individually reared buffaloes was 16.5% and in buffaloes reared in herds 66.6%. Prevalence was higher in males (25%) than in females (12.9%)	Padilla and Romero[1297]

(Continued)

Table 8.3 (*Continued*)   Prevalence of *Eimeria* Species in Water Buffaloes Worldwide

Country/Region	Age Range	Number Tested	Number Positive (%)	Number of *Eimeria* spp.	*Eimeria* Species and Remarks	Reference
Turkey						
Different regions	Different	130	124 (95.3)	11	*E. alb* 10.3%, *E. ank*, *E. aub*, 43.8%, *E. bov* 34.8%, *E. brs* 1.6%, *E. can* 20%, *E. cyl* 4.6%, *E. elp* 53%, *E. sub* 15.3%, *E. wym* 0.7%, *E. zur* 48.8%	Sayin[1504]
Ankara	NS	50	1 (2)	1	***E. bar***	Sayin[1505]
Afyon	Different	104	78 (75)	11	*E. alb* 11.5%, *E. ank* 16.7%, *E. aub* 44.9%, ***E. bar* 5.1%**, *E. bov* 44.9%, *E. brs* 3.8%, *E. can* 5.1%, *E. cyl* 10.5%, *E. elp* 28.2%, *E. sub* 16.7%, *E. zur* 55.1%; 40 buffaloes were <1 yr, while 64 were >1 yr	Nalbantoglu et al.[1232]
Venezuela						
Zulia	Different	512	311 (60.7)	5	*E. alb*, *E. bov*, *E. elp*, *E. sub*, *E. zur*	Ramírez et al.[1389]
Falcon	8 or more	64	30 (46.8)	NS	NS	Bethencourt et al.[112]

Source: Modified from Dubey, J.P. 2018. *Vet. Parasitol.* 256, 50–57.
Abbreviations: *E. alb*, *E. alabamensis*; *E. ank*, *E. ankarensis*; *E. aub*, *E. auburnensis*; ***E. bar*, *E. bareillyi*; *E. bov*, *E. bovis*; *E. brs*, *E. brasiliensis*; *E. can*, *E. canadensis*; *E. cyl*, *E. cylindrica*; *E. elp*, *E. ellipsoidalis*; *E. gok*, *E. gokaki*; *E. ill*, *E. illinoisensis*; *E. ovo*, *E. ovoidalis*; *E. sub*, *E. subsoherica*; *E. wym*, *E. wyomingensis*; *E. zur*, *E zuernii*. d, day old; wk, week; mo, month; yr, year; NS, not stated.

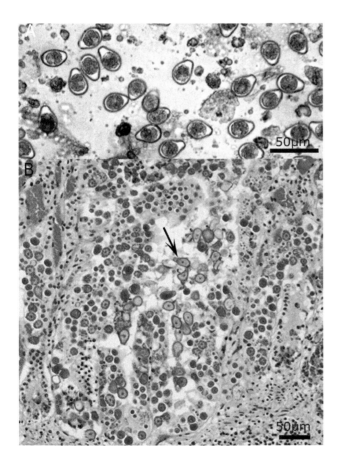

Figure 8.1   Stages of *E. bareillyi* in a 22-day-old naturally infected buffalo. (A) Pear-shaped oocysts in feces. Unstained. (B) Severe parasitization in jejunum, from tip of the villus to tunica muscularis mucosae. Note gamonts and oocysts obliterating host tissue (arrow). Hematoxylin and eosin stain. (From Dubey, J.P. 2018. *Vet. Parasitol.* 256, 50–57.)

born in November to December 2007 died after clinical illness with diarrhea. The calves were born on slatted floor and then separated from dams. For 1 month, calves were housed individually in an igloo and then housed with other calves. Each calf received colostrum from its dam for the first 2 days and then was fed milk replacer. Diarrhea was noticed in 3- to 6-week-old calves, and the calves died after 1–20 days after the farmer noticed diarrhea. The following findings are from the 22-day-old calf. Extensive diagnostic testing did not reveal viral, bacterial, or other parasites other than *E. bareillyi* in an index case. Numerous *E. bareillyi* unsporulated oocysts were identified in colon contents (Figure 8.1A). Lesions were seen in jejunum and ileum but not in colon. The small intestines were severely congested, edematous, twisted, and had fibrous deposits on the serosal surfaces. Parasitic stages were seen throughout the villus, but crypts of Lieberkühn were most severely parasitized (Figure 8.1B). The intestinal lumen, particularly crypts, were packed with oocysts, desquamated host tissue (Figure 1.12B, Chapter 1). More than two generations of schizonts were seen. Details of asexual and sexual multiplication from this calf were recently published.[426]

Gamonts and oocysts of *E. bareillyi* have also been noted in ileum of naturally infected buffaloes in samples obtained at a slaughter in Mathura, India.[1320] Polyp-like whitish, raised 3–6 mm diameter areas were noted in small intestine. Numerous gamonts and oocysts but no schizonts were seen in these lesions. Oocysts in these gross lesions were 23.3–27 × 13.3–17 μm in histological sections versus 27–31 × 20–22 μm in fresh smears. Microgamonts were 20–37 × 18–25 μm, and macrogamonts were 23–35 × 14–17 μm. These animals also had concurrent infections with *E. ellipsoidalis* and *E. bovis*–like oocysts.[1320]

Clinical status of these animals was unknown because samples were obtained at an abattoir.

8.2.2 *Eimeria ankarensis* Sayin, 1968

This species has been reported from Turkey[1232,1504] and Brazil.[1691] Sayin[1504] proposed this name because it was first found in Ankara, Turkey. Oocysts are elongate-ovoid, yellowish brown, with two walls 3.0–5.0 μm thick. The outer layer is punctated. The micropyle is 6 μm wide. Oocysts are 39.2 × 26.4 μm (32–43 × 25–29), and sporocysts are 21.4 × 8.7 um (18–23 × 8–10). It was found in 9.9% of 130 buffaloes from the Ankara region[1504] and 16.7% of 104 buffaloes from the Afyon region.[1232] Three cattle calves fed 50 *E. ankarensis* oocysts from buffaloes did not excrete oocysts, but the same calf fed 10 times or higher oocysts of four *Eimeria* species from buffaloes did excrete oocysts (Table 8.2). Nothing is known of the competition for patency of *Eimeria* species simultaneously infected with five species.

Confirmation of this species from other parts of the world is awaited. It most closely resembles *E. auburnensis* from cattle.

8.2.3 Other Species of *Eimeria*

At least 11 *Eimeria* species originally described from cattle have been reported in buffaloes (Table 8.1). Currently, it is uncertain if *Eimeria* species in cattle are the same as in buffalo. I am not aware of any reports of *Eimeria* species listed in Table 8.1 causing clinical coccidiosis in naturally infected buffaloes. However, endogenous stages (schizonts, gamonts) thought to be *E. bovis*, *E. subspherica*, *E. cylindrica*, *E. canadensis*, *E. auburnensis*, and *E. ellipsoidalis* were found in intestines of buffaloes in India[119,1320,1328]; the intestines were obtained at an abattoir without any available clinical history—the diagnosis was based on literature on *Eimeria* species in cattle.

Experimentally, *E. ellipsoidalis* and *E. zuernii* were pathogenic to buffaloes.[1490,1491] Three cattle and three buffalo calves were each orally inoculated with oocysts of *E. zuernii* and *E. ellipsoidalis* of the buffalo origin (Table 8.2). The buffaloes fed *E. ellipsoidalis* developed diarrhea starting at 15 DPI and excreted large numbers of oocysts (60,000 oocysts per gram of feces [OPG]), whereas the cattle had only soft feces and excreted relatively fewer oocysts (16,200 OPG). Endogenous stages of *E. ellipsoidalis* (schizonts and gamonts) were seen both in cattle and buffaloes; however, morphology of these stages was not described.

All calves (cattle and buffaloes) fed *E. zuernii* developed dysentery starting at day 18 (buffalo) or 20 (cattle) postinoculation (PI). In another report, six 15- to 30-day-old buffaloes were each inoculated orally with 50,000 *E. zuernii* oocysts, of buffalo origin[1490]; three animals were killed 7, 14, and 21 DPI (it is not stated if these were the same buffaloes as reported by Sanyal and colleagues[1491] (Table 8.2).

These calves developed diarrhea on day 15 and dysentery on day 18 PI. Two calves were recumbent on day 20 and died day 24 PI. Schizonts were seen in the lamina propria of the ileum on day 7 PI. Gamonts were seen in ileum and colon of the calf euthanized day 14 PI.

8.3 EPIDEMIOLOGY

Epidemiological investigations revealed that buffaloes can acquire *Eimeria* infection soon after birth.[72,306,346,567,632] The acquisition and severity of symptoms varied with management and climate. In one of the early studies, feces of 24 buffalo calves in São Paulo, Brazil, were tested for parasite stages starting the first week of birth. *Eimeria* sp. oocysts were detected in 2 calves during the second week, in 13 calves by the third week and in all 24 calves by the sixth week of life. In a more recent study, a herd of 40 buffaloes on pasture were sampled for *Eimeria* species.[346] The calves born in February through March (summer in Brazil) were kept with their dams, and the buffaloes were not milked. In the first phase of the study, feces of 18 calves born in 2000–2001 were tested for *Eimeria* from birth to 12 months of age. Oocysts were first detected in feces on day 6 of birth. Prevalence increased with age, 6%–17% of 22- to 156-day-old calves were positive, compared with 28%–78% positive in 157- to 367-day-old calves. These authors critically described morphology of oocysts and identified *E. ellipsoidalis*, *E. zuernii*, *E. auburnensis*, and *E. cylindrica*–like oocysts. All buffaloes appeared healthy. Compared with these studies in pastured buffaloes in Brazil mentioned earlier, infection rates were higher in stall-fed animals in Italy.[306,567,632] Infection rates were higher in stall-fed (96.6%) versus those in stalls with limited pasture (84%). Prevalences were higher in calves (50.3%) than in adult buffaloes (8.7%).[632] In a longitudinal study, 80 dams and 42 calves in two herds from Southern Italy were tested for *Eimeria* infection. The dams were tested twice weekly from February to September 1996, and calves were tested weekly from birth to 13 weeks. Two of the 80 buffaloes were consistently negative, and in the remaining 78 buffaloes, prevalence fluctuated between 19.5% and 50.6%.[306] *Eimeria* oocysts were seen beginning the first week of life. Prevalence increased from 30.3% to 100% between week 2 and week 13.[306] Oocysts were seen in 5-day-old buffaloes.[567] Seven species of *Eimeria* were identified in decreasing order of prevalence; *E. bareillyi*, *E. zuernii*, *E. ellipsoidalis*, *E. subspherica*, *E. auburnensis*, *E. bovis*, *E. pellita*. *E. bareillyi* was the most prevalent and earliest to be detected.[306] *E. zuernii* was the second most prevalent. Apparently, all animals were healthy.

The prevalence of *Eimeria* species in 500 buffalo fecal samples collected at slaughter in Pakistan were 8.8% in summer, 30.2% in autumn, 16.9% in winter, and 27.3% in spring; prevalence was higher in animals younger than 6 months of age.[689]

There appears to be a discrepancy concerning the identity of oocysts found in calves less than 1 week old. In nursing buffaloes fed as many as 1 million *E. bareillyi* oocysts, the minimum prepatent period was 12 days.[1492,1543,1546] In naturally exposed buffaloes, *E. bareillyi*–like oocysts were reported to be present in feces of 5-day-old animals in Italy[567] and in 7-day-old buffaloes in Brazil.[86] Whether oocysts were passing through gut of buffaloes ingested from the environment or different species of *Eimeria* were involved needs further investigation.

8.4 TREATMENT

Several anticoccidial drugs are effective in treating coccidiosis in buffaloes.[128,147,588,1492] Sulfadimidine (30 mg/kg body weight, orally) and amprolium (10 mg/kg body weight, orally) prophylaxis were effective against experimentally induced *E. bareillyi* coccidiosis.[1492] Similar results were obtained in buffaloes experimentally infected with *E. bovis* and *E. zuernii*[588] and medicated prophylactically with toltrazuril (20 mg/kg body weight, twice orally) at 1-week intervals.[147]

REFERENCES

17, 44, 58, 72, 84–86, 112, 119, 120, 128, 147, 306, 323, 345, 346, 423, 426, 449, 474, 475, 479, 551, 567, 577, 588, 595, 632, 647, 679, 689, 756, 772, 775, 853, 861, 875, 949, 1120, 1187, 1230, 1232, 1255, 1259, 1297, 1320, 1328, 1388–1390, 1399, 1400, 1415, 1489–1493, 1504, 1505, 1543–1547, 1680, 1681, 1691, 1841

CHAPTER 9

Coccidiosis in Sheep

J. M. Molina and A. Ruiz

CONTENTS

9.1 INTRODUCTION

Eimeria spp. are the only intestinal coccidia of sheep. Coccidiosis can cause considerable morbidity and mortality, especially when lambs are reared in production systems that involve a high stocking rate.[713] Additionally, subclinical coccidiosis can affect production of infected animals.[247]

9.2 ETIOLOGY

Species of the genus *Eimeria* affecting sheep and goats were considered the same for many years due to the morphological similarity of their oocysts. Cross-infection studies have shown that coccidia in small ruminants are host specific.[1163] Currently, 13 *Eimeria* spp. are recognized affecting sheep worldwide (Table 9.1). Two of these, *E. crandallis* and *E. ovinoidalis,* are the most pathogenic.[187,822,979]

9.2.1 Morphology and Life Cycle

Morphological characteristics of 13 ovine *Eimeria* spp. oocysts are summarized in Table 9.1 and Figures 9.1 and 9.2.

After the excretion of unsporulated oocysts in feces, sporulation can be completed under ideal conditions in 1–4 days (Table 9.2) but may be delayed several weeks in cold weather. Oocysts are also sensitive to low humidity and temperatures above 40°C or below −30°C.[546] Excystation of sporozoites

Table 9.1 Morphological Characteristics of *Eimeria* Species of Sheep

| *Eimeria* spp. | Size (μm) | | Oocyst Shape/ Color | Micropile | Polar Cap | Residual Body | | Polar Granules |
	Oocyst	Sporocyst				Oocyst	Sporocyst	
E. ahsata Honess, 1942	29–37 × 17–28 (33.4 × 22.6)	18–20 × 6–10	Ellipsoidal/ yellowish-green to yellowish-brown	+	+	−	+	+
E. bakuensis Musaev, 1970	23–33 × 18–24 (31 × 20)	11–17 × 6–9	Ellipsoidal/light green to brown	+	+	−	+	+
E. crandallis Honess, 1942	18–25 × 15–23 (21.9 × 19.4)	8–11 × 5–8	Ellipsoidal/colorless to yellowish-brown	+	+	−	+	+
E. faurei (Moussu and Marotel, 1902) Martin, 1909	28–37 × 21–27 (32 × 23)	14–16 × 8–9	Ovoid/colorless or yellowish-brown	+	−	−	−	+
E. granulosa Christensen, 1938	22–35 × 17–25 (29.4 × 20.9)	13–16 × 8–9	Urn-shape/ yellow-greenish	+	+	−	+	−
E. intricata Spiegel, 1925	40–56 × 30–41 (48 × 34)	16–18 × 8–10	Ellipsoidal/dark brown	+	+	−	+	−
E. marsica Restani, 1971	15–22 × 11–14 (19 × 13)	8–11 × 4–6	Ellipsoidal/colorless to light yellow	+	+	−	+	+
E. ovinoidalis McDougald, 1979	17–25 × 13–20 (23 × 18)	5–6 × 3–4	Ovoid-spherical/ colorless to light greenish-gray	−	−	−	+	−
E. pallida Christensen, 1938	12–20 × 8–15 (14 × 10)	6–9 × 4–6	Ellipsoidal/colorless to light yellow	−	−	−	+	±
E. parva Kotlán, Mócsy and Vajda, 1929	13–22 × 11–13 (16.5 × 14)	6–13 × 5–8	Subspherical- spherical/colorless or slightly brownish yellow	−	−	−	+	−
E. weybridgensis Norton, Joyner and Catchpole, 1974	17–30 × 14–19 (24 × 17)	13–15 × 6–8	Ellipsoidal- subspherical/ colorless and dark inner membrane	+	+	−	−	+

Source: Hidalgo Argüello, M.R., Cordero del Campillo, M. 1999. In Cordero del Campillo, M. and Rojo-Vázquez, F.A. (Ed.), *Parasitología Veterinaria*. Madrid: McGraw-Hill, 195–212; Taylor, M.A. et al. 2007. In Taylor, M.A., Coop, R.L., and Wall, R.L. (Ed.), *Veterinary Parasitology*. Oxford, UK: Blackwell Publishing, 3rd ed., 152–258.

occurs in intestinal lumen, and sporozoites invade intestinal cells, where they undergo two rounds of schizogony. One of the characteristics of ovine coccidia is that the first-generation schizonts are large, approaching being macroscopic and contain thousands of merozoites. The second-generation schizonts and gamonts are typically small, and they are site specific. The prepatent period depends on the *Eimeria* sp. and is 12 days or more (Table 9.3).

9.3 EPIDEMIOLOGY

9.3.1 Transmission and Epidemiology

The ingestion of sporulated oocysts from the environment is the only known mode of transmission.[247,620,683,1495]

Environmental contamination or oocysts excreted by adult sheep or lambs of the last season may be the initial source of infection in lambs. Later, given the high multiplication rate of the parasite in susceptible animals, lambs become the most important source of infection for younger

and susceptible animals, resulting in a rapid spread of the disease.[585,1683] Oocyst excretion peaks around the period of weaning, and then excretion of oocysts declines with age of lambs, suggesting the development of a specific immune response.[712,1401]

Transmission may be favored by some management factors in indoor reared lambs such as those related with poor hygiene and overcrowded conditions; thus, a high concentration of animals kept on dirty and damp bedding are more at risk than those on slatted floors or clean bedding.[1494,1688] The use of pens to house different age groups is also considered a risk factor. In this respect, bottle feeding of lambs can prevent infection, but transmission may occur during colostrum intake from ewes or by contamination of equipment.[713] Clinical coccidiosis may also occur in extensive management systems, particularly when there is a high population density and a reduction in pasture availability.[348] In this case, a marked seasonality is usually observed. In many cases, the times of greatest risk coincide with spring grazing with symptoms appearing 2–3 weeks after turnout. However, depending on geographical factors or different

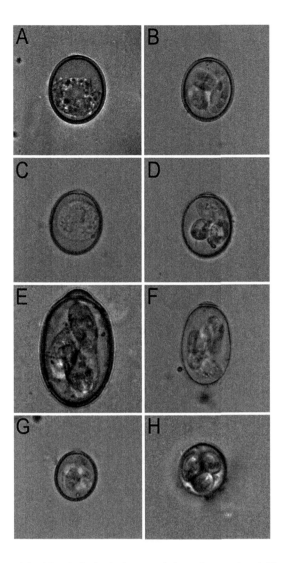

Figure 9.1 Morphological characteristics of oocysts of *Eimeria ovinoidalis* (A = unsporulated, B = sporulated), *E. crandallis* (C = unsporulated, D = sporulated), *E. ahsata* (E), *E. bakuensis* (F), *E. marsica* (G), and *E. parva* (H).

grazing routines, cases of clinical coccidiosis in lambs are also described in summer or even in autumn.[1109,1263,1583]

9.3.2 Immunity and Predisposing Factors

The role of passive immunity in ovine coccidiosis is controversial. Some authors consider that feeding colostrum protects lambs from coccidiosis during the first weeks of life. This is supported by studies that showed significantly increased growth rates in lambs born from hyperimmunized ewes (by inoculation with high doses of *Eimeria* spp. oocysts during pregnancy) compared with lambs born from unimmunized animals.[618,621]

The susceptibility and the dynamics of oocyst excretion are clearly related to the development of specific and

effective immune responses. The absence of such protective responses makes young animals more susceptible, and it is in this age group where clinical coccidiosis is most frequently observed. The onset of clinical disease varies within an age range depending mainly on the farming system, the immune status of each animal, or both. The excretion dynamics of oocysts increases progressively until reaching a peak, in which some animals excrete up to 10^6 oocysts per gram of feces (OPG). As a result of active immunity after exposure to the parasite, the animals acquire resistance showing a progressive reduction in oocyst excretion. However, the protective immunity is not absolute, and the animals may continue to harbor a small number of coccidia throughout their lives.[186,333,1359,1683,1872]

The achievement of an immune status against homologous infections, as well as the maintenance of such protection over time, may be affected by several factors, most of them stress-related factors such as inadequate nutritional intake, weaning, dietary changes, transport, or drastic changes in climatic conditions. Other possibilities that have been considered responsible for the loss of resistance to infection are the presence of concomitant infections, the alteration of complex interactions with intercurrent digestive parasites, or even sex-related factors. Thus, some authors reported that females are more susceptible to *Eimeria* infection than males during pregnancy, birth, and lactation.[175,184,247,1688,1840]

9.3.3 Prevalence and Geographical Distribution

Coccidial infections in sheep are ubiquitous. Although differences in prevalence were observed in different regions, they could generally be more closely related to the factors mentioned in the previous section. Obviously, some environmental or climatological conditions may favor the accumulation of sporulated oocysts in certain periods of the year with higher humidity and higher temperatures. For this reason, the sampling period and even the characteristics of the epidemiological study such as the sample size could affect the prevalence obtained in each case. Some reviews on the epidemiology of ovine coccidiosis during the last decades have shown this worldwide distribution and wide ranges of prevalence mentioned previously.[247,348,880]

9.4 PATHOGENESIS, CLINICAL SIGNS, AND LESIONS

9.4.1 Pathogenesis

The pathogenesis of coccidiosis in sheep is affected by all factors inducing changes in parasite-host interaction, such as all those considered in some previous sections. In addition, other factors related to the parasite itself, such as the predominant species or the infective dose, or factors

Eimeria species from sheep

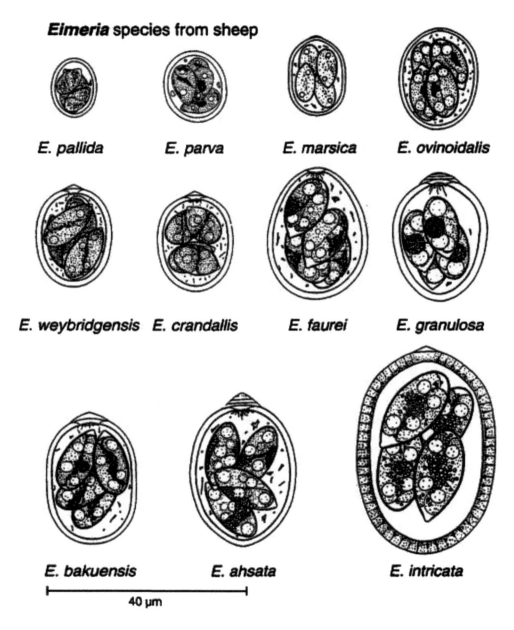

E. pallida   E. parva   E. marsica   E. ovinoidalis

E. weybridgensis   E. crandallis   E. faurei   E. granulosa

E. bakuensis   E. ahsata   E. intricata

|——————————————————|
40 μm

Figure 9.2 Sporulated oocysts of ovine *Eimeria* spp. (From Eckert, J. et al. 1995. *COST 89/820 Biotechnology: Guidelines on Techniques in Coccidiosis Research*. 306. European Commission Directorate-General XII, Science, Research and Development Environment research programme.)

associated with the host, such as the different genetic susceptibilities and earlier exposure to the parasite, may also be considered.[837]

Another important factor of clinical signs that characterize coccidiosis is the strong interaction of coccidia with the intestinal flora, as well as the infective dose, establishing a clear relationship between the severity of the clinical signs/ mortality, and the number of sporulated oocysts ingested by the susceptible animals. The pathogenicity of *Eimeria* may also be modified if coccidiosis is associated with concomitant infections caused by parasites or even other pathogenic agents such as viruses or bacteria.[87,247,348,1822]

All species of *Eimeria* in sheep affect the small and/or large intestines except *E. gilruthi*, which is detected in the abomasum of sheep;[707,1124] its life cycle is unknown. In general, two species (*E. crandallis* and *E. ovinoidalis*) affecting the distal half of the intestines are considered major pathogens, while the remaining *Eimeria* spp. are thought to be of negligible importance. In any case, they are usually present leading to mixed infections.[822,1252]

Damage in large intestines as a result of parasite proliferation can lead to both severe hemorrhage and water reabsorption disorders. One hypothesis proposed that the fact that the species that develop their endogenous cycle in

Table 9.2 Sporulation Time at 20°C and 27°C of Ovine *Eimeria* spp. Oocysts

Eimeria spp.	Sporulation Time at 20°C (Hours)	Sporulation Time at 27°C (Hours)
E. ahsata	48–72	16–32
E. bakuensis	48–96	24–42
E. crandallis	24–72	41–65
E. faurei	24–72	24–41
E. granulosa	72–96	36–41
E. intricata	72–168	68
E. marsica	72	72
E. ovinoidalis	24–72	24–44
E. pallida	24–72	24–44
E. parva	72–120	48–68
E. weybridgensis	24–72	45

Source: Hidalgo Argüello, M.R., Cordero del Campillo, M. 1999. In Cordero del Campillo, M. and Rojo-Vázquez, F.A. (Ed.), *Parasitología Veterinaria*. Madrid: McGraw-Hill, 195–212; Engidaw, S. et al. 2015. *Afr. J. Basic Appl. Sci.* 7, 311–319.

the large intestines are more pathogenic was explained by the shorter length of this intestinal part. In addition, the rate of cellular turnover is much lower here, so that the damage caused is more difficult to compensate than in the small intestines. Subsequent diarrhea, dehydration, and emaciation may produce the death of the affected animals.[879] In the most severe forms, inflammation of the intestinal mucosa

causes a significant loss of fluid and electrolytes as well as plasma and lacteal constituents leading to acidosis and serum electrolyte derangement.[494] In contrast, the *Eimeria* spp. that develop more superficially in the small intestines are usually less pathogenic. The reduction of the surface area available for absorption affects feed efficiency. In addition to all digestive disorders, an increase in plasma levels of some hormones that are associated with anorexia, such as cholecystokinin and somatostatin, has also been described.[1020]

9.4.2 Clinical Signs

Lambs with severe coccidiosis may die without prompt and appropriate treatment. In these cases, the mortality percentage can reach up to 10% of infected animals or more. Clinical signs may appear fairly suddenly, and lambs only mildly ill the day before may be very sick the next day. In other cases, before death occurs, some lambs may have a tucked-up and open-fleeced appearance, showing fecal staining of the perineum and hindlegs, reflecting the first cases of diarrhea. The change in fecal appearance coincides with the first detection of oocysts, which varies according to the prepatent period of each species.[247,880,1020,1092,1683]

Acute signs of coccidiosis include different degrees of yellow to dark watery diarrhea (with or without blood). In many cases, the feces have clumps of mucus and intestinal tissue. As a result, the lambs may be dehydrated with pale

Table 9.3 Endogenous Stages, Site of Infection, and Prepatent Period of Most Prevalent *Eimeria* spp. in Sheep

Eimeria spp.	Site of Infection	Prepatent Period (days)	Meronts/Schizonts, Merozoites	Gamonts
E. ahsata	Small intestine	18–30	1G: 256 × 162 μm. Thousands merozoites	Macro: 35–45 μm
			2G: 52 × 30 μm; 48 merozoites approximately (1.6–5 μm)	Micro: 26–36 μm
E. bakuensis	Small intestine	18–29	1G: 122–146 μm. Thousands merozoites (2 × 9 μm)	NS
			2G: 10 × 15 μm	
E. crandallis	Ileum and cecum, colon	15–20	1G: 250 μm. 250,000 merozoites approximately (1.7 × 10 μm)	NS
			2G: 5–9 merozoites	
E. faurei	Small and large intestine	13–15	1G: 45–100 μm. Large merozoites (4 × 19.5 μm)	Macro: 25–54 μm; Micro: 36–71 μm
E. granulosa	NS	NS	NS	NS
E. intricata	Small intestine	23–27	1G: 37.5–75.0.400 merozoites (1.7 × 12 μm)	Macro: 29–32 μm; Micro: 34–52 μm
E. marsica	NS	14–16	NS	NS
E. ovinoidalis	Ileum and cecum, colon	12–15	1G: 290 μm. Thousands of merozoites (2 × 12 μm)	Macro: 12 × 16 μm
			2G: 12 μm. 24 merozoites (1.4 × 5.5 μm)	Micro: 12 × 15 μm
E. pallida	NS	NS	NS	NS
E. parva	Small intestine	12–14	1G: 128–256 μm. Thousands of merozoites (12 μm)	Macro: 10–19 μm
			2G: 60 μm	Micro: 10–19 μm
E. weybridgensis	Small intestine, Mesenteric lymph node	23–33	NS	NS

Source: Data compiled and adapted from Levine, N.D., Ivens, V. 1986. *The Coccidian Parasites (Protozoa, Apicomplexa) of Artiodactyla*. Urbana, IL: University of Illinois Press, 120–141; Hidalgo Argüello, M.R., Cordero del Campillo, M. 1999. In Cordero del Campillo, M. and Rojo-Vázquez, F.A. (Ed.), *Parasitología Veterinaria*. Madrid: McGraw-Hill, 195–212; Taylor, M. 1995. Diagnosis and control of coccidiosis in sheep. In *Practice*. 172–177; Taylor, M.A. et al. 2007. In Taylor, M.A., Coop, R.L., and Wall, R.L. (Ed.), *Veterinary Parasitology*. Oxford, UK: Blackwell Publishing, 3rd ed., 152–258.

Note: 1G, First-generation schizonts; 2G, second-generation schizonts; Macro, macrogamonts; Micro, microgamonts; NS, not stated.

mucous membranes, and hematological evaluation shows a decrease in levels of erythrocytes, hemoglobin, and iron. They will invariably be depressed, but fever is not always present. When this occurs, it is usually during the early stages of the disease. Other clinical signs that have been seen in some coccidiosis outbreaks are related to abdominal pain and bloating.[546,879,903,1092,1822]

In other cases, coccidiosis is manifested by subacute or chronic clinical forms, with less obvious clinical signs, and affects the animals for a longer period of time. Lambs with chronic coccidiosis may have had acute severe coccidiosis earlier or may not ever have been noticed ill. The animals that develop these clinical forms of the disease have different levels of digestive disorders, which determine nutrient and electrolyte losses, as well as absorption alterations, with the consequent reduction of mineral and vitamin levels.[1020,1476] Poor body condition score and weight loss are often the most common findings in these cases. It is also common that the perianal regions may be dirty due to intermittent diarrhea. Recovery time can be long depending on the severity of intestinal tissue damage, and some lambs with chronic coccidiosis may never fully recover.[41,1020]

In lambs with mild coccidiosis, there is some degree of inappetence, a reduction in weight gain, uneven lamb size, and higher food conversion ratio. Sometimes, feces are softer or nonpelleted. Subclinical coccidiosis is also considered to increase the susceptibility of animals to other infections.[36,344]

9.4.3 Lesions

9.4.3.1 Gross

The most important lesion is catarrhal enteritis that affects the jejunum, ileum, cecum, and possibly the colon. The bowel may appear congested, edematous, thickened, and have petechiae.[713,879,1091,1687]

In lambs, coccidiosis usually results in enterocyte hyperplasia, which in addition to thickening of the intestinal wall, leads to the development of whitish 1–2 mm diameter nonpedunculated plaques/polyps or nodules (Figure 9.3, also see Figure 1.28F, Chapter 1), which are a coalescence of different stages of the parasite (schizonts, gamonts, oocysts). These lesions may have certain morphological characteristics and a variable distribution pattern throughout the intestine depending on the species of *Eimeria* involved, although it seems that they do not develop in *E. faurei* and *E. weybridgensis* infections.[713,880]

The presence of polyps may not reflect the severity of coccidiosis. In *E. bakuensis* infections, more prolific polyps can also be observed, whose pathogenic role is unknown. Similarly, in advanced cases of coccidiosis, progressive thickening, folding, or corrugating to pseudoadenomatosis of the intestinal mucosa associated to numerous well-raised nodules is seen. These nodules sometimes are pedunculated reaching 0.3–1.5 cm in diameter and are composed of hypertrophic crypt-villus units in which epithelial cells are infected by the parasite. For some authors, these polypoid lesions are the result of the mitotic stimulation of some parasitic stages (progamonts). When these proliferative lesions are projected toward the serosa of the intestines, they determine a lesion pattern that has been denominated cerebraliform, which could have diagnostic value in coccidiosis.[247,623,879,1687] Lesions in abomasum are associated with macroscopic schizonts of *E. gilruthi* (Figure 1.28G, Chapter 1).

9.4.3.2 Microscopic

Histopathologically, lesions are associated with loss of surface epithelial cells, villous atrophy (mainly during the first asexual stages of the parasite), and crypt destruction or compensatory hyperplasia (associated with gamonts). Destruction of the mucosa may result in the presence of ulcerations. Hemorrhages and edema may also be noticed in the mucosa and submucosa. Hyperplastic reactions used to be more manifest in older animals, and hemorrhages are more common in younger animals. Intense inflammatory cell infiltration may be noted in the hyperplastic areas. The infiltrations are generally composed of eosinophils, lymphocytes, neutrophils, and macrophages. In some cases, proliferation of connective tissue is observed due to chronic inflammatory reactions. Likewise, analysis by immunohistochemical methods of cytokine and chemokine expression at the gut lesions reveals that the most expressed mediators are interleukin-1α and interferon-γ.[247,1295,1687]

Enteritis may vary in severity, affecting the lamina propria and even the submucosa. As a result of all these morphological alterations, the function of the epithelial cells can be compromised, at the same time as intestinal motility and intercellular signaling, triggering the clinical signs mentioned previously.[617,837]

Of the two most pathogenic species, *E. ovinoidalis* causes lesions in the terminal ileum, cecum, and proximal colon inducing edema and thickened wall. Minimal lesions are associated with large (300 μm in diameter) first-generation schizonts that develop in cells deep in the lamina propria of the terminal ileum. The second-generation schizonts infect epithelial cells lining the colonic crypts, and subsequently, gamonts attack the remaining crypt epithelium, leading to destruction of most of the cells, including stem cells. Various degrees of lymphocyte depletion have been observed present in the ileal lymphoid follicles in *E. ovinoidalis*–infected lambs 3 weeks after infection, showing decreased follicle size and reduced staining for leukocyte common antigen (CD45) and B-cell markers.[617,880]

Similarly, *E. crandallis* first-generation large (250 μm in diameter) schizonts are located in the lamina propria of the jejunum. The development of first-generation schizonts is associated with the infiltration of eosinophils and

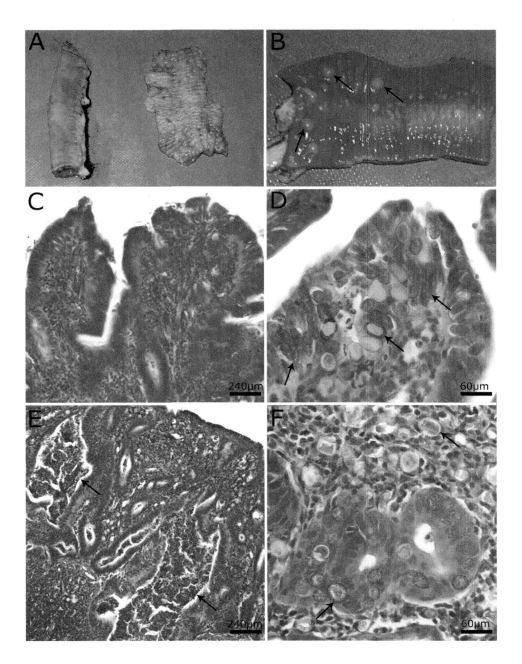

Figure 9.3 Lesions in lambs infected with *Eimeria* spp. (A) Thickened ileum. (B) Thickening of the mucosa with scattered whitish nodules (arrows). (C) Blunt ileal villi: hyperemia and hemorrhage were observed below the epithelium. Hematoxylin and eosin (HE) stain. (D) Ileal villi with many *Eimeria* spp. (arrows) in both the epithelium and the lamina propria. HE stain. (E) Crypt abscesses (arrows) in the ileum; note the infiltration of inflammatory cells in the lamina propria. The surface epithelium is flat and villi are absent. HE stain. (F) *Eimeria* spp. stages in the crypt epithelium and lamina propria of the cecum (arrows). There is hypertrophy of the crypt epithelium and infiltration of inflammatory cells in the lamina propria. HE stain. (From Odden, A., 2018. Coccidiosis in lambs: Treatment and control. PhD thesis. Thesis number 2018:54, Norwegian University of Life Sciences. With permission.)

lymphocytes into the lamina propria as well as the appearance of areas of focal necrosis, destruction of crypts, and hypertrophy of the surrounding crypts. Second-generation schizonts are observed within the cytoplasm of jejunal and ileal epithelial cells. The lamina propria then shows an inflammatory response associated with the development of the second asexual stage of the parasite. There is resulting villous atrophy and loss of crypts. Finally, pro-gamonts are seen within epithelial cells of the crypts and villi of the small intestines and cecum, differentiating subsequently into micro- and macrogamonts. The presence of gamonts results in congestion and inflammation of the mucosa. This inflammatory response seems to be related with the presence of increased numbers of inflammatory cells (lymphocytes and macrophages) within the lamina propria. In heavy infections, the cecum and colon may be similarly affected, showing hyperplastic crypts with large enterocytes and an increased number of goblet cells. Under experimental conditions, lambs infected with a high number of oocysts also showed schizonts in enlarged mesenteric lymph nodes. These parasite stages presented similar characteristics to those observed at the intestinal wall.[619,622,1094,1687,1688]

9.5 DIAGNOSIS

9.5.1 Coproscopical Methods

Although oocysts can be detected by microscopic examination of diarrheic feces in heavily infected lambs, concentration methods are often necessary for the detection of oocysts.[1726]

Flotation methods using solutions with densities >1.18 are useful in the detection of *Eimeria* spp. oocysts from feces. Among them, one of the most widely used is the saturated sodium chloride solution, although some authors suggest the use of sodium chloride solutions with higher specific gravity (1.27 g/mL) by adding glucose or sucrose flotation fluids to increase the sensitivity of this technique on ovine fecal samples.[199,307,1262]

The detection of large numbers of oocysts alone is not sufficient for diagnosis of clinical coccidiosis. Additional data on epidemiology (age, number affected, mortality) and clinical signs (diarrhea in young animals) as well as postmortem findings (thickening cecum, inflammation of the intestine, or detection of different parasitic stages in scrapings of the intestinal mucosa) can aid diagnosis. Likewise, this diagnosis should be focused on the general situation of the herd and not on an individual basis.[351,713,1688]

Quantitive data on oocyst excretion are useful for diagnosis. One of the classic procedures includes various modifications of the McMaster method. Nevertheless, the observation of large oocysts numbers in fecal samples is not always indicative of coccidiosis, especially when the species involved have a low pathogenicity, so numerous oocysts can be observed in apparently healthy animals.[1683] On the contrary, a moderate number of oocysts of pathogenic species could be a significant indicator of coccidiosis. It should also be considered that oocysts may not be observed in animals with clinical signs during the early stages of infection.[1822]

As indicated earlier, in addition to the information provided by quantitative fecal analysis, it is of great interest to collect information on the *Eimeria* species involved, given the different degrees of pathogenicity that can be observed among species.[1020] To achieve this objective, the most feasible and widely used procedure is stool culture in a thin layer of 2.5% potassium dichromate for 7–10 days at 20°C–27°C. *Eimeria* species of each oocyst were determined by light microscopy according to the characteristics of the oocysts

after sporulation (size; shape; color; presence or absence of micropyle and its cap; presence or absence of residual, polar, and Stieda bodies) described by Eckert and colleagues[459] (Figures 9.1 and 9.2), Hidalgo Argüello and Cordero del Campillo,[713] and Taylor and colleagues[1688] (Table 9.1). After sporulation, it is possible to differentiate between species whose nonsporulated oocysts are very similar (*E. crandallis* and *E. weybridgensis*), taking into account the size and shape of the sporozoites.[459] The same has been described by Engidaw and colleagues[494] for *E. parva* and *E. pallida*.

Based on the data obtained by quantitative coprological analysis and the identification of *Eimeria* spp., the participation of this protozoan in the development of intestinal diseases should be considered with counts from 50,000 OPG or higher, if a predominance of pathogenic species is found. However, a differential diagnosis has to be performed with other diseases that cause ovine diarrhea.[41,247,713]

9.5.2 Molecular Methods

Limited molecular data are available concerning molecular characteristics of ovine *Eimeria* and the usefulness of polymerase chain reaction (PCR) for differential diagnosis of ovine *Eimeria* species. It could be highlighted by a quantitative PCR (qPCR) based on the amplification of a fragment of the 18S rRNA locus and subsequent sequencing, which allows speciation and quantification of *Eimeria* spp. oocysts from fecal samples. This method is able to detect the two most pathogenic species *E. ovinoidalis* and *E. crandallis* in addition to differentiating between species with oocysts of similar size and shape (*E. crandallis/E. weybridgensis*).[1229,1850]

9.6 TREATMENT

Many anticoccidials (see Chapter 6) used for poultry coccidiosis have also been used to treat ovine coccidiosis (Table 9.4).

During an outbreak of coccidiosis, all sheep (ill and healthy) should be treated. The aim of this measure is to reduce the damage caused by the parasite to the intestinal mucosa and to ensure that subsequent recovery takes place more quickly. In these cases, if a large number of animals need to be treated, lambs may be group treated through feed or drinking water. However, in some cases, treatment must inevitably be applied on an individual basis, for example, when the animals are very young, unweaned, or extremely ill and do not have regular consumption of feed or water.[41,1688] Sulfonamides, amprolium, ionophores, and various triazines have been used to control coccidiosis in sheep.[494,1331,1811]

Triazines commonly used in veterinary species include toltrazuril, diclazuril, ponazuril (toltrazuril sulfone), clazuril, and nitromezuril, the first two being the most commonly used in control and treatment of ovine coccidiosis. With regard to diclazuril, although its mechanism of action

Table 9.4 Drugs Used in the Treatment of Coccidiosis in Lambs

Chemical Group	Active Principle	Dosage/Remarks
Nitrofurans	Amprolium	40–50 mg/kg BW. Orally for 5–7 days.
Sulfonamides	Sulfaguanidine	100–280 mg/kg BW. Orally for 4–7 days.
	Sulfadimethoxine	20–75 mg/kg BW. Orally for 3–5 days.
	Sulfadimidine	135–200 mg/kg BW. Orally for 3–5 days.
	Sulfadoxine	16–24 mg/kg BW. Intramuscular. 3 days.
Triazines	Diclazuril	1 mg/kg BW. Orally.
	Toltrazuril	20 mg/kg BW. Orally.

Source: Grilo, M.L., de Carvalho, L.M. 2014. *Vet. Med.* 34–48; Engidaw, S. et al. 2015. *Afr. J. Basic Appl.* Sci. 7, 311–319.
Abbreviation: BW = body weight.

is not fully known, in lambs infected with *Eimeria* spp., its activity appeared to have a direct effect on several stages of the parasite life cycle, in particular, the large, first-generation schizont, but also against other specific endogenous stages such as second-generation schizonts and gamonts.[368,1217,1687]

Several studies have been performed in sheep testing the effect of either toltrazuril or diclazuril in reducing oocyst excretion and clinical signs. In general, these studies show that clinical efficacy of toltrazuril against *Eimeria* spp. under field conditions appears to be superior to diclazuril in naturally infected lambs, as evidenced by a greater decrease in oocyst shedding, decreased diarrhea duration, and increased weight gain. However, it should be noted that the toltrazuril dose was 20 times that of diclazuril (20 mg/kg toltrazuril versus 1 mg/kg diclazuril).[368,950,1495,1689] According to the reviews carried out by Grilo and de Carvalho[628] and Engidaw and colleagues,[494] Table 9.4 contains information on the dosage and certain properties of all these active principles for the treatment of coccidiosis in lambs, which as indicated earlier should be subject to the corresponding sanitary legislation in each country.

When the treatment of infected animals is inevitable in coccidiosis outbreaks and the proper treatment protocols have been selected, the first control measure to be implemented should be isolation of diarrheic animals from the group to stop environmental contamination. Lambs should be treated and moved as soon as possible to uncontaminated pasture or clean and dry pens to prevent reinfection.[41,1688]

In very ill animals, in addition to individual coccidiosis therapy, supportive care should be taken into account in order to correct dehydration and electrolyte imbalances and reestablish homeostasis. Additionally, broad-spectrum antibiotics have been shown to prevent secondary bacterial infections in the digestive system or respiratory complications that are frequently associated with coccidiosis in lambs. The treatment of septicemia due to alteration of the intestinal mucosal barrier induced by parasites is another complication that should be considered in more severe cases.[1640]

9.7 CONTROL

9.7.1 Management

A hygienic measure that seems to provide good results in housed lambs is the deep cleaning of facilities before lambing. For this purpose, a blowtorch designed to avoid fecal contamination can be used on flooring, feeders, and drinkers. If the pens do not have slatted floors, the animals should be provided with clean and dry bedding that is regularly replaced and disinfected.[494,546,1088,1495,1688]

Another measure used to prevent coccidiosis outbreaks in lambs is nutritional management. It is recommended that ewes receive good nutrition before lambing, and newborns get enough colostrum as well as vitamin and mineral supplements. Other management practices that can contribute to an environment with little oocyst contamination have already been considered in previous sections (see Section 9.3), among them the rearing of animals of similar age and avoiding overcrowding are considered the most important.[36,1683]

Some of these approaches can be applied to lambs outdoor in pastures. In this case, adequate turnout, grazing period, composition by age of flocks, as well as duration of pasture rotations have to be established. Given the specificity of *Eimeria* spp., other animal species could be included in rotation programs to optimize grazing resources.[921]

9.7.2 Chemoprophylaxis/Metaphylaxis

In sheep production, management measures are generally not sufficient to prevent either the development of coccidiosis outbreaks or production losses caused by subclinical disease, so anticoccidial drugs are commonly used for preventive purposes.[950,1263,1359,1495,1689]

The chemoprophylactic treatments with this class of drugs are usually applied in feed or drinking water for a sufficiently long time to cover the period in which there is a risk of clinical outbreaks or economic losses.[1685]

a. *Decoquinate*: Although it can be used for curative purposes, there are several studies reporting the benefits of feeding lambs with decoquinate to control coccidiosis. The treatments may include dosing of ewes 28 days before lambing (0.5 mg/kg body weight/day), as well as lambs for at least 1 month from 2 weeks of age at a daily dosage of 1 mg/kg body weight. Decoquinate should not be administered to sheep used to produce milk for human consumption.[41,1685]

b. *Other chemoprophylactic drugs*: Clopidol, robenidine, and sulfonamides included in sustained-release intraruminal boluses may be used to control ovine coccidiosis.[628,649]

Some preventive protocols in which all these products are used have been reviewed.[494,628]

When anticoccidial agents develop an activity against all parasitic stages, they are usually applied as therapeutic agents or in a metaphylactic basis before the clinical signs of the disease develop, to further allow the generation of protective immune responses against later reinfections. In these cases, application of the drug at a more specific time (one or two treatments, 2 or 3 weeks apart), which usually coincides with the prepatent period, is established on the basis of the history of the farm as well as the management and rearing systems carried out, aiming for the desired effect in terms of reducing the negative impact of the disease and also enabling the development of protective immune responses. Therefore, the same pharmacological groups considered in the treatment of ovine coccidiosis, for example, the triazines, could also be used for metaphylactic purposes, even at the same dose.[41,347,1217,1460,1689]

9.7.3 Anticoccidial Drug Resistance

Testing for anticoccidial efficacy is not standardized for sheep as in other species, so the most advisable method would be a controlled efficacy test based on experimental infections with both suspected resistant and known sensitive strains. These procedures also could demonstrate that in sheep, the intensive long-term use of anticoccidial drugs can contribute to the emergence of resistant *Eimeria* spp. strains, although the number of reported cases is still low.[822,1263,1264]

9.7.4 Alternative Control Methods

There is a current interest in the use of "natural" products, which include fungal extracts, plant extracts, and probiotics, to reduce problems caused by coccidiosis. Accordingly, there are many studies that have been conducted, especially in the control of avian coccidiosis, which have resulted in the use of dietary supplements with anti-inflammatory, antioxidant activities, or immune system stimulating effects. Among these supplements are some fats, natural antioxidants, essential fats, and herbal extracts or medicinal plants.[1379]

In relation to the control of coccidiosis in sheep, most of the information available on the use of natural supplements focuses on the use of medicinal plants. That is the case with tanniferous plants such as sainfoin (*Onobrychis viciifolia*) or sericea lespedeza (*Lespedeza cuneata*). These plants, which have also shown anthelmintic activity, have demonstrated their effect to control coccidiosis when used as a supplement in ewes (from before lambing to weaning) or in lambs.[164,1496,1497]

Some other extracts from curcuma or from some citric fruits have also been preliminarily evaluated in the control of ovine coccidiosis, which have shown interesting results but require further research to confirm a possible use as natural supplements in the control of coccidiosis in this ruminant species. Similarly, given the role that some minerals play in generating immune responses, and that some of them are affected in the course of infection, mineral supplementation could also be a future alternative.[199,342,1352]

In contrast to avian coccidiosis, where vaccination is a control alternative to the use of anticoccidial drugs, only a few preliminary trials have been carried out for the development of vaccines against *Eimeria* spp. in small ruminants, so the use of vaccines in sheep does not seem feasible in the short term.[186,1462]

REFERENCES

36, 41, 87, 164, 175, 184, 186, 187, 199, 247, 307, 333, 342, 344, 347, 348, 351, 368, 459, 494, 546, 585, 617–623, 628, 649, 683, 707, 712, 713, 822, 837, 879, 880, 903, 921, 950, 979, 1020, 1088, 1091, 1092, 1094, 1109, 1124, 1163, 1217, 1229, 1252, 1262–1264, 1295, 1331, 1352, 1359, 1379, 1401, 1460, 1462, 1476, 1494–1497, 1583, 1640, 1683, 1685, 1687–1689, 1726, 1811, 1822, 1840, 1850, 1872

CHAPTER 10

Coccidiosis in Goat (*Capra hircus*)

A. Ruiz and J. M. Molina

CONTENTS

10.1 INTRODUCTION

During the last two decades, the number of goats has increased to more than 1 billion worldwide. Thus, goat production is currently not only the livelihood of small farmers in developing countries but also an important economic opportunity in a world with a continuously growing population. Goat coccidiosis is a cosmopolitan disease, but with special relevance in semiarid geographical areas that depend economically on goat production, such as the Mediterranean basin, North Africa, and certain regions of Asia or Latin America, where *Eimeria* infections may affect animal health and thus the profitability of goat production.[188] Coccidiosis can affect up to 100% of goats between 4 and 10 weeks of age, depending on the type of housing, the distribution and sanitary conditions of the farm, the immune status of the animals, and the climatic conditions, as has already been considered in some studies.[1459] The mortality rate from this disease can be as high as 50% of kids, and those who do not die suffer significant stunting, resulting in significant economic losses.[777,1592] These huge losses could be prevented with a correct diagnosis of the *Eimeria* species involved and their adequate prophylactic control as discussed here.

10.2 ETIOLOGY

Based on cross-infection studies showing high host specificity in coccidia of small ruminants, goat *Eimeria* species are now accepted to be different than those of sheep. Currently, 13 species of *Eimeria* in goats are recognized[1093,1536] (Table 10.1). Of these, *E. ninakohlyakimovae* and *E. arloingi* are considered the most pathogenic and often the most prevalent.[1459,1576]

Morphological characteristics are summarized in Tables 10.1 and 10.2. Like *Eimeria* in other hosts, oocysts are excreted unsporulated, and sporulation occurs in the environment 2 or more days later (Table 10.1).

Of the 13 species of goat *Eimeria,* more is known of the life cycle of *E. ninakohlyakimovae* than others. It has two generations of schizonts. The first-generation schizonts develop 10–12 days post-inoculation (DPI) and may have a diameter of up to 166×124 μm.[1748] They contain thousands of merozoites and are in the endothelium of lymphatic vessels (Table 10.2).[1688,1747] Presumably, the sporozoites initially enter enterocytes and are then carried to lymphatic endothelial cells by an unknown mechanism. The *in vivo* development of first-generation schizonts was confirmed by *in vitro* studies using ruminant cell lines[1458] (Figure 10.1). In contrast, second-generation schizonts are smaller (average size 17×12 μm) and develop around 13 DPI in epithelial cells of the crypts of the cecum and colon. Gamonts also develop in the large intestine, and oocysts are excreted 14–15 DPI.[1461,1748] Ultrastructural studies of second-generation schizonts revealed that development occurs in enterocytes above the host cell nucleus.[1748] The merozoites are formed at the periphery leaving a prominent residual body.

The second most pathogenic *Eimeria* species, *E. arloingi* follows the same life-cycle pattern as *E. ninakohlyakimovae.* It also has two generations of schizonts, the first one very large (300 μm) and the second generation small (10–20 μm).[681] The gamonts are formed as early as 7 DPI, and ultrastructurally, gametogony is like other *Eimeria* species.[681]

E. christenseni and *E. alijevi* also have two asexual generations preceding gamonts, but full details are unknown. Relatively little is known of the endogenous stages of other *Eimeria* in goats (Table 10.2). First-generation schizogony in other *Eimeria* species generally occurs in epithelial cells of a different part of the small or large intestine. The location of the different asexual and sexual stages of most prevalent *Eimeria* species in goats is summarized in Table 10.2; their prepatent periods vary from 7 to 23 days.

10.3 EPIDEMIOLOGY

10.3.1 Prevalence and Geographical Distribution

Coccidiosis is one of the most ubiquitous and widespread enteric diseases in goat production systems. It has been described in several regions and countries in Europe, Africa, Asia, and America (Table 10.3).[15,60,513,1349] As an example, in a Brazilian study, 92.1% of the goats were positive; eight species were identified, of which *E. alijevi, E. arloingi,* and *E. hirci* were the most prevalent.[188] Also in North America (southwestern Montana), *Eimeria* oocysts were observed in 97.2% of the total Cashmere goat feces; nine *Eimeria* species were identified, of which *E. arloingi, E. ninakohlyakimovae,* and *E. alijevi* accounted for 88.3% of the total oocysts identified.[1349] In Tanzania, a high prevalence (94.7%) was found in some climatic areas, but in general the infection rates were slightly lower than that described on the American continent, around 80%.[928] In this study, the predominant species were *E. arloingi* (91.7%), *E. alijevi* (80.3%), *E. ninakohlyakimovae* (71.4%), and *E. christenseni* (45.2%). A high prevalence of *Eimeria* infections (97.3%) was also reported in Shaanxi province, northwest China, in Saanen and Guanzhong breeds.[1900] The authors mentioned that mixed infections by several species of *Eimeria* were common; in this case, the most frequent species were *E. jolchijevi, E. arloingi, E. alijevi, E. caprina, E. hirci,* and *E. christenseni,* with different prevalence per breed. Several studies have also shown a high prevalence of coccidiosis in Europe. For instance, in Central Europe (Ukraine and Poland), the prevalence of *Eimeria* infection in goats was estimated at 74%, particularly, *E. arloingi, E. christenseni, E. jolchijevi,* and *E. ninakohlyakimovae.*[61]

The prevalence and intensity of *Eimeria* infections in goats also seem to be influenced by the age of the animals as reported in several geographical locations worldwide, such as Brazil,[188] Tanzania,[891] or Europe,[61,343a] with young having a higher degree of infection than adults. Fecal oocyst counts range from about 1000 to 2000 oocysts per gram (OPG) in adults, while in young animals counts as high as 10^6 OPG can be found.[713,1459] Age-related differences have even been found in relation to the frequency of presentation of the different *Eimeria* species. For example, in Brazil a study found that *E. ninakohlyakimovae* was the most prevalent in young animals (97%), while *E. alijevi* (77%) was the most frequently found in adult goats.[188]

10.3.2 Predisposing Factors and Transmission

Variation in prevalence and distribution of *Eimeria* species may be attributed to factors related to differences in management and hygienic conditions, temperature, agroecology, climate, weather conditions, the immune state of the host, sample size, breed, sex, sampling period, or breed susceptibility to coccidia.[60,510,678,680,880,1459,1463,1924] Little is known of strain-dependent pathogenicity of *Eimeria* in all hosts, including goats. Even a high dose (10^6 sporulated oocysts) of *E. ninakohlyakimovae* induced only mild coccidiosis, and no deaths.[316] In contrast, in experimental infections with *E. ninakohlyakimovae* GC strain using an infective dose five times lower, goats developed such a severe clinical disease that an immediate emergency treatment was necessary to prevent death.[1142]

Table 10.1 Morphological Characteristics of the Oocysts of *Eimeria* Species of Goats

Eimeria spp.	Shape	Size (μm)	Shape Index	Wall Color	Micropyle	Micropylar Cap	Shape	Size (μm)	Shape Index	Stieda Body	Sporocyst Residuum	Sporulation Time (hours) at 25°C–28°C
E. alijevi Musaev, 1970	Subspherical	16–23.7 × 14–22 (19.9 × 18.0)	1.10–1.44 (1.27)	Yellowish green	–	–	Broadly ovoid	7–13 × 4–9	1.1–2.00	–/+	+	48
E. apsheronica Musaev, 1970	Ovoid	24–37 × 18–27 (30.5 × 22.5)	1.14–1.70 (1.31)	Yellowish pink	+	–	(10 × 6.5)	1.1–2.00	(1.55)	–/+	+	60
E. arloingi (Marotel, 1905) Martin, 1909	Ellipsoid	22–36 × 16.2–26 (29 × 21.1)	1.10–1.72 (1.41)	Yellowish brown	+	+	(1.55)	NS	1.2–2.20	–	+	48
E. caprina Lima, 1979	Ellipsoid	27–40 × 20–26 (33.5 × 23)	1.2–2.1 (1.7)	Brownish yellow	+	–	Pear shaped	11–17 × 7–11	(1.7)	+	+	68
E. caprovina Lima, 1980	Broadly ellipsoid	26–36 × 20–28 (31 × 24)	1.10–1.5 (1.3)	Light pink	+	–	(14 × 9)	1.2–2.20	1.2–2.3	+	+	72
E. christenseni Levine, Ivens, and Fritz, 1962	Pear shaped	34–43.8 × 23–28.5 (38.9 × 25.8)	1.4–1.70 (1.55)	Yellowish brown	+	+	(1.7)	NS	(1.75)	–/v	+	104
E. hirci Chevalier, 1966	Roundish oval	18–27 × 14–20ss (22.5 × 17)	1.09–1.5 (1.3)	Greenish	+	+	Elongate ovoid	10.9–17 × 6–10	1.60–2.25	–/+	+	72
E. jolchijevi Musaev, 1970	Ovoidal to ellipsoid	25–37 × 18–26 (31 × 22)	1.25–1.69 (1.47)	Brownish green	+	+	(14.0 × 8.0)	1.2–2.3	(1.9)	+	+	84
E. ninakohlyakimovae Yakimoff and Rastegaieff, 1930; amend. Levine,1961	Subspherical to ellipsoid	19–28 × 14–23 (23.5 × 18.5)	1.0–1.62 (1.31)	Greenish brown	+	–	Elongate ovoid	12.6–17 × 7–10	(1.80)	+	+	96
E. pallida Christensen, 1938	Ellipsoid to ovoid	13–18 × 10–14 (15.5 × 12)	1.2–1.6 (1.3)	NS	–	–	(15 × 8)	1.60–2.25	1.3–2.27	–	+	NS
E. punctata Landers, 1955	Truncated ellipsoid	20–31 × 15–23 (25.5 × 19)	1.2–1.7 (1.45)	Yellowish brown	+	+	(1.9)	NS	(1.79)	NS	NS	60

Source: Alyousif, M.S. et al. 1992. *Int. J. Parasitol.* 22, 807–811. Soe, A.K., Pomroy, W.E. 1992. *Syst. Parasitol.* 23, 195–202.
Note: Figures in parenthesis are average.
Abbreviation: NS, not stated; v = vestigeal (see Ref. 1594).

Table 10.2   Endogenous Stages, Site of Infection, and Prepatent Period of *Eimeria* spp. in Goats

Eimeria spp.	Location	Prepatent Period (days)	Schizont Generations	Schizonts	Gamonts
E. alijevi	Small and large intestine	7–12	2	1G: 260 × 180 μm 2G: 15–18 × 9–12 μm	Macrogamonts: 14–18 × 9–14 μm Microgamonts: 20–25 × 15–20 μm
E. apsheronica	NS	14–17	NS	NS	NS
E. arloingi	Small intestine	14–17	2	1G: 140–360 × 65–240 μm, thousands merozoites (9–12 × 1–2 μm) 2G: 11–44 × 9–20 μm, 8–24 merozoites (4–10 μm long)	Macrogamonts: 12–28 × 8–20 μm Microgamonts: 11–34 × 8–29 μm
E. caprina	Small and large intestine	17–20	NS	NS	NS
E. caprovina	NS	14–20	NS	NS	NS
E. christenseni	Small intestine	14–23	2	1G: 100–227 × 81–130 μm, thousands merozoites (6–8 × 1–2 μm) 2G: 9–20 × 8–12 μm, 8–24 merozoites	Macrogamonts: 19–35 × 13–25 μm Microgamonts: 19–50 × 12–40 μm
E. hirci	NS	13–16	NS	NS	NS
E. jolchijevi	NS	14–17	NS	NS	NS
E. ninakohlyakimovae	Small and large intestine	10–13	2	1G: 165.5 × 123.6 μm 2G: 16.8 × 11.6	Microgamonts: 16.1 × 13.0 μm, Macrogamonts: 14.7 × 12.5 μm

Source: Data are compiled and adapted from Levine, N.D., Ivens, V. 1986. *The Coccidian Parasites (Protozoa, Apicomplexa) of Artiodactyla.* 120–141. Urbana, IL: University of Illinois Press; Vieira, L.S. et al. 1997. Mem. Inst. Oswaldo Cruz 92, 533–538; Taylor, M.A. et al. 2007. In Taylor, M.A., Coop, R.L., and Wall, R.L. (Ed.), *Veterinary Parasitology.* Oxford, UK: Blackwell Publishing, 3rd ed., 152–258.
Abbreviations: 1G, first-generation schizonts; 2G, second-generation schizonts; NS, not stated.

The initial infection usually occurs in the first weeks of life, when goat kids ingest oocysts attached to the udders of their dams but generally acquire low numbers to trigger clinical signs. From the second to the fourth weeks onward, kids start excreting oocysts in feces, which is the most important risk period for environmental contamination because they can excrete millions of oocysts in a period when animals are very susceptible to disease.[859] Later on, infection may result from oocysts that survive from the previous breeding period or even from the previous year. The infection pressure can be high if goat kids are kept in pastures with their mothers and even higher if they are maintained in confined pens.[713] The changes in diet and the stress suffered by the kids during weaning are the reasons why this period is especially critical for the appearance of clinical coccidiosis in most goat production systems.[1459]

10.4   IMMUNE RESPONSE

As mentioned earlier, previous exposure to *Eimeria* spp. in goats can lead to protective immunity against subsequent infections[316,1461] (Table 10.4). Under field conditions, natural exposure to the parasite ensures continuous contact that allows the development of immunity, which would explain why adult goats have significantly lower OPG than kids.[61,1459]

Accordingly, primary infections with the *E. ninakohlyakimovae* GC strain led to a significant reduction of OPG counts in challenge-infected goat kids compared to infection controls as well as the amelioration of clinical disease. However, immunoprotection induced was only partial, as some clinical signs—although milder—still occurred after challenge infections.[1461] Comparable partial protection was also achieved when applying high infections and challenge doses.[316] Challenge infections can be lethal if dose is high (around 10^6 oocysts), a circumstance that may occur in highly contaminated environments.[1459]

As previously referred, some *Eimeria* species such as *E. arloingi*, *E. ninakohlyakimovae*, and *E. christenseni* first parasitize endothelial cells of the lymphatic vessels of the intestine,[1458,1578] and there is some evidence in literature that *Eimeria* first-generation schizonts represent a major target for protective immune reactions.[1611] In agreement, it has been recently reported that protective immune responses during prepatency in goat kids experimentally infected with *E. ninakohlyakimovae*, which probably result from a complex framework of molecular mechanisms, effector cells, and cytokines involving both innate and adaptive immune responses, can be addressed to first-generation schizonts.[1142]

Several immunocompetent cells have been found within the mucosa of goat kids experimentally infected with *E. ninakohlyakimovae*, including polymorphonuclear

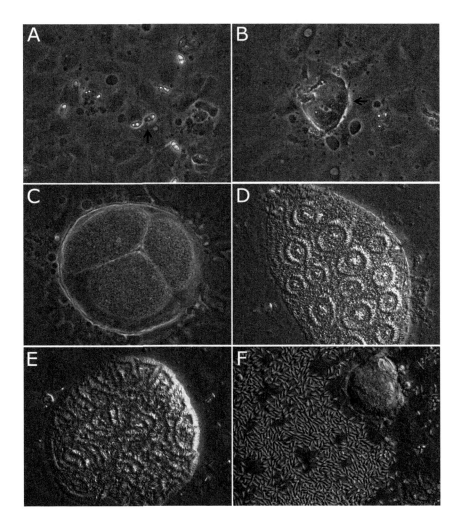

Figure 10.1 Infection and development of *E. ninakohlyakimovae* in caprine umbilical vein endothelial cells (CUVECs). CUVECs were grown to confluency and infected with freshly isolated *E. ninakohlyakimovae* sporozoites. Infection and development were monitored daily for up to 22 days. (A) Four DPI, intracellular sporozoites are indicated by an arrow; (B) 7 DPI, immature schizont (arrow); (C) 16 DPI, mature schizont; (D) 19 DPI, rosette-type schizont with merozoites; (E) 20 DPI, periphery-type schizont with merozoites; (F) 22 DPI, merozoite I release.

cells (PMNs), mast cells, eosinophils, globular leukocytes, and lymphocytes.[1142,1143,1462,1463] In agreement to increased mean lymphocyte counts in the intestinal mucosa, goat kids challenge infected with *E. ninakohlyakimovae* had a higher number of TCD4+ and TCD8+ cells, and increased relative gene expression of interleukin (IL)-2, IL-4, IL-10, and interferon (IFN)-γ, which suggests that both Th1- and Th2-mediated responses could be most probably generated against *E. ninakohlyakimovae*.[1142] Besides, in relation to the involvement of the innate immune response in caprine coccidiosis, the circulatory levels of most systemic inflammatory markers, e.g., proinflammatory cytokines (IFN-γ, tumor necrosis factor [TNF]-α, IL-4, IL-6), acid glycoprotein (AGP)-α1, and adenosine deaminase (ADA), increased significantly in goat kids infected with sporulated oocysts of three *Eimeria* species, including *E. caprina* (57%), *E. ninakohlyakimovae* (28%), and *E. arloingi* (15%).[1660] In addition,

E. ninakohlyakimovae sporozoites and soluble oocyst antigen (SOA) significantly upregulated proinflammatory cytokines and chemokines in a stimulated caprine PMN and induced caprine NETosis in a NOX-independent way, and the same was found in goats infected with *E. arloingi*.[1576] Early innate reactions of monocytes against *E. ninakohlyakimovae* also induce NADPH oxidase-dependent monocyte extracellular trap and additionally upregulate gene transcription of critical immunoregulatory molecules including IL-12 and TNF-γ, in addition to IL-6 and CCL2.[1351]

Humoral immune reactions are also triggered in response to *Eimeria* infections in goats. The detailed analyses of T-cell subpopulations of *E. ninakohlyakimovae*–infected goat kids showed that CD45+ T cells were increased in the ileum of challenge-infected animals, and negative correlations to the number of immature schizonts were recorded both in the ileum and colon, which could be related to the mild increase

Table 10.3 *Eimeria* spp. Prevalence in Goats Using Fecal Examinations (Last 20 Years)

Country	Number of Goats Tested	Percentage (%) Positive	Most Prevalent *Eimeria* spp.	References
Brazil	202	(77.2% animals)	*E. ninakohlyakimovae* (28.7%), *E. alijevi* (25.2%), *E. jolchijevi* (11.4%), *E. caprovina* (10.4%)	Coelho et al.[282]
Brazil (Northeast)	215	(88.1% adults) (100% kids)	*E. alijevi* (26.7%), *E. arloingi* (20.6%), *E. hirci* (18%), *E. ninakohlyakimovae* (16.2%),	Cavalcante et al.[188]
Brazil (Western Santa Catarina)	217	(68.2% animals)	Not determined	Radavelli et al.[1381]
China (Northeast)	199	(87.9% animals)	*E. christenseni* (78.3%), *E. alijevi* (73.7%), *E. caprina* (62.3%), *E. arloingi* (44.6%)	Wang et al.[1776]
China (Shaanxi province)	584	(97.3% animals)	*E. arloingi* (83.9%), *E. alijevi* (73.8%), *E. jolchijevi* (63%), *E. caprina* (48.5%)	Zhao et al.[1900]
Egypt (Suez Governorate)	135	(60% animals)	*E. ninakohlyakimovae*, *E. hirci*, *E. caprina*, *E. christenseni*, *E. jolchijevi*, *E. apsheronica*, *E. arloingi*	Mohamaden et al.[1195]
India (Meghalaya)	834	(23% animals)	*E. christenseni*, *E. hirci*, *E. caprina*, *E. jolchijevi*, *E. ninakohlyakimovae*, *E. arloingi*, *E. kocharii*	Das et al.[323]
Italy (Lombardy)	2554	(8.3–100% farms)	Not determined	Di Cerbo et al.[366]
Iran (Southeast)	208	(89.91% animals)	*E. arloingi* (68.26%), *E. christenseni* (50.9%), *E. ninakohlyakimovae* (41.8%), *E. caprina* (31.7%)	Kheirandish et al.[878]
Papua New Guinea	55	(17.3% animals)	Not determined	Koinari et al.[904]
Poland	110	(81% adults) (100% kids)	*E. arloingi* (80%), *E. christenseni* (39.3%), *E. ninakohlyakimovae* (40%), *E. caprina* (20%)	Balicka-Ramisz[60]
Poland (Western Pomerania) and Ukraine (West region)	311	(87% adults) (100% kids)	*E. arloingi* (36.4%), *E. christenseni* (46.8%), *E. ninakohlyakimovae* (33.5%), *E. alijevi* (30.6%)	Balicka-Ramisz[60]
Portugal (South)	144	(98.61% animals)	*E. ninakohlyakimovae* (88%), *E. arloingi* (85%), *E. alijevi* (63%), *E. caprovina* (63%)	Silva et al.[1576]
Spain (Gran Canaria)	2646	(96.1% animals)	*E. ninakohlyakimovae* (30.0%), *E. arloingi* (28.6%), *E. alijevi* (20.5%), *E. caprina* (9.1%)	Ruiz et al.[1459]
Sri Lanka	203	(87% adults) (80% kids)	*E. ninakohlyakimovae* (31%), *E. alijevi* (29%), *E. arloingi* (21%), *E. christenseni* (7%)	Faizal and Rajapakse[513]
South Africa	824	(88.7–100% animals)	*E. arloingi* (97.47%), *E. hirci* (84.34%), *E. caprovina* (61.11%), *E. ninakohlyakimovae* (45.95%)	Harper and Penzhorn[678]
Switzerland	148	(100% animals)	Not determined	Marreros et al.[1131]
Tanzania	81	(64.2% animals)	Not determined	Kimbita et al.[891]
Turkey (Igdir province)	212	(82.55% animals)	*E. arloingi* (47.43%), *E. christenseni* (45.14%), *E. ninakohlyakimovae* (36%), *E. alijevi* (26.85%)	Gül[640]
Turkey (Van province)	242	(73.6% animals)	*E. arloingi* (40.9%), *E. christenseni* (34.3%), *E. alijevi* (32.6%), *E. pallida* (31.0%)	Deger et al.[353]
Zimbabwe	580	(43% animals)	Not determined	Zvinorova et al.[1924]

of specific IgA in mucus samples.[1142] In agreement, the analysis of IgA levels in gut mucus samples of *E. ninakohlyakimovae*–infected animals revealed significantly enhanced levels of this immunoglobulin both in challenge-infected and challenge-control goat kids in comparison to uninfected controls.[1141] The authors also demonstrated that IgG and IgM levels in serum samples were significantly increased in infected animals, and a wide range of peptides of SOA was recognized by specific IgG as determined by immunoblotting.[1141] However, no correlations were found between

Table 10.4 Clinical, Pathological, and Immunological Studies on Experimental Infections with *Eimeria* spp. in Goats

Eimeria spp.	Age	Infection Dose (SP)	Samples	Method/Analysis	Main Findings	Reference
E. ninakohlyakimovae	20 days	1×10^4, 1×10^5, 1×10^6	Blood	Biochemistry	• No significant differences in serum AST, ALT, tutal protein, albumin, globulin, Na+, K+, Cl– • No serum indication of liver damage	Dai et al.[316]
			Intestinal mucosa, liver	Pathology (postpatency)	• Mild subacute to chronic proliferative enteritis in small and large intestine	
				Clinical inspection	• Clinical signs more severe at higher doses	
E. arloingi	15 days	1×10^3, 1×10^5	Blood	Biochemistry: haptoglobin (Hp), serum amyloid A (SAA), TNF-α, and IFN-γ	• Hp ↑, SAA ↑ • Significant correlations for TNF-α and IFN-γ with SAA and Hp, respectively	Hashemnia et al.[680]
			Small and large intestines, liver, spleen, pancreas, and mesenteric lymph nodes	Pathology (postpatency)	• Thickened mucosa due to mucosal hyperplasia and adenomatous-like changes • Proliferative enteritis with the developmental stages of parasites • Mild lymphoid hyperplasia of the Peyer's patches	
				Clinical inspection	• Clinical and pathological changes more severe at higher doses	
E. caprina (65%), *E. ninakohlyakimovae* (33%), *E. arloingi* (2%)	14 days	2×10^3	Blood	Biochemistry	• ↓ Activities of the main erythrocyte antioxidant enzymes • ↓ Total antioxidant capacity • ↑ Serum levels of malondialdehyde • ↑ Total homocysteine	Rakhshandehroo et al.[1386]
E. ninakohlyakimovae	4 weeks	2×10^5	Blood	Hematology	• ↓ Total protein, ↑ PCV, ↑ eosinophils • Differences not statistically significant	Ruiz et al.[1461]
			Intestinal mucosa	Pathology (postpatency)	• Moderate hyperplasia of the intestinal epithelium • Hypertrophy of the mesenteric lymph nodes and Peyer's patches • Eosinophilic enteritis + diffuse infiltration of mast cells, lymphocytes, and neutrophils	
				Clinical inspection	• Moderate to severe clinical disease • Important immunoprotection after challenge	
E. ninakohlyakimovae	4 weeks	2×10^5, 1×10^6	Blood	Hematology	• Decrease in PCV and Hb • Leukocytosis with neutrophilia and eosinophilia • Differences not statistically significant	Ruiz et al.[1463]
			Intestinal mucosa, mesenteric lymph nodes, spleen	Pathology (patency and postpatency)	• Inflammatory cellular infiltration • Hyperplasia of goblet cells • Hyperplasia of Peyer's patches • Infiltration of eosinophils • Reactive hyperplasia in mesenteric lymph nodes and spleen • ↑ Eosinophil, lymphocyte,0 and neutrophil counts	
				Clinical inspection	• Severe to fatal clinical disease, particularly in goat kids challenged with the higher dose	

(Continued)

Table 10.4 (Continued) Clinical, Pathological, and Immunological Studies on Experimental Infections with *Eimeria* spp. in Goats

Eimeria spp.	Age	Infection Dose (SP)	Samples	Method/Analysis	Main Findings	Reference
E. arloingi	14 days	1×10^3, 1×10^5	Blood	Hematology and biochemistry	• ↓ ALP • ↑ PCV and Hb • ↓ Na⁺, Cl⁻, and K⁺ • No significant differences in AST, ALT, GGT, albumin, and total proteins • No hepatic damage	Hashemnia et al.[682]
E. ninakohlyakimovae (vaccination with attenuated oocysts)	5 weeks	2×10^5	Blood	Hematology	• Slight ↑PCV and Hb • Nonsignificant changes in leukocyte subpopulations	Ruiz et al.[1462]
			Intestinal mucosa, mesenteric lymph nodes	Pathology (postpatency)	• Moderate hyperplasia and hypertrophy of the mesenteric lymph nodes and Peyer's patches • Moderate to severe enteritis • ↑ Eosinophils, ↑ lymphocytes, ↑ globular leukocytes, ↑ mast cells, ↑ neutrophils	
				Clinical inspection	• In association to ↓ OPG, animals vaccinated with attenuated oocysts had ↓ clinical signs	
E. ninakohlyakimovae	5 weeks	2×10^5	Intestinal mucosa, mesenteric lymph nodes	Pathology (prepatency)	• Moderate hyperplasia and hypertrophy of the mesenteric lymph nodes and Peyer's patches • Eosinophilic enteritis with diffuse infiltration of mast cells, lymphocytes, neutrophils, and globular leukocytes • Less immature schizonts in challenged animals	Matos et al.[1142]
			Ileal mucus	ELISA	• ↑IgA	
			Ileal and colonic mucosa	IHC	• ↑CD4⁺, ↑CD8⁺, ↑CD45⁺, mainly in challenged animals • ↑MCHII and myeloid/histiocyte markers, mainly in primary infected goat kids	
			Ileal and colonic mucosa	Real-time PCR	• ↑IL2, ↑IL4, ↑IL10 IFN-γ without changes	
				Clinical inspection	• Clinical signs only during the patency of primary infection	
E. ninakohlyakimovae	5 weeks	2×10^5	Blood	ELISA	• ↑IgG, ↑IgM	Matos et al.[1141]
				Immunoblotting	• Most proteins appeared in the range of 54–108 kDa • Polypeptides of smaller mw (16–38 kDa) were also detected • Most prominent bands: 74, 54, 23, and 20 kDa	
			Ileal mucus (postpatency)	ELISA	• ↑IgA	
Eimeria spp. (vaccination with attenuated oocysts)	5 weeks	2×10^6		Clinical inspection	• In association to ↓OPG, animals vaccinated with attenuated oocysts had ↓ clinical signs	Guedes et al.[633]

(Continued)

Table 10.4 (*Continued*) Clinical, Pathological, and Immunological Studies on Experimental Infections with *Eimeria* spp. in Goats

Eimeria spp.	Age	Infection Dose (SP)	Samples	Method/Analysis	Main Findings	Reference
E. ninakohlyakimovae	3, 4, 5 weeks	2×10^5	Blood	Hematology	• Hematologic changes were very mild in all groups: moderate increase in the total number of leukocytes, neutrophilia, and temporary monocytosis • Moderate eosinophilia	Matos et al.[1143]
			Intestinal mucosa, mesenteric lymph nodes	Pathology (postpatency)	• Moderate hyperplasia and hypertrophy of the mesenteric lymph nodes and Peyer's patches • Moderate to severe enteritis • ↑Eosinophils, ↑ lymphocytes, ↑ globular leukocytes, ↑ mast cells, ↑ neutrophils • Youngest age group was the only one in which no statistical differences were observed on lymphocyte counts in challenge infection	
				Clinical inspection	• Three age groups develop patent infections • Slightly longer prepatent periods in goat kids primary infected at younger age • Three age groups develop patent infections • Slightly longer prepatent periods in goat kids primary infected at younger age • Severity of the disease was milder in challenged animals of all age groups	

Abbreviations: ALT, alanine transaminase; AST, aspartate transaminase; ALP, alkaline phosphatas; ELISA, enzyme-linked immunosorbent assay; GGT, gamma-glutamyl transferase; Hb, hemoglobin; IHC, immunohistochemistry; OPG, oocysts per gram; PCR, polymerase chain reaction; PCV, packed cell volume; SP, sporulated oocysts; ↑, increased in comparison to uninfected control; ↓, decreased in comparison to uninfected control.

immunoglobulin levels and OPG counts after challenge infection, which agrees with controversial data on whether specific humoral responses against ruminant *Eimeria* species may convey immunoprotection or not.

Finally, some antimicrobial peptides that are produced by leukocytes and epithelial cells, known as defensins, have been recently involved in important innate immune responses against caprine eimeriosis.[762]

10.5 PATHOGENESIS, CLINICAL SIGNS, AND LESIONS

10.5.1 Pathogenesis

The pathogenicity of different *Eimeria* species is particularly related to the location of replication of the parasite in the host and may influence the clinical outcome of the disease. Table 10.2 shows the locations of the main *Eimeria* species affecting goats. In general, the most pathogenic species in goats, that is, *E. ninakohlyakimovae*, *E. arloingi*, and *E. christenseni*, must pass through the intestinal epithelium and invade the endothelial cells of the central lymphatic capillaries of the intestinal villi. Once in endothelial cells, they form macroschizonts, a process that requires a prolonged replication time and, therefore, modulation at a larger scale of the host cell.[1458] Because of large-size schizonts, the cellular damage produced in the intestinal mucosa may be severe.[1458,1461,1463] Furthermore, the enormous numbers of first-generation merozoites resulting from the first schizogony consequently lead to an exponential destruction of the epithelium during the second schizogony and, finally, during the phase of sexual reproduction or gametogony. In general, the severity of coccidiosis is determined by the proliferation capacity of the pathogenic *Eimeria* species, which is defined as the number of schizogonies and the number of merozoites produced by schizonts, and is closely related to the number of cells destroyed by each sporulated oocyst ingested. Therefore, the primoinfective dose (number of viable oocysts ingested) and the magnitude of reinfection may influence the development and course of the disease.[1463]

The extensive damage to the intestinal mucosa during the development and proliferation of intracellular stages of the parasite clearly interferes with both digestion and homeostasis. Such events cause negative effects on animal health and production performance, and thus substantial economic losses may occur, even when the typical clinical signs of the disease are absent.[1459] The destruction of epithelial cells in different parts of the intestine, and endothelial cells in some cases, can affect large enteric sections, exposing the mucous membrane itself.[1463] Because of fluid loss from diarrhea and malabsorption, animals often suffer a dehydration process, especially in long-term infections with pathogenic species such as *E. ninakohlyakimovae*.[316] Probably because mucosal damage in the ileum prevents reabsorption of bile

in the small intestine, serum bile acids are decreased, as reported for other ruminant hosts. Increased serum bilirubin and decreased liver enzyme activity are more complex to explain but may reflect anorexia and transient alteration of liver metabolism.[731] Anorexia associated with dehydration can lead to a state of prostration and death of affected animals if urgent fluid therapy is not instituted.[1463]

The pathogenic effect of *Eimeria* spp. can be complicated by concomitant infections with gastrointestinal nematodes affecting different parts of the digestive tract.[15,344,1383] Goat *Eimeria* spp. may all coexist and exacerbate the clinical course of other pathogens such as viruses or bacteria.[247] Thus, an outbreak of intestinal coccidiosis increased susceptibility to bronchopneumonia by *Pasteurella haemolytica* in experimentally vaccinated goat kids against sarcocystosis.[418]

10.5.2 Clinical Signs

When optimal conditions for the development of pathogenic species occur, common clinical signs of coccidiosis are usually observed: anemia, weakness, depression, abdominal pain, lethargy, anorexia, dehydration, coarse hair, poor weight gain, low conversion of food, and pasty stools without blood streaks. In addition, in animals heavily infected with species that develop gamonts in the large intestine, such as *E. ninakohlyakimovae*, accompanying all clinical signs previously mentioned, a severe liquid diarrhea can be observed, sometimes hemorrhagic, capable of dragging portions of intestinal mucosa.[316,1461] The acute phase may last 3–4 days, but diarrhea with elimination of liquid stools, with mucus, with or without blood, and color changes from brown to dark yellow or tarry may persist for several days or weeks, usually until turnover of the affected intestinal mucosa takes place.[316] Animals weaken, suffer from ataxia, and may not be able to stand, although they usually recover, and mortality of more than 10% is not frequent, even with high infection doses.[1461,1463] The mortality rate can reach 30% in farms where *E. arloingi* and *E. ninakohlyakimovae* are the predominant species.[910] If the animals do not die within 7–10 days, they recover slowly but remain unthrifty.[1142]

Under certain conditions, coccidiosis may be associated with sudden death with absence of clinical signs, especially in young animals, which has been related to the damage on the intestinal mucosa produced by some *Eimeria* species during the prepatent period due to first schizogony.[1142,1463]

10.5.3 Biochemical and Hematological Findings

Despite the severity of the clinical signs, hematological alterations are not as striking as would be expected in experimental infections with *E. ninakohlyakimovae*.[316,682,1461] Similarly, only slight increase of packed cell volume (PCV) values have been observed in *E. ninakohlyakimovae*–infected animals, which would be explained as a decrease of the total blood volume in circulation because of fluid losses during the phase of diarrhea.[316,1461] The same pattern was also demonstrated in experimental infections with *E. arloingi*.[682]

Several serum enzymes and electrolytes have also been evaluated in *E. ninakohlyakimovae* experimentally infected goats, showing a slight fall in alkaline phosphatase (ALP) levels, while plasmatic concentrations of albumin, globulin, Na$^+$, K$^+$ and Cl$^-$ exhibited no pattern and no significant differences were found between inoculated and non-inoculated groups.[316] In experimental infections with *E. arloingi*, diarrhea was also associated with a reduction in ALP activity, while decreased levels of Na$^+$, K$^+$, and Cl$^-$ were proved in this occasion.[682] Although endogenous stages in livers and gallbladders of goats naturally and experimentally infected with *E. ninakohlyakimovae* have been found, changes in levels of aspartate aminotransferase (AST) and alanine aminotransferase (ALT), two enzymes that reflect liver damage, could not be demonstrated.[316]

With respect to blood leukocyte counts, a transient increase in eosinophil and monocytes counts was recorded for challenged animals in *E. ninakohlyakimovae* primary-infected goat kids,[1463] while lymphocytes and neutrophils varied irregularly.[1461,1463] Finally, responses of the enzymatic antioxidant systems during experimental coccidiosis indicate that infections with pathogenic species of *Eimeria* in goats can significantly reduce the major erythrocyte antioxidant mechanisms and enhance the blood levels of lipid peroxidation and total homocysteine.[1386]

10.5.4 Lesions

In animals that die due to experimental *E. ninakohlyakimovae*, the perianal area is soiled by diarrheal feces, which may be liquid and of a variable color, from yellow to reddish. Gross lesions differed per the period when the animal was necropsied and whether they were primary of challenge-infected animals.[316,1142,1461] Thus, in challenge-infected goat kids euthanized during prepatency (7 DPI), macroscopic lesions included various degrees of congestion and thickening of the intestinal mucosa, particularly affecting the ileum, colon, and cecum, while primary-infected animals did not have gross lesions. No relevant macroscopic alterations were observed in the intestines of *E. ninakohlyakimovae* experimentally infected animals when slaughtered during postpatency, when no oocysts were observed in feces or the counts were close to zero.[316,1461] But when the animals are subjected to continuous infections under field conditions, macroscopic pathological changes in goat kids have been reported, including mucosal hemorrhages and whitish nodular polyps in the jejunum, most probably due to coinfection by *E. arloingi* and *E. ninakohlyakimovae*.[910]

Numerous developmental stages of *Eimeria* are microscopically found in enterocytes and lacteals of intestinal villi in naturally infected animals.[910,1142,1461] Histopathological changes found in goat coccidiosis are further characterized

by local hypertrophy and hyperplasia of intestinal villi, villus blunting, and inflammatory infiltration in the lamina propria.[910] Hypertrophy of the mesenteric lymph nodes and Peyer's patches has also been found in *E. ninakohlyakimovae* experimentally infected goat kids and, in some cases, mild villous atrophy in the lower small intestine.[316,1461] Futhermore, clear eosinophilic enteritis and a diffuse infiltration of mast cells, lymphocytes, and PMN cells have also been demonstrated.[1461] A mild inflammatory cell infiltration involving different immune cells is already observed during prepatency of *E. ninakohlyakimovae*–infected goat kids. Eosinophils and lymphocytes were significantly increased both in challenge-infected and challenge-control animals with respect to uninfected controls, while PMN were predominantly increased in challenge controls both in ileum and colon samples.[1142] Interestingly, cellular immune responses and histopathological alterations in the gut mucosa of fatal *E. ninakohlyakimovae* challenge-infected goat kids showed severe eosinophilic enteritis in affected animals, with an extensive infiltration of intraepithelial lymphocytes and neutrophils.[1463]

10.5.5 Biliary-Hepatic Coccidiosis and Other Atypical Locations

Isolated cases of biliary-hepatic coccidiosis associated with unknown *Eimeria*-like parasites have been reported in goats from different areas.[419,1290] Schizonts, gamonts, and unsporulated oocysts were present in biliary epithelium. In the cases reported from China, oocysts from bile were morphologically like *E. ninakohlyakimovae*.[315] In another case from the United States, the oocysts fit the size range of *E. pallida* (Table 10.1).[419]

An atypical location of *Eimeria* in goats has been described within epithelial cells of a Brunner's gland in the duodenum.[1119] Light microscopic appearance of the oocysts in histological sections was considered compatible with *E. ninakohlyakimovae*, suggesting that this *Eimeria* species might be more ubiquitous than others.

10.6 DIAGNOSIS

10.6.1 Coproscopical Methods

Qualitative analysis using the flotation concentration method, e.g., with saturated NaCl solution, is probably the most common routine method for the detection of goat *Eimeria* spp. However, a quantitative method is generally preferred to estimate the degree of infection in goat kids and establish a more rational administration of anticoccidials, both for therapeutic and prophylactic purposes.[247,771,1460] McMaster's technique is probably the most commonly used method to quantify *Eimeria* oocyst counts. With different modifications, this technique has been employed in many epidemiological studies involving goat herds from diverse geographical areas.[513,878,1459] Results are usually expressed as OPG, and when the parasitic load is very high, it is necessary sometimes to make fecal dilutions 1:10, 1:100, etc., to facilitate the counting.[1460]

Most probably, different *Eimeria* spp. are present in all animals of the herd, but not all of them may be pathogenic species, so the simple presence of oocysts in feces is not a sufficient reason for the diagnosis of goat coccidiosis, even though very high OPG are found.[910] Therefore, a specific diagnosis trying to determine whether the pathogenic *Eimeria* species are or are not a major component of the samples taken in that farm is required. For this purpose, fecal oocysts are routinely incubated with 2% potassium dichromate to facilitate oocyst sporulation and then have more morphological and structural parameters available for characterization.[35,979,1459,1594] For illustration, Figure 10.2 depicts drawings of sporulated oocysts of the main *Eimeria* species in goats, and Figure 10.3 provides pictures of sporulated oocysts of the most prevalent species.

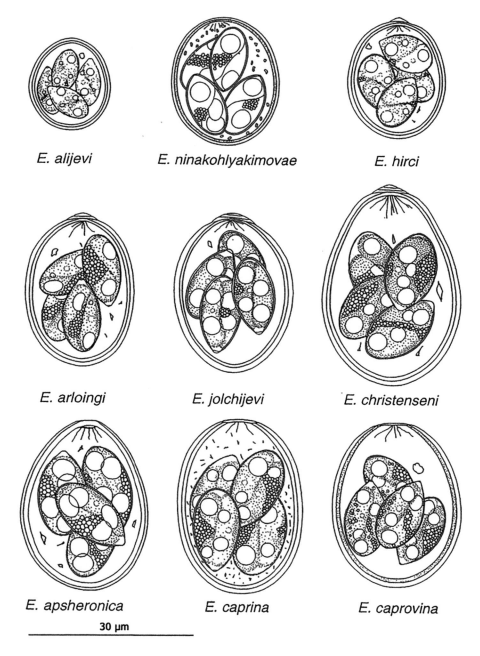

E. alijevi   E. ninakohlyakimovae   E. hirci

E. arloingi   E. jolchijevi   E. christenseni

E. apsheronica   E. caprina   E. caprovina

30 µm

Figure 10.2 Sporulated oocysts of *Eimeria* spp. in goats. (From Eckert, J. et al. 1995. *COST 89/820 Biotechnology: Guidelines on Techniques in Coccidiosis Research*. 306. European Commission Directorate-General XII, Science, Research and Development Enivironment research programme.)

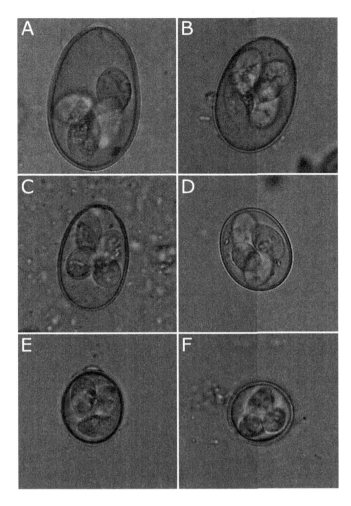

Figure 10.3 Sporulated oocysts compatible with some of the most frequent *Eimeria* species in goats: (A) *E. christenseni*, (B) *E. caprina*, (C) *E. arloingi*, (D) *E. ninakohlyakimovae*, (E) *E. hirci*, (F) *E. alijevi*.

10.6.2 Lesions

Postmortem examination may include histopathological evaluation of the intestinal mucosa.[316,1461,1463] Goat kids with high burdens of pathogenic *Eimeria* species may be ill before oocysts are excreted in feces. In such cases, diagnosis is only possible by visualizing the endogenous stages of *Eimeria* by observation of intestinal tissues in necropsies of recently dead animals or in fragments of intestinal mucosa removed with feces.[1463]

10.6.3 Molecular and Other Diagnostic/ Complementary Methods

Molecular techniques have been applied to *Eimeria* of goats for diagnosis and phylogenetic relationships. For this purpose, different loci have been employed, such as 18S rRNA, mitochondrial cytochrome oxidase gene (COI), and ITS-1.[20,881,1195,1577]

Different isotypes of immunoglobulins (IgG, IgM, and IgA) specifically increase after *E. ninakohlyakimovae* experimental infections when using antigens from sporulated oocysts; therefore, serological diagnosis for the detection of *Eimeria* soluble antigens in feces or in tissue biopsies could also be used for the detection of *Eimeria* infections in goat kids.[1141–1143] However, these methods are not standardized currently for routine identification of coccidiosis in this ruminant species.

Some experimental studies have demonstrated changes in patterns of acute phase proteins and inflammatory mediators in serum from goat kids infected with *E. arloingi*. The magnitude and duration of the haptoglobin (Hp) and serum amyloid A (SAA) responses correlated well with the inoculation doses and the severity of the clinical signs and diarrhea in kids, and significant correlations were also observed with TNF-α and IFN-γ. Accordingly, Hp and SAA have been suggested as nonspecific diagnostic indicators in caprine coccidiosis.[680]

Finally, a differential diagnosis must be made with respect to other gastrointestinal diseases including parasitosis, bacteriosis (colibacillosis, enterotoxemia, salmonellosis), viral infections (viral enteritis), or even diarrhea produced because of inadequate diets.[1592]

10.7 TREATMENT

Most of the anticoccidials have been mainly registered for cattle and sheep but not for goats, and in certain parts of the world such as Europe, there are no anticoccidials specifically registered for caprine. In other countries, e.g., the United States, some compounds (ionophores and decoquinate) are approved for prevention and control of coccidia in goats when premixed in feed, but there are no drugs approved for treatment. Table 10.5 summarizes anticoccidials described either for treatment or prevention, specifying which are referred to as extralabel drug use (ELDU) or experimental tested used (EXTU). Some data on the effect of some anticoccidials experimentally tested in goats are described in the following sections. Anticoccidials used for treating coccidiosis in ruminants are discussed in Chapter 6.

10.8 PREVENTION

Currently, coccidiosis prevention focuses on improving management practices in combination with prophylactic/ metaphylactic chemotherapy using specific anticoccidials. Other control alternative strategies are under investigation.

10.8.1 Pharmacological Control

Coccidiosis prophylaxis by coccidiostats in drinking water or feed is commonly employed to control the

Table 10.5 Anticoccidial Agents for Use in Treatment and Prevention of *Eimeria* Infection in Goats

Agent	Treatment	Prevention	Comments
Amprolium[a] (Corid)	25–40 mg/kg BW for 5 days (ELDU)		Available in multiple forms: • 9.6% oral solution • 20% soluble powder • 1.25% or 2.5% crumbles/pellets
Decoquinate (Deccox)		0.5 mg/kg BW for at least 28 days	Feed additive For prepartum use in sheep and goats • 1 kg of 13% premix in 22 kg of trace mineralized salt
Lasalocid (Bovatec)		1 mg/kg BW continuously (ELDU)	Feed additive For prepartum use in sheep and goats: • 1 kg of 6% premix in 22 kg of trace mineralized salt
Monensin (Rumensin)		20 g/ton of feed	Feed additive May be best choice for goats
Sulfaquinoxaline	10–20 mg/kg BW for 3–7 days (SLDU)		As a 0.015% solution in water
Toltrazuril		20, 30, 40 mg/kg BW oral, single dose (EXTU)	No adverse effects were found (Chartier et al.[248])
Ponazuril	10 mg/kg BW oral, single dose		Well absorbed (Gibbons et al.[593], Love et al.[1095])
Diclazuril		1–2 mg/kg BW oral, single or double treatment (EXTU)	Adapt treatment to risk of clinical disease (Ruiz et al.[1430])

Source: Adapted from Keeton, S.T.N., Navarre, C.B. 2018. *Vet. Clin. Food Anim.* 34, 201–208.
Abbreviations: BW, body weight; ELDU, extralabel drug use; EXTU, experimental tested use.
[a] Amprolium is a thiamine analog that can cause polyencephalomalacia, especially at high doses.

disease, particularly in intensive goat production systems.[880] Although there is no registered drug for pharmacological treatment of coccidiosis in goats in many areas, in certain countries (e.g., the United States), there are some compounds that can legally be used in prevention of the disease. For example, as depicted in Table 10.5, decoquinate (0.5 mg/kg) in feed mixtures for at least 28 days is a safe and very effective coccidiostat in goats.[868] Besides, monensin at 20 mg per ton of feed controls shedding of oocysts and increases feed conversion in goats. Monensin could be considered the best choice for prevention of coccidiosis in goats; however, high levels of monensin render the feed unpalatable and toxic.[288]

When a drug is administered either prophylactically or metaphylactically, a major concern is whether continuous or repeated treatments may interfere with immunity. In general, a primary infection exposure sufficient to trigger acquired immunity has to be ensured; accordingly, in metaphylactic treatments with diclazuril (extralabel drug use), it is recommended that (1) the timing of the first dose should be set at 4 weeks of life, once goat kids have already had contact with *Eimeria* species and thereby had the chance to develop immune reactions; (2) for the same reason, treatments at an interval of 3 weeks (instead of 2 weeks) would be a better option in case an additional dose is necessary to control goat coccidiosis in a particular herd.[1460]

The continued use of coccidiostats reduces the number of oocysts passed in the feces over time, but it may also lead to selection for resistance, so that a regular monitoring of

the treated animals is needed. There are no data currently available in literature on anticoccidial resistance in goats, but based on recently published results in sheep, it is not discarded that this should be an issue to investigate in detail in the future.[1264]

10.8.2 Management

General hygienic and management practices can also be applied to control goat coccidiosis. As an example, high density and corresponding overcrowding have been correlated to an increased risk of clinical coccidiosis in large goat farms, something that can be overcome by regular prophylactic/metaphylactic treatments with anticoccidials.[1459]

10.8.3 Alternative Control Methods

10.8.3.1 Phytotherapy

Several studies have been performed to evaluate the effect of different plant extracts against goat coccidiosis. For example, the exposure of *Melia azedarach* fruits to *Eimeria* lowers oocyst output in yearling Tswana goats[1110] and *Aloe ferox* and *Leonotis leonurus* caused significant reduction in *Eimeria* spp. oocysts.[1123] Similarly, less clinical signs were found in goats fed dried pelleted sericea lespedeza (*Lespedeza cuneata*) in comparison with the control group, in addition to a decrease in OPG counts.[905]

10.8.3.2 Strategic Nutrient Supplementation

In goat production systems with nutritional limitations of forages and other feed resources, supplementation with leguminous fodders, cactus during periods of severe drought, or energy sources such as molasses, cereal grains, and by-products, apart from minerals and vitamin A, are suggested as an alternative.[865] Another nutrition-related control strategy in sustainable animal production has been the use of probiotics. In investigating the effects of kefir on coccidial oocysts excretion and performance of dairy goat kids following weaning, reduced numbers of positive samples and lower OPG counts were recorded, but the frequency of diarrhea, level of highest oocyst excretion, and performance of the kids remained unaffected.[322]

10.8.3.3 Vaccines

Immunization of kids with oocysts attenuated by X radiation developed protective immune responses against coccidiosis produced by *E. ninakohlyakimovae*.[1462] The immunization protocol was based on the use of oocysts attenuated by irradiation X, following a methodology previously described for the attenuation of oocysts in avian vaccines (Chapter 4). Immunized animals showed no apparent symptomatology during the primary infection and released fewer oocysts than animals infected with unattenuated oocysts. Furthermore, during challenge infection, the immunoprotection conferred on the vaccinated group (in terms of reduction of fecal oocysts counts and general improvement of the clinical picture of coccidiosis) was comparable to that obtained on kids challenged with nonirradiated oocysts.[1462] Similar results have been obtained when using a mixture of *Eimeria*

spp. in the vaccination protocol, although the response to multispecies infection was more complex than when using the monospecific *E. ninakohlyakimovae* strain.[633]

Recombinant vaccines have not yet been tested against ruminant coccidiosis, but some attempts have been performed to identify target candidates. Interesting results were obtained by using a phage display library to identify surface proteins of caprine umbilical vein endothelial cells (CUVECs).[1464] The authors could identify two peptides that specifically bind to the surface of CUVEC (PCEC2 and PCEC5) and selectively reduced the infection rate by *E. ninakohlyakimovae* sporozoites.

Recently, age-related studies on immune response to experimental infection with *E. ninakohlyakimovae* in goat kids have demonstrated that goat kids of either 3, 4, or 5 weeks of age can develop patent infections and immunoprotective responses against *E. ninakohlyakimovae*. Nevertheless, detailed analysis of immunological data showed some differences among the three age groups, related both to the *Eimeria* infection outcome and the resulting immune response, suggesting that the youngest goat kids are not fully immunocompetent. These findings may be of interest for the design of immunoprophylactic approaches.[1143]

REFERENCES

15, 20, 35, 60, 61, 188, 247, 248, 282, 288, 315, 316, 322, 323, 343a, 344, 353, 366, 418, 419, 459, 510, 513, 593, 633, 640, 678, 680, 681, 682, 713, 731, 762, 771, 777, 859, 865, 868, 878, 880, 881, 891, 904, 905, 910, 928, 979, 1093, 1095, 1110, 1119, 1123, 1131, 1141–1143, 1195, 1264, 1290, 1349, 1351, 1381, 1383, 1386, 1458–1464, 1536, 1576–1578, 1592, 1594, 1611, 1660, 1688, 1747, 1748, 1776, 1900, 1924

CHAPTER 11

Coccidiosis of Pigs

A. Joachim and A. Shrestha

CONTENTS

11.1 INTRODUCTION

In pigs, two genera of intestinal coccidia are recognized, *Eimeria* and *Cystoisospora*. While members of the genus *Eimeria* are of limited clinical importance, *C. suis* is a major cause of diarrhea in suckling piglets, and its presence is highly associated with intensive pig production worldwide.

It is generally accepted that the domestic pig, *Sus scrofa domestica*, and wild boar, *Sus scrofa scrofa*, share the same species of coccidia.

11.2 SPECIES OF *EIMERIA* AND *CYSTOISOSPORA*

Currently eight species of *Eimeria* are considered valid in pigs (Table 11.1).[325,460] Since their first descriptions, some of these species were redescribed or renamed.[1343,1745] *E. guevarai* Romero-Rodriguez and Lizcano-Herrera, 1971, was described from a pig in Spain,[1343] but this species is now considered invalid. This is also the case for *E. scrofae*

Galli-Valerio, 1935, from Switzerland, *E. betica* Martinez-Gomez and Hernandez-Rodriguez, 1973, and *E. residualis* Martinez-Gomez and Hernandez-Rodriguez, 1973.[455,1343] *E. romaniae* Donciu, 1962, and *E. ibrahimovae* Musaev, 1970, are considered synonyms of *E. scabra*; *E. cardonis* Vetterling, 1965, a synonym of *E. polita*; *E. brumpti* Canchemez, 1921, *E. almaataensis* Musaev, 1970, and *E. jalina* Krediet, 1921, are synonyms of *E. debliecki* or *E. neodebliecki*.[455,1343] *E. yanglingensis* from China[1890] is not described in sufficient detail to be considered a valid species.

In pigs, four species of *Cystoisospora* have been described: *C. almaataensis* Paichuk, 1953; *C. neyrai* Romero-Rodriguez and Lizcano-Herrera, 1971; *C. sundarbanensis* Ray and Sarkar, 1985; and *C. suis* Biester and Murray, 1934.[455,1343] The existence of *Cystoisospora* in pigs was first questioned and considered as contaminants with feces from passerine birds.[1343] Of the four described species, *C. almaataensis*, *C. sundarbanensis*, and *C. neyrai* are now considered invalid,[455] whereas *C. suis* has been known to be a pathogen of suckling piglets since the 1970s.[105,1487]

Table 11.1 Stages of Porcine *Eimeria* spp. and *Cystoisospora suis*

(A) Exogenous stages

Species	Oocyst Form	Oocyst size (μm) [average]	Micropyle	Outer Layer	Color	OR	SR	Stieda Bodies	Sporocyst (μm)	Sporozoite (μm)	Prepatent Period (days)	Sporulation Time (days)
C. suis Biester and Murray, 1934	(Sub-) spherical	17–25 × 16–22 [20.6 × 18.1]	No	Smooth, single layer	Colorless or light yellow	No	Yes	No	13.4 × 9.2	8.9–11.1 × 3.1–3.6	5–6	1–2
E. debliecki Douwes, 1921	Ellipsoid or ovoid	15–23 × 11–18 [18.2 × 14.3]	No	Smooth	Colorless or yellowish	No	Yes	Yes	11.5 × 5.3	17.8–3.2	6.5	5–7
E. neodebliecki Vetterling, 1965	Ellipsoid or ovoid	17–26 × 13–20 [21.2 × 15.8]	No	Smooth, bilayered	Colorless	No	Yes	Yes (prominent)	12.9 × 6.3		10	13
E. perminuta Henry, 1931	Ovoid-subspherical	12–15 × 10–13 [13.7 × 11.7]	No	Rough	Yellow	No	Yes	Yes	6.9 × 5.0			10–12
E. polita Pellérdy, 1949	Ellipsoid or broad ovoid	20–33 × 14–22 [25.9 × 18.1]	No	Slightly rough (may be missing)	Yellowish-brown or pink	No	Yes	Yes	16.3 × 6.6	17–18	8–9	8–9
E. porci Vetterling, 1965	Ovoid	18–27 × 13–18 [23.2 × 15.7]	Yes (not distinct)	Smooth	Colorless to yellowish-brown	No	Yes (fine granules)	Yes	9.7 × 6.5		7	9
E. scabra Henry, 1931	Ovoid or ellipsoid	24–42 × 20–24 [31.2 × 11.8]	Yes	Thick, coarse, (can be missing)	Brown	No	Yes	Yes	17.1 × 7.8		8–9.5	9–12
E. suis Nöller, 1921	Ellipsoid	15–23 × 12–18 [18.2 × 14.0]	No	Smooth	Colorless	No	Yes	Yes	8.4 × 5.8		10	5–6
E. spinosa Henry, 1931	Ovoid	17–24 × 12–19 [20.6 × 16.2]	No	Rough, with long spines	Brownish	No	Yes	Yes	11.1 × 5.6		8–9	9–12

(B) Endogenous stages

Species	Location	Merozoite Generations	Meronts/Schizonts, Merozoites	Gamonts
C. suis	Jejunum, ileum	Types of meronts/ merozoites described instead	Type I meronts: 8–13 × 4–6 μm, binucleated (2–7 merozoites; 10 × 3.6 μm) from 24 hours postinfection; Type II meronts: 9–18 × 4–14 μm, multinucleated (6–8 merozoites; 6.3 × 2.1 μm) from 3 days postinfection (DPI) Type III meronts: length 12.7 μm, multinucleated (8–10 merozoites; 8.0 × 2.8 μm), 4–6 DPI	Microgamonts: 7–13 × 6–9.5 μm; Macrogamonts: 6.5–14 × 4–9 μm (immature?)
E. debliecki	Small intestine	2	1G: 8–12 μm with 16 merozoites (12–13 × 1.8 μm) 2G: 13–16 μm with 32 merozoites (6–8 × 1.8 μm)	Microgamonts: 7–22 μm in diameter, with 70 microgametes (2–3 × 0.5–0.7 μm) Macrogamonts: 10 × 16 μm Macrogametes: 12–16 × 10–12 μm
E. polita	Schizonts in jejunum, gamonts in jejunum/ileum	2	1G: 17.2 × 14.5 μm in diameter, with 16–30 merozoites (14 × 2.3 μm) 2G: 14–23 μm with 15–30 merozoites (12 × 2 μm)	Microgamonts: 16–29 × 13–29 μm, with 60–150 microgametes (2.2 × 0.6 μm) Macrogamonts: 14 × 11.5 μm, with 16–29 macrogametes Macrogametes: 16–29 × 15–25 μm
E. scabra	Jejunum and ileum	3	1G: 12–19 × 11–17 μm, with 14–22 merozoites (9–17 × 2–4 μm), 3G: 16–27 × 13–27 μm with 14–28 merozoites (12–19 × 2.4 μm)	Microgamonts: 17–34 × 14–22 μm Microgametes: 2.5–4.4 × 0.6–1 μm, two flagella Macrogametes: 14–23 × 9–16 μm
E. spinosa	Small intestine	3	Schizonts: 8–10 μm, around 20 merozoites (4–6 × 1–1.5 μm)	Microgamonts: 6–8 μm, microgametes 3 μm Macrogamont: 7–9 μm, macrogametes 10–12 μm

Source: Data compiled from Pellérdy, L.P. 1974. *Coccidia and Coccidiosis.* 2nd ed., Germany: Parey; Lindsay, D.S. et al. 1980. *J. Parasitol.* 66, 771–779; Matuschka, F.R., Heydorn, A.O. 1980. *Zool. Beitr.* 26, 405–476; Harleman, J.H., Meyer, R.C. 1983. *Vet. Quart.* 5, 178–185; Harleman, J.H., Meyer, R.C. 1984. *Vet. Parasitol.* 17, 27–39; Ernst, J.V. et al. 1986. *Vet. Parasitol.* 22, 1–8; Eckert, J. et al. 1995. In Eckert, J., Braun, R., Shirley, M.W., and Coudert, P. (Ed.), *COST Biotechnology—Guidelineson Techniques in Coccidiosis Research.* European Commission Directorate-General XII Science, Research and Development: Agriculture Biotechnology. Luxembourg, 103–119; Daugschies, A. 2006. Protozoeninfektionen des Schweines. In Schnieder, T. (Ed.), *Veterinärmedizinische Parasitologie.* Berlin, Germany: Parey, 6th ed., 359–368.

Abbreviations: OR, oocyst residuum; SR, sporocyst residuum; 1G, first-generation schizonts; 2G, second-generation schizonts; 3G, third-generation schizonts.

Table 11.2 Prevalences of *Eimeria* spp. in Pigs (Larger Studies Selected from Recent Literature, Only Reports Differentiating the Species)

Country	Examined Population	*Eimeria* Species Found, Infection Rates	Reference
China	779 litters (1–4 weeks) 80 herds	*E. debliecki* (46.9% of litters) *E. suis* (20.8%) *E. polita* (13.9%) *E. perminuta* (13.9%) *E. scabra* (4.6%) *E. yanglingensis* (1.5%)	Zhang et al.[1890]
India	341 piglets <4 months 228 growers (4–8 months) 227 adults (>8 months)	*Eimeria* spp.[a] 12.9% 7.0% 7.0%	Sharma et al.[1540]
Germany	1204 sows 54 herds	8.6% *Eimeria* spp.[b] 52% *Eimeria* spp.	Daugschies et al.[331]

[a] *E. debliecki, E. neodebliecki, E. perminuta, E. polita, E. porci, E. scabra, E. spinosa, E. suis.*
[b] *E. debliecki, E. polita*: 100%, *E. suis* 84%, *E. scabra* 60%, *E. porci* 52%, *E. perminuta* 49%, *E. spinosa* 20% of samples.

Its role as a primary pathogen was experimentally confirmed later,[1425] and from then on it was frequently used in experimental infections of suckling piglets to study various aspects of the parasite. First described as *Isospora suis*, in 2005, it was moved to the genus *Cystoisospora*.[80]

11.3 PREVALENCE AND DISTRIBUTION

Swine coccidia are ubiquitous. The exact geographical distribution of the species of *Eimeria* is not known,[1343] and only a few studies describe the discrimination of *Eimeria* oocysts by species. As with other domestic ungulate hosts, mixed infections are the rule (Table 11.2). In previous studies, *E. debliecki* and *E. polita* were described as the most common species in Europe (Austria: Supperer[1651]; Switzerland: Indermühle[766]; Germany: Daugschies et al.[331]), while in the United States, *E. neodebliecki* seemed to prevail, and *E. polita* was rare.[1745] *Eimeria* species can occur in all age groups. Weaners, fatteners, and breeding stock, especially sows, appear to be frequently infected; the prevalence rates vary with age, reproductive cycle, and production systems. In China, 12.6% of samples from intensive and 19.7% of samples from extensive swine herds (2971 samples from 14 herds) were positive for *Eimeria*.[936] In Poland 2.6% of 780 litters, 6% of 267 sows, and 11.5% of 104 farms were positive.[860] In Northern Germany, 8.6% of 1204 sows from 54 farms (52% herd prevalence) were positive[331]; in central Germany (southern Hessia), 44.5% of the 110 farms and 12.6% of the 2745 sows excreted *Eimeria* oocysts[318] (Table 11.2).

In suckling piglets, *C. suis* is the most common coccidian.[764,766,1179,1291,1391,1428,1502] Both the endogenous and the exogenous development of *C. suis* is faster than that of any porcine *Eimeria* species (see Table 11.1A for prepatent periods and sporulation times), which favors the fast spreading of *C. suis* within and among litters of suckling piglets in the first 4 weeks of life. In addition, a distinct age resistance

(and probably stable immunity due to constant reinfections) largely prevents oocyst excretion in older animals (see later).

Investigations on the prevalence of *C. suis* revealed a wide distribution of the parasite on the farm level. The first described infections were detected in 1967 (minimal disease herd in the United Kingdom; O'Neill[1257]) and 1974 (Danish SPF herd; Greve[627]). In 1983 the parasite was already known in 14 countries, Austria, Belgium, Canada, England, France, Germany, India, New Zealand, Nigeria, Poland, Russia, Switzerland, the United States, and Yugoslavia (see Harleman and Meyer[675]). In Australia, an early study revealed a farm prevalence of 70%, making *C. suis* the most common enteropathogen in suckling piglets.[400] Studies from Europe revealed a similar picture. Herd prevalences of 50% and more were reported for 12 countries[860,1700] (Table 11.3). In Asia, reports are scarce; a recent study revealed coccidia prevalences of 66% in China in different provinces, with *C. suis* (53% of the farms) being the most prevalent.[1890] From the Americas, only a few recent data are available. In the 1970s–1980s, numerous prevalence studies were conducted in the United States and Canada, mostly in relation to enteral disease. In diarrheic suckling pigs, infection rates ranged between 10% and 21% in studies involving between 749 and 1975 animals.[105,106,509,1207,1485,1486] A more recent study on 50 farms (709 litters) from Canada (Ontario) revealed 70% prevalence on farm level and 26% litter prevalence.[25] Older reports from South and Central America (Brazil, Chile, Cuba), Asia (Korea, Singapore, India, Japan), Africa (Zimbabwe), and Oceania (Australia, Papua New Guinea) from the 1980s and 1990s confirm the presence of coccidia in pigs, especially *C. suis* in suckling piglets.[22,207,211,260,400,497,856,911,1021,1502,1732]

Although detailed longitudinal studies over time are missing, it does not seem that *C. suis* prevalences have significantly decreased over the last 20–30 years despite the introduction of highly effective hygiene management and chemotherapeutics (see Section 11.9).

Table 11.3   Prevalence of *Cystoisospora suis* in Pigs (Larger Studies Selected from Recent Literature)

Country	Examined Population	Infection Rates	Reference
Austria	32 farms Suckling piglets	100%	Mundt et al.[1214]
Belgium	10 farms 10 litters/farm	40% 6% (0–50%)	Maes et al.[1112]
Canada	50 farms 709 litters	70% 26.4%	Aliaga-Leyton et al.[25]
China	80 farms 779 litters, 1–4 weeks	52.5% 63.9%	Zhang et al.[1890]
China (Chongqing)	14 farms 2971 pigs 160 breeding boars 605 breeding sows 916 fatteners 972 growers 318 weaners	(Overall, 6.1% in intensive and 5.0% in extensive herds) 5.6% 4.8% 4.1% 4.2% 10.1%	Lai et al.[936]
Czech Republic	8 farms 2996 litters (2–7 days)	24%	Hamadejova and Vítovec[657]
Germany	53 farms 1204 sows	18.5% 1%	Daugschies et al.[331]
Germany	18 farms 327 litters	83% 42%	Niestrath et al.[1240]
Germany	111 farms 2745 sows	0%	Damriyasa[318]
Germany	71 farms Suckling piglets	65.9%	Mundt et al.[1214]
Poland	780 litters 104 farms 267 sows	27.8% 66.7% 6.7%	Karamon et al.[860]
Switzerland	9 farms Suckling piglets	69.2%	Mundt et al.[1214]
Switzerland	74 farms 125 animals 39 suckling piglets 60 weaners 26 fatteners	8.1% 8.8% 12.8% 6.7% 7.7%	Schubnell et al.[1519]

11.4 MORPHOLOGY AND LIFE CYCLE

Oocysts of porcine *Eimeria* spp. can readily be discerned morphologically (Table 11.1A), and this was also used to develop an algorithm for semiautomated differentiation of porcine *Eimeria* species.[330,1360] *C. suis* oocysts are characterized by the lack of a Stieda body and their spherical shape. Upon sporulation, the two sporocysts allow for easy discrimination from *Eimeria*, even for less-experienced examiners (Figure 11.1). Occasionally, the formation of two sporocysts within *C. suis* oocysts can already be noticed upon fecal examination, which can aid the diagnosis.[1040]

Endogenous stages have not been described for all *Eimeria* species. *E. debliecki* and *E. polita* have two and *E. scabra* and *E. spinosa* have three schizogonic generations. Micro- and macrogamonts have been described (Table 11.1B). For *E. neodebliecki*, *E. perminuta*, *E. porci*, and *E. suis*, no information on endogenous stages is available. Asexual development of *C. suis* is not characterized by generations but by types of stages subsequently arising that

can be discerned by their size and number of nuclei.[1051,1155] Transmission electron microscopic analysis of *in vitro* cultured merozoites of *C. suis* showed intracellular structures like those of other apicomplexan parasites.

Upon ingestion of oocysts, infection is initiated for both *Eimeria* spp. and *C. suis*. Sporozoites subsequently released in the intestinal tracts invade primarily enterocytes of the small intestines; predilection sites depend on species and stage of development. Information on asexual and sexual is summarized in Table 11.1B. Compared with the asexual cycle, gamogony is generally more synchronized, and rapid.[1764]

The endogenous development of *C. suis* is very rapid with a prepatent period as short as 3.5 days[1751] but is commonly 5 days (Table 11.1). This enables infection of the villous epithelium despite the rapid cell turnover in the intestine.[615] Unsporulated oocysts are excreted in both *Eimeria* and *C. suis* infections, and sporulation takes place in the environment. Table 11.1A gives an overview on the published sporulation times, but variations have been reported

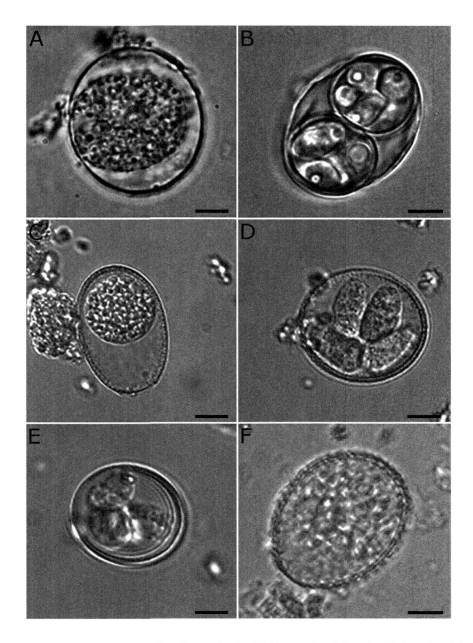

Figure 11.1 Oocysts of *Cystoisospora suis* and *Eimeria* spp. in pig. (A) Unsporulated *C. suis*. (B) Sporulated *C. suis*. (C) *E. scraba*. (Ɔ) *E. polita*. (E) *E. debliecki*. (F) *E. spinosa*. Bar in all figures = 20 μm.

(compiled by Meyer[1180]; Ernst et al.[502]) and may be due to different temperature profiles, as the different publications do not always state the exact conditions for sporulation *in vitro*. It is worth noting that *Eimeria* spp. require 5 days or more to sporulate, while *C. suis* can sporulate in 12 (24–48) hours (Figure 11.2A through H) under suitable conditions prevailing in a farrowing unit.[502,1039,1155,1630] *C. suis* seems to be able to tolerate higher temperatures greater than 30°C for sporulation compared to *Eimeria* spp. but does not sporulate at temperatures greater than 37°C–40°C.[1039,1630] Fast sporulation time in combination with pig behavior, i.e., coprophagy, promotes the spread of the parasite within a litter.[844]

The duration of oocyst shedding varies among species. For porcine *Eimeria* spp., patent periods of 5–11 days have been described.[1432,1433,1754,1792] *C. suis* excretion can be as short as 1 day,[1218] with an average of 2.25 to 3.06 days in different infection models with high variability, independent of the infection dose or the age of the piglets.[826] When excretion of *C. suis* is monitored, a second period of shedding can be observed around 10 days after the onset of oocyst discharge (see Section 11.4.1).

Eimeria stages are confined to the intestines. Only a single report describes gamonts and oocysts in the bile ducts of pigs experimentally infected with *E. debliecki*.[363] For other

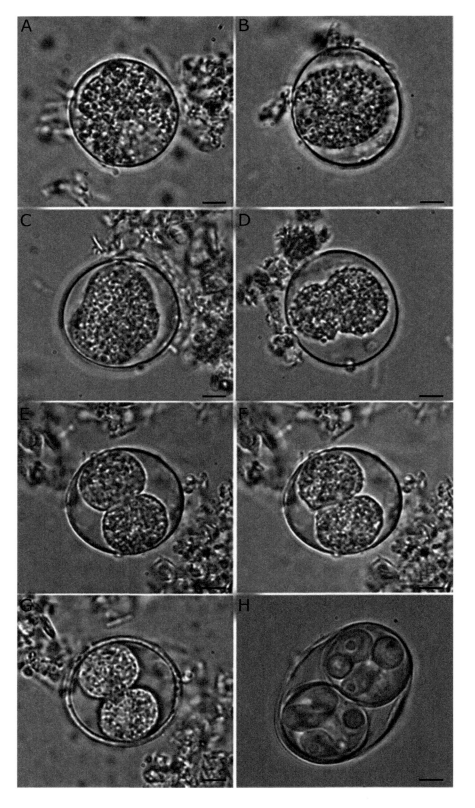

Figure 11.2 Sporulation of *Cystoisospora suis*. Unsporulated oocyst contains a uninucleate sporont (A and B) that undergoes a series of nuclear divisions resulting in two uninucleate sporoblasts (C–G), and subsequently in two sporocysts each containing four sporozoites (H). Bar in all figures = 20 μm.

species of *Eimeria*, extraintestinal stages were not found (*E. polita*; Koudela and Vítovec[914]) or not investigated.

11.4.1 Extraintestinal Stages and Search for Tissue Cysts of *Cystoisospora suis*

As per definition of the genus, *Cystoisospora*, a tissue cyst is expected in members of this genus. The ability of *C. suis* to form extraintestinal stages has not been unequivocally demonstrated. In one report, intraperitoneal inoculation of homogenates of liver, spleen, and intestinal lymph nodes from piglets resulted in the discharge of *C. suis* oocysts 10–11 days later; the donor piglets were dosed with high numbers of oocysts, and the extraintestinal tissues were harvested 24 and 48 hours later. From these results, the authors proposed the extraintestinal stages in the life cycle of *C. suis*.[676] However, other studies could not detect extraintestinal stages in mice or pigs fed *C. suis* oocysts, and so far, their presence in pigs is limited to molecular detection of parasite DNA in tissue except for gamonts and oocysts in Peyer's patches.[1357,1569,1628,1750] The authors argued that other *Cystoisospora* species also develop as monozoic tissue cysts in nonintestinal organs, both in definitive and paratenic hosts, which are difficult to detect, and that *C. suis* displays a biphasic oocyst excretion that may be due to two rounds of the endogenous cycle.[676] This cycle is too short to be attributable to reinfection with merogony 3–4 days and 8–10 days post-inoculation (DPI), followed by gamogony (5 and 11–14 DPI) and oocyst excretion (Figure 11.3). Re-excretion of

oocysts after weaning was also attributed to the reactivation of dormant extraintestinal stages.[1242]

One can argue that these findings of the observed long prepatent period of 10–11 days, compared to 5 days in piglets infected with oocysts,[676] contrast with findings in *C. felis* of cats where the prepatent period is shorter (4 days) when cats are infected with tissue cysts compared to oocysts (7 days; Dubey[421]). Arguably, the presence of dormant tissue stages is of high importance for the epidemiology of the parasite, but conclusive evidence is lacking.

11.5 CLINICAL SIGNS AND LESIONS

Eimeria species of pigs parasitize the small intestine (Table 11.1). Their distribution varies with species, developmental stage, and infection dose. Most species are considered only mildly pathogenic because they mostly parasitize the superficial epithelia; however, animals reared coccidia-free succumbed to infection after transfer to a contaminated environment.[704] An exception is *E. debliecki*, which leads to degradation of host cells shortly after invasion of the lamina propria and the submucosa.[141] *E. debliecki* infections leading to diarrhea, anorexia, and even death have been described in weaners and fatteners with corresponding pathological changes like edema and hemorrhages of the intestinal wall[141,1254]; however, this could not be reproduced.[1870a] High doses of *E. debliecki* did not induce clinical disease in suckling piglets,[1752] in contrast to *C. suis* that can cause clinical

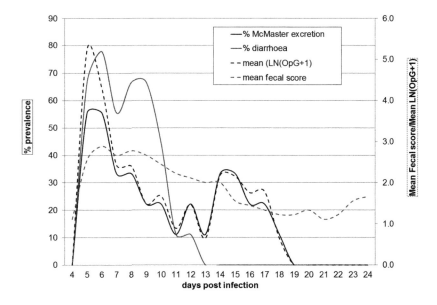

Figure 11.3 Course of oocyst excretion and diarrhea after experimental *Cystoisospora suis* infection of piglets (*n* = 9) on the fourth day of life. Oocyst excretion (black lines: full line, mean prevalence of McMaster-countable excretion; broken line, mean LN[OPG + 1]) follows a biphasic pattern, while diarrhea is seen mostly during the first peak of excretion and the fecal consistency (given as fecal scores 1–4 with 3 and 4 as diarrhea[822]) reaches normal values after that (gray lines: full line, diarrhea prevalence; broken line, average fecal score). (Adapted from Joachim, A. et al., 2014. *Parasitol. Res.* 113, 1863–1873.)

disease in neonatal piglets, even in low doses.[826] *E. sca-bra* infections can lead to diarrhea and anorexia with signs of nonhemorrhagic (rarely hemorrhagic) enteritis.[1433,1754] Natural infections with fatal outcome have been described for *E. scabra*[719] and for *E. spinosa*.[1049] Experimental *E. spinosa* infections caused diarrhea and death in weaners,[1798] but like for *E. debliecki*, this could not be reproduced by other authors.[914] Evident differences during experimental infections of pigs with *Eimeria* spp. may be attributable not only to the parasite species but also to infection dose, parasite strain, age of the animals, and accompanying enteropathogens. It seems that suckling piglets are less susceptible to clinical disease upon experimental infection than weaners.[914,1432,1752]

C. suis is the most important parasitic enteropathogen of suckling piglets.[210,832,1465,1519] In susceptible pigs, it causes nonhemorrhagic diarrhea of pasty to watery (typically "after-sun lotion") consistency and whitish-gray to yellow color (Figure 11.4), which is unresponsive to most antibiotic treatments.[1036,1042,1155,1216,1291,1488] Some authors describe

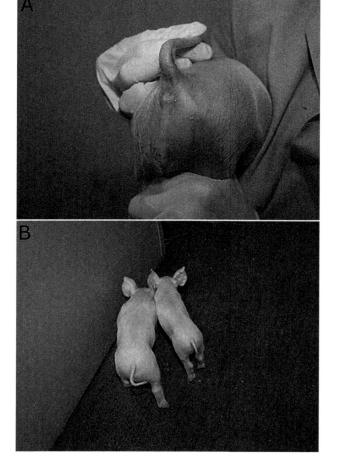

Figure 11.4 Clinical hallmarks of cystoisosporosis. (A) Characteristic watery-to-pasty yellowish diarrhea. (B) Uneven weaning weights in littermates.

a frothy appearance of the feces[1488], and after experimental infection with very high doses, heavy diarrhea with blood and tissue in feces was observed.[1155,1630] Not all piglets of the same litter and in different litters of the same herd are equally affected.[917,1036,1042,1133,1179,1216,1632] Due to the high performance of modern pig production, however, diarrhea in young piglets is receiving much attention as a factor influencing productivity at later phases of life, and even subclinical cystoisosporosis is now recognized as an economically important issue.[1112] The reduced weight gain is the economically most important result of *C. suis* infection and can occur with or without diarrhea.[400,1042,1218,1420,1485]

The clinical outcome of cystoisosporosis in pigs is strongly age-dependent. Piglets younger than 1 week are most severely affected, while older animals are only mildly diseased or show no clinical signs[826,912,913,1033,1042,1629,1819]—as for every rule, however, exceptions have been noted: weaned piglets can also succumb to infection, probably due to contributing factors such as weaning stress or concurrent viral infections.[83,140,627,1242] In parallel to clinical signs, the highest prevalences of oocyst excretion are usually observed in suckling piglets less than 3 weeks of age.[312,400,844,915,916,1031, 1036, 1133,1135,1179,1206,1391,1425, 1485,1488,1502,1628,1630–1632] Rarely, later time periods are reported.[1240,1292] *C. suis* oocyst shedding by older pigs has been observed but is not accompanied by clinical illness, and excretion rates are low.[140,318,331,719,1179,1242,1424,1732]

The small intestines of affected piglets are edematous and filled with yellow, smelly fluid. Lymph nodes are frequently enlarged, and tissue of Peyer's patches can be hyperplastic. The most prominent microscopic lesions include atrophy, fusion, and necrosis of the villi in the small intestines (mostly the medial and distal jejunum), accompanied by crypt hyperplasia (Figure 11.5C). The desquamation of the intestinal lining can be extensive despite low numbers of parasites; villous atrophy and fusion can persist for up to 2 weeks after infection until the epithelial integrity is fully restored and inflammation of the underlying lamina propria is cleared.[312,677,1155,1218,1219,1240,1630,1750,1751] The comparatively strong pathogenic effect of *C. suis* was also attributed to the ability of type I merozoites to penetrate cells several times during their development as demonstrated *in vitro*.[1037] Both meronts and gamonts are responsible for lesions.[1240] Malabsorption caused by the intestinal alteration leads to a significant reduction of weight gain and even emaciation in affected animals.[823,826,1042,1218,1519] It may be due to the relatively slow regeneration of the intestinal epithelium in suckling piglets that causes prolonged stunting of the villi resulting in reduced absorption of nutrients.[715,1216] The pathogenesis is unclear since *C. suis* primarily resides in the villi and not the crypt epithelium, unlike other coccidia that cause prolonged villous damage and atrophy (Figure 11.5C).[715,1425]

Early experimental studies (refer to Table 11.5 for an overview on experimental infections) used very high doses of 200,000 oocysts and more to induce clinical disease.[913,1631]

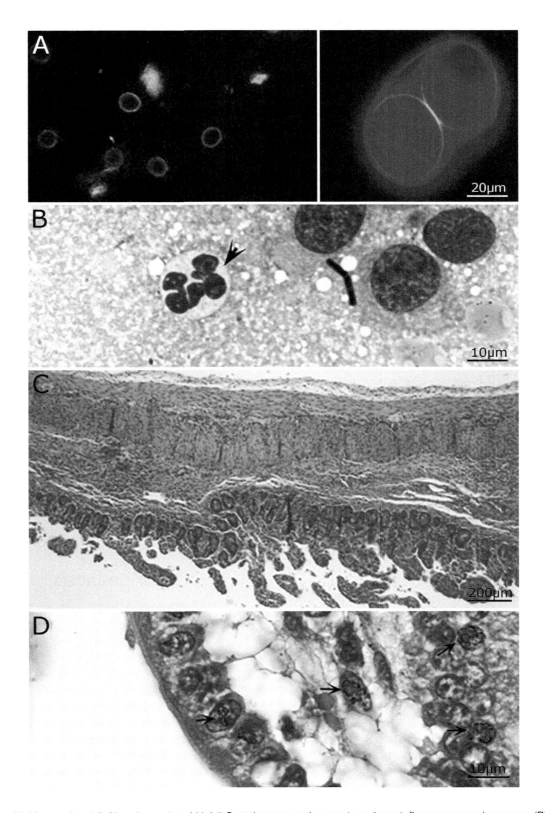

Figure 11.5   (A) Unsporulated (left) and sporulated (right) *Cystoisospora suis* oocysts under autofluorescence microscopy. (B) Merozoites
in intestinal mucosal smears, Giemsa stain. (C and D) Histological sections of piglet jejunum 5 days postinocuation with
C. suis (hematoxylin and eosin stain). Infection resulted in stunted and atrophied villi (C) with numerous asexual endogenous
stages (arrows, D).

However, it could be shown that doses of 100–1000 oocysts can also cause clinical signs in most piglets in the first 3 days of life.[56,826,827] Although the outcome of infection is determined most likely by a strong litter or genetic influence, differences in strain virulence are conceivable.

In some instances, fibrinous masses or fibrinous to necrotic membranes lining the mucosa of affected piglets are described (see Figure 1.28H, Chapter 1), especially in young animals infected with high doses of oocysts[509,1486,1628,1630,1631]; these may probably be attributable to overgrowth and/or invasion of *Clostridium perfringens* or other opportunistic bacteria.

11.6 INTERACTIONS WITH INTESTINAL MICROBIOTA

Although *C. suis* can cause disease on its own,[677] other intestinal pathogens have been implicated in increased morbidity and mortality of *C. suis* infections.[1630] Especially rotavirus, transmissible gastroenteritis virus, clostridia, and *Escherichia coli* were present in coinfections.[400,1207,1420,1421,1488] Rotavirus coinfections have a synergistic effect, most likely because both pathogens inhabit the same site and induce similar lesions.[1753] However, the exact mode of the influence of coinfections (mutual or one-sided, competitive versus synergistic influence, etc.) is only poorly understood. Lately, a focus has been on the interactions not only between two pathogens but between coccidia and enteral bacterial communities.

Despite the fact that the majority of enteric bacteria reside extracellularly, whereas coccidia cherish primarily an intracellular lifestyle, interactions between intestinal parasites and the gut microbiota have been demonstrated in chickens and mice, indicating that coccidial infection disrupts the microbiome of the gut, and that the resulting dysbiosis (microbial imbalance) can contribute to the clinical and pathological outcome of coccidiosis.[684,749,750,1108] More specifically, in chickens, infections with *Cl. perfringens* and *Eimeria* lead to necrotic enteritis.[33,1710] For porcine *Eimeria* spp. infections, the synergistic effect of dysbiosis has not yet been investigated experimentally. A group of gilts that had been moved from a clean to a dirty environment suffered from necrotic enteritis from what was suspected to be a combination of *Eimeria* infection and an overgrowth of *Cl. perfringens*,[704] but this topic was not pursued further. In *C. suis* infections, early epidemiological studies already showed that while the control of cystoisosporosis in piglets cannot be achieved with antibiotics, adequate chemoprophylaxis with anticoccidials leads to reduced use of antibiotics against bacterial enteropathogens[400,631] but not against other bacterial diseases,[917] indicating that *C. suis* promotes enteric disease caused by bacteria. In suckling piglets, *Cl. perfringens* type A and C (*Cp*A, *Cp*C) and enterotoxigenic (ETEC) or enteropathogenic (EPEC) *E. coli* are considered the main

bacterial enteropathogens. *Cp*C is primarily pathogenic and the cause of neonatal hemorrhagic and necrotic enteritis, whereas *Cp*A and *E. coli* are part of the intestinal microbiota of swine.[1921] Synergistic effects between *C. suis* and virulent *E. coli* could not be demonstrated unambiguously. A recent case report from Japan describes the fatal outcome of coinfection[1150]; however, ETEC or EPEC are not always present in cases of piglet coccidiosis.[207,1207,1620] In contrast, enhancing effects of experimental *C. suis* infections on *Cl. perfringens* are well described, and metaphylactic control of parasite infection can relieve bacterial enteritis.[177] In chickens, it could be shown that mucogenesis (as part of the proinflammatory response to parasite invasion of the gut) induced by infections with *E. maxima* and *E. acervulina* promotes the massive growth of *Cl. perfringens* and α-toxin production with the consequence of necrotic enteritis.[285] It can be assumed that in piglets the pathomechanism is similar and might also explain why younger piglets are often most heavily affected by clinical coccidiosis. During the first days of life, the porcine gut flora is rich in *Cl. perfringens*, which is only later displaced during an increase of microbial diversity.[770] Dysbiosis caused by coccidial enteritis is therefore likely to be more pronounced in the first days of life when only a few bacterial species prevail. Conversely, *C. suis* is not affected by the gut microbiota and develops both in gnotobiotic and conventionalized piglets in the same manner.[676,677,1751]

Interestingly, infection with *C. suis* seems to inhibit the establishment of *Salmonella typhimurium* in the intestines as well as in mesenteric lymph nodes (MLNs) in pigs when parasite infection takes place shortly after bacterial inoculation. However, the mechanism of this interference remained unexplored.[53]

11.7 DIAGNOSIS

Detection of oocysts in the feces of animals is the most widely used method of diagnosis. Porcine *Eimeria* species can readily be differentiated by their morphology (see Table 11.1) and are easily distinguished from *C. suis*. Species-specific features were used to create an algorithm for semiautomated detection and differentiation.[330,1360] In *C. suis* infections, the high fat contents of feces can impair the detection of oocysts due to the formation of grease plugs during floatation, and detection without concentration is preferable. Since unstained oocysts are difficult to detect in light microscopy, different staining methods have been used by various authors,[1031,1135] but by far the most sensitive method for the detection of *C. suis* oocysts in piglet feces is autofluorescence.[329,824,918] This method utilizes the properties of the oocyst (and, in sporulated oocysts, the sporocyst) wall to emit a blue light upon excitation without the use of antibodies or additional staining of the sample (Figure 11.5A), permitting a sensitive diagnosis of oocyst shedding.

For quantification, McMaster protocols adapted to the available amount of fecal matter can be used for counting of *C. suis* oocysts, often with saturated sugar or sugar-salt solutions to reduce the number of lipid bubbles in the counting chamber.[702,1042,1180,1218]

Under practical conditions, the detection of oocysts in single samples from an affected herd can be negative because diarrhea and oocyst excretion are only poorly correlated, and oocyst excretion can be as short as 1 day in infected piglets.[1218] Repeated and multiple sampling is therefore necessary for reliable detection of the pathogen.[824] For the decision whether to treat or not, the detection of oocysts in combination of the clinical signs should be considered. If oocysts are excreted despite toltrazuril treatment, this must be evaluated carefully, in single cases animals may simply not have received treatment[917]; however, the occurrence of antiparasitic resistance must be considered (see Section 11.3; Table 11.2).

In postmortem examinations, intestinal stages of *Eimeria* spp. or *C. suis* can be detected in histological sections of the small intestines[715] (Figure 11.5D; Table 11.1B) or in stained impression smears[1616] (Figure 11.5B–D). This method is superior to the detection of oocysts in acute cases (e.g., in the presence of other enteropathogens) when animals succumb to infection without previous shedding of oocysts.[715,1467] Determination of infection as the cause of clinical signs can be achieved when the presence of intestinal stages is accompanied by macroscopical and microscopical signs of tissue damage and even bacterial invasion (see Mundt et al.[1219]).

Conventional polymerase chain reaction (PCR) for the detection of *Eimeria* spp. and *C. suis* is highly sensitive and specific.[825,1466] Recently, a quantitative PCR assay for the detection of *C. suis* was developed.[748] With increased availability of sequence information on different species of *Eimeria* of swine,[1540] multiplex assays may become available for practical use.

Serological detection of *C. suis* antibodies has been developed as indirect fluorescent antibody test (IFAT) or enzyme-linked immunosorbent assay (ELISA) for experimental applications.[1522,1523,1571] Due to the ubiquitous nature of the coccidia, the qualitative detection of specific antibodies is of little diagnostic value for the diagnosis of acute coccidiosis.

11.8 IMMUNITY

Very little is known about the immunity against *Eimeria* of pigs. Early studies assumed that *Eimeria* infections routinely induce a stable immunity primarily directed against early invasive stages (sporozoites).[152] However, the age distribution of infected pigs hints at a rather ephemeral immunity; pigs of all age groups can excrete oocysts of *Eimeria* with high prevalence in sows (see Section 11.3; Table 11.2), indicating that immunity is either very short-lived and wanes quickly or is not protective against reinfection with oocyst shedding. Experimental primary infections of suckling piglets and weaners with *E. scabra* or *E. polita* induced a stable but short-lasting immunity with some cross-immunization effect between the two species[1432] that, once established, could not be influenced by immunosuppressing drugs.[914,1431] In other studies, several rounds of infection induced a low level of immunity or no immunity at all.[124,141] It must be assumed that primary infections with high doses can induce disease at least in the more pathogenic species of *Eimeria* in swine (see earlier) and that constant reinfection leads to a reduced oocyst excretion in adult animals without clinical signs but does not completely suppress oocyst shedding. This is supported by the observation that gilts shed more oocysts than sows.[331]

In contrast to porcine *Eimeria* spp., in *C. suis* infections a strong age influence is observed that is not directly related to acquired immunity. While piglets experimentally infected in the first 3 days of life show significant clinical signs, in older animals this effect quickly declines (see Table 11.5 for an overview).[823,826,912,913,1218,1425,1628] The reasons for this phenomenon are not clear. It may in part be due to the maturation of the immune system of the growing piglet, the changing physiology of the gut, or both.[1817–1819]

Since age resistance and acquired immunity cannot readily be dissected, early studies described the absence of oocyst shedding in previously exposed piglets and concluded that this is due to the development of acquired immunity.[675,1121,1629,1682] However, it is conceivable that this is not the only (and maybe not even the primary) reason for the age restriction of cystoisosporosis in pigs.

It is generally accepted that cellular immunity is more important than humoral immunity for controlling intracellular pathogens. In studies on the immunity against coccidia, this view is supported; especially dendritic cells, cytotoxic T lymphocytes (CTLs) as well as CD4+ T-helper and CD8+ (memory?) T cells are essential. A Th1-driven proinflammatory T-helper cell response involving interleukin (IL)-2, IL-12, interferon (IFN)-γ, and tumor necrosis factor (TNF)-α as cytokines can either directly or indirectly inhibit parasite invasion and replication or promote killing of parasites.[31,139,563,706,1402,1678,1736,1854] When considering the role of the humoral immune system in the acquired immunity against coccidia, however, there is no consensus on the importance of specific antibodies. Their production upon infection has been demonstrated in coccidial infections, but their protective role in parasite elimination is unclear.[510,563,1141,1401,1766] The development of a novel subunit vaccine against avian *Eimeria* spp. has sparked this discussion as it is applied as a maternal vaccine that confers passive protection to broiler chicks, which implies a (direct or indirect) protective role for specific antibodies, either via direct binding to the pathogen or indirectly by stimulation of cell-mediated immune responses.[178,179,1542,1766]

When evaluating the role of the innate and the acquired immune system in the control of *C. suis* infections, species-specific features should be considered. Newborn piglets are agammaglobulinemic and require passive immunization via colostrum from the sow as a first line of defense against pathogens before they can develop active immunity.[1479] This process is delayed as piglets are born with an immature immune system and the intestinal tract is almost void of functional T cells for the first weeks of life.[1204,1614] When considering the early time point of infection under natural conditions, the role of active immunity against *C. suis* must carefully be evaluated. Although immune responses are detectable upon infection as described later, application of immunosuppressive steroids did not induce oocyst excretion upon challenge.[1629] This indicates that protection against reinfection may not only be based on adaptive immunity. In experimental models for porcine cystoisosporosis, both the peripheral (systemic) and the local cellular immune responses and the expression of effector molecules were investigated in suckling piglets as well as in weaners (Table 11.4). The most significant findings include a decrease of T cells in the periphery and an increase in the mucosa at the site of infection, especially of T-cell receptor-γδ+ (TcR-γδ+) T cells upon infection of young piglets. This implies a shift of these cells from the periphery to the site of infection and their involvement in the immune response to the parasite.[568,1816] Four days after infection, a relative increase of TcR-γδ+ T cells was observed in the mucosa (with a simultaneous decrease in MLNs). Cells of this phenotype make up a large proportion of total peripheral lymphocytes in swine but are only present in low numbers in the gut mucosa of healthy pigs. They are supposed to be involved in protection against

both intra- and extracellular pathogens and are, among others, important producers of IFN-γ, TNF-α, and IL-17.[1527] TNF-α was also increased in jejunal mucosa of infected piglets and weaners.[561,568] Blood-derived lymphocytes of *C. suis* infected and reinfected weaners could be stimulated by specific antigen to produce proinflammatory IFN-γ, but the fraction of stimulated cells was too small for further phenotyping.[1820] By contrast, a weak systemic cytokine response of peripheral blood mononuclear cells (PBMCs) could be observed upon stimulation with *C. suis* recombinant antigen with increased anti-inflammatory IL-4, IL-6, and IL-10 but decreased proinflammatory IFN-γ, IL-2, and transforming growth factor beta (TGF-β) in comparison to uninfected controls.[561] A subpopulation of CD4+ T cells in blood that is considered to be of regulatory function was decreased in *primo* infected piglets 1 week after infection.[568,1816]

Other cells and factors possibly involved in the immune reaction to *C. suis* include cytotoxic T lymphocytes (CTLs) that were increased in the small intestines of *C. suis*–infected piglets 9–15 DPI after they had previously expanded in the MLNs. The expression levels of TNF-α were also increased in the acute phase 4 days after infection.[568] TNF-α is a proinflammatory cytokine and may act as an activator for specific cellular immune responses to *C. suis*, but it also induces mucin production in enteric infections. In addition, expression of toll-like receptor (TLR)-2 and nucleotide-binding oligomerization domain (NOD2) were also increased. TLR-2 had been shown to bind to different protozoan ligands, but the role of NOD2 in protozoal infections is not yet clear.[568] A proinflammatory cascade

Table 11.4   Immune Responses in *Cystoisospora suis*–Infected Piglets

Infection Model	Organ/Tissue	Detection Method	Parameter Change: Cells	Parameter Changes: Cytokines, Receptors	Reference
Suckling piglets, first infection	PBMC, MLN, spleen	Flow cytometry	T cells ↓ (resting Th cells, TcR-γδ+ T cells, Treg)		Worliczek et al.[1816]
	PBMC, MLN		Treg ↓		Gabner et al.[568]
	Spleen		NK cells ↑		Worliczek et al.[1816]
	Spleen		Treg ↑		Gabner et al.[568]
	MLN, Spleen		T cells ↓ (CD4+ T cells, resting Th cells)		Gabner et al.[568]
	MLN		CTL ↑		Gabner et al.[568]
Suckling piglets, first infection	Jejunal mucosa	IHC	γδ+ T cells ↑↑		Worliczek et al.[1816]
			T cells ↑↑, CTL ↑, TcR-γδ+ T cells ↑		Gabner et al.[568]
		qPCR		TLR-2 ↑, NOD2 ↑, TNF-α ↑	Gabner et al.[568]
Weaners, reinfected	PBMC + Ag	ELISpot assay		IFN-γ ↑	Worliczek et al.[1820]
	PBMC + Ag	qPCR, MFI		IL-4 ↑, Il-6 ↑, IL-10 ↑ IFN-γ ↓, IL-2 ↓, TGF-β ↓	Freudenschuss et al.[561]
	MLN +Ag			IL-10 ↑, TNF-α ↑	Freudenschuss et al.[561]
	MLN			IL-12 ↑, IFN-γ ↓	Freudenschuss et al.[561]

Abbreviations: ELISpot, enzyme linked immunospot; IHC, immunohistochemistry; MFI, multiplex fluorescent immunoassay (Luminex); MLN, mesenteric lymph node; PBMC, peripheral blood mononuclear cell; qPCR, quantitative reverse-transcription real-time PCR; +Ag, stimulated with specific *C. suis* antigen; ↑, increased in comparison to uninfected control; ↑↑, strong increase; ↓, decreased in comparison to uninfected control.

initiated by the binding of pathogen-specific molecules to TLR-2 can lead to NOD2 expression, which in turn induces IFN-γ production,[1698] so it seems reasonable that this is also involved in the immune response against *C. suis*.

It seems that immunocompetent weaners show immune reactions to *C. suis*, which include pro- as well as anti-inflammatory components. Lymphocytes derived from the MLNs of immunocompetent weaners experimentally infected with *C. suis* produced IL-12,[561] supporting the concept of a Th1-directed immune response to coccidial infections with IL-12 as a key cytokine.[32,1854] However, IFN-α, but not IFN-γ, was also increased upon stimulation, and unstimulated MLN cells from infected animals already expressed higher levels of IL-10, which drives Th2-directed immune responses,[561] and could induce the proliferation of B cells in the MLNs.[1816]

The humoral responses to infection were addressed under varying aspects. One of the first studies on *C. suis* described that animals in a minimal disease herd appeared to be protected against reinfection when exposed at an early age, and the authors put this down to maternal immunity.[1257] *C. suis*–specific colostral antibodies were shown to be transferred to piglets.[1522,1523,1682] Their role in immunity was refuted in early studies.[56,675,1633,1682] However, in experimental studies, a significant negative association of anti–*C. suis* IgA (and in part also IgG) in the blood and colostrum of sows with the corresponding immunoglobulin serum titers, oocyst shedding, and diarrhea in their experimentally infected offspring could be demonstrated.[1522] In addition, superinfection of sows with high doses of *C. suis* oocysts antepartum led to a marked temporary increase of specific IgG and IgA in blood and milk also associated with amelioration of clinical and parasitological outcome of experimental infection of the piglet, indicating at least partial maternal protection against cystoisosporosis.[1523] Maternal antibodies in piglet serum quickly decline and are only replaced by actively produced immunoglobulins from the third week of life onward,[1522] when they can be detected by IFAT or ELISA.[1522,157] Interestingly, antibody titers not only in colostrum but also in milk were negatively correlated with disease in the piglets, indicating that even after the closure of the intestinal barrier, milk antibodies may retain a local function in the gut. In addition, specific *C. suis* antibodies could also be detected in the intestinal mucus of infected weaners.[561] Their role in the protection against *C. suis*, whether direct – by binding to extracellular (invasive) parasite stages–or indirect – by regulation of the local cellular immune defense, remains to be elucidated.

11.8.1 Role of the Sow in *Cystoisospora suis* Infections

Increased oocyst excretion of oocysts by sows around the time of parturition was described and interpreted to play a primary role for the infection of piglets, and sow treatment was therefore recommended in early studies.[277,675,936,1420]

However, due to the usually rather low infection rates and limited oocyst excretion in sows, this age group is usually not considered to be essential in maintaining the parasite in a litter.[1047,1523,1630] Transmammary or even intrauterine transmission of stages does not appear likely since shortened prepatent periods compared to infections with oocysts have never been observed for *C. suis*, and stages of *C. suis* were not detected by light microscopy in milk or placenta[1630]; however, experimental infections of pregnant sows and examination of their piglets have not been published. Field observations on the population dynamics of *C. suis* did not reveal any obvious influence of the sow on the course of infection in the piglets.[1599] However, *C. suis*-specific antibodies, especially IgA, transferred from the sows to their litters, were correlated with reduced diarrhea and oocyst excretion in experimental infections of the piglets.[1522] Furthermore, increased IgA and IgG titers in blood, colostrum and milk after superinfection of sows with high doses of *C. suis* antepartum ameliorated the effects of infections of the piglets compared to offspring from uninfected sows.[1523] It can be concluded that sows play a minor role in the transmission but possibly a significant one in conveying maternal immunity in the first weeks of life.

11.9 CONTROL OF PORCINE COCCIDIOSIS

11.9.1 Treatment of Coccidiosis

Treatment of coccidiosis after the onset of clinical signs is futile, since damage to intestinal epithelium has already taken place. Prevention and control are therefore of paramount importance to minimize the impact of coccidiosis in the pig farming industry. Successful control of porcine coccidiosis on a farm can be achieved by minimizing the source of infection by combined approaches of chemotherapy and strict sanitation and disinfection.[1630]

In the past, only a few works have reported treatment of *Eimeria*-associated enteritis in weaned piglets and gilts under natural and experimental conditions.[704,1049,1752] In sow feed, it used to be common to mix amprolium at 20 mg/kg in 2 weeks pre- and postfarrowing to control oocyst shedding of *Eimeria* spp.[597] Buquinolate at 330 mg/kg feed and sulfaguanidine at 0.22 g/kg body weight were also shown to diminish oocyst production in pigs infected with mixed *Eimeria* infections.[26,1280] However, *Eimeria* infection in pigs is seldom pathogenic; thus, therapeutic interventions are usually unwarranted.[331,1034]

For the control of piglet cystoisosporosis, treatment options are limited. Farrowing units contaminated with oocysts from previous litters are the main source of infection. The addition of anticoccidials in feed or drinking water is no option as suckling piglets do not eat or drink sufficiently to attain proper dosing. Since piglets must be handled individually for dosing, anticoccidials should be cost-effective and have minimum treatment frequencies to make treatment attractive and feasible even on large farms. A wide variety of anticoccidial drugs have been introduced and tested experimentally since the 1970s for treatment of piglet coccidiosis. However, for effectiveness, most drugs must be administered at the time of exposure or shortly thereafter.

For an overview on experimental infections to evaluate treatment efficacy, see Table 11.5. The prophylactic use of chlortetracycline in combination with sulfamethazine and penicillin at 375 mg/kg feed and lincomycin hydrochloride at 330 mg/kg feed were described as effective as coccidiostat against *C. suis*.[1280] The use of these antibiotics in the feed of weaned piglets resulted in decreased oocyst output and improved body weights. The antibiotics appeared to retard the process of schizogony, but it was difficult to pinpoint whether these therapeutic effects were solely due to specific inhibition of *C. suis* or due to control of secondary bacterial pathogens.

Amprolium has been widely used as coccidiostat in farm animals and birds. Piglets treated with 2 mL of amprolium hydrochloride (9.6%) solution orally for 5 days after farrowing comparatively had lower oocyst output and slightly improved body weights compared to untreated animals. However, treatment did not have any effect on occurrence of diarrhea.[597]

Quinolines are thought to block the mitochondrial respiratory chain in coccidian species and prevent development of first-generation meronts.[42,564,1772,1800] The quinoline decoquinate in combination with amprolium given to sows at 1 kg/ton of feed for 3 weeks pre- and postfarrowing reduced the incidence of neonatal diarrhea in their piglets.[123,1486] Halofuginone, a natural quinazolinone alkaloid, used as coccidiostat at 6 mg/kg of feed in early weaned piglets experimentally infected with *C. suis* inhibited oocyst excretion but resulted in reduced weight gain due to poor feed intake.[1156]

Ionophores such as monensin and lasalocid have been used in sow feed 1 week before and after entry to the farrowing unit to control cystoisosporosis in litters.[1419] However, monensin failed to prevent diarrhea, oocyst output, and intestinal lesions caused by *C. suis* in piglets when used at 15 mg/kg/day, every alternate day, for 9 days.[398] Early weaned piglets infected with *C. suis* and fed lasalocid incorporated feed at 150 mg/kg excreted oocysts throughout the patent period although there was no difference in the body weight gain between infected and control piglets. These piglets, however, seemed to develop strong immunity to reinfection with *C. suis*.[1156]

The nitrofuran derivatives furazolidone and nitrofurazone have been used as coccidiostats in chickens and goats.[741,1677] Preventive therapy of suckling piglets with 1 mL furazolidone for 3 days after infection with *C. suis* and then every other day for 6 days delayed the appearance of clinical signs but failed to reduce oocyst excretion, occurrence of diarrhea, and intestinal lesions.[597] Additionally, the use of nitrofuran derivatives is restricted in many countries owing to persistent residues as well as mutagenic and carcinogenic effects.[159,1157]

Sulfonamides were the first synthetic anticoccidials used successfully for prevention and control of coccidiosis in farm animals including chicken. They interfere with the ability of coccidia to utilize folic acid and thereby block parasite replication.[115] Coccidiostatic activity of sulfonamide and its derivatives was established as early as 1940 when it was found to be effective against coccidiosis in chickens, cattle, sheep, and calves.[148,550,663,982] However, only limited information is available about their efficacy against *C. suis* in piglets. Oral formulation of sulfonamides (sulfadimidine and sulfamethoxypyrimidine) administered orally for 3–7 days following infection with *C. suis* in suckling piglets had no effect on the reduction of oocyst excretion and diarrhea.[823,1219] An injectable formulation of sulfamethoxypyrimidine administered repeatedly for 6–7 days following infection efficiently reduced oocyst excretion and occurrence of diarrhea, while short-term treatments, either during early prepatency or after the onset of excretion, had no effect on clinical and parasitological outcomes of infection.[823] However, the use of injectable sulfonamides seems to be impractical as preventive therapy against cystoisosporosis owing to multiple animal handling, labor-intensiveness, and the risk of development of resistance.[823]

The triazinone derivative toltrazuril was used as a coccidiocidal drug in chickens and turkeys before it was introduced for use against cystoisosporosis in piglets (see Chapter 6). Toltrazuril is a highly effective broad-spectrum anticoccidial drug active against both sexual and asexual stages of coccidia, including *E. debliecki, E. perminuta, E. spinosa,* and *C. suis*.[651] The exact mode of action of toltrazuril is not clear, but light and electron microscopic studies suggested that it interferes with protozoal nuclear division and mitochondrial activity.[674] In 1991, the prophylactic and therapeutic efficacy of toltrazuril in piglets naturally infected with *C. suis* was reported.[916] A significant reduction of oocyst excretion and occurrence of diarrhea in piglets treated with toltrazuril at 20 mg/kg body weight on 6 and 8 days of life was noted. A single oral dose of toltrazuril at 20 mg/kg body weight was effective in suppressing oocyst excretion and diarrhea in piglets experimentally infected with *C. suis*[54,400,1111,1216] and under field conditions.[9,7,1361,1507,1581] The first commercial use of toltrazuril in piglets started in the year 1998 under the trade name of Baycox (5% toltrazuril), which is the first and only licensed coccidiocidal drug for the prevention of porcine cystoisosporosis.[1171] At present, several generic toltrazuril products have been approved for use in piglets as prophylactic treatment against porcine cystoisosporosis. In addition, injectable formulations of toltrazuril have been tested and reported to be as effective as the oral application in preventing cystoisosporosis.[827] Another compound of the same triazinone group, diclazuril, however, was ineffective in preventing clinical signs and

Table 11.5 Studies Employing Experimental Infections with *Cystoisospora suis*

Number of Piglets (If Not Stated Otherwise)	Age Upon Infection (days)	Infection Dose/Animal	Course of Infection		Other Observations	Reference
			Clinical and Parasitological Outcome	Pathohistological Observations		
10	1	1.5–2×10^5	Killed 12 hours to 7 DPI or 8–14 DPI (higher dose).	Developmental stages throughout the small intestine.	No extraintestinal stages.	Lindsay et al.[1051]
5 litters, 6–9 piglets each	Litters 1: 2; Litters 3–5: 1	Litter 1: 3×10^3; Litter 2: 10^4; Litters 3: 1.5×10^5; Litter 4: 2×10^5; Litter 5: 4–10^5	Litters 1, 2: mild diarrhea. Litters 3, 4: diarrhea from 72 Litter 4: lethargy, emaciation, diarrhea. Litter 5: Severe clinic, 10 piglets died or had to be euthanized.	Litters 1, 2: no stages, mild lesions. Litter 4, 5: NE, pronounced VA and VN.		Stuart et al.[1631]
Group I: 26 + 6; Group II: 27 + 6; Group III: 13 + 11; Group IV: 5 (71 infected, 23 uninfected)	I: 1; II: 3; III: 2 weeks; IV: 4–6 weeks	I: 2–4×10^5; II: 2–4×10^5; III: 4×10^5; IV: 1–2×10^6	Group I: severe diarrhea, high mortality (up to 70%). Group II: yellow diarrhea for 2–4 days, weight loss, dehydration. Two piglets comatose 7 and 10 DPI with very high OPG (758,000). Group III: mild to moderate diarrhea for 3–4 DPI for 4–6 days. OPG up to 160,044. Group IV: mild diarrhea, mean OPG: 50,000.	Severe NE in groups I and II. Severe VA in group II, mild to moderate in group III and mild in group IV.	Strong age relation of diarrhea and excretion, crowding effect with high infection doses.	Stuart et al.[1628]
56; 7; 7; 20	14–28; 0.5–1; 18–21; 21 (10 challenged 6 weeks later)	1×10^4–10^6	Prepatent period 132–144 hours, patency 10–18 days, two peaks of excretion 1–3 and 7–9 of patency. Inoculation with high doses caused vomiting. Piglets infected at 21 days all survived; newborns died within 3–5 days. Anorexia 3–7 DPI, heavy diarrhea from 3 DPI for 3–4 days or longer/intermittent, in two peaks. Loss of fluid, reduced body weight gain, reduced feed conversion in weaners.	Sacrifice 24–168 hours postinfection; catarrhalic to hemorrhagic enteritis, stages only in small intestines. Description of endogenous development.	No extraintestinal stages.	Matuschka and Heydorn[1155]
28 SPF piglets, artificially reared	3	5×10^4–1×10^5	Diarrhea in 78.6% of the animals from 4–6 DPI. 82% of piglets: anorexia, depression, dehydration, growth retardation. Oocyst excretion in 80% of piglets 4 DPI. Max. OPG: 558,000.	VA and sexual stages peaked 4 DPI.		Robinson et al.[1425]
21 (gnotobiotic)	2	2.4×10^5 (eight piglets conventionalized second–third DOL); four germ-free and four conventionalized uninfected controls	Excretion 5–9 and 11–14 DPI, peak 5–6 DPI, patent period max. 3 days in most piglets.	3–14 DPI: detailed description of stages. Most stages in distal half of the small intestine.	Two piglets infected with high doses and killed 24/48 hours later; no extraintestinal stages in different organs.	Harleman and Meyer[676]
10 (gnotobiotic)	15–23	2.1×10^5 (six piglets conventionalized); two germ-free and two conventionalized uninfected controls	Excretion and diarrhea biphasic in both groups (see Harleman and Meyer[676]).	VA and VN 4–6 and 8–12 DPI.	Adding bacteria does not alter the course of infection or histopathology.	Harleman and Meyer[677]
49 (51 uninfected controls)	3	3×10^5	Diarrhea 3–5 DPI, watery 1–2 days after onset, duration 6–10 days, 20.4% mortality, loss of condition, significantly reduced weight gain.	VA.		Lindsay et al.[1042]
6 (feral piglets, 1 litter)	3	1.5×10^4–1×10^5	Diarrhea 4–10 (12) DPI.	VA, sexual stages in impression smears.	Feral pigs are susceptible to *C. suis*.	Lindsay et al.[1042]
6 minipigs + 4 conventional	7 (minipigs), 5 (conventional)	1×10^5	Oocyst excretion 6–10 (11) DPI with peak on 6–7 DPI. Diarrhea 5–8 (10) DPI.	VA in both groups.	No difference between conventional and miniature pigs.	Blagburn et al.[129]
47	4–11	1×10^2–5×10^4	Excretion 5–7 DPI, patency 8–16 DPI in 2–3 peaks, low infection dose: higher excretion in the second peak, third peak visible, higher doses: in the first peak, third peak not distinct.	n.d.		Christensen and Henriksen[288]

(Continued)

Table 11.5 (Continued)   Studies Employing Experimental Infections with Cystoisospora suis

Number of Piglets (If Not Stated Otherwise)	Age Upon Infection (days)	Infection Dose/Animal	Clinical and Parasitological Outcome	Pathohistological Observations	Other Observations	Reference
4	5	1×10^3–6.6×10^4	Diarrhea 6–14 DPI, prepatent period 6–9 days, excretion 3–10 days, two peaks.	No alteration 21 DPI in epithelial cells.		Sayd and Kawazoe[1503]
50	3	1×10^4	Oocyst shedding from 5 DPI, second lower peak 10 DPI. Max. OPG 251,501. Excretion for 5–6 days in most animals, highly variable. Diarrhea peak 6 DPI, duration 1–3 days in most animals; watery diarrhea in 25% of infected animals 4 DPI. Diarrhea and weight gain negatively correlated. Body weight gain markedly reduced from 14 DOL compared to 17 uninfected control animals. Fecal score correlated negatively with OPG on the same day but positively with the OPG the following day.	VN followed by VA; VA still present 14 DPI.		Mundt et al.[1218]
9 25 40 50	1 4 4 4	1×10^3 1×10^3 1.5×10^3 1×10^4	Weight depression and watery diarrhea most prominent after early infection. Higher doses lead to earlier excretion peaks but early infection correlated with higher excretion rates.	n.d.	Strong age effect.	Worliczek et al.[1819]
52 93 20 8	4 4 1 4	1×10^3 1.5×10^3 1×10^3 5×10^3	Acute phase 5–9 DPI: 2.2–2.9 days (out of six) with diarrhea (80%–95% of piglets), 2.3–3.1 days of excretion. Steep increase in excretion 5 DPI, drop on eighth DPI, second peak 12–16 DPI. Second excretion peak lower in all models, most pronounced in model with 1.5×10^3 oocysts/fourth DOL. Highest excretion rates in infections on the first DOL.	n.d.	No influence of infection time point or age at infection. No difference between small and large litters. No breed influence. OPG values higher in samples of firmer faces. Diarrhea onset more sudden in models with higher infection doses.	Joachim et al.[826]

Course of Infection/Immunity

Number of Piglets (If Not Stated Otherwise)	Age Upon Infection (days)	Infection Dose/Animal	Clinical and Parasitological Outcome	Pathohistological Observations	Other Observations	Reference
(a) 8 (pre-exposed between 14 and 35 DOL) (b) 13 (4 piglets in each group treated with steroid before second challenge)	(a) 12–30 Second challenge 16–28 days later (b) 19–31	(a) First challenge: 2–4×10^5 Second challenge: 4×10^5–2×10^6 (b) Initial infection: 5×10^4–4×10^5 First and second challenges: 2–4×10^5 (1 animal: 2×10^6)	Piglets challenged 1–2× after natural exposure (a) or experimental infection (b). Challenge induced only low OPG (<2000), while *primo* infection at the age of 14 days resulted in mean excretion for 4.4 days and mean OPG of 127,254. Second challenge leads to excretion for 2 days in one piglet.	n.d.	Steroids after second challenge had no effect on re-shedding.	Stuart et al.[1629]

Immunology/Immunity

Number of Piglets (If Not Stated Otherwise)	Age Upon Infection (days)	Infection Dose/Animal	Clinical and Parasitological Outcome	Pathohistological Observations	Other Observations	Reference
No details given	No details given		First infection induces massive shedding which is greatly decreased in reinfections.	n.d.		Biester and Schwarte[124]
4 sows 88 piglets	2×/week from 10 weeks antepartum 2	Each dose: 1×10^5 8.2×10^4	Diarrhea 5–7 DPI in 79% of piglets from superinfected sows, 89% of piglets from control sows. Oocyst excretion in 60%–100% of the piglets, peak 5–7 DPI, 10^5 OPG. Reduction in mean daily weight gain from 5 DPI. From the 12th DOL mean daily weight gain higher in piglets from superinfected sows.	n.d.	No maternal immunity observed.	Baekbo et al.[56]

(Continued)

Table 11.5 (Continued) Studies Employing Experimental Infections with *Cystoisospora suis*

Number of Piglets (If Not Stated Otherwise)	Age Upon Infection (days)	Infection Dose/Animal	Clinical and Parasitological Outcome	Pathohistological Observations	Other Observations	Reference
11 10 11	3 19 3+19	2×10^5	Early infection: excretion from 5 DPI in all animals (max OPG 223,400, DPI 7), lithiasic excretion. Diarrhea from 2–4 DPI until 10–11 DPI. Hairy, dirty, smelly piglets. (Re-) challenge: prepatent period 5 days, lower prevalence (60%), max OPG 23,700, no cyclic pattern, pasty feces 3–5 DPI. Birth weights reduced in all infected groups after 5 weeks, especially in double infections. Weight depression lower in animals inoculated only at 19 DOL.	n.d.	Nonacquired immunity important for susceptibility/resistance (age-resistance). Maternal immunity not important.	Koudela and Kučerová[912,913]
34 (15 infected, 19 uninfected)	3	10^3	Excretion 5–15 DPI, diarrhea 6–10 DPI.	n.d.	Infection led to significant reduction in leukocyte and lymphocyte counts compared to uninfected controls.	Worliczek et al.[1816]
12 uninfected and 14 infected piglets	3	1×10^3	Oocyst excretion 5–18 DPI, max. 5 DPI and 11 DPI. Diarrhea from 5 DPI for max. 4 days in 71% of the piglets. Body weight gain higher in uninfected controls.	n.d.	Transfer of specific maternal anti-*C. suis* antibodies, IgA and IgM for 2–3 weeks in blood, IgG for 6 weeks, active antibody production 2–3 weeks postinfection. Neg. correlation of IgA with OPG but pos. correlation of IgG and IgM with OPG (AUC). Infected animals had higher jejunal Ig titers against merozoites.	Schwarz et al.[1522]
94 (from 12 sows, 6 of them superinfected with 100,000 *C. suis* antepartum)	3	1×10^3	Excretion and diarrhea from 5–6 DPI, peak 6 and 12 DPI for excretion, 8–9 DPI for diarrhea.	n.d.	Piglets nursed by superinfected sows excreted fewer oocysts and had less diarrhea. No effect on weight gain. Neg. correlation of excretion and diarrhea with colostral and serum IgG.	Schwarz et al.[1523]
51 (25 infected, 26 uninfected)	3	1×10^4	Excretion from 5 DPI in two peaks (7 and 12 DPI), diarrhea from 4 DPI, peak 9 DPI.	n.d.	Increase of IgG and IgA in serum and intestinal mucosa upon infection, correlation with oocyst shedding.	Gabner et al.[568]
50, 10/group	10–11 weeks (weaners)	5 groups: uninfected control, 6×10^2 oocysts once, 3×200 oocysts, 6×10^3 oocysts once, 3×2000 oocysts	No clinical presentation, low oocyst excretion in single animals for 1–6 days.	n.d.		Freudenschuss et al.[561]
Coinfections						
5	9	5×10^4	Diarrhea 4–5 DPI, in some cases until 10 DPI, severe.	n.d.	*C. suis* infection inhibits intestinal *Salmonella*.	Baba and Gaafar[63]
42 conventional, 26 gnotobiotic	1–2 (5–6)	$1 \times 10^3 – 2 \times 10^5$	Prepatent period 4.5–5 days (single observation of 3.5 days).	Alterations 3–4 and 8–9 DPI.	Conventional piglets: earlier onset of clinical and histopathological signs and quicker resolution but no quantitative differences.	Vitovec and Koudela[1751]
63 conventional, 51 gnotobiotic (plus 15 and 10 uninfected controls)	1–4	$1–2 \times 10^5$	Infection with/without rotavirus.	Both induce VA, synergistic effect.		Vitovec et al.[1753]

(Continued)

Table 11.5 (Continued)   Studies Employing Experimental Infections with *Cystoisospora suis*

Number of Piglets (If Not Stated Otherwise)	Age Upon Infection (days)	Infection Dose/Animal	Clinical and Parasitological Outcome	Pathohistological Observations	Other Observations	Reference
Coinfection/Treatment Efficacy						
31, 15 treated with toltrazuril 12 hours postinfection Natural coinfections with *Clostridium perfringens* type A	4 hours	1×10^3	Oocyst excretion in untreated piglets, 59.2% of the samples from untreated piglets were diarrheic. 30.8% mortality (NE).	*C. perfringens* present in tissue, increased in infected untreated piglets.	In treated animals only 12% of samples diarrheic; in untreated animals, no mortality, no excretion.	Mengel et al.[1177]
Treatment Efficacy (see also Chapter 6, Section 6.4)						
10/group (uninfected, infected, infected and treated with halofuginone or lasalocid)	22–23	1×10^5	Prepatency 6 days; diarrhea 4–14 DPI. Reduction of daily body weight gain by 19.7%–27.2% and 18.6% higher food intake in the infected untreated group compare to the uninfected controls.	Destruction of the lamina epithelialis in infected animals.	Lasalocid treatment alleviated clinical signs but did not reduce oocyst excretion. No excretion upon reinfection. Halofuginone treatment reduced oocyst excretion but also feed intake (which leads to reduced weight gain), and oocysts were shed upon challenge 6 weeks after first infection.	Männer et al.[1121]; Matuschka and Männer[1156]
15 (7 controls, 8 monensin-treated in feed)	3	5×10^4	Excretion from 3 DPI for ca. 4 days. Max. OPG 2×10^5. Anorexia, poor growth, diarrhea 3–7 DPI for a mean of 3.8 days (1.8 in treated piglets).	VA, crypt hyperplasia in lower jejunum and ileum.	Monensin not effective.	Doré and Morin[398]
30 (SPF), 23 infected (8 treated with amprolium, 7 with furazolidone from the day of infection), 7 uninfected controls	4	5×10^5	Growth retardation in all infected animals, anorexia and diarrhea from 5 DPI, furazolidone group 7–8 DPI. Max. OPG 38,950.	VA in jejunum, ileum.	No efficacy of amprolium/furazolidone.	Girard and Morin[597]
50	3	1×10^4	Diarrhea, reduced body weight gain and oocyst excretion in all but the toltrazuril-treated groups.	Villi sign. longer in in toltrazuril-treated animals.	Treatment with toltrazuril (20 mg/kg, 2 DPI), diclazuril (2 mg/kg, 2 and 3 DPI or 15 mg/kg, 2 DPI or 2 and 9 DPI), sulfadimidine (200 mg/kg, 5, 6, 7 DPI). Only toltrazuril effective.	Mundt et al.[1216,1219]
96 (7–9/group), treated with sulfonamides in different formulations and application schemes or with toltrazuril (1×20 mg/kg of body weight)	4	1.5×10^3	Control animals: excretion onset and peak 5 DPI until the end of the study (15 DPI), diarrhea 6 DPI in two peaks, 6 and 11 DPI. Ca. 50% of samples positive for oocysts and 32% diarrheic.	n.d.	Toltrazuril and repeated parenteral sulfonamide treatment effective in suppression of excretion and diarrhea, oral or single application of sulfonamides ineffective.	Joachim and Mundt[823]
34 (5 groups)	4	1×10^3	Controls: excretion from 6–15 DOL, mean duration 4.2–4.4 days. Max. OPG 365,301 9 DPI. Peak excretion 7–8 DPI. Diarrhea: 25%–60% of piglets, peak 9 DPI.	n.d.	Strain Holland-I was resistant to toltrazuril (20 and 30 mg/kg body weight).	Shrestha et al.[1570]
10 controls, 12 toltrazuril oral, 13 toltrazuril parenteral	4	1.5×10^3	Control: excretion by 90% of piglets, 22.1% samples positive, all piglets had diarrhea for at least 1 day, 35.7% of samples diarrheic.	n.d.	Both toltrazuril formulations highly effective.	Joachim et al.[827]

Note: Conventional pigs if not stated otherwise. Age upon infection is in days if not stated otherwise.

Abbreviations: DOL, days of life; DPI, days post-inoculation; n.d., not determined; NE, necrotic enteritis; OPG, oocysts per gram of feces; VA, villous atrophy; VN, villous necrosis.

oocyst excretion in piglets infected with *C. suis*.[1219] In the United States, toltrazuril was never licensed, and in 2005, Canada repealed the submission process of toltrazuril for use in piglet coccidiosis, leaving the North American pig farming industry without an effective registered therapeutic approach for cystoisosporosis.[1033]

In the absence of other treatment alternatives including vaccines, toltrazuril has constantly been in use for almost two decades now. Once introduced on a farm, eradication of *C. suis* cannot be achieved despite high efficacy of toltrazuril, leaving farmers with the only option of continuous treatment of all piglets. Consequently, anti-toltrazuril resistance has arisen, and a toltrazuril-resistant field isolate of *C. suis* has recently been described from a Dutch pig farm.[1570] The genetic basis of toltrazuril resistance in *C. suis* remains to be elucidated. However, continuous use of a drug over an extended period, underdosing, as well as treating piglets at the wrong time point favor an increase in the frequency of resistant genes by selection of resistant mutants, inevitably leading to the emergence of strains that are resistant to the drug.[1684] The high reproductive potential of *C. suis* and subsequent genetic variation can also increase the probability of selection of resistant strains from the parasite population. Toltrazuril-resistant *C. suis* are a potential threat to pig farming, as no other effective and economically sustainable alternative treatment is available. Therefore, monitoring of resistance should be incorporated in every farm, and strict sanitation and disinfection should be taken into consideration to prevent the spread of cystoisosporosis.

11.9.2 Prevention

With limited prophylactic treatment options, good sanitation and hygiene measures are important aspects in controlling porcine coccidiosis. Rather than eradication, these measures are targeted to reduce infection pressure in a farm environment sufficiently enough to combat clinical disease and production losses that can be caused by a few existing infectious oocysts.

Daily removal of manure and bedding materials followed by high-pressure or steam cleaning of the farrowing pen between litters is one of the most efficient methods to prevent *C. suis* infection[25,1043,1630,1713] but is nowadays no option in intensive piglet production on (semi-) slatted floors without bedding. Nevertheless, in all-in–all-out systems, thorough cleaning and disinfection between farrowings can be applied, and are still an important factor for reducing clinical coccidiosis.[25,1581,1599] However, high humidity promotes oocyst survival in the environment, whereas low humidity, combined with relatively high temperatures prevailing in farrowing units, are detrimental to oocysts.[941] Given that coccidian oocysts are quite robust and resistant to commonly available disinfectants, selection of an appropriate disinfectant is crucial. Application of ammonia, bleach, and phenol-based disinfectants for several hours were shown to be effective in killing oocysts upon contact.[277,501,1040,1627,1630] Commercially available cresol-based disinfectants were also reported to be effective to reducing contamination of farrowing crates when applied at 4% concentration for 2 hours after thorough cleaning.[1621] Additionally, strict farm biosecurity measures should be maintained to prevent crate-to-crate spread of infectious oocysts via farm equipment and workers' boots and clothes. Mechanical transport and transmission of viable oocysts by flies, cockroaches, and other insects should be controlled as well. However, *C. suis* is prevalent even in herds with superior hygiene standards,[627,715,1133,1179,1180,1257] so even rigorous measures do not seem likely to eradicate the parasite.

11.9.3 Novel Control Options

Due to their limited pathogenicity, little research on the control of porcine *Eimeria* spp. has lately been undertaken. Therapeutic options against cystoisosporosis are limited and utterly challenged by the emergence of resistant parasite strains. Detailed knowledge about the mode of action of a drug is imperative to understand the mechanism of resistance development. The only licensed drug, toltrazuril, acts by unresolved mechanisms, and action is needed to either develop alternative compound for therapy or to move toward alternative strategies such as immunoprophylaxis. A vaccine would be an ideal alternative to combat emerging anticoccidial drug resistance. Although probably effective, live and virulent vaccines are impractical in cystoisosporosis, since even very low doses can cause clinical disease in suckling piglets.[268] Attempts to develop a recombinant vaccine against *C. suis* derived from sporozoite and merozoite proteins showed initially promising results[1378,1790] but did not result in a commercial product, and in 2003 the vaccine patent was withdrawn. Currently, there are no commercial vaccines available against cystoisosporosis. Superinfection of sows with high numbers of live *C. suis* antepartum resulted in partial protection of their offspring against experimental challenge,[1523] so maternal immunization appears to be a promising option, but the use of high numbers of live parasites is both impracticable and risky in terms of contamination of the piglet environment, and alternatives must be developed.

The complex life cycle of apicomplexan parasites and gaps in the understanding of the pathobiology of these parasites inhibit the development of new control options.[1639] Research gaps in identifying genes regulating the transition of life cycle stages, molecular mechanisms involved in host cell invasion, and shunning of host immunity are critical for the design of novel drugs and vaccines. Recent advances in parasite genomics, biotechnology, and bioinformatics have facilitated virtual screening of a large number of candidates using rapid and cost-effective *in silico* approaches. Genetic information on porcine *Eimeria* spp.

Table 11.6 Genetic and Genomic Information on Porcine Coccidia

Species, Strain	Genetic Locus	Size (Bp)	Genbank[a] Accession Number	Reference
	Ribosomal RNA Genes			
E. porci	18S rRNA (= small subunit rRNA), partial	1318	AF279666	Ruttkowski et al.[1466]
E. polita	18S rRNA, partial	1318	AF279667	Ruttkowski et al.[1466]
E. scabra	18S rRNA, partial	1316	AF279668	Ruttkowski et al.[1466]
E. debliecki, E. neodebliecki, E. perminuta, E. spinosa, E. suis	18S rRNA, partial	509–511	BioProject: PRJEB23344	Sharma et al.[1540]
C. suis, Guelph-I	18S rRNA, partial, plastid	1822	U97523	Carreno et al.[177]
C suis Guelph, 2008	16S rRNA, partial; plastid	509	JN181040	Ogedengbe et al.[1270]
C. suis YZ	18S rRNA, partial; ITS1; 5.8S rRNA, ITS 2; 26S rRNA, partial	1633	KR139985	Samarasinghe et al.[1480]
C. suis	ITS1, partial	353	LC212985	Kanamori et al.[857]
C: suis	Large subunit rRNA, partial	572	AF093428	Ellis et al.[487]
C. suis	18S rRNA, partial	169	AJ877043	Gualdi et al.[631]
C. suis Kumamoto-1	ITS-1	436	LC085519	Matsubayashi et al.[1150]
	Cytochrome c Oxidase I Subunit Gene (Mitochondrial), Partial			
C. suis		158	AIQ84265	Ogedengbe et al.[1268]
C. suis MEO2010-CS1 to CS4		475	KF854262-KF854265	Ogedengbe et al.[1268]
C. suis Kumamoto-1		426	LC212986	Kanamori et al.[857]
C. suis Shizuoka-1		441	LC212987	Kanamori et al.[857]
	Other Loci			
C. suis Wien-I	Whole genome, merozoite transcriptome	n/a	MIGC00000000.1 (Master entry)	Palmieri et al.[1318]

Abbreviations: C., Cystoisospora; E., Eimeria; ITS, internal transcribed spacer.
Note: Complete sequences if not stated otherwise.
[a] GenBank: https://www.ncbi.nlm.nih.gov/bioproject/?term=PRJNA341953; ToxoDB: . https://toxodb.org/toxo/

and *C. suis* is currently scarce. Single loci are described for various *Eimeria* spp. and *C. suis*. A whole genome annotation (including a transcriptomic annotation of merozoites derived from *in vitro* cultures) is only available for *C. suis*, strain Wien I (Table 11.6).

The reference genome of *C. suis* with ~84 Mb sequence assembly is available and can be used in vaccine discovery using a reverse vaccinology approach. Vacceed, a tool based on reverse vaccinology, was used to screen the predicted *C. suis* proteome, which identified 1168 candidate proteins with high immunogenicity scores.[1318] This genome-based approach of drug discovery seems very attractive; however, it is still a challenge to pinpoint appropriate candidates, as the designated function of a protein does not always reflect its protective potential.[45] Therefore, epitope mapping and protein identification should be combined with proteomic, biotechnological, and *in vitro* culture studies to define cell specificity, subcellular localization, and expression patterns to provide a more complete picture of the immune response evoked by a parasite.

More than 50% of the identified possible vaccine candidates of *C. suis* have unknown functions.[1318] Therefore, the need for an optimal protein expression platform for production of recombinant protein is crucial to facilitate

structure-function studies and screening *in vitro* and *in vivo*. Keeping up the pace, a *C. suis*–specific uncharacterized merozoite protein, CSUI_005805, was cloned, and its molecular characteristics, expression patterns, and immunological potential were demonstrated *in vitro*.[1572] Expression of gene encoding protein CSUI_005805 was almost 20-fold higher in merozoites compared to sporozoites and might thus be crucial for survival and establishment of merozoites inside porcine epithelial cells. Immunogenic proteins expressed in other developmental stages, e.g., in gamogony, should also be identified, screened, and combined with other complementary antigens to design a robust vaccine against *C. suis*. To attain this, *in silico* and *in vitro* methods for predicting and evaluating putative candidates can be helpful, such as genomic and transcriptomic data in combination with *in vitro* cultivation of *C. suis*.[1318,1821] *In vitro* culture for *C. suis* supports the complete life cycle, promoting access to defined developmental stages.[1050,1821]

11.10 CONCLUSION

In pigs, two genera of coccidia are described, which occur worldwide in varying prevalences; *Eimeria* (with currently eight valid species) and *Cystoisospora* (with one valid species). They all develop in a direct, one-host life cycle. While porcine *Eimeria* occur mostly in weaners and adult pigs and only have a limited clinical relevance, *C. suis* is one of the most important enteral pathogens of suckling piglets. It causes creamy to watery diarrhea, mostly in the second to third weeks of life, with considerable morbidity. In the presence of toxigenic *Clostridium perfringens*, exacerbated disease with increased mortality is seen. In contrast to other *Cystoisospora* species, *C. suis* has not been shown to have extraintestinal stages in pigs or other hosts. Sporulated oocysts of all nine species can be differentiated by morphology and detected by classical or modified copro-microscopical techniques, including autofluorescence detection. Immunity against the different *Eimeria* species seems to be short-lived and unstable; however, *C. suis* induces a strong age-related resistance that largely prevents oocyst excretion and disease in weaned and adult pigs. Immune reactions against primary infections with *C. suis* are limited to an increase of γδ-T cells in the intestine, since no other T-cell population is present in larger numbers in young piglets. The effect of IgA in maternal immunity has been implied for experimental *C. suis* infections. The treatment options for porcine coccidiosis are very limited; some compounds have been tested against *Eimeria*, but only sulfonamides are available. The only registered drug effective against *C. suis*

in suckling piglets is toltrazuril, but continuing use for decades has led to the development of resistance in the field. In situations where toltrazuril is not available or not effective, the only remaining control options are strict hygiene and reduction of environmental contamination. Alternative control measures are still under scrutiny.

REFERENCES

22, 25, 26, 31–33, 42, 45, 53, 54, 56, 80, 83, 105, 106, 115, 123, 124, 129, 139–141, 148, 152, 159, 177–179, 207, 210, 211, 260, 268, 277, 285, 312, 318, 325, 329, 330, 331, 363, 398, 400, 421, 455, 460, 487, 497, 501, 502, 509, 510, 550, 561, 563, 564, 568, 597, 615, 627, 631, 651, 657, 663, 674–677, 684, 702, 704, 706, 715, 719, 741, 748–750, 764, 766, 770, 822–827, 832, 844, 856, 857, 860, 911–918, 936, 941, 982, 1021, 1031, 1033, 1034, 1036, 1037, 1039, 1040, 1042, 1043, 1047, 1049–1051, 1108, 1111, 1112, 1121, 1133, 1135, 1141, 1150, 1155–1157, 1171, 1177, 1179, 1180, 1204, 1206, 1207, 1214, 1216, 1218, 1219, 1240, 1242, 1254, 1257, 1268, 1270, 1280, 1291, 1292, 1318, 1343, 1357, 1360, 1361, 1378, 1391, 1401, 1402, 1419, 1420, 1421, 1424, 1425, 1428, 1431–1433, 1465–1467, 1479, 1480, 1485–1488, 1502, 1503, 1507, 1519, 1522, 1523, 1527, 1540, 1542, 1569–1572, 1581, 1599, 1614, 1616, 1620, 1621, 1627–1633, 1639, 1651, 1677, 1678, 1682, 1684, 1698, 1700, 1710, 1713, 1732, 1736, 1745, 1750–1754, 1764, 1766, 1772, 1790, 1792, 1798, 1800, 1816–1821, 1854, 1870a, 1890, 1921

CHAPTER 12

Coccidiosis in Old World Camels

J. P. Dubey and R. K. Schuster

CONTENTS

12.1 HISTORY AND SPECIES OF COCCIDIA

The literature on camel coccidia is very confusing. One reason for this confusion is that different groups of researchers reported on *Eimeria* infections in camels from different countries at about the same time, and there are no archived specimens for verification. Recently, we reviewed in detail the history, bibliography, taxonomy, life cycles, and biology of coccidiosis and coccidia in camels and concluded that there are three valid species of *Eimeria, E. cameli, E. dromedarii*, and *E. rajasthani*, and one species of *Cystoisospora, C. orlovi*.[447] Here, we summarize essential information and add references missed in our review.

12.2 *EIMERIA* INFECTIONS

12.2.1 *Eimeria cameli* (Henry and Masson, 1932) Reichenow, 1952

This species is morphologically distinct from other species of *Eimeria* of camels (Figure 12.1). There is a high variability in size of oocysts, varying from 67 to 108 μm in length and 57 to 94 μm in width (see Table 1 in Dubey and Schuster[447] and Table 1 in Abbas et al.[3]). The most complete description is provided by Yagoub.[1837] Unsporulated oocysts are truncate, ovoid, and dark brown to black. The oocyst wall

consists of three layers, a pitted brown outer layer up to 14 μm thick, the middle layer 1.5 μm thick and light yellow to brown, and a third layer that is black and 3–4.5 μm thick. Micropyle is up to 28 μm wide and 6–9 μm high; the micropylar cap is absent. A recent paper reported variability of structures in *E. cameli* oocysts from Egypt including a polar cap–like structure and a transparent capsule in some oocysts.[3] Polar granule and oocyst residuum were also absent. The sporulation time is up to 25 days, depending on the temperature. Sporocysts are elongated with tapering ends, 37.4 × 18.6 (30–40 × 18–20) μm. Stieda bodies and residual bodies are absent. Sporozoite size is uncertain but estimated at 30 μm long.

E. cameli infections were widely prevalent in surveys reported from several countries (Table 12.1). Overall, *E. cameli* was the most prevalent species, and its prevalence was highest in spring and summer in Dubai.

Until recently, there was great uncertainty concerning endogenous stages of *E. cameli*. Previously, many authors reported asexual and sexual stages of *E. cameli* in camels.[145,262,495,703,866,877,1233,1387] A recent review concluded that asexual stages are unknown and that microgamonts were most likely misidentified as schizonts.[446] They described the development of microgamonts, macrogamonts, and oocysts in camels naturally infected with *E. cameli*.[446] Based on a review of the literature, and their findings, development occurred in the lamina propria of the small intestine. Stages were located throughout the villus, up to the tunica

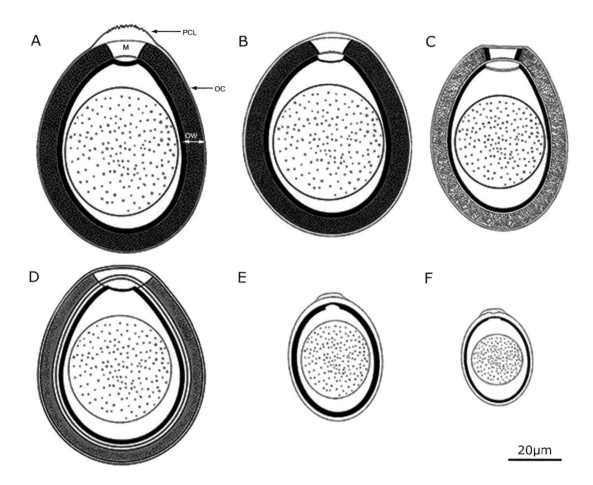

Figure 12.1 Unsporulated *Eimeria* oocysts from *Camelus dromedarius*. (A) *E. cameli* morphotype 1, note the dome-shaped polar cap–like structure (PCL) with serrated top (arrow). (B) *E. cameli* morphotype 2, note the PCL which resembles a small thickening with a smooth top (arrow). (C) *E. cameli* morphotype 3, note the flat anterior end with no PCL (arrow). (D) *E. cameli* morphotype 4, note the divided middle wall layer (arrow). (E) *E. rajasthani*. (F) *E. dromedarii*. Unstained. Scale bar applies to all images. (From Abas, L.E. et al. 2019. *J. Parasitol.* 105, 395–400.)

muscularis mucosae. The parasitized host cell nucleus was indented but not hypertrophied. The parasitophorous vacuoles containing gamonts were up to 360 μm long, and the parasitophorous vacuolar membrane was up to 3 μm thick. The microgamonts were macroscopic (339×309 μm).[866] Oocysts in sections were up to 88×60 μm.

There is uncertainty concerning the pathogenicity of *E. cameli*. Although *E. cameli*–associated coccidiosis has been reported by several authors,[760,894,1233,1387,1392] evidence for a cause-and-effect association is lacking, and other causes of enteritis in natural infections were not excluded.[447]

Experimentally, *E. cameli* was only mildly pathogenic. In an experiment, 10 camels were inoculated orally with *E. cameli* 15,000–63,000 oocysts and observed for 2 months for oocyst excretion and clinical signs. All inoculated camels developed patent infections. Overall, the inoculated camels were not severely ill. None of the camels given 17,000 oocysts had clinical signs.[587] At higher dosages of 63,000 oocysts, lethargy and faintness over 2 days in one of six camels and mild diarrhea lasting 1 day in two others were noted. Six of these

experimentally infected camels were treated with toltrazuril (Baycox 5%, 20 mg/kg of body weight) on different days. One animal infected with the high dose received treatment 6 days postinfection and one treatment on days 6 and 12 after infection. Animals in the low infection group received treatment 22 days after infection. Four camels infected with the high infection dose remained as untreated controls. Animals from the low infection group were observed for 63 days and those of the high infection group for 77 days. Prepatent periods ranged from 30 to 37 days irrespective of treatment or infection dose. Patent periods ranged from 18 to 38 days in the treated and 32 to 46 days in the untreated animals without appreciable differences. One untreated animal started to excrete oocysts 16 days after infection; this was considered an accidental previous infection.

12.2.2 *Eimeria dromedarii* Yakimoff and Matschoulsky, 1939

Kasim et al.[863] and Yagoub[1837] provided the most complete description of 270 oocysts from 24 camels. Oocysts

Table 12.1 Prevalence of *Eimeria* Species in Old World Camels

Country	Region	Number Sampled	Percentage (%) Positive	Remarks	Reference
Bahrain		223	15.2	*E. dr*, only species reported	Abubakr et al.[8]
Chad		204	7.0	*E. ca*	Gruvel and Graber[630]
China	Inner Mongolia	321	50.0	*E. ra, E. dr, E. ca, E. ba, E. pe.* Samples collected 1982–1987 from Bactrian camels	Wei and Wang[1789]
Egypt	Cairo	820	8.2	*E. ra* 1.9%, *E. ba* 6.1%	Sakr[1478]
Egypt	Cairo	800	19.7	*E. dr* 9.2%, *E. no* 5.5%	El-Manyawe and Iskander[477]
Egypt	Cairo	205	40	*E. ra* 36.7%, *E. dr* 2.9%, *E. ca* 2.4%, *E. ba* 35.1%	Morrsy[1209]
Egypt	Assiut	113	27.6	*E. dr* 10.6%, *E. ca* 19.5%	El-Salahy et al.[472]
Egypt	Red Sea	530	27.2	*E. ra* 7.6%, *E. dr* 1.5%, *E. ca* 13.2%	Mahran[1115]
Egypt	Cairo	105	46.6	*E. ra* 6.7%, *E. dr* 8.6%, *E. ca* 31.4%	Wahba and Radwan[1760]
Egypt	Assiut	174	33.3	*E. ra* 6.9%, *E. dr* 16.1%, *E. ca* 18.4%	Elbadr et al.[485]
Egypt	Assiut and El-Wadi Elagded	460	9.9		Abdel-Rady[6]
Egypt	Zagazig	420	24.3	*E. ra* 8.6%, *E. dr* 11.4%, *E. ca* 22.1%, *E. bac* 4.5%, *E. pe* 7.2%	Mohammed[1196]
Egypt	Beheira	120	13.3	*E. dr* 4.2%, *E. ca* 6.7%, *E. pe* 2.5%	Khedr[876]
Egypt	Cairo	200	38	*E. ra* 18%, *E. dr* 14%, *E. ca* 31%	Abbas et al.[3]
Egypt	Aswan	120	28.3	*E. ca* 15.8%, *E. dr* 6.7%, *E. ra* 5%, *E. pe* 0.8%	El-Khabaz et al.[476]
India	Rajasthan	45	62.2	*E. ra* in 28 (62%) *E. dr* in 20 (44%) *E. ca* in 1 (2.2%) No clinical signs, rectal samples from calves <10 months old from one farm	Dubey and Pande[442,445]
India	Rajasthan	103	8.7	Histologically diagnosed coccidiosis found in 9 of 110 intestines	Kumar et al.[923]
India	Rajasthan	34	6.8		Kumar et al.[922]
India	Rajasthan	509	13.5	*E. ca, E. dr*	Pravinbhai[1365]
India	Punjab	321	24.0	*E. ra* in 13 (4%) Other species in 64	Gill[596]
India	Rajasthan	897	25.1	*E. dr, E. ca, E. pe, E. ra*	Partani et al.[1325]
Iran	Miandoab region	125	12.8	33.3% of Bactrian camels versus 14.3% of dromedary camels infected. *Eimeria* species reported: *E. ra* 15.6% (only Bactrian camels), *E. ca* 11.1%, *E. dr* 4.4%. Diarrhea in young calves	Yakhchali and Cheraghi[1839]
Iran	Mashhad	306	18.6	Samples collected at an abattoir. Lesions associated with *E. ca* detected in 29 camels	Borji et al.[145]

(Continued)

Table 12.1 (Continued) Prevalence of *Eimeria* Species in Old World Camels

Country	Region	Number Sampled	Percentage (%) Positive	Remarks	Reference
Iran	Tabriz	164	20.7	*E. ba* 52.4%, *E. ca* 19.3%, *E. pe* 15.6%, *E. dr* 12.6%	Yakhchali and Athari[1838]
Iran	Kerman	100	29	Samples collected at an abattoir. Lesions associated with *E. ca* detected in 29 camels	Kheirandish et al.[877]
Iran	Yazad province	305	9.5	*E. ca* 14 (47.5%), *E. dr* 13 (42.5%), *E. ba* 2 (10.0%)	Sazmand et al.[1506]
Iraq		200	NS	30 samples from northern Iraq were negative for oocysts. Of 170 samples from central Iraq, *E. ca* was found in 68 (40%) and *E. dr* in 86 (50.65%)	Mirza and Al-Rawas[1188]
Saudi Arabia	Hofuf, eastern province	960	14	*E. ca* oocysts found in 146 of 960 samples of feces collected twice weekly from an unspecified number of camels for 12 consecutive months	Kawasmeh and Elbihari[866]
Saudi Arabia	Four regions	500	41.6	Prevalence reported for four different regions in 6-month-old to 5-year-old camels; *E. dr* 28.4%, *E. ra* 22.2%, *E. ca*	Kasim et al.[863]
Saudi Arabia	Five regions	385	40	*E. dr* was the most prevalent, followed by *E. ra*, and the least prevalent was *E. ca*, but relative figures were not stated. Clinical signs observed in young camels	Hussein et al.[760]
Saudi Arabia	Gassim region	240	12.8	Intestines and feces from camels at an abattoir, 15.7% of 83 adults and 10.2% of calves infected. In adult camel *E. ca* 2.4%, *E. ra* 7.2%, *E. dr* 12%. In calves, *E. ca* 1.3%, *E. ra* 5.1%, *E. dr* 6.3%	Mahmoud et al.[1114]
Saudi Arabia		203	4.9	*E. ca*	Al-Afaleq et al.[19]
Sudan		230	17.4	*E. ra* in 21 (9.1%) *E. dr* in 15 (6.5%) *E. ca* in 9 (3.9%)	Yagoub[1837]
Turkey	Maramara	10	7	*E. ca*	Cirak et al.[273]
United Arab Emirates	Dubai	13,301		*E. ca* in 1469 (13%) *E. ra* in 578 (6%) *E. dr* in 452(4%)	See Dubey and Schuster[447]
Uganda	Karamoja	82	11	*E. ca* 100%	Nakayima et al.[1231]
USSR		467	74.4	*Eimeria* species	Tsygankov[1711]

Abbreviations: E. ba, E. bactriani; E. ca, E. cameli; E. dr, E. dromedarii; E. pe, E. pellerdyi; E. ra, E. rajasthani.

are subspherical to ellipsoidal, 23–33 × 19–25 µm; most oocysts were ovoidal (Table 2 in Dubey and Schuster[447]). The oocyst wall is 2–3 µm thick, smooth with two layers, the outer light yellow and the inner brownish green. The oocyst cap is 4–8 µm wide and 1–3 µm high. Micropyle is absent. Sporocysts are ovoid, 7–11 × 5–9 µm without Stieda body and residuum. Sporozoite size is unknown.

12.2.3 *Eimeria rajasthani* Dubey and Pande, 1963

Oocysts are ellipsoidal 34–39 × 25–29 µm with a length-to-width ratio of 1.3–1.4 (Table 3 of Dubey and Schuster[447]). There is remarkably low variability in dimensions of oocysts. The oocyst wall is 2–3 µm thick with the outer layer yellowish green and the inner layer light brown. The micropylar end is covered with a dome-shaped cap, 4–11 µm wide and 1–3 µm high. Oocyst residuum and polar granule are absent. Sporocysts are ovoid, 12–16 × 8–11 µm. Polar granule and oocyst residuum, with an indistinct Stieda body, are present at the narrow end. Sporozoites are curved, approximately 10 µm long.

12.3 *CYSTOISOSPORA ORLOVI* (TSYGANKOV, 1950; AMEND. KINNE, ALI, WERNERY, AND DUBEY, 2002) FRENKEL, 1977

Unsporulated oocysts are excreted in feces, and they are 25–35 µm long.[146,893,1384,1521,1711] They are usually ovoid. Sporulation occurs rapidly, and some sporulate in host if postmortem is delayed (Figure 1.9, Chapter 1). Sporulated oocysts might be slightly larger than unsporulated oocysts. Sporocysts are 20 × 15 µm, and they contain elongated or ovoid sporozoites. Endogenous development occurs in the large intestine. Asexual stages are unknown. Microgamonts are big and contain hundreds of microgametes. A micropyle, oocyst residuum, and Stieda bodies are absent.

Cystoisospora-associated infections have been reported from India, Kenya, and the United Arab Emirates (Table 12.2). Cystoisosporosis is a clinical infection of nursing camels from 9 to 35 days old,[1521] but occasionally older calves may also suffer. Oocysts are most commonly detected in camels with diarrhea and in younger camels. Infections occur both in stall-fed as well as pastoral camels. In a comprehensive investigation of dairy camels, most infections were in winter and spring (coinciding with calving period), and most infections were seen in 14- to 29-day-old calves.[1521]

Many aspects of transmission of *C. orlovi* infections are unknown. One hypothesis is that oocysts sporulate rapidly and calves become infected soon after birth; excretion of oocysts in newborn camels is probably the source of infection to other camels. Currently, there is no evidence for an arrested stage of the parasite in camel tissues or intrauterine or lactogenic transmission.

Affected calves develop diarrhea and dehydration and can die within a short time. The lesions are confined to the large intestine, and consist of diphtheroid to hemorrhagic colitis with erosions or elevated areas (Figure 1.28B, Chapter 1). Massive numbers of gamonts and oocysts might be present, especially in elevated areas (Figure 1.27, Chapter 1).

12.4 DIAGNOSIS OF COCCIDIOSIS

Fecal examination and histopathology can aid diagnosis. Of the three common species of *Eimeria*, in camel feces, *E. cameli, E. rajasthani,* and *E. dromedarii* are morphologically distinctive (Figure 12.1). *E. cameli* oocysts are the largest and the heaviest. It is important to use sedimentation techniques or flotation solutions higher than 1.3 specific gravity to float *E. cameli.* Oocysts of *E. rajasthani* have a prominent micropylar cap and are larger in size than *E. dromedarii* (Figure 12.1). *Eimeria* oocysts are excreted unsporulated, and sporulation requires more than 2 days. Histologically, *E. cameli* stages are big in size and occur in

Table 12.2   Reports of *Cystoisospora orlovi* in Old World Camels

Country	Region	Remarks	Reference
USSR		Oocysts detected in 10 calves, 10- to 35-days-old.	Tsygankov[1711]
Kenya	Lakipia District	*C. orlovi*–associated diarrhea diagnosed in four herds. Oocysts were seen in 13 calves, 12–30 days old. Two calves died. Postmortem revealed ulcerative colitis in one calf with intralesional coccidian stages.	Younan et al.[1868]
Kenya	Rift Valley	Oocysts were detected in feces of 21 of 253 calves. 19 of 21 calves excreting oocysts had diarrhea. Oocysts were not found in healthy calves and in calves older than 8 weeks of age.	Bornstein et al.[146]
India		Oocysts found in feces of a 6-month-old calf with diarrhea.	Raisinghani et al.[1384]
United Arab Emirates	Dubai	Outbreak of diarrhea on two farms. 22 calves that died were necropsied. Colitis was found in eight calves. Endogenous stages of *C. orlovi* were detected in large intestine.	Kinne et al.[892a,893]
United Arab Emirates	Dubai	Oocysts were found in feces of 72 of 2885 samples from calves, and 13 of 76,969 adult camels tested between 2005 and 2016.	Schuster et al.[1521]

the small intestine, mostly in the ileum. Endogenous stages of *E. rajasthani* and *E. dromedarii* are unknown.

Oocysts of *C. orlovi* are often excreted sporulated, and they contain two sporocysts, compared with four sporocysts in *Eimeria* species (Figure 1.9, Chapter 1). In some cases of cystoisosporosis, calves die before oocysts are detectable in feces. *C. orlovi* stages are found in the large intestine. Scrapings of intestinal mucosa can reveal numerous coccidian stages. Histologically, there is enteritis with occasional inflammation in submucosa.

12.5 TREATMENT

Little is known regarding the treatment of coccidiosis in Old World camels. Sulfadimidine given as an aquatic suspension orally for 10 days in a dose 30 mg/kg body weight was used to treat dromedary calves.[760] Gerlach[587] attempted to examine the efficacy of toltrazuril in experimentally infected dromedaries. Although toltrazuril showed promising high serum levels in a pharmacokinetic study, it failed to prevent patent infections when given 6, 12, or 22 days postinoculation.

REFERENCES

3, 6, 8, 19, 145, 146, 262, 273, 442, 445–447, 472, 476, 477, 485, 495, 587, 596, 630, 703, 760, 863, 866, 876, 892a, 893, 894, 922, 923, 1114, 1115, 1188, 1196, 1209, 1231, 1233, 1325, 1365, 1384, 1387, 1392, 1478, 1506, 1521, 1711, 1760, 1789, 1837–1839, 1868

CHAPTER 13

Coccidiosis in South American Camelids

J. P. Dubey

CONTENTS

13.1 INTRODUCTION AND HISTORY

The South American camelids (SACs) consist of four species – llamas (*Lama glama*), alpacas (*Lama pacos*), guanacos (*Lama guanicoe*), and vicuñas (*Lama vicugna*); their generic nomenclature is controversial. I have used the genus *Lama* for all four species. Traditionally, they are distributed at high altitudes (3600–5400 m) in South America where they are sources of meat, hide, fiber, and transport, and their feces are used for fuel and fertilizer. In many countries, such as the United States, they are reared for recreation, and the commercial product is a live animal. Oocysts of one of the species of *Eimeria* of SACs, *E. macusaniensis*, are morphologically distinctive; its oocysts are up to 110 μm long, piriform, and have a very thick brown wall. Examination of coprolites and llama mummies dating about 10,000 years in South America found *E. macusaniensis*–like oocysts; shapes and sizes of these oocysts were remarkably preserved.[566]

I recently reviewed coccidiosis in SACs in detail listing complete bibliography up to 2018, history, taxonomy, life cycles, and diagnosis.[422] Here essential information is summarized, and citations missed earlier are provided.

13.2 SPECIES OF *EIMERIA* IN SOUTH AMERICAN CAMELIDS

There are five common species of *Eimeria* in SACs (Table 13.1). They are morphologically so different in size and shape that species can be identified without the need of sporulation (Figure 13.1).

13.3 MORPHOLOGY AND LIFE CYCLE

13.3.1 *E. macusaniensis* Guerrero, Hernandez, Bazalar, and Alva, 1971

Its oocysts are the largest among all *Eimeria* species, distinctively resembling watermelon seed or a cut avocado and up to 110 μm long (Table 13.1). It has long sporulation time; 9 days at 30°C, in 21 days at 18–25°C, but oocysts did not sporulate at 6°C–7°C.[1429] Its prepatent period is 36–41 days, and it was transmissible between lama, guanaco, and alpaca.[194,547,786,1429]

Its asexual stages are unknown.[425] Sexual stages are in the villar epithelium and lamina propria of small

Table 13.1   Common Species of *Eimeria* in South American Camelids

Character	*E. macusaniensis*	*E. lamae*	*E. alpacae*	*E. punoensis*	*E. ivitaensis*
Oocyst shape	Ovoid, piriform	Ellipsoidal, ovoid	Ellipsoidal, ovoid	Ellipsoidal, ovoid	Ellipsoidal
Size[a]	81–107 × 61–80 **100–110 × 77–84**[b]	30–40 × 21–30 **35–38 × 26–30**	22–26 × 18–21 **24–27 × 22–24**	17–22 × 14–18	83–98 × 49–59
Mean	93.6 × 67.4 **106.6 × 80.5**	35.6 × 24.5 **36.7 × 28. 9**	24.1 × 19.6 **25.8 × 22.9**	19.9 × 16.4	88.8 × 51.8
Wall thickness	8.3–11.4	1.4–1.8	1.2–1.6	0.8–1.1	4.0–4.5
Micropylar cap	2–5 high, 9–14 wide	1.5–2.2 high, 8.8–11.4 wide	0.7–1.3 high, 4.4–7.5 wide	0.4–0.8 high, 3.5–5.5 wide	Absent[c]
Sporocyst shape	Elongate	Elongate, ovoid		Elongate, ovoid	Elongate
Size range	33–40 × 16–20 **44–48 × 20–23**	13–16 × 8–10 **17–20 × 9–12**	10–13 × 7–8 **10–12 × 7–9**	8–11 × 5–7	32–41 × 12–13
Mean	36.3 × 18.3 **45.2 × 22.6**	15.2 × 8.5 **18.6 × 10.7**	11.0 × 6.8 **11.3 × 7.8**	9.2 × 6.1	35.4 × 13.1
Stieda body	Faint	Present	Faint	Faint	Not described
Original host	*Lama pacos*	*Lama pacos*	*Lama pacos*	*Lama pacos*	*Lama pacos*
Reference	Guerrero et al.[638]	Guerrero[635,636]	Guerrero[635,636]	Guerrero[635,636]	Leguía and Casas[966]

Source: From Dubey, J.P. 2018. *Parasitol. Res.* 117, 1999–2013.

a   The measurements are in micrometers. Guerrero measured 50 or more oocysts and sporocysts; the number of specimens measured by Leguía and Casas and Schrey et al. was not stated.

b   Values in bold are from oocysts in *Lama glama*.

c   Absent in original description of Leguía and Casas but present in some oocysts (see Figure 13.1).

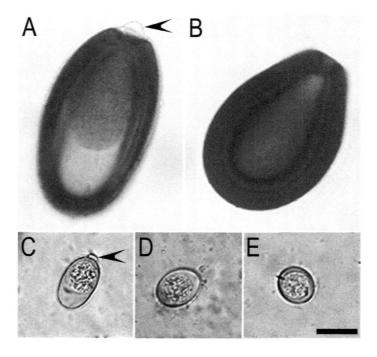

Figure 13.1   Unsporulated oocysts of five common species of *Eimeria* in South American camelids. Unstained. (A) *E. ivitaensis*; (B) *E. macusaniensis*; (C) *E. lamae*; (D) *E. alpacae*; (E) *E. punoensis*. Note micropylar caps (arrowheads). The scale bar = 20 μm and applies to images. (From Dubey, J.P. 2018. *Parasitol. Res.* 117, 1999–2013.) (Courtesy of Dr. M. M. Cafrune.)

and large intestine, and the ileum is the most affected region. Occasionally, stages are found even in submucosa. Microgamonts can be very large, up to 199 μm long. Gamonts are located in large parasitophorous vacuoles; even the earliest macrogamonts were seen in the parasitophorous vacuoles that were 68 × 45 μm (Figure 1.16D, Chapter 1).

13.3.2 *E. ivitaensis* Leguia and Casas, 1998

Its oocysts are ellipsoidal and are up to 98 μm long. Its endogenous stages are unknown. A study reported schizonts and gamonts in the jejunum and ileum of an alpaca, but results need confirmation.[1316]

13.3.3 *E. alpacae* Guerrero, 1967

Its oocysts are ellipsoidal and measure 22–27 × 18–24 μm (Table 13.1). Its prepatent period is 16–18 days.[547] Nothing is known of its endogenous stages.

13.3.4 *E. lamae* Guerrero, 1967

Its oocysts are ovoid to ellipsoidal and measure 30–40 × 21–30 μm (Table 13.1). Its prepatent period is 10 days and was reported to be pathogenic, but details of endogenous stages are not known.[637]

13.3.5 *E. punoensis* Guerrero, 1967

Its oocysts are ovoid to ellipsoidal and smallest among the SAC *Eimeria*, measuring 17–22 × 14–18 μm (Table 13.1). Nothing is known of its life cycle.

13.4 PREVALENCE OF *EIMERIA* SPECIES

Prevalence data in llamas (Table 13.2), alpacas (Table 13.3), guanacos (Table 13.4), and vicuñas (Table 13.5) indicate SACs are commonly infected with *Eimeria* species. In general, *E. lamae* was the most prevalent, and *E. ivitaensis* was the least prevalent. Infections were most common in nursing animals. Up to 90% of crias younger than 2 months old were found infected.[638] It is noteworthy that despite excretion of as many as 411,600 oocysts per gram (OPG) of feces, all vicuñas were asymptomatic.[167]

13.5 CLINICAL INFECTIONS

Little is known of SAC coccidiosis in the wild. However, *Eimeria* infections can be pathogenic in SAC dependent on age, concurrent infections, environmental conditions, stress of captivity and transportation, and nutrition in general.[369]

Except for a report of coccidiosis in a captive guanaco from the United States,[726] all clinical reports were in llamas and alpacas.[422] *E. macusaniensis* was considered the main cause.[195,261,425,634,672,829,970,1314–1316,1397,1430,1436,1437,1513,1518]

Clinical coccidiosis usually occurs in very young (3-week-old) but sometimes in old SACs.[195] Lethargy, diarrhea, abdominal distention, anorexia, weight loss, constipation, and colic have been reported in SACs with uncomplicated coccidiosis.[195,298,829] Animals can die suddenly without obvious clinical signs.[970,1316,1437,1513] Diarrhea is an inconsistent finding, especially in adult

Table 13.2   Prevalence of *Eimeria* in Llama (*Lama glama*)

Country, Region	Number Tested	Number Positive (%)	*Eimeria* Species	Remarks	Reference
Argentina					
Jujuy	478	233 (48.7)	*E. macusaniensis* in all, mixed with *E. ivitaensis* in 2	1 llama with mixed *E. macusaniensis* and *E. ivitaensis* had diarrhea	Cafrune et al.[166]
Salta	48	17 (35.4)	*E. macusaniensis* in 17		
Catamarca	100	65 (65)	*E. macusaniensis* in all, mixed with *E. ivitaensis* in 2		
Austria	160	132 (82.5)	*E. alpacae/punoensis* = 82.5% (these species were not differentiated); *E. lamae* = 31.3% and *E. macusaniensis* = 6.3%	Samples include 145 lamas, 13 alpacas, and 2 guanacos	Pichler[1356]
Switzerland	293 from 38 farms	(68)	*E. macusaniensis*	Only herd prevalence stated	Hertzberg and Kohler[709]
United States	189 adults	69 (37)	*E. alpacae* (27%), *E. macusaniensis* (1%) *E. punoensis* (17%), *E. lamae* (9%)	1 species in 58%, 2 species in 38%, 3 species in 4% in adults	Rickard and Bishop[1416]
Oregon	50 crias	30 (60)	*E. alpacae* (52%), *E. macusaniensis* 0, *E. punoensis* (40%), *E. lamae* (32%),	In crias, 47% contained 2 species, 30% had 3 species, 23% had 1 species; all animals were healthy	
10 states	301	36 (12)	*E. macusaniensis*	<1 year 19 of 86 (22.1%), >1 year 17 of 200 (8.5%)	Jarvinen[785]
Colorado and Wyoming	121 Colorado	76 (62.8)	*E. alpacae* 75, *E. macusaniensis* 0, *E. lamae* 1	4 herds surveyed	Schrey et al.[1518]
	23 Wyoming	15 (65.2)	*E. alpacae* 5, *E. macusaniensis* 2, *E. lamae* 8		

Source: Modified from Dubey, J.P. 2018. *Parasitol. Res.* 117, 1999–2013.

Table 13.3   Prevalence of *Eimeria* in Alpacas (*Lama pacos*)

Country/region	Number Tested	Number Positive (%)	*Eimeria* Species (%)	Remarks	Reference
Bolivia	54	42 (76)	*E. punoesis* 67.3, *E. alpacae* 16.4, *E. macusaniensis* 12.7		Fabian et al.[511]
Ecuador Cotopaxi	204	165 (81.0)	*Eimeria* spp. 81 *E. macusaniensis* 25.0		Valdivieso[1727]
Ecuador Five regions	285	150 (52.5)	*E. macusaniensis* 7.2, *E. ivitaensis* 0.4		Gareis-Waldburg[583]
Japan Kanto	53	42 (79.2)	*E. lamae* 1.9, *E. macusaniensis* 7.5, *E. punoensis* and/or *E. alpacae* 69.8	53 of 390 alpacas from one farm tested	Hyuça and Matsumoto[761]
New Zealand	460	15 (3.2)	*E. macusaniensis*	Five farms were surveyed	Rawdon et al.[1397]
Peru Cuzco	160	67 (58.1)	*E. lamae* 60.4, *E. punoesis* 30.0, *E. alpacae* 45.6, *E. macusaniensis* 50.4	90% of 2-month-old alpacas were positive with an oocyst burden of 1.016 oocysts per gram of feces	Guerrero et al.[637]
Southern Peru	316	145 (46.2)	*E. macusaniensis* 56.5%	22 herds surveyed	Cordero Ramirez et al.[291]
Puno	478	418 (87.5)	*E. lamae* 15.6, *E. punoesis* 20.0, *E. alpacae* 16.9, *E. macusaniensis* 25, *E. ivitaensis* 6.2	<90-days-old healthy cria, infection with multiple species was common	Rodríguez et al.[1427]
Puno	350	224 (64.3)	*E. lamae* 91, *E. macusaniensis* 35, *E. punoensis* 78, *E. alpacae* 87, *E. ivitaensis* 13	Unweaned alpacas from 23 herds	Díaz et al.[369]
Switzerland	72	Not stated	*E. macusaniensis*	Present in 68% of farms, no individual animal data	Hertzberg and Kohler[709]
United Kingdom	Not stated	Not stated	*E. ivitaensis*	Present in two herds. Zinc sulfate sp. gr. 1.36 used for flotation	Twomey et al.[1714]
United States—10 states	115	8 (7.0)	*E. macusaniensis*		Jarvinen[785]
Maryland	61	14 (26.2)	*E. alpacae* in 7, *E. punoensis* in 5, mixed in 2	Two farms. Cesium chlorite sp. gr. 1.4 used for flotation	Trout et al.[1708]

Source: Modified from Dubey, J.P. 2018. *Parasitol. Res*. 117, 1999–2013.

Table 13.4   Prevalence of *Eimeria* in Guanaco (*Lama guanicoe*)

Country/Region	Number Tested	Number Positive (%)	*Eimeria* Species	Remarks	Reference
Argentina Salta	4	1 (25.0)	*E. macusaniensis*	Semicaptive	Cafrune et al.[166]
Mendoza, San Juan	35	Not stated	*E. macusaniensis, Eimeria* sp.	Wild guanaco surveyed; only published as abstract	Borghi et al.[144]
Patagonia	12	10 (80.3)	*E. macusaniensis* in 9, *Eimeria* spp. in 10	Mortality due to starvation in wild population; feces were from animals necropsied	Baldomenico et al.[99]
Chile Magallanes	15	6 (40.0)	*E. macusaniensis*	Semicaptive	Correa et al.[295]
Peru—9 districts	132	43 (33.3)	*E. punoensis* 21.2%, *E. alpacae* 13.6%, *E. lamae* 4.5%, *E. macusaniensis* 15.9%	Wild population	Castillo et al.[183]
United States—10 states	27	2 (7.4)	*E. macusaniensis*		Jarvinen[785]

Source: From Dubey, J.P. 2018. *Parasitol. Res*. 117, 1999–2013.

Table 13.5   Prevalence of *Eimeria* in Vicuñas (*Lama vicugna*)

Country/Region	Number Tested	Number Positive (%)	*Eimeria* Species	Remarks	Reference
Argentina					
Jujuy	81 juveniles	81 (100.0)	*E. punoensis* 100.0%, *E. alpacae* 85.1%, *E. lamae* 48.1%, *E. macusaniensis* 82.7%, and *E. ivitaensis* 3.7%	Born and raised at an experimental station. Prevalence was higher in May versus in November 2011. All were asymptomatic. Mixed infections were common.	Cafrune et al.[167]
	154 adults	143 (92.8)	*E. punoensis* 89.6%, *E. alpacae* 66.8%, *E. lamae* 27.2%, *E. macusaniensis* 15.5%, and *E. ivitaensis* 1.2%		
Bolivia					
Apolobamba	25 adults	22 (88.0)	*E. alpacae* 88.0%, *E. puneonsis* 80.0%, *E. lamae* 12.0%, and *E. macusaniensis* 8.0%	Wild population.	Beltrán-Saavedra et al.[101]
	7 juveniles	7 (100.0)	*E. alpacae* 100.0%, *E. puneonsis* 100.0%, *E. lamae* 42.9%, and *E. macusaniensis* 14.3%		
Peru					
Pampa Galeras	39 adults	15 (41.0)	*E. punoensis/E. lamae*	Wild population. Oocysts per gram (<48).	Bouts et al.[149]

Source: From Dubey, J.P. 2018. *Parasitol. Res.* 117, 1999–2013.

camelids.[191] Coccidiosis predisposes SACs to other microbial infections, especially *Clostridium perfringens*. and enterotoxemia was associated with mortality in newborn alpacas.[1314]

Concurrent coccidial infections with other enteropathogens such as *Escherichia coli*, Coronavirus, Rotavirus, *Giardia*, or *Cryptosporidium* have been reported, but their relative role in causing diarrhea in SACs has not been assessed.[192,1314,1430, 794]

Housing in close quarters and poor nutrition are some of the complicating factors in coccidiosis. Stress of transportation, shows or change of ownership/location can predispose SACs to coccidiosis. Adult alpacas were reported to develop fatal coccidiosis within 5 weeks after transportation to a new farm.[261,829]

13.6 PATHOLOGY AND CLINICAL SIGNS

Gross lesions are most common in ileum, although any region of small intestine, cecum, and colon may be affected.[195,829,1316,1437] Mucosal thickening, congestion, plaques, and severe hemorrhagic enteritis may be seen in primary lesions. Secondary bacterial infection can lead to severe necrotic enteritis.[195,829,1436,1513] The bowel may also appear grossly normal, even with severe infection.

Microscopically, there is hyperplasia (Figure 1.28D, Chapter 1), nonsuppurative enteritis, depending on concurrent infections. Blunting, fusion, and necrosis of villi, particularly at the tips, have been reported.[829,1437] Although developmental stages of SAC *Eimeria* spp. occur in the mucosal epithelium and lamina propria (Figure 1.26, Chapter 1), occasionally *Eimeria* and associated changes have been noted in the tunica muscularis mucosae.[829]

Little is known of pathogenesis of coccidiosis in SACs. As stated earlier, of the five most prevalent species of *Eimeria* in SACs, *E. macusaniensis* has been most commonly identified in lesions. Pathogenesis is apparently related to gamonts because its schizont stage is unknown.[425] Experimentally infected SACs generally remained asymptomatic despite excreting large numbers of oocysts.[547] However, two of five llama crias fed 20,000 *E. macusaniensis* oocysts had pulpy or watery or bloody diarrhea 3–10 or 9–16 days postinoculation (DPI).[1429]

E. macusaniensis was mildly immunogenic because llamas excreted *E. macusaniensis* oocysts after reinoculation; in challenged llamas, the prepatent period was longer (37–40 days versus 32–36 days after primary infection), patency was shorter (39–43 days versus 20–23 days after challenge), and fewer oocysts were excreted after challenge.[1429]

In a few cases, *E. ivitaensis* had been associated with clinical coccidiosis in alpacas in Peru[1316] and the United States.[190,191] *E. lamae* is another pathogenic species. It was reported to develop in surface epithelium versus in crypts parasitized by *E. macusaniensis* and *E. ivitaensis*[634]; however, its endogenous stages are unknown.[422]

13.7 DIAGNOSIS

The detection of oocysts in feces can help diagnosis. Although most coccidian oocysts float in sugar or salt solutions with specific gravity (sp. gr.) of 1.28, *E. macusaniensis* oocysts are large and heavy and do not float well in these solutions.[193] Therefore, solutions of sp. gr. >1.28 are recommended for flotation. Supersaturated sugar solution (sp. gr. 1.33, Johnson et al.[829]), saturated zinc sulfate solution (sp.gr. 1.36, Twomey et al.[1714]), cesium chlorite solution (sp. gr. 1.4,

Trout et al.[1708]) or mixed salt solutions (zinc chloride 105 g, NaCl 20 g, water to 100 mL, sp. gr. 1.59, Cafrune et al.[166]) are some examples of flotation solutions. The sedimentation methods used for trematode ova are as effective as the flotation method.[1429] The number of oocysts detected does not correlate with clinical signs.[99,167,195,298,547,786,1429] Some cases of coccidiosis may be missed because of the development of clinical signs before oocysts are excreted in feces (prepatent phase). To alleviate this problem, a polymerase chain reaction test has been described[194] for *E. macusaniensis* and *E. lamae* diagnosis.[194] In experimentally infected alpacas, oocyst DNA was detectible up to 7 days before oocyst detection in feces. The internal transcriber spacer primers were species-specific without cross-detection of *E. macusaniensis* and *E. lamae*. Finding *Eimeria* oocyst DNA 7 days before prepatent period is intriguing.

Smears made from biopsied material can reveal the parasitic stages.[195] However, histological examination is needed to evaluate lesions.[195,261,829]

13.8 TREATMENT

There are no anticoccidial drugs approved specifically for SACs.[422]

Efficacy of various drugs for treating clinical coccidiosis is unknown. None of the anticoccidials have any measurable effect on late stages of gamonts and oocysts that have been commonly related with clinical coccidiosis associated with *E. macusaniensis* and *E. ivitaensis*.

Treatment for coccidiosis included amprolium hydrochloride (10 mg/kg) in a 1.5% solution orally daily up to 15 days, or sulfadimethoxine (110 mg/kg) orally daily for 10 days, and supportive therapy. However, some camelids died despite this therapy and had confirmed coccidiosis histologically.[195] In one instance, an entire herd of 30 alpacas that developed coccidiosis 20 days after introduction to a new farm was treated with amprolium hydrochloride, two died and four were euthanized. Two of four alpacas that died had histologically confirmed coccidiosis.[195]

The benzene acetonitrile compounds in general have low toxicity. They are used extensively to treat coccidiosis in camelids in countries where they are readily available in a convenient treatment form. Prophylactic treatment should be considered during winter when outbreaks of coccidiosis are common. Decoquinate may be added to feed at 0.5 mg/kg/day for 4 weeks.[191] In summary, therapeutic treatment for coccidiosis in South American camelids needs validation.

ACKNOWLEDGMENTS

I would like to thank Drs. R.J. Bildfell, C. Bauer, M.M. Cafrune, C.K. Cebra, A. Daugschies, P. Díaz, G. Leguía, G.A. Perkins, and R.H. Rosadio for their help in preparation of this review.

REFERENCES

99, 101, 144, 149, 166, 167, 183, 190–195, 261, 291, 295, 298, 369, 422, 425, 511, 547, 566, 583, 634–638, 672, 709, 726. 761, 785, 786, 829, 966, 970, 1314–1316, 1356, 1397, 1416, 1427, 1429, 1430, 1436, 1437, 1513, 1518, 1708, 1714, 1727, 1794

CHAPTER 14

Coccidiosis in Rabbits (*Oryctolagus cuniculus*)

M. Pakandl and X. Liu

CONTENTS

14.1 INTRODUCTION AND HISTORY

Coccidiosis in rabbits is of historical and economic importance. Historically, *Eimeria stiedai*, the causative agent of rabbit liver coccidiosis, is thought to be the first protozoan recognized in 1674.[976] Coccidiosis causes economic losses to rabbit growers worldwide.

14.2 ETIOLOGY

All rabbit coccidia belong to the genus *Eimeria*. Currently, 11 *Eimeria* species are considered valid (Table 14.1).

Four other *Eimeria* species are considered invalid, including *E. nagpurensis* (Gill and Ray, 1960), *E. oryctolagi* (Ray and Banik, 1965), and *E. matsubayashi* (Tsunoda, 1952) because of similarities with recognized species. Descriptions of two other species, *E. roobroucki*[626] and *E. kongi*,[309] need

additional information before being accepted as valid species. *E. roobroucki* was first named from a wild rabbit in France with a very low intensity of infection. *E. kongi* was described from China. Its oocysts resemble those of *E. irresidua*, but the prepatent period (132 hours) and its sequence of 18S rDNA are different; its endogenous stages are unknown.

Morphological features of recognized species were summarized[459] (Table 14.1).

Oocyst morphology, prepatent period, endogenous stages, and DNA characteristics are helpful in the diagnosis of different *Eimeria* species in rabbits. Figure 14.1 shows sporulated oocysts of rabbit coccidia. Concerning the prepatent period, caution is needed for using it as a reliable criterion because of the peculiar physiology of the rabbit; oocysts in feces can be detected only during a certain time (afternoon until next morning), while in the cecum and stomach they can be observed earlier.[301] Oocyst morphology, prepatent period, and sporulation time of these 11 *Eimeria* species

Table 14.1 Oocyst Morphology, Prepatent Period, and Sporulation Time

Species	Oocyst Shape	Measurements (μm)	Average Size	Oocyst Residuum	Micropyle	Prepatent Period (days)	Sporulation Time (hours)[a]
E. coecicola Cheissin, 1947	Elongate-ovoid	27–40 × 15–22	34.5 × 19.7	Yes	Yes, surrounded by slight collar-like thickening	9	85
E. exigua Yakimoff, 1934	Spherical or subspherical	10–18 × 11–16	15.1 × 14.0	No	No	7	23
E. flavescens Marotel and Guilhon, 1941	Ovoid	25–35 × 18–24	30.0 × 21.0	No	Yes, very large at broad end	9	80
E. intestinalis Cheissin, 1948	Piriform	22–30 × 16–21	26.7 × 18.9	Yes, large	Yes	8.5	70
E. irresidua Kessel and Jankiewicz, 1931	Ovoid, barrel shaped or subrectangular	31–44 × 20–27	39.2 × 23.1	Hardly visible, only few granules[b]	Yes	9	85
E. magna Pérard, 1925	Ellipsoid, ovoid, truncated at micropylar end	31–42 × 20–28	36.3 × 24.1	Yes, very large	Yes, surrounded by collar-like thickening	6.5	80
E. media Kessel, 1929	Ellipsoid or ovoid	23–30 × 15–20	31.1 × 17.0	Yes	Yes, with a pyramidal-shaped protuberance	4.5	41
E. perforans (Leuckart, 1879) Sluiter and Swellengrebel, 1912	Ellipsoid to subrectangular	15–27 × 11–17	22.2 × 13.9	Yes, small	No or difficult to detect	5	30
E. piriformis Kotlán and Pospesch, 1934	Piriform, often asymmetric	25–33 × 16–21	29.5 × 18.1	No	Yes	9	90
E. stiedai (Lindermann, 1865) Kisskalt and Hartmann, 1907	Slightly ellipsoid (often asymmetric, note of M. Pakandl)	30–41 × 15–24	36.9 × 19.9	Hardly visible, only few granules[c]	Almost inapparent	14	63
E. vejdovskyi Pakandl, 1988	Elongate or ovoid	25–38 × 16–22	31.5 × 19.1	Yes	Yes	10	50

[a] At 22°C, at lower temperature, it is longer; at 26°C it is shorter.
[b] Norton, C.C. et al., 1979. *Parasitology* 79, 231–248.
[c] Norton, C.C. et al., 1977. *Parasitology* 75, 1–7.

are also summarized in Table 14.1. Additionally, molecular characteristics are helpful in the diagnosis of rabbit *Eimeria* as summarized in Table 14.2. Phylogenetic analysis grouped rabbit *Eimeria* species into two sister lineages, corresponding to the presence/absence of the oocyst residuum.[931] For nine *Eimeria* species, random amplified polymorphic DNA (RAPD) method as a genetic tool was found valuable for the diagnosis.[197] A 750 bp fragment derived from RAPD could be used for *E. media* identification by polymerase chain reaction (PCR) with primers specific for this fragment, and the detection threshold is 10 oocysts purified or 30 oocysts in fecal matter.[196] The differentiation of 11 *Eimeria* species by PCR was established using primer pairs against internal transcribed spacer (ITS)-1 ribosomal DNAs of each species. The detection limit ranges from 500 fg to 1 pg (0.8–1.7 sporulated oocysts).[1273] More recently, multiplex PCR

was developed for the simultaneous identification of three *Eimeria* species (*E. stiedai*, *E. intestinalis*, and *E. flavescens*).[1843] Disruption of oocysts is necessary for successful extraction of DNA from oocysts. Treatment of oocysts with sodium hypochlorite or saturated sodium solution has been attempted to break up the oocysts' wall for the sufficient release of the DNA.[1668]

To detect DNA from a few oocysts, whole genome amplification (WGA) could be an alternative strategy before the DNA extracts were subjected to PCR. In a study, a single oocyst was directly used for random amplification of the whole genomic DNA, and then PCR was successful for the amplification of ITS-1, 18S rDNA, and 23S rDNA from a single oocyst of *E. stiedai* or *E. media*. This work showed the value of WGA when combined with nested PCR in molecular diagnosis of eimerian parasites at the single-oocyst level.[1781]

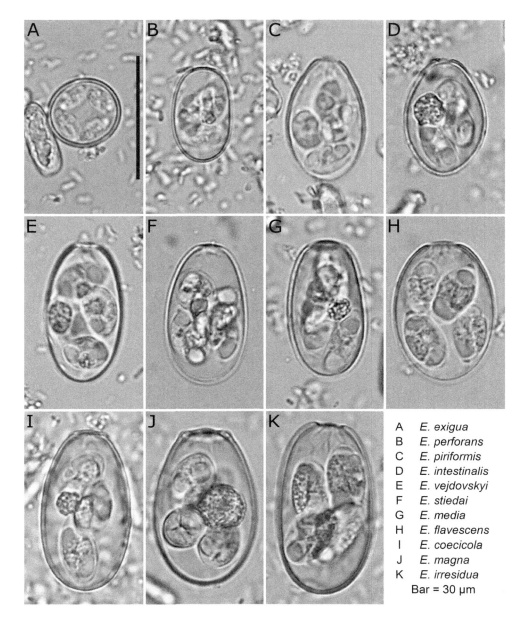

A   *E. exigua*
B   *E. perforans*
C   *E. piriformis*
D   *E. intestinalis*
E   *E. vejdovskyi*
F   *E. stiedai*
G   *E. media*
H   *E. flavescens*
I   *E. coecicola*
J   *E. magna*
K   *E. irresidua*
Bar = 30 µm

Figure 14.1   Sporulated oocysts of 11 *Eimeria* species infecting rabbits.

Mitochondrion-derived genes (such as COI and cytoB) are also used for molecular diagnosis and phylogenetic analysis of *Eimeria* species infecting domestic rabbits.[1058] In addition, COI is a suitable DNA barcoding target for species-level diagnostic and phylogenetic studies of rabbit coccidia.[1269]

An example of the advantage of molecular analysis of rabbit coccidia is a recent study showing that an isolate of coccidia from Zhangjiakou, Hebei Province of China shares very low similarities (27.1%–30%) in ITS-1 sequence with the 11 valid rabbit *Eimeria* species. This isolate, together with its morphological characteristics, was thought to be a new *Eimeria* species and named as *E. kongi*.[309] Accessible sequences of rabbit coccidia are summarized in Table 14.2.

14.3 EPIDEMIOLOGY AND PREVALENCE

Coccidia infection is common in rabbits worldwide. Morphological survey of coccidia infection in many countries or regions showed that the infection rate ranges from about 20% to more than 80% (Table 14.3). Most of the published data deal with the prevalence of rabbit coccidiosis in a specific period of one region or even several farms, but these are not comprehensive surveys of the disease and its control.

With the rapid development of the rabbit industry in China, publications are increasing concerning prevalence studies of coccidia infection. A survey of coccidia infection in 48 farms in 14 provinces of China conducted from July to October 2010 found that the overall infection rate

Table 14.2 Genetic Information Regarding Rabbit Coccidia

Species, Strain	Genetic Locus	Size (bp)	GenBank Accession Number
E. media	18S rRNA, partial	1467	EF694013
E. media	18S rRNA gene, 5.8S rRNA, partial; ITS-1	468	HM768887
E. media	18S SSUrRNA, partial	1738	HQ173834
E. media	23S LSUrRNA, partial	986	HQ173848
E. media LCED1	ITS-1, partial	153	KX379239
E. media YW006	18S rRNA, 28S rRNA, partial; 5.8S rRNA; ITS-1; ITS-2	1070	JX406877
E. media Hebei	18S rRNA, 5.8S rRNA, 28S rRNA, ITS-1, ITS-2, region	440	JQ071392
E. vejdovskyi	18S rRNA, partial	1346	EF694010
E. vejdovskyi	18S SSUrRNA, partial	1739	HQ173838
E. vejdovskyi	23S LSUrRNA, partial	984	HQ173856
E. vejdovskyi	18S rRNA, 5.8S rRNA, partial; ITS-1	406	HM768891
E. vejdovskyi LCEV1	ITS-1, partial	167	KX379242
E. flavescens	18S SSUrRNA, partial	1738	HQ173830
E. flavescens	23S LSUrRNA, partial	984	HQ173843
E. flavescens	18S rRNA, 5.8S rRNA, partial; ITS-1	463	HM768883
E. flavescens	18S rRNA, partial	1419	EF694011
E. flavescens YW002	18S rRNA, 28S rRNA, partial; ITS-1; 5.8S rRNA; ITS-2	1061	JX406873
E. flavescens LCEF1	ITS-1, partial	199	KX379235
E. magna	ITS-1, partial	213	KX379238
E. magna	ssrRNA, partial, ITS-1, complete, 5.8SrRNA, partial	430	MH843654
E. magna	cytb, complete	1080	HQ173882
E. magna	18S rRNA, partial, IST-1, 5.8S rRNA, ITS-2, complete, 28S rRNA, partial	1107	JX406876
E. magna	18S rRNA, IST-1, 5.8S rRNA, ITS-2, 28S rRNA	424	JQ071391

Table 14.3 Prevalence of Coccidia in Domestic Rabbits, Investigated by Morphological Methods

Country/Region	Sample Numbers	Number Positive (%)	Remarks (Most Prevalent Species)	Reference
China	480 fecal samples	41.9	E. perforans	Jing et al.[818]
China, Northwest	1622 fecal samples	78.11	E. perforans	Qiao et al.[1369]
China, Wenzhou	595 fecal samples	77.1	E. irresidua	
China, Sichuan Provence	110 fecal samples from 11 farms	56.4	E. perforans	Yin et al.[1857]
Slovakia	137 farms	63.5		Bukovszki and Kocisova[161]
Egypt	298 fecal samples	33.9	E. perforans and E. magna	Elshahawy and Elgoniemy[488]
Egypt	100 rabbits	70	E. intestinalis and E. coecicola	El-Shahawi et al.[478]
Germany	434 fecal samples	21.2		Raue et al.[1394]
Kenya	61 rabbits and 302 fecal samples	85% in fecal samples and 90.2% in individual rabbits		Okumu et al.[1271]
Nigeria, Southeastern	Intestines and livers of 274 rabbits	78.83		Szkucik et al.[1658]
Saudi Arabia	100 fecal samples	75	E. coecicola (70%)	Abdel-Baki and Al-Quraishy[4]
Estonian	65 fecal samples and 15 dead animals		E. media and E. magna	Järvis et al.[787]
Northwestern Iran	320 rabbits	26.87% for E. stiedai		Tehrani et al.[1690]
India, Haryana	2703 rabbits	23.3% overall morbidity and 16.7% overall mortality		Gupta et al.[648]
India, Gujarat	431 fecal samples	29		Hirani and Solanki[720]
India, Andaman	10 fecal samples	80		Jeyakumar et al.[808]

was 41.9%, with *E. perforans* as the most prevalent species.[818] Local studies of the prevalence of rabbit coccidiosis also show that mixed infection of 2–10 *Eimeria* species is common in China.[815] In a study with samples from Sichuan Province of China, the overall prevalence of *Eimeria* infection was 56.4% (62/110), and coinfection with two to seven *Eimeria* species was detected, with which *E. perforans* was the most prevalent species (42.73%).[1857] In the Wenzhou area of Zhejiang Province, the overall prevalence of infection from 595 fresh fecal pellets was 77.1%.[812]

A few studies reported molecular or serological diagnosis of coccidia infection in rabbits. Enzyme-linked immunosorbent assay using oocyst antigen proved to be the best tool for early diagnosis of hepatic coccidiosis and can be used in field studies to assess coccidiosis seroprevalence in rabbit farms.[7]

14.4 ENDOGENOUS CYCLES AND BIOLOGY

Data on endogenous development of *Eimeria* species parasitizing intestines are summarized in Table 14.4. Salient features are summarized in the following sections.

14.4.1 Migration of Sporozoites

The small intestine, especially the duodenum, seems to be a universal gate for rabbit coccidia, regardless of the specific sites of their further development. The sporozoites of *E. intestinalis* were found within 10 minutes after inoculation in the duodenal mucosa, and 4 hours later the sporozoites reached ileum, the specific site of parasite development.[405] Similar results were obtained after infection with *E. magna*, the sporozoites of which migrate from the duodenum to the jejunum and, more abundantly, to the ileum.[1304] In both instances, sporozoites were often seen in intraepithelial lymphocytes (IELs).

Unusual localization of parasites in different endogenous stages was observed in *E. coecicola*.[1303,1306] Although its first asexual generation develops in gut-associated lymphoid tissue (GALT) in distinct parts of the intestine (appendix, *sacculus rotundus* and Peyer's patches), and following stages in the epithelium covering these parts of intestine, the sporozoites first penetrate the small intestine and were found in their specific site of multiplication as late as 48 hours postinoculation. One of the hypotheses is that transport of *E. coecicola* sporozoites is via lymphatic circulation because large numbers of sporozoites were found in mesenteric lymph nodes and spleen.[1313,1408] In contrast, sporozoites of *E. intestinalis* were not found extraintestinally,[1313] although they have been observed in IELs and in lymphocytes in lamina propria.[998,1313] The route of migration seems different in *E. coecicola* and other intestinal coccidia. The migration of sporozoites can be affected by immune response of the host.[1313]

The life cycle of *E. stiedai* is intriguing and has been the subject of research for more than a century because of its exclusive location in bile ducts. After the excystation in the small intestine, *E. stiedai* sporozoites reach bile ducts in 1–2 days by an unknown mechanism, most likely through lymphatic circulation. They have also been detected in bone marrow and mesenteric lymph nodes.[452,1294,1344] From the mesenteric lymph nodes, the sporozoites are likely distributed throughout the body via ductus thoracicus and consequently infect the liver.[452] Although infection can be transmitted to coccidia-free recipients with blood, a direct transportation of the sporozoites with portal blood to the liver probably plays minor, if any, role.[452,539,1344]

14.4.2 Phenomenon of Multinucleated Merozoites

Although polynucleate merozoites were reported previously in a few *Eimeria* species (see Chapter 1), they are a regular feature in *Eimeria* of rabbits. The only exceptions are the first and second generations of *E. coecicola*.[1303]

Polynucleate merozoites differ from uninucleate ones in number of nuclei and in the presence of some structures belonging to newly formed merozoites, namely, inner membranous complex, rhoptry anlage, and sometimes, conoid.[320,1306] In some species, such as *E. magna*, *E. media*, *E. vejdovskyi*. and *E. flavescens*, even "sporozoite-like schizonts" were found, but this is not limited to rabbit coccidia.[1299,1302,1305,1307] The exact role of polynucleate merozoites in the life cycles is not quite clear, but we consider them as an integral part of the life cycle.

Some authors believe that the presence of two types of schizonts reflects sexual dimorphism.[1344,1622] It was postulated that there are two lines in the endogenous development of *E. perforans*: the male, represented by meronts forming polynucleate merozoites in which endomerogony (formation of daughter merozoites inside the cells) occurs, and the female, which is characterized by uninucleate merozoites arising by ectomerogony (merozoites are formed in contact with plasmalemma of the meront, type B merozoites). The last male (polynucleate, type A) merozoites give rise to microgamonts, and the female (uninucleate, type B) ones to macrogamonts. The life-cycle study showed that as the endogenous development progresses, the proportion of type A meronts decreases in subsequent generations.[1622] Because the microgamonts are fewer than macrogamonts, such observation supports the hypothesis mentioned. The same is applicable for other species of rabbit coccidia.[998,1301,1302,1305,1307]

14.4.3 Infection of Suckling Rabbits

Suckling rabbits until the age of about 16–19 days are naturally resistant to infection with low oocyst doses of intestinal coccidia *E. flavescens* (200 oocysts) and *E. intestinalis* (2000 oocysts). By 1 month of age, rabbits are fully susceptible to coccidiosis.[1308,1309] However, this age-related immunity is relative as rabbits of any age can be infected with large doses of oocysts.[453,1517] The rate of excystation

Table 14.4 Overview of Endogenous Cycles of Enteric *Eimeria* of Rabbits (Generation of Schizonts[a])

Species	Intestinal Segment	Localization in the Mucosa	Number of Asexual Generations	Number of merozoites					Number of Nuclei in Type A Merozoites
				First Generation	Second Generation	Third Generation	Fourth Generation	Fifth Generation	
E. coecicola	Appendix, sacculus rotundus, Peyer's patches	First a.g. GALT; second–fourth a.g. and gamogony epithelium of domes and mushrooms in vermiform appendix, sacculus rotundus, and Peyer's patches	4	Up to 12	2	A: 2–10 B: 10–200	Like third generation		2–3 (3,4)[a];1303,1306
E. exigua	Duodenum-ileum; successively moves from proximal to distal parts of the small intestine	Tops of the villi	4	2	A: 2 B: 3–7	A: 2–4 B: 4–16	A: 2 B: 4–13		2 (2,3,4)[797]
E. flavescens	First a.g. small intestine, second-fifth a.g. cecum	First a.g. crypts, second—fourth a.g. superficial epithelium, fifth a.g. and gamonts crypts	5	16	12–20	12–20	12–24	Approximately 50	Not given (5)[1247]
				A: 4–8 B: 20–40	A: 2 B: 2–4	A: 2 B: 2–4	A: 2–4 B: 8–25	A: 2–4 B: 30–150	2–4 (1,2,3,4); up to 9 (5)[1301]
E. intestinalis	Lower jejunum and ileum	First and second a.g. crypts, third and fourth a.g. and gamonts crypts and wall of the villi	3–4	A: 3–5 B: 15–25	A: 5–8 B: 10–20	A: <30 B: 60–120	A: not found B: <30		2–5 (1,2,3)[998]
E. irresidua	Jejunum and ileum	First a.g. in crypts, second a.g. in lamina propria, third a.g., fourth a.g. and gametocytes in the villous epithelium	4	?	Approximately 50	40–50	40–50		Type A meronts not observed[1247]
E. magna	Jejunum and ileum, in a lesser extent duodenum	First a.g. crypts, other stages villi	At least 5	4–12		A: 2–8 B: 12–100; generations not distinguished	A: 2–8; generations not distinguished		2–6 (generations not distinguished)[1473]
E. media	Duodenum-jejunum, low concentration of the parasite in the ileum	All stages villi except third a.g., which is in crypts	4	A: 8–12 B: 18–20	A: 2–8 B: 20–30	A: 4–10 B: 20–60	A: 4–20 B: 20–60		2–3 (1,2,3), up to 8 (4)[1305]
		Intestinal villi (walls and tops)	3	A: none B: 8–20	A: 2–6 B: 10–20	A: 2–6 B: 10–40			2–3 (2), 4–8 (3)[1307]
E. perforans	Maximal parasite concentration in the duodenum, but also in the jejunum and ileum	Both villi and crypts	2	A: 2–8 B: 12–24	A: 2–12 B: 20–36				2–8 (1,2)[1622]
E. piriformis	Colon	Crypts	4	A: 2 B: 2	A: 2 B: 10–32	A: 2 B: 2	A: 2 B: 18–45		2 (1), 4–8 (2), 2 (3), 4–10 (4)[1311]
E. vejdovskyi	Ileum	First–third a.g. crypts, fourth and fifth a.g. villi	5	A: none B: 20–50	A: 2–8 B: 2–8	A: 4–20 B: 10–40	A: 25–70 B: 50–200	A: 2–4 B: 4–20	2–3 (2,3,4,5)[1302]

Abbreviations: a.g., asexual generation(s); GALT, gut-associated lymphoid tissue.

[a] The figures in brackets mean the generations in which the polynucleate merozoites were found.

is minimal in very young animals and increases gradually with age. Perhaps inefficiency of excystation, physiological and biochemical properties of the intestine, and absence of para-aminobezoic acid in the mother's milk contribute to the innate resistance to coccidia in very young mammals.[1517]

14.4.4 Transmission to Hares

Rabbit coccidia are typically strictly host specific, but *E. stiedai* was experimentally transmitted to European hares (*Lepus europaeus*) in which it completed its development and caused macroscopic lesions and clinical signs of coccidiosis.[1516,1731] The oocysts isolated from hares were infective for both rabbits and hares.[1731] However, under natural conditions, this coccidium is extremely rare in hares.[150,1343]

14.5 PATHOGENESIS

Under natural conditions, young rabbits after weaning are the most susceptible to coccidiosis. Because coccidia are ubiquitous, older animals become less sensitive due to acquired immunity. Nevertheless, age of animals itself may play a role in pathogenesis of liver coccidiosis.[601]

Rabbit coccidia can be grouped per their pathogenicity: nonpathogenic (*E. coecicola*), slightly pathogenic (*E. perforans*, *E. exigua*, and *E. vejdovskyi*), mildly pathogenic or pathogenic (*E. media*, *E. magna*, *E. piriformis*, and *E. irresidua*), or highly pathogenic (*E. intestinalis*, *E. flavescens*, and potentially *E. stiedai*).[300–302,1001]

In the two most pathogenic enteric species, *E. intestinalis* and *E. flavescens*, infective doses of 2000–5000 oocysts per animal lead to mild disease, and 10,000 to 13,000 oocysts cause severe disease with high mortality. In contrast, only doses of 100,000 or more oocysts of *E. perforans*, *E. exigua*, *E. coecicola*, and *E. stiedai* can elicit an obvious disease.[300–303]

Pathogenicity may differ even among strains/isolates of the same species, as a strain of *E. intestinalis* isolated in China could only cause clinical symptoms when the inocula were more than 5×10^4 oocysts.[1554]

There is no correlation between oocyst excretion and severity of the disease. For example, infection of a naïve rabbit with 100 oocysts of *E. flavescens* is sufficient to give maximum oocyst yield ($1–2 \times 10^8$), and increasing the infective dose does not result in enhanced oocyst output. However, this dose does not cause any symptoms of a disease.[301]

Weight loss or retardation of growth is simple, but the most reliable criterion of health status of rabbits and way to measure the severity of infection in growing animals.

14.5.1 Intestinal Coccidiosis

Typical signs of intestinal coccidiosis are growth depression, reduced food and water consumption, lethargy, weakness, and in some cases mortality, namely, after infections with *E. intestinalis* and *E. flavescens*. During the acute phase of coccidiosis, a short period of diarrhea, during which feces are more hydrated (*E. magna*, *E. intestinalis*) or watery (*E. flavescens*), can be observed. Lesions, although spectacular, are rather transient. Their localization is characteristic for individual species[301] (Figure 14.3).

Although the most pathogenic species, *E. intestinalis* and *E. flavescens*, parasitize in different parts of the intestine, the crucial point seems to be the destruction of stem cells in crypts that subsequently fail to keep the integrity of the epithelium. In rabbits infected with *E. flavescens*, denudation of mucosa results in tissue invasion by bacteria and severe inflammation.[616] After infection with *E. intestinalis*, severe villus atrophy occurs, and some biochemical parameters, such as significant hypokalemia and uremia indicating protein catabolism were changed.[1338] The disease is accompanied by a significant increase in fecal *Escherichia coli* output.[1004,1338]

The changes in water and hydromineral metabolism were observed in diarrheal rabbits infected with *E. intestinalis*. Total water loss in infected rabbits was just slightly significant, though hematocrit decreased in infected rabbits and resulted in hemodilution.[1002] In the same trial, disturbances of electrolytes, such as Na^+ and K^+, were obvious since day 5 postinoculation, resulting in hyponatremia, hypochloremia, and hypokalemia, and indicating the lessened efficiency of intestinal absorption, while the increase of uremia greater than twofold was often detected in infected animals.[1003] A subsequent study using rabbits with diarrhea caused by infection with *E. intestinalis* or *E. flavescens* showed that sodium reabsorption was against potassium secretion in the colon, resulting in excessive loss of potassium and thus obvious hypokalemia.[1005]

14.5.2 Hepatic Coccidiosis

Liver coccidiosis causes a slight depression of growth in standard rabbit breeding, but more severe disease can be observed after experimental doses with 10^4 or greater than 10^5 oocysts per animal; these are controversial data.[76,301] Typical clinical signs are meteorism, inappetence, diarrhea, or in contrast, constipation, and icterus.[1343] Characteristic macroscopic lesions are shown in Figure 14.2D.

As a result of functional disorder, changed blood parameters such as hyperproteinemia, bilirubinemia, lipemia, and increased activity of liver enzymes (sorbitol dehydrogenase, glutamate oxalate transaminase, glutamate pyruvate transaminase, glutamate dehydrogenase, γ-glutamyl transferase, glutamic oxalacetic transaminase, alanine aminotransferase, aspartate aminotransferase, and lactate dehydrogenase) are characteristic for the infection.[76,77,600,693,819]

14.6 TREATMENT

14.6.1 Chemotherapy

To date, preventive chemotherapy with anticoccidial drugs is the main strategy to control rabbit coccidiosis.

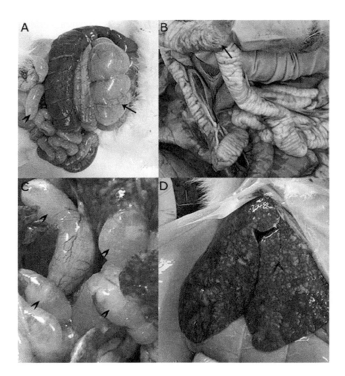

Figure 14.2 Gross lesions in rabbits with coccidiosis. (A) Tympany of the cecum (arrowhead) and thin wall of the jejunum (arrow) in a rabbit heavily infected with *E. magna*. (B) Hemorrhage of the mucosal surface on jejunum in a rabbit infected with *E. magna*. (C) *E. stiedai* infection with dilated bile ducts (arrowheads) near the gallbladder. (D) Necrosis in the liver of rabbit infected with *E. stiedai*.

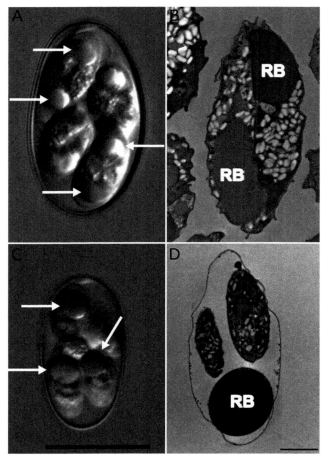

Figure 14.3 Oocysts and sporocysts of the parent strain (A, B) and precocious line (C, D) of *E. media*. (A and C) Light microscopy; while two refractile bodies (RBs) can be seen in each sporocyst of the parent strain, only one RB is visible in sporocysts of the precocious line (arrows). (B and D) Transmission electron microscopy; in the parent strain, RBs are only within sporozoites. In the precocious line, only one huge RB is outside the sporozoites. Bars: (A and C) = 20 μm; (B and D) = 2 μm. (Images provided by Dr. Xiaolong Gu.)

Several reviews or monographs have detailed the anticoccidial drugs currently used for the rabbit industry.[454,1300] As most anticoccidial drugs were first tested and used in chickens, fewer effective ones are available for rabbits.

In the 1940s–1950s, sulfonamides, such as sulfathalidine, sulfamezathine, and sulfaquinoxaline were introduced for treating coccidiosis in rabbits.[245,738,1100] Sulfonamides are still widely used for the treatment of rabbit coccidiosis where this disease emergently occurs.

Several ionophore drugs are effective for the prevention of rabbit coccidiosis. In a study with experimental infection, salinomycin was shown as the most effective ionophore drug against spontaneous infection of *Eimeria* when compared to lasalocid and monensin.[1298] The addition of narasin at 12–24 mg/kg in the feed was shown to be effective to reduce oocyst shedding.[1341] For maduramicin, its safety dose is too close to the effective dose and can easily cause toxicity in rabbits even when administrated in 2 mg/kg.[1134]

Triazine is another category of effective drugs for the control of chicken coccidiosis. Diclazuril and toltrazuril were soon proven effective against rabbit coccidiosis.[1339,1729] These two drugs are currently widely used as a feed additive for the prophylaxis of rabbit coccidiosis. For ponazuril, a recently developed triazine, its anticoccidial effect was tested with positive results.[995] As an alternative way, improving the bioavailability by complexation could increase the effect of existing drugs.[1880]

Though diclazuril-resistant strains of *Eimeria* species were reported in chickens, no publication from the rabbit industry was found to date. However, as robenidine-resistant *Eimeria magna* was reported,[1340] the potential occurrence of drug resistance should be taken into consideration and is valuable for further study in farms with long-term drug application but with outbreaks of coccidiosis.[1836]

14.6.2 Precocious Lines

Since it is desirable to avoid continuous medication with anticoccidial drugs, live attenuated vaccine is a promising and relatively feasible method; hence, attenuated lines of rabbit coccidia have been derived using the same method as in chicken coccidia—that is, selection for precociousness.[790] Reproductive potential and pathogenicity in precocious lines (PLs) are substantially reduced. These lines of E. intestinalis, E. media, and E. magna were characterized. In E. intestinalis, the reproductive potential was reduced 1000 times and in E. magna and E. media 500 times.[999,1000,1001]

Infection with 1000 or 2500 oocysts of attenuated lines of E. media or E. magna, respectively, protected rabbits from challenge with high doses of the parent strains.[1000,1001] The same can be expected in E. intestinalis, since this species is highly immunogenic and infection with even six oocysts leads to protection against challenge.[302] E. flavescens, which besides E. intestinalis is the most pathogenic rabbit coccidium, is weakly immunogenic; therefore, an appropriate method of vaccination is to be tested.[1247]

The pathogenicity of original E. flavescens and precocious line derived in China was compared. The relative weight gain rate (from day 7 to day 21 postinfection) of rabbits inoculated with 10^3 oocysts/animal of the parental strain was 42.15%, while this value in the group infected with PL was 90.48%. Hence, the pathogenicity of the precocious line of E. flavescens was reduced, but the immunogenicity of PL was maintained (unpublished data from Jiao et al.).

14.6.2.1 Changes in the Life Cycles and Oocyst Morphology

By definition, PLs means lines with shortened prepatent periods. The shortening of the prepatent period is caused by the absence or reduction of one or more asexual generations. It happens after several passages under selection pressure, during which first excreted oocysts are picked up and in the next passage rabbits are infected with them. The genetic background of this phenomenon remains unclear. The changes in life cycles and prepatent periods are summarized in Table 14.5.

Unlike chicken coccidia, the oocysts of PLs, with exception of E. flavescens, can be recognized by the oocyst morphology. Using a light microscope, two refractile bodies (RBs), each of them belonging to one of two sporozoites, can be seen within each sporocyst in parent strains. In the oocysts of the PL of E. intestinalis, two sporocysts lack RB,

and two remaining sporocysts possess one huge RB.[999] In PL of E. magna, E. media, and E. piriformis, each sporocyst contains a large RB.[1000,1001,1311] Electron-microscopic study of oocysts of E. magna, E. media, and E. piriformis revealed that the extremely large RB (Figure 14.3) can be found either inside one of the sporozoites, or free inside the sporocyst.[1312] In E. piriformis, RB, when outside the sporozoites, is included in the sporocyst's residual body.[1311]

Sporozoites of attenuated lines of E. intestinalis, E. magna, and E. media contained no or very small RB after in vitro excystation and hence they must lose RB during excystation.[1312] Consequently, merozoites of the first and second generation of E. magna and E. media do not harbor any remnants of RB like the parent strains.[1305,1307]

14.6.2.2 Vaccination Trials

Vaccination with a precocious line of E. magna elicits immunity sufficient to protect young rabbits against challenge with a wild strain. The individual vaccination with 3500 oocysts/rabbit gave total protection against challenge with vaccination between 25 and 29 days of age. Vaccination of a whole litter by spray dispersion with 40,000 oocysts at 25 days of age was totally effective on oocyst output and weight gain after challenge at 36 days of age.[402,403] The protection is related to immune response elicited in young rabbits and not by transfer of immunity from does.[404]

14.6.2.3 Commercial Vaccines

Although attenuated lines of rabbit coccidia were already derived or new such lines may be obtained, the commercialization of precocious lines of rabbit coccidia did not step into the final stage. Recently, precocious lines of several pathogenic and prevalent species were selected and a trivalent live vaccine is under testing for its efficacy and safety in China.

14.7 CONCLUSION

In our overview, we listed valid species of Eimeria in rabbits. However, discovery of new species cannot be

Table 14.5 Precocious Lines of Rabbit Coccidia

Species	Shortening of the Prepatent Period	Number of Passages Needed	Changes in the Endogenous Development	Reference
E. coecicola	3.5 days	a	a	Coudert et al.[301]
E. flavescens	67 hours	19	Second (or third) and fourth a.g. are absent	Pakandl[1299]
E. intestinalis	71 hours	6	Probably the third a.g. is absent	Licois et al.[999]
E. magna	46 hours	8	Last (fourth) a.g. is absent	Licois et al.[1001,1305]
E. media	36 hours	12	Last (third) a.g. is absent	Licois et al.[1000,1307]
E. piriformis	24 hours	12	Last (fourth) a.g. is absent	Pakandl and Jelínková[1311]

Abbreviation: a.g., asexual generation.
a No details were published.

excluded. For example, in a wild rabbit that excreted many oocysts of *E. exigua*, endogenous stages were found in host nuclei. However, it is unlikely that these stages belong to *E. exigua*, since *E. exigua* does not parasitize host nuclei.[625,797] Therefore, this may be a new coccidian parasite. Taxonomic status of the species that are currently considered to be valid may not be definitive, as they may include more sibling species or an analogy of operational taxonomic units found in chicken coccidia.

Several precocious lines of rabbit coccidia were derived, but commercial vaccines are, to our knowledge, under development only in China.

New trends and methods have been recently applied in the research of rabbit coccidia. A transgenic line of *E. magna* (EmagER) expressing enhanced yellow fluorescent protein (EYFP) and red fluorescent protein (RFP) was constructed. Specific immune response was induced by the exogenous protein expressed by EmagER and favored future studies on application of transgenic rabbit coccidia as recombinant vaccine vectors.[1676] A transfected line of *E. intestinalis* was also obtained.[1555] Immunoproteomic analysis revealed 41 parasite proteins that elicited humoral response.[1595] and thus a new approach is applied in research aimed on rabbit coccidia as well.

REFERENCES

4, 7, 76, 77, 150, 161, 196, 197, 245, 300–303, 309, 320, 402–405, 452–454, 459, 478, 488, 539, 600, 601, 616, 625, 626, 648, 693, 720, 738, 787, 790, 797, 808, 812, 815, 818, 819, 931, 976, 995, 998–1005, 1058, 1100, 1134, 1247, 1248, 1269, 1271, 1273, 1294, 1298–1309, 1311–1313, 1338–1341, 1343, 1344, 1369, 1394, 1408, 1473, 1516, 1517, 1554, 1555, 1595, 1622, 1658, 1668, 1676, 1690, 1729, 1731, 1781, 1836, 1843, 1857, 1880

CHAPTER 15

Coccidiosis in Chickens (*Gallus gallus*)

B. Jordan, G. Albanese, and L. Tensa

CONTENTS

15.1 INTRODUCTION AND HISTORY

More than 60 billion chickens are produced in the world each year, resulting in the production of more than 1.1 trillion eggs and 90 million tons of meat.[136] In 2018 in the United States, 9.04 billion broilers and 249 million turkeys were raised and 109 billion eggs were produced, and the combined value of poultry production (broilers, turkeys, and eggs) was $46 billion (https://www.nass.usda.gov/Charts_and_Maps/Poultry/index.php, 2019). There are many diseases that impact the commercial poultry industry, with coccidiosis being the costliest on a yearly basis. The total global economic impact of coccidiosis is estimated to be in excess of $3 billion per year, due to poor feed conversion, reduced egg production, failure to thrive, treatment, and prevention costs.[317] Approximately 80% of these costs are associated with the subclinical effects including the loss of performance parameters, and the final 20% of costs are associated with the cost of prophylaxis and treatment.[1802] Coccidiosis causes further loss and concerns of zoonotic foodborne disease as it is associated with increased intestinal colonization of bacteria *Clostridium perfringens* and *Salmonella enterica* serovars Typhimurium and Enteritidis.[285,1372] In the United Kingdom, more than 40% of all antimicrobials sold for the use of food animals are classified for the control of coccidial parasites.[136]

Although bloody coccidiosis in chickens was known for two centuries, its etiology was not properly understood until the early 1930s, and control programs were not developed until a decade later.[228,230a] Through the pioneering

studies by W.T. Johnson, E.E. Tyzzer, and P.P. Levine in late 1929 through the 1930s, the life cycles of *Eimeria* species in chickens were described. Of the seven species of *Eimeria* in chickens universally recognized (Table 15.1), Johnson named two species (*E. necatrix, E. praecox*), Tyzzer[1717] named three (*E. acervulina, E. maxima, E. mitis*), and Levine named *E. brunetti*. We had great difficulty locating the original description of *E. necatrix* and *E. praecox*, because they were named not in an official journal but in a report of the Institute.[834] The descriptions of *E. praecox* and *E. necatrix* are buried on page 119 of the 142-page report; most of the report does not concern coccidiosis. A formal description of these species was promised but never published, probably because of the author's untimely death. The name *E. necatrix* signifies "murderess," and *E. praecox* signifies precocity—short prepatent period of 4 days—this was explained in a paper written posthumously by his wife, Mrs. W.T. Johnson.[835a] The following information is from that publication[835] and is quoted here for the benefit of future researchers.[834]

This investigation has resulted in the recognition of six species of coccidia, two of which are new and for which names *Eimeria praecox* and *Eimeria necaltrix* are proposed.

The average size of fifty oocysts of *E. praecox* was found to be 20.6 × 23.8 microns, or a shape index (width divided by length) of 0.87. The oocysts prove infective after twenty-four to thirty-six hours sporulation at room temperature. New oocysts appear in the feces on the fourth day after feeding sporulated oocysts, a few hours sooner than with *E. acervulina* (Tyzzer). *E. praecox* attacks the small intestine,

Table 15.1   Summary of Life Cycle of Common *Eimeria* Species in Chickens

Species	Oocyst Size	Region Parasitized	Asexual Generations	Pathogenicity	Reference
E. acervulina (Tyzzer, 1929)	Avg. 18.3 × 14.6 μm	Duodenum		++	Tyzzer[1717]; Vetterling and Doran[1746]
E. brunetti (Levine, 1942)	Avg. 24.6 × 18.8 μm	Ileum/colon	4	+++	Levine[983]; Boles and Becker[143]
E. maxima (Tyzzer, 1929)	Avg. 30.5 × 20.7 μm	Small intestine	2–3	++	Tyzzer[1717]; Dubey and Jenkins[437]
E. mitis (Tyzzer, 1929)	Avg. 15.6 × 14.2	Ileum/jejunum		+	Tyzzer[1717]; Joyner[842]
E. necatrix (Johnson, 1930)	Avg. 20.4 × 17.2 μm	Ileum/jejunum		+++	Johnson[834]; Tyzzer et al.[1718]; Van Doornenck and Becker[1723]
E. praecox (Johnson, 1930)	Avg. 21.3 × 17.1 μm	Duodenum/ upper ileum		+	Tyzzer et al.[1718]; Long[1074]
E. tenella (Railliet and Lucet, 1891) Fanthom, 1909	Avg. 22.0 × 19.0 μm	Ceca	3	++++	Tyzzer[1717]; Tyzzer et al.[1718]

beginning near the gizzard. Failure in cross-immunization has been established between *E. praecox*, *E. mitis* (Tyzzer), *E. acervulina* (Tyzzer), and *E. maxima* (Tyzzer).

E. necatrix attacks the small intestine, beginning near the gizzard, and in severe infections produces marked hemorrhages and dilation of the intestine. The schizonts are the largest of any species attacking the duodenum and free portion of the small intestine. The average size of nine schizonts selected from a large number was 49.2 × 63.1 microns, and included a minimum of 42.0 × 44.0 microns and a maximum of 62.7 × 84.7 microns.

In a 114-page monograph, Tyzzer[1717] described the life cycles of *E. maxima*, *E. mitis*, and *E. acervulina* that he named and also the other species of *Eimeria* in chickens.

P. P. Levine first advocated the use of an antibiotic, sulfonamide, for the treatment of coccidiosis in chickens.[980]

15.2 MORPHOLOGY AND LIFE CYCLE

In chickens, coccidiosis is caused by species in the genera *Eimeria*. Chicken *Eimeria* are host specific, and most invade specific regions of the gut. There is still some uncertainty concerning the species of *Eimeria* present in chickens. Seven species (*E. acervulina*, *E. brunetti*, *E. maxima*, *E. mitis*, *E. necatrix*, *E. tenella*, and *E. praecox*) are universally recognized (Table 15.1). These species were characterized using classic methodology that included defined prepatent periods, oocyst morphology, location of infection, and cross-protection from challenge, before molecular techniques were available. These species have been found in multiple countries across all six continents that raise poultry.[275] The status of two species, *E. hagani*[981] and *E. mivati*[470], remains uncertain, and original samples are not available for verification.[1758] Additionally, with the increasing use of molecular tools, recent studies suggest the presence of three additional species currently referred to as operational taxonomic units (OTUs) X, Y, and Z, in the southern hemisphere.[172,275] When compared to the classically

described species, they most closely match with *E. maxima*, *E. brunetti*, and *E. mitis*, respectively.[1205]

Data on life cycles and biology are summarized in Table 15.1.

Five of the generally accepted seven *Eimeria* species infecting chickens have an ovoid shape (*E. acervulina*, *E. brunetti*, *E. maxima*, *E. praecox*, and *E. tenella*), while the remaining two are subspherical (*E. mitis*) or oblong ovoid (*E. necatrix*). *E. maxima* has the largest oocyst with an average length multiplied by width measurement of 30.5 × 20.7 μm. *E. brunetti* has the second largest oocyst size, with an average measurement of 24.6 × 18.8 μm followed by *E. tenella* (22.0 × 19.0 μm), *E. praecox* (21.3 × 17.1 μm), *E. necatrix* (20.4 × 17.2 μm), *E. acervulina* (183. × 14.6 μm), and *E. mitis* (15.6 × 13.4 μm) (reviewed in McDougald and Fitz-Coy[1165]). Other than *E. maxima*, many of the *Eimeria* infecting chickens overlap in average oocyst size, making species differentiation by microscopy difficult to the untrained observer (Figure 15.1). Each species also differs, but overlaps, in the region of the intestinal tract parasitized. Site of infectivity for each species is predetermined, as the greatest number of sporozoites for each species are found at that site as compared to other places within the intestine following excystation.[1559] The zone of parasitism for each species is as follows: *E. acervulina* is focused in the duodenum but will move into the upper jejunum during heavy infection; *E. brunetti* can be found throughout the intestinal tract but is most associated with the lower ileum, colon, and ceca; *E. maxima* is concentrated in the jejunum but can move up into the duodenum or down into the ileum during heavy infection; *E. mitis* is focused in the lower jejunum and ileum; *E. necatrix* is found in the lower duodenum, jejunum, and upper ileum; *E. praecox* is found in the duodenum and upper jejunum; and *E. tenella* is isolated to the ceca. Clinical signs and disease states from infection are related to the region of the intestinal tract parasitized, the pathogenicity of the species and strain, and where in the epithelium (villus tips versus crypts) development takes place.

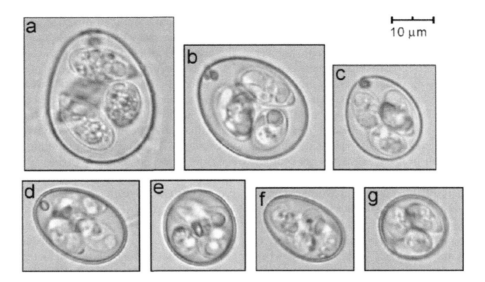

Figure 15.1 Photomicrographs of oocysts of the seven *Eimeria* species of chickens. (a) *E. maxima*, (b) *E. brunetti*, (c) *E. tenella*, (d) *E. neca-trix*, (e) *E. praecox*, (f) *E. acervulina*, and (g) *E. mitis*. (From *Pattern Recognition*, 40 (7), César, A.B. et al., Biological shape characterization for automatic image recognition and diagnosis of protozoan parasites of the genus *Eimeria*. 1899–1910. Copyright 2007, with permission from Elsevier.)

The major species to cause pathogenicity differ depending on the type of chicken being raised, and the pathogenic effects of *Eimeria* species can vary depending on the host infected. Broilers are most often impacted by *E. acervulina*, *E. maxima*, and *E. tenella*. Long-lived birds such as breeders and layers face challenge from those three in addition to *E. necatrix* and *E. brunetti*.[1139] The most pathogenic strains causing significant mortality in chickens include *E. tenella*, *E. necatrix*, and *E. brunetti*. Other species, such as *E. maxima*, are an economical problem, causing significantly impaired weight gain, increased feed conversion ratios, or predisposition to other disease states, such as necrotic enteritis. *E. mitis* and *E. praecox* are typically considered the least pathogenic and may not cause overt lesions but in high enough numbers can impact the growth and health of birds leading to decreased performance of the flock.[1525] Within the zone of parasitism described earlier, infection with each species causes a specific lesion or presentation as well: *E. acervulina* produces whitish, round lesions, sometimes in ladder-like streaks in light infections and plaques will coalesce and cause intestinal wall thickening in heavy infections; *E. brunetti* causes necrosis and bloody mucoid enteritis; *E. maxima* causes diarrhea, thickened intestinal walls, mucoid exudate, and petechiae; *E. mitis* causes lesions similar to *E. acervulina* though in a less organized (not ladder-like) pattern; *E. necatrix* causes ballooning of the intestine, petechiae, and mucoid blood-filled exudate; *E. praecox* causes an increase in mucoid exudate but no defining lesions; and *E. tenella* causes thickening of the cecal wall, hemorrhage, and cecal cores.[289] The severity of the lesion caused by each species is also influenced by the location of the parasite in the intestinal cells.

E. acervulina, *E. mitis*, and *E. praecox*, the least pathogenic species, all replicate in the epithelial layer of cells in the intestinal tract, while *E. brunetti*, *E. maxima*, *E. necatrix*, and *E. tenella* replicate in the subepithelium and cause more cellular damage during the process. More specifically, for the five species that are of most concern for commercial poultry, *E. tenella* in the ceca causes dilation and necrosis of the submucosal glands, multifocal areas of severe inflammatory hemorrhage, and foci of hemorrhage (Figure 1.28C, Chapter 1). Parasitic stages are found in the submucosal glands and can be located transmurally throughout the mucosa in more severe cases. *E. acervulina* in the duodenum causes villus atrophy, fusion of the villi, proliferation of epithelial cells, interstitial edema, and mononuclear infiltrate at the submucosa membrane. Parasitic stages are intracellular and found clustered at the tips of the villi. *E. maxima* causes villus blunting and fusion (Figure 1.25A, Chapter 1), discrete hemorrhage, and mononuclear infiltrate in the lamina propria. Parasitic stages are found in submucosa and lamina propria.[1165] *E. brunetti* causes the tips of the villi to break off, coagulating necrosis, and a caseous eroded surface over the entirety of the mucosa. *E. necatrix* causes large areas of the mucosa to be sloughed off due to submucosa and lamina propria being crowded with large clusters of schizonts. Lesions may also extend through the muscle layers to the serosal membranes.

All *Eimeria* species that infect commercial poultry have the same general life cycle, with primary differences between the species arising in host predilection and the target tissue described earlier. Most *Eimeria* species that infect domestic fowl undergo three cycles of asexual replication (~3–4 days post-inoculation).[1159] Upon completion of asexual replication, a sexual cycle occurs as described (Chapter 1 and illustrated in Figure. 1.7 for *E. maxima*). Sexual differentiation in *Eimeria* is not predetermined, and male and female gamonts can be formed from a clonal strain of merozoites. Within this general description of the life cycle of *Eimeria*, differences in minimum prepatent period and minimum sporulation time do exist among species. These differences, along with average size and shape, were used to differentiate between species when initially classifying the parasites. *E. praecox* has the shortest minimum prepatent period at 83 hours, while *E. necatrix* has the longest at 138 hours. The minimum prepatent periods for *E. maxima* (121 hours), *E. brunetti* (120 hours), *E. tenella* (115 hours), *E. acervulina* (97 hours), and *E. mitis* (93 hours) fall in between. Minimum sporulation times do not follow the same time hierarchy as minimum prepatent periods; *E. praecox* does have the shortest sporulation time (12 hours), but *E. maxima* has the longest (30 hours). Minimum sporulation times for *E. brunetti* (18 hours), *E. necatrix* (18 hours), *E. tenella* (18 hours), *E. acervulina* (17 hours), and *E. mitis* (15 hours) fall in between.

15.3 IMMUNITY

Each species of *Eimeria* induces a specific host response at their respective site of infection in the intestinal tract. T cells play a major role in the development of immunity. CD4+ T cells and intraepithelial lymphocytes are involved in primary infections, while CD8 T-helper cells are involved in secondary infections.[317] The role of cellular and humoral immunity to *Eimeria* infections in chickens is reviewed in detail in Chapter 3.

Chickens are considered to have developed partial immunity when they have decreased oocyst excretion following challenge, decreased feed conversion ratios, decreased lesion scores, and most importantly, increased body weight gains when compared to nonimmunized birds.[1808] *E. maxima* is the most antigenic and requires a single oocyst or even sporocyst infection to confer a partial immune response, as measured by an increase in average weight gain following a challenge compared to previously unexposed birds. *E. acervulina* and *E. tenella* are also capable of infecting birds and allowing for oocyst excretion, with as little as a single sporocyst.[953,954]

15.4 DIAGNOSIS AND ENUMERATION

To diagnose coccidiosis, defined as the presence of clinical disease in birds, three procedures are traditionally used: gross lesions, oocyst count scores, and microscopic lesion scores. Additionally, to detect the presence of oocysts on farms, there are two methods of detection: fecal or litter oocyst counts and polymerase chain reaction (PCR).

The most commonly used method to diagnose clinical coccidiosis is to examine for the presence of gross lesions during necropsy. Each species has a predilection for infection of specific sites of the intestinal tract, and most cause distinct lesions as described earlier. Limitations to this method include the lack of gross lesions in light infections

or with nonpathogenic strains. Chickens are often infected with multiple species in field cases, confounding and skewing gross lesion scores for the species of interest.[1166]

Oocyst count scores (OCSs or microscores) have also been used to characterize infection and are more rewarding for species and strains that do not cause severe gross lesions. To perform an OCS, a mucosal scraping of the area of interest is taken and the number of oocysts per high power field is counted, assigning a score ranging from 0 (no oocysts seen) to 4 (too numerous to count).[603,1165] Microscores can be affected by the virulence of the strain, with more oocysts present with more virulent strains.[1164]

The gold standard for detecting and diagnosing active coccidiosis infections is through histopathology and microscopic lesion scores. Samples are collected, fixed in formalin, sectioned, and stained for examination for the presence of *Eimeria* species, inflammatory response, and disruption of the normal tissue using hematoxylin and eosin stain.[603,763] The use of the three scoring systems simultaneously can reveal inconsistencies, as the lesion scores assigned based on the gross lesion scores underestimate the prevalence when compared with the damage and corresponding microscopic lesion scores.[763]

Other recognized methods to diagnose coccidial infections rely on litter or fresh feces instead of performing a necropsy on dead birds or euthanizing when ill. Fecal and litter oocyst counts are used to quantify the number of oocysts that a bird is excreting or that are found in the litter of infected flocks. Morphological distinction of the oocysts can be made to determine the number of species excreted.[181,289,1084] Care must be taken with this approach as many of the size measurements and morphologies overlap between the species. Additionally, strains within a species can have different morphologies present, making interpretation of the morphological differences inaccurate.[1080,1362] Many factors influence the litter oocyst counts including season, litter quality, and number of previous flocks raised on the litter, as well as the use of a synthetic drug in combination with an ionophore.[242,1413,1613] In most flocks, oocyst counts increase at 3 weeks, with a sharp peak at 4 weeks and a sharp decline by weeks 5 and 6.[233,1413]

Many different methods of oocyst enumeration have been used for litter and fecal samples. The most common method of enumeration is to use a McMaster chamber.[289,1084] However, there are multiple methods for this technique. The most traditional technique is labor intensive to get to the stage where samples can be read. These steps include adding water, potentially diluting out small counts, having to filter out the large debris, and adding additional steps including centrifugation and the addition of a saturated sodium chloride solution before the oocysts are ready to count. Another method of counting removes the majority of the preparation steps and uses a mini-shaker to homogenize the fecal mixture before adding the saturated sodium chloride allowing for a much faster processing while still keeping the sensitivity of the test.[686] Other techniques add a specific amount of fecal matter and use sugar floatation with success.[1725]

Another method is the use of a hemocytometer to count, although this method can be more variable with different oocyst numbers.[1334]

PCR can also be utilized to identify and differentiate the species present. Depending on the region amplified, it is a highly sensitive and specific technique that minimizes the margin for error. It can also easily detect the presence of multiple species, even in low numbers or in strains with low pathogenicity. Primarily, it is used to identify species present in litter and fecal samples but can also be utilized with tissue samples, both fresh and formalin fixed.[1245] PCR allows for the rapid and precise identification of *Eimeria* species, without bias. Two techniques, standard PCR and real-time (quantitative) PCR, are most often used to identify the *Eimeria* species present in the litter on different farms in poultry production regions around the world.

For standard PCR, four regions of the genome are presently used to distinguish species: ITS-1, ITS-2, 18s rDNA, and cytochrome c oxidase subunit 1 gene (COI). Both species-specific and universal primers have been developed for the ITS1 and COI genes.[78,984,1512] Recent attention has been focused on using the COI gene, as it is highly conserved within a species but is clearly identifiable between species,[1366] as compared to the ITS-1 region that can be highly variable between different strains of the same species. Using the ITS-2 region, three additional populations, OUT-X, Y, and Z, have been isolated in the southern hemisphere only. They were originally described in Australia but have since been found in high prevalence in Africa as well.[275,788]

Real-time PCR has also been developed to quantify the number of oocysts of each species using different regions of the genome from standard PCR. Nonpolymorphic sequence-characterized amplification regions (SCARs) have been used, which are advantageous due to the lack of cross-reactivity between species.[1755] One drawback to quantitative polymerase chain reaction (qPCR) is that the method of DNA extraction and starting number of oocysts can affect the efficiency of the reaction, potentially skewing the results.[200] Another drawback is the variability of the detection limit with qPCR, which can result in underrepresenting the presence of coccidiosis.[1337] Other real-time assays have been developed using the ITS-1 region and can detect as few as 100 oocysts from purified samples but require 1000 oocysts when concentrating oocysts from fecal samples.[802]

15.5 CONTROL

Coccidiosis control in poultry relies predominantly on the use of anticoccidial drugs and vaccination. Prior to 2000, anticoccidial drugs were utilized in ~95% of flocks where anticoccidial control was employed, including ~99% of commercial broiler flocks.[239] The first drug with demonstrated coccidiostatic activity was sulfanilamide in 1939, and it first began to have widespread commercial application

in 1947.[980] The history and application of different anticoccidial drugs are reviewed in detail in Chapter 6. It should be noted here, however, that the improper use of drugs can encourage the parasite to develop resistance. These include inadequate mixing of drugs, underdosing, use of the same anticoccidials for an extended time, and frequency and timing of treatments.[223] Recently, depending on the time of year, usage of anticoccidial drugs falls to as low as 60% or lower, driven by legislative and consumer pressure.[239,598,1566] Nonattenuated vaccines are included in the coccidiosis prevention program of at least 35%–40% of broiler companies, and use is growing each year.[239]

Use of live oocyst vaccines containing *Eimeria* species has been available in the United States since 1952.[469] The live vaccines are given or applied to chicks shortly after hatch. Different methods of vaccination have evolved throughout time and include the application of gel beads to the feed, the introduction of vaccine in the water line, vaccination *in ovo*, ocular vaccination, and vaccination with a spray cabinet at the hatchery.[236] Currently, vaccines administered in the hatchery are given in a water-based or gel-based diluent;[21,1694] this subject is reviewed in detail in Chapter 4. Vaccines differ on the number of oocysts present, the different species present, and the attenuation status of the oocysts. All major commercial vaccines for chickens contain strains of *E. acervulina*, *E. maxima*, and *E. tenella*, representing the most common species found on broiler farms. The presence of additional strains varies with manufacturer, with some choosing to include *E. necatrix* and *E. brunetti* in vaccines designed for layers, as these strains tend to cause clinical signs in older birds. Other companies choose to include novel strains, including *E. mivati* and *E. mitis*.[236] One vaccine contains all seven species.[317]

15.6 CONCLUSION

Coccidiosis in chickens is a major disease with extreme negative economic impacts for the worldwide commercial poultry industry. Much research has been performed to understand the basic biology of the parasite, but gaps still exist in our knowledge of genomics, host interactions, and control of the disease. Further research is needed to elucidate these mechanisms and develop novel control strategies to ensure the longevity and sustainability of poultry production.

REFERENCES

21, 78, 136, 143, 172, 181, 200, 223, 228, 230a, 233, 236, 239, 242, 275, 285, 289, 317, 437, 469, 470, 598, 603, 686, 763, 788, 802, 834, 835, 835a, 842, 953, 954, 980, 981, 983, 984, 1074, 1080, 1084, 1139, 1159, 1164, 1165, 1166, 1205, 1245, 1334, 1337, 1362, 1366, 1372, 1413, 1512, 1525, 1559, 1566, 1613, 1694, 1717, 1718, 1725, 1728, 1746, 1755, 1758, 1802, 1808

CHAPTER 16

Coccidiosis in Poultry in China

X. Suo

CONTENTS

16.1 INTRODUCTION AND COCCIDIOSIS RESEARCH IN CHINA BEFORE 1991

In China, poultry coccidiosis caused by *Eimeria* parasites was first reported in the early 1950s. The poultry production emerged in China in the late 1950s.[1059] At the same time, coccidiosis became prevalent and persisted as a major barrier. Thus, research on basic parasite biology, isolation and propagation, epidemiology, drugs, and vaccines began in the 1960s, although research papers were published only from 1976.[1023,1059] The research encompassed biology, epidemiology, pathogenicity, and immunogenicity. Scientists in China synthesized zoalene (3,5-dinitro-o-toluamide) in 1977,[1912] studied the anticoccidial activity of artemisinin,[1059,1669,1920] which was discovered by Youyou Tu in 1972,[284,1669,1712] and developed live and killed vaccines in 1985.[1059,1669]

The first coccidiosis control symposium was organized in 1985 at Laohekou, Hubei Province, by scientists to communicate and discuss epidemiology, control, and species-specific immunity and educate the poultry industry on control strategies.[1865]

Coccidiosis research in China before 1991 was mainly driven by field problems, viz., mortality, poor performance, and lost productivity caused by *Eimeria* infection.[1917] Since 1991, research has evolved into two paths: one is still applied research, addressing treatment and prevention, and the other is basic research utilizing molecular technology for a better understanding of the *Eimeria* life cycle and infection with the goal of controlling coccidiosis.

16.2 NATURAL INFECTIONS

16.2.1 Prevalence

Microscopic examination and polymerase chain reaction (PCR) tests of fecal samples revealed a high prevalence of *Eimeria* spp. in Chinese chicken farms of all regions with some regional differences (Table 16.1). For example, the overall prevalence of *Eimeria* species in chickens in Anhui Province was 87.75% (150/171), with *E. tenella* the most prevalent species (80.67%, 121/150), followed by *E. necatrix, E. mitis, E. maxima, E. brunetti,* and *E. acervulina* (68% [102/150], 55.33% [83/150], 54.67% [82/150], 44.67% [67/150] and 2.67% [4/150], respectively).[985] In Zhejiang Province, the overall prevalence of *Eimeria* spp. was 30.7% (95 of 310), with *E. tenella, E. acervulina, E. maxima, E. necatrix,* and *E. mitis* common [985] Mixed infections were common, with *E. tenella, E. maxima, E. necatrix, E. brunetti,* and *E. mitis* (26.67%, 40/150) coinfection being most prevalent.[985]

16.2.2 Clinical and Subclinical Infection

Clinical and subclinical infections are very common, especially in small-scale farms. Microscopic and postmortem examinations of samples from 545 farms across nine provinces over a 5-year period revealed the highest coccidiosis morbidity rate in Guangdong, low morbidity in the Inner Mongolia Autonomous Region, Fujian and Liaoning provinces, with moderate morbidity in the Beijing, Sichuan, Zhejiang, and Shandong provinces, and the Xinjiang Uygur Autonomous Region.[1879] Microscopy and PCR analysis of feces from broilers with subclinical signs (viz. with low feed efficiency) at 50 small-scale farms with a stock size of 2000–6000 in the Shandong Province of eastern China detected more than one *Eimeria* species in most fecal samples, and infection rates of 90%, 88%, 72%, 68%, 60%, 26%, and 8% for *E. tenella, E. praecox, E. acervulina, E. maxima, E. mitis, E. necatrix,* and *E. brunetti,* respectively.[1648] With widespread and rapidly increasing drug resistance, it is envisaged that clinical and subclinical infections will become more prevalent, causing considerable reductions in chicken meat and egg production.

16.3 EXPERIMENTAL INFECTIONS

16.3.1 Development

16.3.1.1 Invasion

Invasion is a critical step in the life cycle of intracellular parasites and involves many proteins. Proteins in *E. maxima* and *E. acervulina* involved in invasion have been studied using the co-immunoprecipitation (co-IP) assay and shotgun liquid chromatography-mass spectroscopy (LC-MS)/MS technique. In *E. maxima*, 35 proteins including microneme proteins 3 and 7 bound with chicken jejunal epithelial cells; 22 (62.86%) were associated with binding activity and 15 (42.86%) are involved in catalytic activity.[751] In *E. acervulina*, 85 proteins bound with chicken duodenal epithelial cells. Of these proteins, 16 were identified only in *Eimeria* parasites, and 9 out of the 16 proteins are involved in binding, catalytic activity, and cellular process.[751,1896] The diversity of proteins involved in invasion suggests a complicated

Table 16.1 Prevalence of Chicken Coccidiosis in China

Area	Time	Province	City or County	Diagnosis	Positive Rate	Species and their Proportions
Northeast	1995–1996	Heilongjinag	Jiamusi	Feces were floated by saturated saline (FFS), intestinal smear (IS)	15.30%	E. tenella, E. acervulina
	1998	Heilongjinag	Harbin	FFS		E. tenella, E. mitis, E. maxima
	2009	Heilongjinag	Harbin	FFS	62.39%	E. tenella, E. acervulina, E. necatrix, E. praecox, E. mitis, E. maxima
	2013–2015	Heilongjinag	Yanshou	FFS, IS. Chickens were inoculated with sporulated oocysts (CISO). Symptoms, lesion, and parasitic sites were detected (SLPD)	44.20%	E. tenella, E. acervulina, E. necatrix, E. maxima
	2010–2011	Heilongjinag	Mudanjiang	FFS, IS. CISO-SLPD	80.58%	E. tenella, E. acervulina, E. maxima
	2003–2005	Jilin	Four cities	FFS, IS. CISO-SLPD	83.13%	The group of E. tenella, E. acervulina, E. maxima accounted for the highest proportion
	2013	Jilin	Jilin	FFS, IS. CISO-SLPD		E. tenella, E. acervulina, E. maxima
North	1981	Beijing		FFS, CISO-SLPD. Coccidia prepatent period was also detected (PP)		E. tenella, E. acervulina, E. maxima, E. praecox, E. mitis, E. hagani, E. necatrix
	2003	Tianjin, Hebei, Shandong		FFS, CISO-SLPD, PP	100.00%	All seven species
	2003	Hebei	Qinhuangdao	FFS, McMaster method	75%–100%	E. tenella, E. acervulina, E. necatrix, E. praecox, E. mitis, E. maxima
	2018	Hebei	Chengde	FFS, McMaster method	66.96%	E. tenella, E. maxima, E. acervulina, E. necatrix
Central	2009	Henan	Wugang	FFS, CISO-SLPD, PP		E. tenella, E. necatrix, E. acervulina, E. maxima, E. mitis, E. brunetti
	2010	Henan	Puyang	Feces were floated by saturated sucrose solution (FFSS)	24.54%	E. tenella, E. acervulina, E. maxima
	2012	Henan	Shangqiu	FFS	93.10%	
	2000	Hunan	Hengyang	FFS	56.2%	E. tenella, E. necatrix, E. acervulina, E. maxima, E. mitis, E. praecox
	2007	Hunan	Yueyang	Feces smear	39.81%–54.48%	
	2011	Hunan	Hengyang	Chickens were inoculated with sporulated oocysts (CISO), and oocyst morphology, prepatent period, sporulation time, parasitic sites, and lesion were detected (MPSPLD)		E. tenella, E. necatrix, E. maxima, E. acervulina, E. praecox
	2012	Hunan	Loudi	FFSS		
East	2005	Shandong	Jiaodong	FFS. McMaster method. Chi-square test	64.60%	E. maxima (31.7%)
	2008	Shandong		FFS. Morphological identification. PCR (ITS-1 rDNA)	65.80%	E. tenella (90%), E. praecox (88%), E. acervulina (72%), E. maxima (68%), E. mitis (60%), E. necatrix (26%), E. brunetti (8%)
	2011	Shandong	Linyi	FFS. Morphological identification	78.00%	E. tenella (52.31%), E. acervulina (43.52%), E. brunetti (30.84%), E. necatrix (18.56%)

(Continued)

Table 16.1 (Continued) Prevalence of Chicken Coccidiosis in China

Area	Time	Province	City or County	Diagnosis	Positive Rate	Species and their Proportions
East	2002	Anhui	Shouxian	FFSS. Morphological identification. Chi-square test	46.10%	*E. acervulina, E. mitis, E. tenella, E. maxima, E. necatrix*
	2004	Anhui	Hefei	FFS. Oocysts were counted. Morphological identification. T test	62.03%	*E. necatrix, E. acervulina, E. maxima, E. tenella, E. mitis, E. praecox*
	2007	Anhui	Five counties	FFS. Oocysts were counted. Sporulated oocysts morphology was identified. Chi-square test	100.00%	*E. maxima, E. mitis, E. acervulina, E. tenella, E. necatrix, E. praecox*
	2009	Anhui	West Anhui	FFS. Oocysts were counted. Sporulated oocysts morphology was identified	100.00%	*E. necatrix* (92.80%), *E. acervulina* (80.84%), *E. mitis* (72.30%), *E. maxima* (71.80%), *E. praecox* (70.20%), *E. tenella* (14%)
	2011	Anhui	Feixi, Changfeng, Fengtai	FFS. Oocysts were counted. Sporulated oocysts morphology was identified. Chi-square test	93.30%	*E. mitis, E. necatrix, E. maxima, E. brunetti, E. tenella, E. praecox, E. acervulina*
	2016	Anhui	Six counties in central Anhui	FFS. Sporulated oocysts morphology was identified. PCR (ITS-1 rDNA)	87.75%	*E. tenella* (80.67%), *E. necatrix* (68%), *E. mitis* (55.33%), *E. maxima* (54.67%), *E. brunetti* (44.67%), *E. acervulina* (2.67%)
	1987–1990	Jiangsu	41 counties	CISO and oocyst morphology, prepatent period, parasitic sites, and lesion were detected (MPPLD)		*E. tenella, E. necatrix, E. acervulina, E. brunetti, E. praecox, E. maxima, E. hagani, E. mitis, E. mivati*
	2009	Jiangsu	Guanyun	CISO-MPPLD		*E. tenella, E. necatrix, E. acervulina, E. maxima, E. brunetti, E. mitis*
East	2010	Jiangsu	Xuzhou	Sporulated oocysts morphology was identified	68.75%	*E. acervulina* (62.5%), *E. maxima* (56.52%), *E. mitis* (56.25%), *E. tenella* (50%), *E. necatrix* (37.5%), *E. praecox* (25%)
	2015	Jiangsu	Jinhu	Morphological identification	39.6%–54.48%	*E. tenella, E. necatrix, E. acervulina, E. maxima, E. mivati, E. praecox*
	1989	Shanghai		CISO-MPPLD		
	2002	Shanghai		FFS. Oocysts were counted. Sporulated oocysts morphology was identified	45%–100%	*E. mivati* (83%), *E. acervulina* (67%), *E. maxima,* (67%), *E. tenella* (58%), *E. necatrix* (33%), *E. mitis* (17%)
	1984–1985	Zhejiang	Hangzhou	CISO-MPPLD		*E. tenella, E. brunetti, E. acervulina, E. maxima, E. mitis, E. hagani, E. praecox*
	2002	Zhejiang	Hangzhou	CISO-MPPLD		*E. tenella, E. maxima, E. necatrix*
	2014	Zhejiang	5 cities	Sporulated oocysts morphology was identified	30.70%	*E. tenella, E. acervulina, E. maxima, E. necatrix, E. mitis*
	1982–1984	Fujian	Fuzhou	CISO-MPPLD		*E. tenella, E. maxima, E. acervulina, E. mitis*
	1984	Fujian	Nanping, Jian'ou	Feces smear		
	2009–2010	Fujian		FFS. Oocysts were counted. Sporulated oocysts morphology was identified	71.50%	*E. tenella* (78%), *E. maxima* (65%), *E. acervulina* (63%), *E. necatrix* (29%), *E. brunetti* (26%), *E. mitis* (23%)

(Continued)

Table 16.1 (Continued) Prevalence of Chicken Coccidiosis in China

Area	Time	Province	City or County	Diagnosis	Positive Rate	Species and their Proportions
South	1980	Guangdong	Guangzhou	FFS. Oocysts were counted. CISO-MPSPLD		E. tenella, E. necatrix, E. acervulina, E. maxima, E. brunetti, E. mitis, E. mivati, E. hagani, E. praecox
	2000	Guangdong	Zhanjiang	FFS. Oocysts were counted. CISO-MPSPLD	93.90%	E. tenella, E. necatrix, E. acervulina, E. maxima, E. mitis, E. praecox
	1984	Guangxi		FFS. Oocysts were counted. CISO-MPSPLD		E. tenella, E. necatrix, E. acervulina, E. maxima, E. brunetti, E. mitis, E. mivati, E. praecox
	2010–2011	Guangxi	Hezhou	FFS. Oocysts were counted. CISO-MPSPLD	51.60%	E. tenella (74.1%), E. necatrix (51.6%), E. acervulina (45.1%), E. maxima (41.9%), E. mitis (35.4%), E. praecox (35.4%)
	2009	Hainan	Haikou, Wenchang, Qionghai	FFS. Oocysts were counted. Morphological identification	Chick, 82.7%	E. tenella, E. necatrix, E. acervulina, E. maxima, E. mitis, E. hagani, E. praecox
Southwest	1986	Guizhou	Tongren	CISO-MPSPLD		E. tenella, E. necatrix, E. acervulina, E. maxima, E. mitis, E. hagani, E. praecox
	2004	Guizhou	Zunyi	CISO-MPSPLD		E. tenella, E. necatrix, E. acervulina, E. maxima, E. brunetti, E. mitis, E. mivati, E. hagani, E. praecox
	1997	Sichuan	Suining	CISO-MPSPLD		E. tenella, E. acervulina, E. maxima, E. mitis
	2000	Sichuan	Chengdu	FFS. Morphological identification		E. tenella, E. necatrix, E. brunetti, E. maxima, E. mitis, E. praecox
	1999	Chongqing		FFS. Morphological identification		E. tenella, E. necatrix, E. acervulina, E. maxima, E. brunetti, E. mitis, E. mivati, E. praecox
	2002	Chongqing		Morphological identification		E. tenella, E. necatrix, E. acervulina, E. maxima, E. brunetti, E. mitis, E. mivati, E. hagani, E. praecox
	2002	Chongqing	Jiangjin	Morphological identification		E. tenella, E. necatrix, E. acervulina, E. maxima, E. brunetti, E. mitis, E. mivati
South	2016–2017	Yunnan	Jianchuan	Morphological identification	21.50%	E. maxima, E. mitis
Northwest	1959	Shaanxi	Xi'an			
	1983–1984	Shaanxi	Eight counties	Morphological identification	74.75%	E. tenella, E. necatrix, E. acervulina, E. maxima, E. praecox, E. mitis, E. mivati
	1998	Shaanxi	Yangling	Morphological identification	58.30%	E. tenella, E. necatrix, E. acervulina, E. maxima, E. mitis, E. hagani, E. praecox
	1980	Gansu	Lanzhou	CISO-MPSPLD		E. tenella, E. necatrix, E. acervulina, E. maxima, E. brunetti, E. mitis, E. mivati, E. hagani, E. praecox, Isospora sp.
	1986	Ningxia	Yinchuan	CISO-MPSPLD		E. tenella, E. necatrix, E. acervulina, E. maxima, E. mitis, E. praecox
	1987	Ningxia	Guyuan	CISO-MPSPLD		E. tenella, E. acervulina, E. maxima, E. mitis, E. hagani
	1989	Qinghai	Xining	FFS. Oocysts were counted. Sporulation time and oocysts morphology was detected (STMD)	Adult, 90%	E. tenella, E. necatrix, E. acervulina, E. maxima, E. mitis, E. praecox

(Continued)

Table 16.1 (*Continued*) Prevalence of Chicken Coccidiosis in China

Area	Time	Province	City or County	Diagnosis	Positive Rate	Species and their Proportions
East	1980	Xinjiang	Urumqi	FFS. STMD		*E. tenella, E. necatrix, E. acervulina, E. maxima, E. mitis, E. hagani, E. praecox*
	1980–1981	Xinjiang	Urumqi	FFS. STMD		*E. tenella* (18.61% for adult and 13%–50% for chick), *E. necatrix, E. acervulina, E. maxima, E. mitis, E. hagani, E. praecox*. The infection rate of *E. tenella* was the highest
	1987	Xinjiang	Urumqi	FFS.STMD. Symptoms and lesion were detected		*E. tenella* (69.1%), *E. necatrix* (48.4%), *E. maxima* (33.4%), *E. acervulina, E. brunetti, E. mitis, E. hagani, E. praecox*
	2003	Xinjiang	Changji	CISO-MPSPLD	35.30%	*E. tenella* (60.6%), *E. acervulina* (16.5%), *E. maxima* (12.6%), *E. mitis* (18.4%), *E. praecox* (9.9%)
	2007	Xinjiang	Aksu	CISO-MPSPLD		*E. tenella* (75%), *E. acervulina* (81%), *E. maxima* (62.5%)
	2013	Xinjiang	Northern Xinjiang	STMD	100.00%	*E. tenella, E. acervulina, E. maxima, E. mitis, E. hagani, E. brunetti*

Source: Summary from Li, C. et al. 2018. *Acta Parasitol. Med. Entomol. Sinica* 25, 230–241 (in Chinese).

molecular basis for distinct host, tissue, and cell tropisms of chicken *Eimeria*.

16.3.1.2 Endogenous Development

16.3.1.2.1 Parasitophorous Vacuole

Intracellular stages of *Eimeria* reside within a membrane-bound parasitophorous vacuole (PV). PVs of apicomplexan parasites like *E. tenella* play important roles in nutrient acquisition, multiplication, and evasion of host immune responses. The dynamic development of the PV of *E. tenella* was studied using transgenic *E. tenella* expressing enhanced yellow fluorescent protein guided by 5' terminal signal sequences derived from *Toxoplasma gondii* GRA8 protein and *Plasmodium falciparum* repetitive interspersed family protein.[1556] Three structurally different types of PVs were observed during the endogenous development of the transfected *E. tenella in vitro*: (1) PVs of sporozoites were characterized by a narrow lumen and few visible subcompartments; (2) PVs of schizonts characterized by three subcompartments, namely, membranous extensions into the host cell cytosol (MEHC), membranous extensions into the vacuolar lumen (MEVL), and particle-like bodies; and (3) in PVs of gametogony, the lumen of the PV was enlarged, MEVLs seem to disappear, and MEHCs are seldom visible. The functions of MEHCs, MEVLs, and particle-like bodies are yet to be elucidated.

16.3.1.2.2 Asexual and Sexual Development

One fascinating feature of parasites in the *Eimeria* genus is the diversified endogenous development and abundance of genes involved in endogenous development. RNA sequencing–based comparative transcriptome analysis has been used to study the mechanisms controlling the switch between different generations of schizogony and from asexual to sexual reproduction. In *E. necatrix*, there were 6977, 6901, and 7983 unigenes in second (MZ2)- and third (MZ3)-generation merozoites and gametocytes (GAM), respectively; 2053 genes were differentially expressed between MZ2 and MZ3, and 95 genes are specifically expressed in MZ2, and 48 genes are specifically expressed in MZ3. Between MZ3 and GAM, 4267 genes were differently expressed with 329 genes specifically expressed in MZ3 and 1289 in GAM.[1636,1637] KEGG pathways in the three stages were very different, although they had a similar number of Gene Ontology (GO) assignments.[1636,1637] The upregulated genes in MZ-2 were mainly enriched for protein degradation and amino acid metabolism, while upregulated genes in MZ-3 are mainly for transcriptional activity, cell proliferation, and cell differentiation.

An ultrastructure study showed that during macrogametogenesis and oocyst formation of *E. tenella* Xiamen strain

in its sexual stage, electron lucent WFB1s appear earlier than the electron denser WFB2 during the process of oocyst wall formation, but WFB2s' proteins are the major components of oocyst wall formation.[1911] Sudan black-B staining revealed that the club-body inside the cytosol is lipoid in nature instead of previously believed amylopectin, suggesting lipo-metabolism is an important energy resource in *E. tenella* development.[1911]

16.3.1.2.3 Precocious and Serotinous Development

Plasticity of the prepatent period and/or oocyst excretion in *Eimeria* is recognized by the fact that precocious and serotinous lines can be selected from their wild-type parental strains. Analysis of subtractive cDNA libraries, derived from sporulated oocysts between the precocious line of *E. maxima* and its parent strain, revealed 21 unique genes downregulated and 11 upregulated in the precocious line. Among these 32 genes, six genes encode proteins homologous with previously reported proteins, including rhomboid-like protein and transhydrogenase of *E. tenella*, serpin and cation-transporting ATPase of *E. acervulina*, a heat-shock protein of *E. maxima*, and a conserved hypothetical protein of *T. gondii*.[745] A line of *E. necatrix* was selected by repeated passages of oocysts that were collected after peak oocyst production from feces or cecal contents of previously infected chickens.[380] When compared with the parent strain, the new line of *E. necatrix* after 16 successive passages had a right-shifted oocyst shedding curve, with its peak of oocyst production delayed by 2 days.

16.3.1.2.4 Egress

Egress is a process that intracellular parasites use to exit from parasitophorous vacuoles and host cells. Parasites exit from consumed host cells and enter new host cells, a process central to *Eimeria* propagation and pathogenesis. Egress or premature egress of parasite stages can be induced by environmental factors surrounding infected cells. The addition of exogenous acetaldehyde, ethanol, or isopropanol induces egress of sporozoites from primary chicken kidney (PCK) cells and stimulates secretion of *E. tenella* microneme 2 protein (EtMic2), a process dependent on the intracellular calcium of the parasites.[1844,1845] Premature egression of sporozoites also occurs when the cells are cocultured *in vitro* with splenocytes from *E. tenella*–infected chickens but not with those from uninfected chickens.[382] Similarly, *Eimeria*-specific antibodies and cytokines (interferon [IFN]-γ, interleukin [IL]-2, and IL-15), derived from *E. tenella*–primed B and T lymphocytes, respectively, can promote premature egress of sporozoites from infected host cells.[382] Both egressed parasites and intracellular sporozoites are viable, although the latter show reduced reinvasion ability. These results suggest a novel, immune-mediated mechanism that the host exploits to interrupt the normal *Eimeria* life cycle *in vivo* and hence block the release of mature parasites into the environment.

16.3.1.2.5 Sporulation

The sporogony process of *Eimeria* is vital for the transmission of coccidiosis. Nitric oxide (NO) donors, such as S-nitroso-glutathione (GSNO), S-nitroso-*N*-acetyl-DL-penicillamine (SNAP), and acidic sodium nitrite (NaNO$_2$), can dose- and time-dependently inhibit the sporogony of *E. tenella* oocysts freshly excreted from feces.[991] The inhibition is irreversible and is mainly limited to the early stage of sporogony within 10 hours after the initial sporulation. Once sporulation is more than 10 hours,[989] GSNO will not interrupt or block the subsequent sporogony process. The NO scavenger hemoglobin can significantly prevent the inhibitory activity of GSNO on the sporogony of oocysts.[991] For infective oocysts or sporocysts, GSNO treatment partially decreases the proportion of sporozoite excystation *in vitro* but has no effects on the infectivity and pathogenicity to chickens.[991] The inhibition of sporogony by NO may be mediated by the complete inhibition of the mRNA expression of EtCRK2 (a cyclin-dependent kinase-related protein-2 in *E. tenella*) in the early stage of sporulation,[989] without affecting the activities of enzymes involved in carbohydrate metabolism, such as lactate dehydrogenase, glucose-6-phosphate dehydrogenase, and aconitase.[990]

Analysis of three subtractive cDNA libraries derived from *E. tenella* unsporulated oocysts, sporulated oocysts, and sporozoites revealed 119 unique sequences, with 31 from sporulated oocysts and 88 from sporozoites. Among the 119 expressed sequence tags (ESTs), 32 genes encode proteins homologous with previously reported proteins including microneme proteins and surface antigen proteins of *E. tenella*, small heat shock proteins, rhoptry proteins of *T. gondii*, and calcium-dependent protein kinase of *Plasmodium* spp., and the remaining 87 ESTs were not reported.[669] The multiplicity of genes involved in sporulation together with the very tough oocyst wall imply the difficulty for searching chemicals blocking transmission of coccidiosis at the sporulation stage.

16.3.1.2.6 Epigenetic Modification in Different Stages of Development

Epigenetic regulation of switching asexual to sexual reproduction has been found in other apicomplexan parasites such as *Plasmodium*. In *Eimeria*, epigenetic modification such as cytosine methylation and histone deacetylation also exists.[381,602] The presence of 5-methylcytosine (5-mC) in genomic DNA of sporozoites and merozoites of *E. tenella* as well as those of *E. maxima, E. necatrix,* and *E. acervulina* and DNA methyltransferase-like activity in *E. tenella* indicates a possible role of genomic DNA methylation in the developmental stages of these parasites.[602]

16.3.2 Immune Responses

16.3.2.1 Innate Immune Response

Signaling by toll-like receptors (TLRs) of intestinal tissues is critical for resistance against intestinal infection. ChTLR4, ChTLR15, and MyD88 expression in heterophils and monocyte-derived macrophages is significantly increased following live or killed *E. tenella* sporozoite stimulation, suggesting the involvement of ChTLR4 and ChTLR15, through MyD88 in response to *E. tenella* infection.[1916] In the cecum of chickens infected on day 21, TLR1LA, TLR4, TLR5, TLR7, and TLR21 expression is upregulated at 12 hours post-inoculation (HPI), and TLR1LA, TLR5, and TLR21 are highly expressed at 72 hpi; while in younger, day-old chicks infected with *E. tenella*, IFN-α, IFN-β, IFN-γ, IL-1β, and IL-12 expression is dramatically upregulated at 3 hpi, indicating an age difference in innate immune response to *Eimeria* infection.[1881] In *E. acervulina*–infected chickens, mRNA expression of innate immunity genes TLR7, IL-1β, IFN-γ, and inducible nitric oxide synthetase (iNOS) in the duodenal epithelium are upregulated.[1645]

16.3.2.2 Adaptive Immune Response

Cellular immune responses are the major force of immunity against intracellular *Eimeria* infection. Sequence analysis of complementarity-determining region-3 (CDR3) of CD8$^+$ T cells isolated from intraepithelial lymphocytes in the jejunum of *E. maxima*–infected chickens showed two possible dominant CDR3, AKQDWGTGGYSNMI and AGRVLNIQY.[1407] Research, using transgenic *E. tenella* as a model, showed that antigen localization influences immune responses, with microneme-targeted antigen elicited a higher level of antigen (Ag)-specific lymphocyte proliferation as well as a stronger IgA response than the same antigen cytoplasm targeted after the second immunization.[754]

16.3.2.3 Dietary Modulation of Immune Responses

Dietary supplementation of fungus or organic zinc products can influence immune responses. Dietary supplementation with *Saccharomyces cerevisiae* fermentation product in feed for *Eimeria*-infected broilers improved immune function and growth performance and increased blood, spleen, and ileum intraepithelial CD3$^+$, CD4$^+$, and CD8$^+$ T lymphocytes.[579] Supplementation of polysaccharide extracts of two mushrooms, *Lentinus edodes* and *Tremella fuciformis*, in conjunction with a live anticoccidial vaccine significantly enhanced body weight gain of infected chickens compared with the vaccine-only group.[642] Another supplement, methionine hydroxyl analog-Zn, reduced oxidative stress and improved secretory IgA production in broilers challenged with *E. tenella*.[162]

16.3.2.4 Antigen Recognition

One most intriguing immunological question is how many of the 5000–8000 proteins expressed by *Eimeria* parasites are recognized by the host immune system. One study using an immunoproteomic approach to identify the antigenic protein repertoire from proteins of unsporulated *E. tenella* oocysts revealed that approximately 101 protein spots out of 656 spots were recognized by sera from chickens infected experimentally with *E. tenella*.[1897] In another report, analysis of sera from *E. tenella*–infected chickens identified 36 putative immunogens, including Mic3, microneme protein precursor EtMic-1, enolase, lactate dehydrogenase, and HSP70 that are shared by sporozoites and second-generation merozoites. Multiple stage-specific immunogens restricted to the second-generation merozoite stage were also evident; these include SAG2, SAG4, SAG, Mic5, SERPINI protein precursor, 14-3-3 protein, tubulin β chain, large subunit ribosomal protein L23, and two hypothetical proteins.

Five proteins, including elongation factor 2 (EF-2), 14-3-3 protein, ubiquitin-conjugating enzyme domain-containing protein (UCE), glyceraldehyde-3-phosphate dehydrogenase (GAPDH), and transhydrogenase from *E. tenella, E. acervulina,* and *E. maxima,* were recognized as immunodominant antigens by sera from *E. tenella*–, *E. acervulina*–, or *E. maxima*–infected chickens.[1669,1888] As these proteins are highly homologous, with amino acid sequence similarity of 92.9%–99%, cross-recognitions are likely.

It is also notable that there are antigenic polymorphisms among strains of *E. acervulina, E. maxima, E. mitis,* and *E. tenella.* An analysis using suppression subtractive hybridization and dot-blot hybridization showed that 10 strain-specific genes exist between the antigenically distinct *E. maxima* SH and NT strains, of which 6 genes from strain SH and 3 from strain NT share significant identities with previously reported proteins of apicomplexan parasites, and 1 gene was presumed to be novel.[1056,1824]

16.3.3 Pathogenesis

E. tenella is the most pathogenic coccidia of chickens. The exact mechanism of cellular damage by *E. tenella* is unclear. Research has shown that multiple factors contribute to *E. tenella*–induced host cell damage. Intracellular calcium overload of host cells is one of the mediators of intestinal epithelial cell death.[310]

Eimeria infection causes apoptosis in both infected cells and noninfected neighbor cells through mitochondria-dependent apoptotic pathways.[996] Mitochondrial permeability transition pore (MPTP) is a key player in the mitochondrial apoptosis pathway in *E. tenella*–infected cells. Inhibitors of MPTP and caspase-9, which are important elements of the mitochondria-dependent apoptotic pathway, decrease DNA injury, apoptosis, and caspase-9 and caspase-3 activities in cecal epithelial cells of chicken embryos after *E. tenella*

infection.[993] In another study, inhibition of MPTP opening by cyclosporin A increased the mitochondrial transmembrane potential and decreased the rate of apoptosis of host cells infected with *E. tenella*.[1836] The opening of mitochondrial ATP-sensitive potassium (mitoKATP) channels by a potassium channel activator, diazoxide, protects infected cecal cells from oocyst-induced mitochondria-dependent apoptosis.[1673]

IL-17 was also found to contribute to intestinal mucosal damage in *E. tenella*–infected chicks.[1882] Robust production of IL-17, as well as STAT-3, IL-1β, and IL-6 in cecal intraepithelial lymphocytes occurs in chickens during early infection, peaking at 6 hpi. Neutralizing IL-17 by anti-IL-17 antibodies reduced cecal lesion scores and fecal oocyst excretion and improved chicken body weight gains associated with enhanced IL-12 and IFN-γ expression and decreased IL-17, IL-6, and TGF-β expression. IL-17 treatment exacerbated intestinal lesions, increased fecal oocyst shedding, and reduced body weight gains. Comparison of apoptosis and cytokines in chickens infected with pathogenic and nonpathogenic species would help elucidate the pathogenesis of coccidiosis.

An analysis employing the Affymetrix chicken genome array combined with transcriptome analysis on cecal epithelia response to *E. tenella* infection at day 4.5 showed that 4033 genes are upregulated and 3066 downregulated in response to infection.[641] Upregulated genes are mainly involved in immunity, responses to various stimuli, apoptosis and cell differentiation, signal transduction, and extracellular matrix production, whereas downregulated genes are those encoding general metabolic enzymes, membrane components, and some transporters. In response to the pathogenesis and damage caused by *E. tenella* infection, chicken cecal epithelia reduce general metabolism, DNA replication and repair, protein degradation, and mitochondrial functions.

16.3.4 Coinfection

Coinfection of chickens with *Eimeria* and viruses and/or bacteria is extremely common. Early studies showed that chickens infected with *E. tenella* have increased populations of *Salmonella enteritidis* in the intestine when challenged with *S. enteritidis* 1 or 4 days after *E. tenella* infection[1376]; chickens previously infected with *S. enteritidis* had significantly higher recrudescence of cecal colonization of *S. enteritidis* when being challenged with *E. tenella* 3–5 weeks later.[1373] As *S. enteritidis* from chickens is a major source for human infection with this zoonotic pathogen, the earlier results indicate a possible role of *Eimeria* infection in heavy contamination of environment with the zoonotic bacterium.

Experimental coinfection of specific-pathogen-free (SPF) white leghorn chickens with avian leukosis virus subgroup J (ALV-J) NX0101 at 1 day of age and *E. tenella* at 14 days of age showed a pathological synergy between ALV-J and *E. tenella*.[308,1673] ALV-J accelerated the disease symptoms induced by *E. tenella*, and *E. tenella* exacerbated ALV-J viremia, resulting in a higher mortality rate and lower body weights of chickens with coinfection compared to a single-pathogen infection. Coinfected chickens had thymus atrophy, suppressed humoral responses to pathogens and the Newcastle Disease vaccine, altered blood lymphocyte sub-populations, and transcriptional cytokine disorders compared to chickens infected with one pathogen and the uninfected controls.[1673] Cecal microbiota examination at 21 days of age by 16S rRNA gene sequencing showed a genus-level opportunistic pathogen enrichment and a decrease in resident probiotics in response to single or dual infection. Interestingly, *E. tenella* sharply decreased the richness and diversity of cecal microflora in infected chickens, while ALV-J infection increased the richness and diversity of the cecal microflora. *E. tenella* and ALV-J coinfected chickens produced a marked enrichment of opportunistic pathogens as well as some other bacteria that may play a role in cecal microbiota carbohydrate transport and metabolic functions.[308]

16.3.5 Microbiota Alteration in *Eimeria* Infection

Eimeria infection alters gut microbiota population. Early studies showed that *E. tenella* infection significantly reduced cecal populations of beneficial normal flora *Bifidobacterium* spp. and *Lactobacillus* spp.[1377], of normal anaerobes *Bacteriodes, Peptostreptococcus,* and *Eubacterium*,[1374] and of facultative anaerobes *Peptostreptococcus* spp. and *Streptococcus* spp.[1375], but significantly increased facultative anaerobes *Enterobacteriaceae* spp.[1375] A recent study showed that *E. tenella* infection perturbs the chicken gut microbiota from the onset of oocyst shedding, characterized by a decline in nonpathogenic bacteria, including *Lactobacillus* and *Faecalibacterium*, and an increase in pathogenic bacteria, including *Clostridium, Lysinibacillus,* and *Escherichia*.[749] Another study revealed that *Bacillus* becomes the dominant microbiota after infection with recombinant *E. tenella* expressing *E. maxima* profilin, whereas, dominant in the microbiota of wild-type infected birds is *Lactobacillus*. The percentage of *Proteobacteria* was increased after reinfection with oocysts of both wild-type and recombinant *Eimeria* parasites infected birds.[1672] As gastrointestinal microbiota is actively involved in the pathogenesis of a variety of pathogens, the influence of microbiota on the course of coccidiosis and on the pathogenicity of the *Eimeria* species merits further investigation.

16.4 MOLECULAR BIOLOGY

16.4.1 Molecular Characterization and Functional Analysis of Genes

The pace of decoding genetic and functional information in *Eimeria* genomes has been slow, with most *Eimeria* genes

remaining "hypothetical or uncharacterized." Fifty genes and/or their proteins were identified and functionally characterized, including those related to invasion, development regulation, metabolism pathway, and structure (Table 16.2). *In vitro* inhibition tests revealed that calcium-dependent protein kinase 4 (EtCDPK4) and EtAMA1 are key sporozoite invasion-related molecules, suggesting two targets for developing antibody-based coccidiosis vaccines.[668,814,1101] Protein-protein interaction analyses showed that *Eimeria* proteins (such as EtAMA1 and EtCDPK4) could interact with several other proteins involved not only in invasion but also in development and metabolic processes, indicating that parasite activities are regulated by complicated protein networks.[668,1101] With advanced genetic tools being established in *Eimeria*, molecular and functional characterization of *Eimeria* proteins will move fast, leading to improved understanding of parasite-host interaction, the discovery of new metabolic pathways, and identification of drug and vaccine targets.

16.4.2 Mitochondrial Genome

Mitochondrial (mt) genome sequences provide mtDNA genetic markers for studying molecular epidemiology, population genetics, and phylogenetics of *Eimeria*. The complete mtDNA sequences of six *Eimeria* species have been sequenced and analyzed, and some novel features of their gene contents and genome organizations were observed.[745,1028] The complete mt genomes of *E. acervulina, E. brunetti, E. maxima, E. mitis, E. necatrix,* and *E. praecox* are 6179 bp, 6148 bp, 6169 bp, 6407 bp, 6214 bp, and 6174 bp in size, respectively. The mt genomes consist of three genes for proteins (*cox*1, *cox*3, and *cyt*b), 12 gene fragments for the large subunit (LSU) rRNA, and 7 gene fragments for the small subunit (SSU) rRNA, with no transfer RNA genes. The gene contents and genome organizations are like that of *Plasmodium* but are distinct from *Babesia* and *Theileria*. The putative direction of translation for three genes (*cox*1, *cox*3, and *cyt*b) is the same in all six *Eimeria* species. In the mt genomes of the six *Eimeria* species, all protein-coding genes have ATT, ATG, GTT, and GTG as their initiation codons, and TAA as their termination codon. The A+T contents of the mt genomes are 65.35% for *E. acervulina*, 65.43% for *E. brunetti*, 64.53% for *E. maxima*, 67.30% for *E. mitis*, 65.04% for *E. necatrix*, and 65.59% for *E. praecox*. The AT bias has a significant effect on both the codon usage pattern and amino acid composition of proteins. Phylogenetic analyses using concatenated nucleotide sequences of the two protein-coding genes (*cyt*b and *cox*1), with three different computational algorithms (Bayesian analysis, maximum parsimony, and maximum likelihood) all revealed distinct groups with high statistical support, indicating that the six *Eimeria* species from domestic chickens represent six distinct but closely related species.

Table 16.2 Molecular and Functional Characterization of Selective Proteins from Chicken *Eimeria* in China

Name	GenBank Accession Number	Approximate Mr in kDa	mRNA Transcription Level	Protein Expression Level	Localization	Proposed function/ Catalytic Substrate	References
Enzymes							
EtLLP1 (lipid phosphate phosphatases 1)	KM880158	38.239	Higher in sporozoites than in unsporulated oocysts, sporulated oocysts, and merozoites	—	—	Substrates: phosphatidate (PA), lysophosphatidate (LPA), sphingosine-1-phosphate (S1P), and ceramide-1-phosphate (C1P)	Hu et al.[745]
EtLLP2 (lipid phosphate phosphatases 2)	KM880159	36.483	Higher in sporozoites than in unsporulated oocysts, sporulated oocysts, and merozoites	—	—	Substrates: PA, LPA, S1P and C1P	Hu et al.[745]
EtLLP3 (lipid phosphate phosphatases 3)	KM880160	34.384	Higher in sporozoites than in unsporulated oocysts, sporulated oocysts, and merozoites	—	—	Substrates: PA, LPA, S1P and C1P	Hu et al.[745]
EtLDH (lactate dehydrogenase)	KJ495733	34.96	Higher in second-generation merozoites than in unsporulated oocysts, sporulated oocysts, and sporozoites. Downregulated in diclazuril-resistant (DZR) strain	Most prominent in second-generation merozoites, moderately in unsporulated oocysts and sporulated oocysts, and weakly in sporozoites. Downregulated by 55.32% in second-generation merozoites of DZR	Anterior region of free sporozoites, and intracellular sporozoites except for the apex	Involved in glycolysis and anticoccidial mechanism of diclazuril. Antibodies inhibit sporozoite invasion into host cells (15.50%)	Hu et al.[745]
EtMDH (malate dehydrogenase)	XM_013377100	33.9	Higher in second-generation merozoites than unpopulated oocysts, sporulated oocysts, and sporozoites. Higher in DZR and maduramicin-resistant strains (MRR) than drug-sensitive strain (DS)	Higher in unsporulated oocysts than in sporulated oocysts, sporozoites, and second-generation merozoites. Upregulated in DZR and MRR	Cytoplasm of free sporozoites and cytomembrane of merozoites	Substrates: Oxaloacetate. Involved in drug resistance. Antibodies inhibit sporozoite invasion into host cells (~40%)	Hu et al.[745]
EtppGalNAc-T2 (polypeptide: *N*-acetylgalactosaminyl transferase 2)	XM_013374265	75.14	Higher in sporozoite than in unsporulated oocysts, sporulated 7 hour oocysts, sporulated oocysts, and second-generation merozoites	—	—	—	Liu et al.[1070]
EtMCAT (malonyl-CoA: acyl-carry protein transacylase)	GU936970	38.8	—	—	Near nuclei of sporozoite	Substrate: Malonyl-CoA	Sun et al.[1647]

(Continued)

Table 16.2 (Continued) Molecular and Functional Characterization of Selective Proteins from Chicken *Eimeria* in China

Name	GenBank Accession Number	Approximate Mr in kDa	mRNA Transcription Level	Protein Expression Level	Localization	Proposed function/ Catalytic Substrate	References
EtCLP (cathepsin-L-like peptidase)	XM_013376589	38	Higher in unsporulated oocysts, merozoites, and gametocytes than in sporozoites	Detected in unsporulated oocysts, sporozoites, merozoites, and gametocytes	—	Substrate: Z-Phe-Arg-AMC. Effective vaccine candidate	Liu et al.[1067]
EtSIR2 (silent information regulator 2A)	KU871068	33.4	Higher in unsporulated oocysts than in sporulated oocysts, sporozoite, and second-generation merozoites	Highest in second-generation merozoites, moderate in unsporulated oocysts and sporulated oocysts, and lowest in sporozoites	Cytoplasm of sporozoites and second-generation merozoites	Involved in parasite cell survival. Effective vaccine candidate	Dong et al.,[381] Zuo et al.[1922]
EtHDAC3 (histone deacetylase 3)	XM_013373580	42.6	Higher in sporulated 7 hour oocysts than in unsporulated oocysts, sporulated oocysts, sporozoites, and second-generation merozoites	—	—	—	Hu et al.[745]
EtHK (hexokinase)	XM_013377068	50.5	—	—	—	Substrates: D-glucose, 2-deoxy-D-glucose, D-fructose, D-mannose. Potential drug target	Sun et al.[1646]
EtCBS (cystathionine β synthase)	JZ905767	68	Higher in sporozoites than in unsporulated oocysts, sporulated oocysts, and second-generation merozoites	—	Surface of sporozoites and merozoites	Involved in invasion and intracellular growth. Antibodies inhibit sporozoite invasion into host cells(~70%)	Hu et al.[745]
EtCDPK3 (calcium-dependent protein kinase 3)	JQ679091	49.26	Higher in sporozoites than unsporulated oocysts, sporulated oocysts, and merozoites	Higher in sporozoites than unsporulated oocysts, sporulated oocysts, and merozoites	Cytoplasm of free sporozoites and apical end of intracellular sporozoites	11 putative interacting proteins. Involved in invasion and survival. Antibodies inhibit sporozoite invasion into host cells(33%~35%)	Hu et al.,[745] Zhang et al.[1888]
EtCDPK4 (calcium-dependent protein kinase 4)	KU925778	68.3	Higher in sporozoites than in unsporulated oocysts, sporulated oocysts, and merozoites	Higher in second-generation merozoites than in sporulated oocysts, unsporulated oocysts, and sporozoites	Cytoplasm of sporozoites except for the refractive body and second-generation merozoites	Interacting with serine protease inhibitor (EtSerpin). Involved in invasion. Antibodies inhibit sporozoite invasion into host cells(52%)	Wang et al.,[1782] Lv et al.[1101]

(Continued)

Table 16.2 (Continued) Molecular and Functional Characterization of Selective Proteins from Chicken *Eimeria* in China

Name	GenBank Accession Number	Approximate Mr in kDa	mRNA Transcription Level	Protein Expression Level	Localization	Proposed function/ Catalytic Substrate	References
EtTRT (telomerase reverse transcriptase)	GU271118	172	Detected in sporozoites and merozoites. Not in unsporulated oocysts	—	—	Interacting with 11-3-3 protein	Yang et al.,[1846] Hu et al.[745]
EtPP5 (serine/threonine protein phosphatase 5)	JX987508	60.82	Downregulated by 51.4% in second-generation merozoites by diclazuril treatment	—	—	Involved in diclazuril-induced apoptosis	Zhou et al.[1910]
EtCDPK4 (calcium-dependent protein kinase 4)	KU925778	68.3	Higher in sporozoites than in unsporulated oocysts, sporulated oocysts, and merozoites	Higher in second-generation merozoites than in sporulated oocysts, unsporulated oocysts, and sporozoites	Cytoplasm of sporozoites except for the refractive body and second-generation merozoites	Interacting with serine protease inhibitor (EtSerpin). Involved in invasion. Antibodies inhibit sporozoite invasion into host cells(52%)	Wang et al.,[1782] Lv et al.[1101]
EtTRT (telomerase reverse transcriptase)	GU271118	172	Detected in sporozoites and merozoites. Not in unsporulated oocysts	—	—	Interacting with 14-3-3 protein	Yang et al.,[1846] Hu et al.[745]
EtPP5 (serine/threonine protein phosphatase 5)	JX987508	60.82	Downregulated by 51.4% in second-generation merozoites by diclazuril treatment	—	—	Involved in diclazuril-induced apoptosis	Zhou et al.[1910]
Microneme Proteins							
EtMIC1 (microneme 1)	KF791866	74.7	—	—	—	Effective vaccine candidate	Chen et al.,[255] Zhang et al.,[1888] Zhang et al.[1878]
EtMIC2 (microneme 2)	AF111839	38	—	—	Anterior region of sporozoites and cytoplasm of merozoites	Interacting with EtAMA1. Involved in invasion. Antibodies inhibit sporozoite invasion into host cells (~20%). Effective vaccine candidate	Hu et al.[745], Wang et al.[1780]
EaMIC2 (microneme 2)	KR063282	29.81	—	Detected in sporozoites and merozoites	Apical tip of sporozoite and become diffused in merozoites	Effective vaccine candidate	Zhang et al.[1894]
EaMIC3 (microneme 3)	KU359773	93.04	—	Detected in sporozoites and merozoites	Apex of sporozoites and become diffused in merozoites	Novel antigen	Zhang et al.[1895]
EaMIC5 (microneme 5)	KF922373	12.18	—	Detected in sporozoites and merozoites	Apical tip of sporozoite, poles of merozoite and become diffused	Involved in invasion. Effective vaccine candidate	Zhang et al.[1893]

(Continued)

Table 16.2 (Continued) Molecular and Functional Characterization of Selective Proteins from Chicken *Eimeria* in China

Name	GenBank Accession Number	Approximate Mr in kDa	mRNA Transcription Level	Protein Expression Level	Localization	Proposed function/ Catalytic Substrate	References
EmitMIC3 (microneme 3)	MG888670	124.9	—	Detected in sporozoites and merozoites	Apex of sporozoites and become diffused in merozoites	Protective antigen	Huang et al.[753]
EbMIC2 (microneme 2)	AB723700	32	—	—	—	Effective vaccine candidate	Hoan et al.[725]
EmaxMIC2 (microneme 2)	FR718971.1	30.5	—	Detected in sporozoites	—	Effective antigen candidate	Zhang et al.[1888]
EmaxMIC7 (microneme 7)	FR718975	18.24	—	—	—	Effective antigen candidate	Zhang et al.[1888]
EtAMA1 (apical membrane antigen-1)	JN032081	58.08	Higher in sporozoites than unsporulated oocysts, sporulated oocysts, and second-generation merozoites	High in sporulated oocysts, sporozoites, and second-generation merozoites, while little in unsporulated oocysts	Membrane of sporozoites and apical end of intracellular sporozoites	14 putative interacting proteins. Interacting with EtMIC2. Involved in invasion and development. Antibodies inhibit sporozoite invasion into host cells(69%)	Jiang et al.,[814] Han et al.,[668] Wang et al.[1780]
EbAMA1 (apical membrane antigen-1)	AB723701.1	59.9	—	—	—	Effective vaccine candidate	Hoan et al.[724]
Gametocyte Proteins							
EnGAM22 (gametocyte protein 22)	KF649255	21.39	—	Detected in gametocyte	Wall-forming bodies of macrogametocytes, and walls of oocysts and sporocysts	Involved in oocyst wall formation	Liu et al.[1055]
EnGAM56 (gametocyte protein 56)	AY129951	53.3	—	—	Wall-forming bodies in macrogametocytes	Involved in oocyst wall formation. Effective vaccine candidate	Zhang et al.,[1888] Hu et al.[745]
EnGAM59 (gametocyte protein 59)	KT119356	52.81	—	—	Wall-forming bodies of macrogametocytes	Involved in oocyst wall formation	Hu et al.[745]
Putative/Conserved Proteins							
EmaxECP (*Eimeria*-conserved protein)	KF372875	25.4	Higher in sporozoites and sporulated oocysts than in unsporulated oocysts, and second-generation merozoites. Downregulated by 70.2% in precocious line	Higher in sporozoites than in sporulated oocysts and unsporulated oocysts, and no expression in second-generation merozoites. Downregulated in precocious line	Refractile bodies of free sporozoites and apical end of intracellular sporozoites	Involved in invasion and development. Antibodies inhibit sporozoite invasion into host cells(15.50%)	Hu et al.[745]
EtCHP559 (conserved hypothetical protein 559)	KT318394	46.04	Higher in sporozoites than in unsporulated oocysts, sporulated oocysts and second-generation merozoites	Detected in sporozoites	Surface of free sporozoites and cytosol of intracellular sporozoites	Involved in invasion. Antibodies inhibit sporozoite invasion into host cells(>70%)	Hu et al.[745]

(Continued)

Table 16.2 (Continued) Molecular and Functional Characterization of Selective Proteins from Chicken *Eimeria* in China

Name	GenBank Accession Number	Approximate Mr in kDa	mRNA Transcription Level	Protein Expression Level	Localization	Proposed function/ Catalytic Substrate	References
EtZB10-E05	ES351395	33.3	Higher in sporozoites than in unsporulated oocysts, sporulated oocysts, and second-generation merozoites	Detected in sporozoites	Apical end of intracellular sporozoites	Antibodies inhibit sporozoite invasion into host cells(>60%)	Hu et al.[745]
Et440	XM_013373244	15.5	—	—	Anterior region of sporozoites and merozoites	Involved in invasion. Antibodies inhibit sporozoite invasion into host cells(~40%)	Tang et al.[1669]
EtCHP317 (conserved hypothetical protein 317)	JZ905773	18	Higher in merozoites than in unsporulated oocysts, sporulated oocysts, and sporozoites	—	Surface of sporozoites and merozoites	Interacting with *Et*AMA1. Involved in invasion. Antibodies inhibit sporozoite invasion into host cells(~70%)	Hu et al.[745]
EacSZ-JN1	JN857359	21.8	—	Detected in sporozoites and merozoites	—	Effective vaccine candidate	Zhu et al.[1918]
EacSZ-JN2	JN857360	5.3	—	Detected in sporozoites and merozoites	—	Effective vaccine candidate	Zhu et al.[1919]
Other Proteins							
EtPDI (protein disulfide isomerase)	EF552214	24.15	Higher in sporulated oocysts than in unsporulated oocysts, sporozoites, and merozoites	Detected in sporulated oocysts, sporozoites, and second-generation merozoites, and not in unsporulated oocysts	Cytoplasm of sporozoites and merozoites	Involved in sporulation, adhesion, invasion, and development. Antibodies inhibit sporozoite invasion into host cells(23%~25%)	Hu et al.[745]
EtROM3 (rhomboid 3)	DQ323509	28	Higher in sporulated oocysts than in unsporulated oocysts, sporozoites, and merozoites	—	—	Interacting with EtMIC4. Involved in microneme protein cleavage	Tang et al.,[1669] Hu et al.[745]
EteIF3s7 (subunit 7 of eukaryotic initiation factor 3)	KP165145	64.925	Higher in second- generation merozoites than in sporulated oocysts, unsporulated oocysts, and sporozoites	Detected in second-generation merozoites, sporulated oocysts, and sporozoites, barely in unsporulated oocysts	Cytoplasm of free sporozoites and anterior region of intracellular sporozoites	Involved in invasion. Antibodies inhibit sporozoite invasion into host cells(21.5%)	Tang et al.[1669]

(Continued)

Table 16.2 (Continued)　Molecular and Functional Characterization of Selective Proteins from Chicken *Eimeria* in China

Name	GenBank Accession Number	Approximate Mr in kDa	mRNA Transcription Level	Protein Expression Level	Localization	Proposed function/ Catalytic Substrate	References
EtTCP-1α (T-complex protein 1 subunit α)	XM_013584691	30.8	Higher in second- generation merozoites than in sporulated oocysts, unsporulated oocysts, and sporozoites. Higher in DZR and MRR than DS	Higher in second-generation merozoites than in sporulated oocysts, unsporulated oocysts, and sporozoites. Upregulated in DZR and MRR	Surfaces of sporozoites and second-generation merozoites	Involved in growth and drug resistance	Tang et al.[1669]
EtHSP90 (heat shock protein 90)	AF042329	82.4	Downregulated by 29.7% in second-generation merozoites by diclazuril treatment	Downregulated by 50.0% in second-generation merozoites by diclazuril treatment	Around nucleus of second-generation merozoites	Involved in anticoccidial mechanism of diclazuril	Shen et al.[1550]
EtTA4	M21004.1	25	—	—	—	Effective vaccine candidate	Zhang et al.,[1888] Zhang et al.[1888]
EtGbp1p (G-strand binding protein)	CDJ37022	25.63	—	—	—	Potentially involved in telomeric DNA binding	Zhao et al.[1902]
EtHSP20.4 (heat shock protein 20.4)	GQ169724.1	20.4	Higher in sporulated oocysts than in sporozoites and second-generation merozoites, barely detectable in unsporulated oocysts	Higher in sporozoites than in sporulated oocysts and second-generation merozoites, but none in unsporulated oocysts	Surface of sporozoites and merozoites	Involved in sporulation and growth	Tang et al.[1669]
EtADF (actin-depolymerizing factor)	EF195234.1	13.18	Higher in merozoites and sporozoites than sporulated oocysts and unsporulated oocysts. Downregulated by 63.86% in second-generation merozoite by diclazuril treatment	—	—	Involved in invasion and anticoccidial mechanism of diclazuril	Xu et al.,[1835] Zhou et al.[1909]
EtIMP1 (immune mapped protein 1)	KC215109	41.75	—	—	Surface of sporozoite, unsporulated and sporulated oocysts	Effective vaccine candidate	Yin et al.,[1858] Zhang et al.[1888]
EtRACK (receptor for activated C kinase)	JQ292804	34.94	Downregulated by 81.3% in second-generation merozoite by diclazuril treatment	—	—	Involved in anticoccidial mechanism of diclazuril	Zhou et al.[1907]
EmaxSAG (surface antigen gene)	XM_013482011	24.73	—	Detected in sporozoite and merozoite	—	Effective vaccine candidate	Zhang et al.[1888]
Emax14-3-3	XM_013480135	33	—	Detected in sporozoite and merozoite	—	Effective vaccine candidate	Liu et al.[1069]

Abbreviations: Ea, *Eimeria acervulina*; Eb, *Eimeria brunetti*; Emax, *Eimeria maxima*; Emit, *Eimeria mitis*; En, *Eimeria necatrix*; Et, *Eimeria tenella*.

16.4.3 *Eimeria* Virus

Double-stranded (ds) RNA viruses and virus-like particles (approximately 30 nm in diameter) were detected in *E. tenella* sporulated oocysts.[670,745] The complete genome sequence of the virus isolate is 6006 bp containing two open reading frames (ORFs) with a five-nucleotide overlap (UGA/UG). The predicted ORF1 is 2367 bp encoding a putative capsid protein of 788 amino acids (84.922 kDa) and ORF2, 3216 bp encoding a putative RNA-dependent RNA polymerase (RdRp) protein of 1071 amino acids (118.190 kDa). The two untranslated regions are 349 bp (5′ UTR) and 78 bp (3′ UTR), respectively. The complete genome sequence of the *E. tenella* virus resembles those of the Totiviridae family. Phylogenetic analysis showed that the virus belongs to the genus Victorivirus. The new isolate was named *E. tenella* RNA virus 1.[670,745] It was further found that the RNA-dependent RNA polymerase of the virus interacts with *E. tenella* ovarian tumor protein-like cysteine protease and enhances the deubiquitinase activity of the protease, which in concert promote host cell growth and proliferation, indicating a symbiosis evolution between *Eimeria* and its virus.[745]

16.4.4 Genetic Manipulation of *Eimeria*

Progress in the transfection of *Eimeria* before 2012 has been reviewed elsewhere.[232,408] In recent studies, electroporation of sporozoites or merozoites with pyrimethamine-mediated selection, FACS of fluorescence reporter proteins, and restriction enzyme mediated integration (REMI) are the gold standard for quickly establishing stable transfection in *Eimeria*.[673,1071,1842] Transgenic *Eimeria* oocysts could be obtained from birds inoculated with transfected sporozoites (e.g., *E. tenella* and *E. mitis*)[1370] via the cloacal routeOne significant advance in genetic manipulation of *Eimeria* is coexpression of multiple genes in a single expression cassette mediated by a short sequence P2A derived from picornavirus.[1670] The P2A sequence mediates ribosome-skipping events and enables the generation of two or more separate peptide products from one mRNA that contains one or more P2A sequences. This mechanism is called "self-cleaving" and works efficiently in various organisms including *Eimeria*. This technique partly mitigates the constraint of construct size and the small number of selection markers in genetic manipulation of *Eimeria*.

16.5 DIAGNOSIS

Acute coccidiosis, especially caused by *E. tenella* and *E. necatrix,* is usually easily diagnosed; however, subclinical infection is common and difficult to diagnose.[1649] Routine monitoring of subclinical infection in flocks under anticoccidial drugs or vaccine prophylaxis should be practiced to prevent losses. A study of 545 poultry farms across nine provinces over a 5-year period on direct association of oocysts per gram (OPG) in litter with the occurrence of coccidiosis showed that the threshold of a coccidiosis outbreak is an OPG level of $>2 \times 10^4$, and when the OPG levels are $\geq 5 \times 10^4$, clinical coccidiosis occurs.[1879] Big data of OPG-level dynamics and occurrence of clinical or subclinical infection in flocks with different prevention programs can improve routine monitoring of coccidiasis or coccidiosis.

16.6 VACCINES

16.6.1 Live Vaccine

Although anticoccidial vaccines have been used in China for more than 30 years, only a few reports are available for their performance in the control of coccidiosis in chicken farms. The first large-scale field trial in China with Supercox, a live vaccine composed of a precocious line of *E. tenella* and naturally less pathogenic strains of *E. maxima* and *E. acervulina*, in 20,330 broilers vaccinated with Supercox and the same number medicated with diclazuril as the comparator showed that the vaccine performed better than drug prevention (Table 16.3).[1650] The study proved the clinical effectiveness and utility of vaccines in the control of clinical coccidiosis, particularly where drug resistance might result in failure to control clinical diseases. Another vaccine containing attenuated monensin-resistant *E. tenella, E. maxima,* and *E. acervulina* combined with drug medication performed better than vaccination or medication alone.[987] As there are antigenic variations among strains of chicken coccidia, a vaccine composed of a hybrid strain from three geographic isolates was developed.[1891] As expected, the hybrid strain provided better protection than their parental strains. The effectiveness of using live vaccines to control coccidiosis depends on the delivery system to ensure an even uptake of vaccinal oocysts by individual chicks.[1649]

Table 16.3 Comparison of Production Performance between Broiler Chickens Vaccinated with Supercox Anticoccidial Vaccine and Those Medicated with an Anticoccidial Drug (Diclazuril)

Groups	Number of Broilers Used	Survival Rate (%)	Weights of Rejected Birds (kg)	Feed/Weight Ratio	Total Profit (US$)
Vaccinated	20330	95.28[a]	284.58[a]	2.126[a]	5716[a]
Medicated	20330	91.98[b]	839.54[b]	2.102[a]	5374[a]

Note: For each column, values between groups with different superscripts (a and b) are significantly different ($P < 0.05$) according to the T test.

16.6.2 Immunogenicity-Enhanced Live Oocyst Vaccines

Generally wild and attenuated anticoccidial vaccines work well for the control of coccidiosis in breeders, layers, and heavy broilers. However, their use is limited in fast-growing broilers, which are marketed before 42 days of age, due to vaccination side effects of medium and/or low immunogenic *Eimeria* spp.[1371] The immunogenicity of *Eimeria* parasites can be improved through genetic manipulation of these parasites. Expression of chicken IgY Fc or IL-2 in transgenic *E. mitis* enhances the immunogenicity of the parasite[997,1371]; expression of profilin, an antigen from highly immunogenic *E. maxima*, in *E. tenella* enhances the immunogenicity of recombinant *E. tenella*.[1672] The clinical efficacy of these recombinant *Eimeria* as vaccine strains is yet to be tested in field trials.

16.6.3 Subunit and DNA Vaccines

More than 30 antigens, delivered either as subunit or DNA vaccines, from most chicken *Eimeria* were documented in their ability to provide partial protection against challenge infection with homologous *Eimeria* species (Tables 16.4 and 16.5). The protective efficiency of the subunit vaccines varies from 11% to 91.11% as measured by parasite replication and/or intestinal lesion scores, and depends on the vaccine and challenge dose (Tables 16.4 and 16.5). Compared with single-valent subunit or DNA vaccines, multivalent vaccines with appropriate adjuvants seem to provide better protection.[381,1597,1669] Commercial utility of the single- or multivalent subunit antigens combined with appropriate adjuvants will need to be evaluated by simulated field trials or clinical trials. In testing subunit and DNA vaccines, one important aspect to consider is the challenge dose, which may range from 10^2 to 10^5 oocysts. Another important consideration is the delivery method using the subunit and DNA vaccines. Egg injection (*in ovo* administration) together with antiviral or antibacterial vaccines may be a possible solution. DNA vaccines have the advantage of eliciting both humoral and cell-mediated immunity. One multiepitope DNA vaccine, constructed by ligating 4 T-cell epitope fragments from the sporozoite antigen SO7 and the merozoite antigen MZ5-7 of *E. tenella*, provided very high protection with an anticoccidial index (ACI, calculated as [relative rate of weight gain + survival rate] – [lesion value + oocyst value]) of 180.39.[1669] Another multiepitope DNA vaccine, composed of protective T-cell epitope fragments of TA4-1 (TA4 from *E. tenella*), NA4-1 (NA4 from *E. necatrix*), LDH-2 (LDH from *E. acervulina*), and EMCDPK-1 (CDPK from *E. maxima*), also induced protection with an ACI of 170 .[1597] Different breeds of chickens have different MHC restrictions—one T-cell epitope with efficacy in a particular breed of chickens may not imply its efficacy in another chicken breed; therefore, efficacy of the previously mentioned multiepitope

DNA vaccines should be tested in different chicken breeds. Another advantage of DNA vaccines is their oral delivery in live bacterial vectors, which is promising for large-scale use in the poultry industry.[406]

16.6.4 Vectored Vaccines

Several vector systems have been tested for presenting and delivering *Eimeria* antigens (Table 16.6). Two related questions must be answered for the development of an anticoccidial vectored vaccine. How many antigens will work well in the chicken farm in a field condition? For broilers, the vectored vaccine should contain antigens effective against at least *E. tenella*, *E. maxima*, and *E. acervulina*; for breeders and layers, antigens against five to seven *Eimeria* species are required. The other question is how many antigens can be stably inserted into a single vector or a small pool of vectors for best efficacy. The ideal vaccination is a single delivery of multiple antigens that will induce a lifelong protection.

Virus-vectored vaccines have two major advantages, one being able to elicit a robust cytotoxic T-lymphocyte response to eliminate pathogens in infected cells, and the other a high level of neutralizing antibodies. The fact that virus-vectored vaccines can elicit much higher neutralizing antibodies than naturally infected animals encourages using virus-vectored vaccines to express and present several *Eimeria* invasion proteins of the sporozoite stage to elicit protective mucosal as well as systemic humoral immunity.[1836]

Attenuated, especially genetically attenuated bacteria have been engineered to deliver heterologous antigens to stimulate mucosal, humoral, and cellular immunity.[1836] Presently, there are no licensed vaccines for infectious diseases based on attenuated bacteria as vectors, and the results of several studies seem promising (Table 16.6). Attenuated bacteria or commensal bacteria like *Lactococcus*[1106] can be orally administered and stimulate immunity to *Eimeria*. Using engineered bacteria to deliver several DNA vaccines that simultaneously express several other protective antigens to enhance immune responses is promising.

Yeast cell wall components such as β-glucans and mannan are recognized by the innate immune system, suggesting the yeast cell surface display system could be a potent vaccine delivery and presentation vehicle. Vaccination with either *Saccharomyces cerevisiae* or *S. boulardi* with surface-expressed *Eimeria* microneme proteins linked to cell wall glucan elicits microneme-specific immune responses and protection against *Eimeria* infection.[1106,1643,1779] Selection of a potent yeast-vectored system delivering *Eimeria* antigens is an active research subject.

16.6.5 *Eimeria* as Vaccine Vectors

One remarkable advance in *Eimeria* research is the successful transgenesis of this economically important group

Table 16.4 Subunit Vaccines: Antigens, Adjuvants, Experimental Designs, and Efficacy

Antigen(s)	Adjuvants	Immune scheme Age (d)	Dosage (μg)	Route	Times	Interval (d)	Immune responses Humoral	CMI	Effector	Challenge information Age (d)	Species	Dosage	Protection criteria	Reference
Et-3-1E	FCA	14	100	I.m.	2	7	—	—	—	28	Et Harbin	5×10^4	LS (1.33)/RGR (89.22%)/OI (1)/ACI (174.92)	Zhang et al.[1888]
Ea-3-1E	AbISCO-300	7	1/5/10	I.m.	2	7	sIgA	CD3-CD4+ CD8+	—	21	Ea BJ	1×10^5	BWG/OO	Zhang et al.[1892]
Et-SO7	—	14	200	I.m.	2	7	—	—	—	28	Et JS	5×10^4	LS(0.43 ± 0.62)/BWG/ODR(20.8%)[b]/ACI (185)	Tang et al.[1669]
Et-SO7	ChIFN-γ	5	100	I.h.	3	7	—	—	—	26	EtYZ	1×10^5	LS(2.35 ± 0.33)/RGR(73.91%)/ODR(50.09%)/ACI (120.41)	Tang et al.[1669]
Et-SO7	—	7	100	I.m.	3	7	—	—	—	29	EtYL	1×10^5	LS(1.4)/RGR(75.8%)/ODR(46.81%)[b]/ACI(160.8)	Tang et al.[1669]
Et-IMP1C terminal	FliC[a]	21	100	I.m.	2	14	IgY(G)	Frequency of secreted IFN-γ T cells	—	49	Et BJ	2×10^3	LS/BWG/ODR (88%)	Yin et al.[1860]
	FCA	14	100	I.m.	2	14	IgY(G)	Frequency of secreted IFN-γ T cells	—	42	Et XJ	5×10^3	LS (1.6 ± 0.3)/RGR(85.37%)/ODR(65.45%)	Yin et al.[1858]
Et-IMP1	CD40L	21	100	I.m.	2	14	sIgA IgY(G)	Frequency of secreted IFN-γ T cells	—	49	Et BJ	5×10^3	LS(1.5 ± 0.2)/BWG/ODR(77.6%)	Zhang et al.[1888]
Et-λMzp5-7	—	7	100	I.m.	3	7/14	IgY(G)	CD4+ CD8+	—	28	Et GZ	3×10^4	LS (3.5 ± 0.2)/RGR (22%)/ODR (11%)[b]	Tang et al.[1669]
Et-Mic1-VD	FCA FIA	7	100	I.m.	3	7	IgY(G)	—	IL-12 IFN-γ	28	Et GD	3×10^4	LS (1.3)/RGR (88.5%)/OI (10)/ACI (165.5)	Tang et al.[1669]
Et-Mic2	HSP70	7	100	I.h.	2	7	IgY(G)	CD4+ CD8+	IL-12/ IL-17/ IFN-γ	21	Et H	3×10^4	LS (2.02 ± 0.1)/BWG/ODR (62%)	Zhang et al.[1883]
Et-Mic2	FCA FIA	7	100	I.m.	3	7	IgY(G)	T-lymphocyte proliferation CD4+ CD8+	IL-6 IL-17 IFN-γ	28	Et SD-01	6×10^3	LS (1.76 ± 0.06)/RGR (88.92%)/ODR (74.66%)[b]/ACI (170.32)	Zhang et al.[1878]
Et-Mic2[c]	—												LS (1.22 ± 0.08)/RGR (93.66%)/ODR (85.01%)[b]/ACI (180.46)	
Et-Mic2[d]	FCA	7	50	I.h.	2	7	sIgA	Blood lymphocyte proliferation CD4+ CD8+	—	21	Et SD-01	3×10^4	LS (1.07 ± 0.99)/BWG/ODR (66.08%)[b]/ACI (172.48)	Chen et al.[257]

(Continued)

Table 16.4 (Continued) Subunit Vaccines: Antigens, Adjuvants, Experimental Designs, and Efficacy

Antigen(s)	Adjuvants	Immune scheme Age (d)	Dosage (ug)	Route	Times	Interval (d)	Humoral	CMI	Effector	Challenge information Age (d)	Species	Dosage	Protection criteria	Reference
Et-Mic4-N[e] terminal	AbISCO-100	7	10	I.m.	2	7	—	CD4+ CD8+	—	21	Et HB	8 × 10⁴	LS (1.10 ± 0.33)/RGR (101.68%)/ODR (67.90%)[b]	Zhou et al.[1913]
Em-Mic2	—	14	200	I.m.	2	7	IgY(G)	—	IL-2/ IL-10/ IL-17/ IL-4/ TGF-β/ IFN-γ	28	Em JS	1 × 10⁵	LS (1.33 ± 0.25)/BWG/ ODR (79.93%)[b]/ACI (165.81)	Zhang et al.[1888]
Em-Mic7	—	14	200	I.m.	2	7	IgY(G)	T-lymphocyte proliferation	IL-2/ IL-10/ IL-17/ IL-4/ TGF-β/ IFN-γ	28	Em JS	1 × 10⁵	LS (1.45 ± 0.18)/RGR/ ODR (75.43%)[b]/ACI (167.10)	Zhang et al.[1888]
Et-TA4/Mic2	—	7	150	I.m.	2	7	—	—	—	21	Et	5 × 10⁴	RGR (88.73%)/ODR (81.96%)	Tang et al.[1669]
Et-TA4/SO7	—	14	400	I.m.	2	14	—	—	—	28	Et JS	5 × 10⁴	LS (1.03 ± 0.81)/RGR (85.99%)/ODR (76.34%)[b]/ACI (174.69)	Zhang et al.[1888]
En-NA4/ NPmz19										28	En JS	5 × 10⁴	LS (1.00 ± 0.83)/RGR (84.10%)/ODR (79.76%)[b]/ACI (173.10)	
Ea-LDH/ MIF/3-1E										28	Ea JS	10 × 10⁴	LS (1.10 ± 0.80)/RGR (83.10%)/ODR (81.08%)[b]/ACI (171.10)	
Em-Em8[f]										28	Em JS	10 × 10⁴	LS (0.87 ± 0.82)/RGR (87.60%)/ODR (80.00%)[b]/ACI (177.9)	
Et-Serpin	—	7	100	I.m.	3	7	—	—	—	35	Et CC	3 × 10⁴	LS (2.36 ± 0.15)/RGR (66.73%)/ODR (30.01%)/ACI (137.13)	Zhang et al.[1888]
Em-Gam56[g]	FCA	5	500	I.h.	3	7	—	—	—	26	Em NT	5 × 10⁴	LS (1.13 ± 0.35)/RGR (93.92%)/ODR (57.04%)/ACI (177.02)	Tang et al.[1669]
Et-Sp	—	ND	100[h]	ND	2	ND	—	CD4+	—		Et BJ	1 × 10³	BWG/ODR (62.46%)	Ding et al.[374]
Ea-TA4											Ea BJ	1 × 10³	BWG/ODR (66.5%)	
Em- Gam56											Em BJ	1 × 10³	BWG/ODR (60.13%)	

(Continued)

Table 16.4 (Continued) Subunit Vaccines: Antigens, Adjuvants, Experimental Designs, and Efficacy

Antigen(s)	Adjuvants	Immune scheme					Immune responses			Challenge information			Protection criteria	Reference
		Age (d)	Dosage (ug)	Route	Times	Interval (d)	Humoral	CMI	Effector	Age (d)	Species	Dosage		
Et-HMGB1	FCA	14	100[h]	I.m.	2	7	IgY(G)	—	—	28	Et FY	1×10^4	LS (1.90 ± 0.18)/BWG/ODR (78.88%)	Tang et al.[1669]
Et-HSP70	—	14	100	I.m.	2	7	—	—	—	28	Et GD	5×10^4	LS (1.20)/RGR (76.92%)/ODR (60.6%)[b]/ACI (164)	Zhang et al.[1888]
Et-5401	Ginsenosides	3	100	I.h.	2	14	IgY(G)	Blood lymphocyte proliferation	—	31	Et ZJ	6×10^4	LS (2.28)/BWG/ODR (62.5%)	Zhang et al.[1888]
Et-EF-1α	—	1	50 / 100	I.h.	2	7	IgY(G)	—	—	14	Et / Em	1×10^4 / 1×10^4	BWG/OO / BWG/OO	Lin et al.[1027]
Em-14-3-3	—	14	200	I.m.	2	7	IgY(G)	CD4+ CD8+	IL-4/ IL-17/ IFN/ TGF-β	28	Em JS	1×10^5	LS (1.27 ± 0.12)/BWG/ODR (75.91%)[b]/ACI (166.96)	Liu et al.[1069]
Et-RH01	FCA FIA	7	100	I.m.	3	7	IgY(G)	CD4+ CD8+	IL-2 IFN-γ	35	Et XJ	3×10^4	LS (1.2 ± 0.20)/RGR (87.03%)/ODR (77.3%)[b]	Zhang et al.[1888]
Et-CHP559	Montanide ISA 71	7	100	ND	2	8	IgY(G)	—	sCD4/ sCD8/ IFN-γ/ IL-17/ IL-10	23	Et SH	1×10^4	LS (1.61 ± 0.86)/BWG/ODR (65.36%)/ACI (160.81)	Hu et al.[745]
Em-SAG	—	14	200	I.m.	2	7	IgY(G)	CD4+ CD8+	IL-4/ IL-17/ IFN/ TGF-β1	28	Em JS	1×10^5	LS (1.22 ± 0.10)/BWG/ODR (75.93%)[b]/ACI (173.07)	Zhang et al.[1888]
Ea-α-tubulin-GST	FCA FIA	10	150	I.h.	2	10	—	T-lymphocyte proliferation	—	30	Ea BJ	1×10^3	BWG/ODR (36.2%)	Ding et al.[373]

Abbreviations: ACI, anticoccidial index; BJ, beijing; BWG, body weight gain; CC, changchun; Ea, *Eimeria acervulina:* Em, *Eimeria maxima;* En, *Eimeria necatrix;* Et, *Eimeria tenella;* FY, fengyang; GD, guangdong; GZ, guangzhou; H, houghton; HB, heibei; JS, jiangsu; LS, lesion score; NT, nantong; ODR, oocyst decrease rate; OI, oocyst index; OO, oocyst output; RGR, relative growth rate SD, shandong; SH, shanghai; XJ, xinjiang; YL, yangling; YZ, yangzhou; ZJ, zhejiang.

a Flic was a truncated flagellin.

b ODR = (the number of oocysts per gram feces or content from control birds − the number of oocysts per gram feces or content from vaccinated birds)/the number of oocysts per gram feces or content from control birds × 100%.

c EtMic2 protein was expressed by *Pichia pastoris.*

d EtMIC2 random mutagenesis was generated using error-prone polymerase chain reaction.

e Protein was expressed by recombinant yeast.

f Multivalent subunit vaccines consisted of Et-TA4, En-NA4, Ea-LDH, and Em-Em8.

g Gam56 was a truncated protein.

h DNA prime protein boost immunization schedule.

Table 16.5   DNA Vaccines: Antigens, Adjuvants, Experimental Designs, and Efficacy

Antigen(s)	Immune Scheme[a]						Immune Responses			Challenge Information			Protection Criteria	Reference
	Adjuvants	Vector	Age (d)	Dosage (ug)	Times	Interval (d)	Humoral	CMI	Effector	Age (d)	Species	Dosage		
Ea-cSZ-2	ChIL-2	pVAX1	14	100	2	7	—	—	—	28	Et JS	5×10^4	LS (0.4 ± 0.69)/RGR (84%)/ODR (78%)[b]/ACI (182.2)	Shah et al.[1537]
Ea-cSZ-2	ChIL-2	pVAX1	7	25	2	7	—	—	—	21	Et JS	5×10^4	LS (1.3 ± 1.03)/BWG/ODR (71%)[b]/ACI (183)	Zhang et al.[1888]
											Ea JS	5×10^4	LS (1.11 ± 0.85)/BWG/ODR (75%)[b]/ACI (188)	
											En JS	5×10^4	LS (1.55 ± 1.05)/BWG/ODR (62%)[b]/ACI (162.4)	
											Em JS	5×10^4	LS (2.2 ± 1.05)/BWG/ODR (38.4%)[b]/ACI (142)	
Ea-cSZ-2	ChIFN-γ	pVAX1	14	100	2	7	—	—	—	28	Et JS	5×10^4	LS (0.8 ± 0.89)/RGR (76.2%)/ODR (57%)[b]/ACI (173)	Tang et al.[1669]
Ea-cSZ-2	ChIL-2	pVAX1	14	100	2	7	—	—	—	28	Ea JS	1×10^5	LS (0.64 ± 0.9)/BWG/ODR (80%)[b]/ACI (192)	Tang et al.[1669]
	ChIFN-γ												LS (0.72 ± 1.3)/BWG/ODR (62.4%)/ACI (171)	
Et-Mic2	ChIL-18	pVAX1	7	100	3	7	IgY(G)	T-lymphocyte proliferation CD4+CD8+	—	28	Et SD-01	6×10^3	LS (1.45 ± 1.37)/RGR (86.67%)/ODR (88.28%)[b]/ACI (171.17)	Zhang et al.[1888]
Et-Mic2	ChIL-2	pcDNA3.0	14	100	2	7	—	—	—	28	Et HB	1×10^4	LS/RGR (81.3%)/OI (5)/ACI (163)	Tang et al.[1669]
Eb-Mic2	—	pVAX1	14	100	2	7	IgY(G)	—	IL-4/IL-10/IL-17/IFN-γ/TGF-β	28	Eb JS	1×10^5	LS (1.03 ± 0.85)/BWG/ODR (77.43%)/ACI (179)	Hoan et al.[725]
Em-Mic2	—	pVAX1	14	100	2	7	IgY(G)	T-lymphocyte proliferation	IL-2/IL-4/IL-10/IL-17/IFN-γ/TGF-β	28	Em JS	1×10^5	LS (1.30 ± 0.85)/BWG/ODR (77.89%)[b]/ACI (170.16)	Tang et al.[1669]
Em-Mic7	—	pVAX1	14	100	2	7	IgY(G)	T-lymphocyte proliferation	IL-2/IL-4/IL-10/IL-17/IFN-γ/TGF-β	28	Em JS	1×10^5	LS (1.31 ± 0.90)/BWG/ODR (75.38%)[b]/ACI (167.84)	Zhang et al.[1888]

(Continued)

Table 16.5 (Continued) DNA Vaccines: Antigens, Adjuvants, Experimental Designs, and Efficacy

Antigen(s)	Adjuvants	Vector	Immune Scheme[a]				Immune Responses			Challenge Information			Protection Criteria	Reference
			Age (d)	Dosage (ug)	Times	Interval (d)	Humoral	CMI	Effector	Age (d)	Species	Dosage		
Et-HSP70	—	pcDNA6	14	100	2	7	—	—	—	28	Et GD	5×10^4	LS (1.50)/RGR (66.15%)/ODR (54.80%)[b]/ACI (150)	Zhang et al.[1888]
Ea-3-1E	mChIL–15	pcDNA3.1	14	100	2	7	—	—	—	28	Ea SH	5×10^4	LS (1.17 ± 0.41)/RGR (96.48%)/ODR (68.35%)/ACI (183.78)	Zhang et al.[1888]
Ea-3-1E	—	pcDNA3.1	7	50	2	7	—	—	—	21	Ea BD	5×10^6	LS (1.13/RGR (88.36%)/ODR (67.67%)[b]/ACI (167.06)	Zhang et al.[1888]
Et-3-1E	ChIFN-γ												BWG/ODR (65.4%)	Tang et al.[1669]
Et-3-1E	ChIFN-γ	proVAX	7	50	2	7	—	—	—	21	Et GS	5×10^4	LS (0.889)/RGR (90.93%)/OI (1)/ACI (181.04)	Zhang et al.[1888]
	ChIL-2	pcDNA3.1	14		2	7	—	—	—	28	Et Harbin	5×10^4	LS (0.778)/RGR (96.08%)/OI (1)/ACI (187.30)	
Et-3-1 E/ CDPK	—	proVAX	7	50	2	7	IgY(G)	T-lymphocyte proliferation	—	21	Et GS	5×10^4	RGR (74%)/ODR (51.46%)[b]	Tang et al.[1669]
Ea-3-1E /ADF	—	pET-32a	7	200	2	7	IgY(G)	T-lymphocyte proliferation	IL-2 IFN-γ	21	Ea BD	4×10^6	LS (1.16)/RGR (88.36%)/ODR (67.88%)[b]/ACI (169.82)	Zhao et al.[1905]
Et-TA4 /Et1A	—	pcDNA3.1/ Zeo(+)	3	50	2	7	—	—	—	17	Et BJ	3×10^4	LS (2.50 ± 0.75)/RGR (95.73%)/ODR (75.73%)[b]/ACI (160.73)	Zhang et al.[1888]
Et-TA4	ChIL-2	pcDNA3.1	14	100	2	7	—	—	—	28	Et JS	5×10^4	LS (0.4 ± 0.66)/RGR (97.3%)/ODR (75.1%)[b] /(192)	Zhang et al.[1888]

(Continued)

Table 16.5 (Continued) DNA Vaccines: Antigens, Adjuvants, Experimental Designs, and Efficacy

Antigen(s)	Adjuvants	Vector	Immune Scheme[a]				Immune Responses			Challenge Information			Protection Criteria	Reference
			Age (d)	Dosage (ug)	Times	Interval (d)	Humoral	CMI	Effector	Age (d)	Species	Dosage		
Et-TA4	ChIL-2	pcDNA3.1	7	25	2	7	—	—	—	28	Et JS	5×10^4	LS (1.57 ± 0.77)/ BWG/ODR (57.13%)[b]/ACI (181.18)	Zhang et al.[1888]
											En JS	5×10^4	LS (1.77 ± 0.77)/ BWG/ODR (56.73%)[b]/ACI (170.26)	
											Ea JS	5×10^4	LS (1.60 ± 0.93)/ BWG/ODR (50.03%)[b]/ACI (164.91)	
											Em JS	5×10^4	LS (2.63 ± 1.00)/ BWG/ODR (4.47%)[b]/ACI (86.82)	
Et-TA4/ Mic4/5401/ pEtk2 Ea-3-1E /LDH En-NA4 Em-EMCDPK[c]	ChIL-2	pVAX1	14	100	2	7	—	—	—	28	Et JS	5×10^4	LS (1.47 ± 0.49)/ RGR (91.28%)/ ODR (75.04%)/ACI (175.91)	Song et al.[1597]
											Ea JS	10×10^4	LS (1.57 ± 0.62)/ RGR (87.12%)/ ODR (79.59%)/ACI (170.40)	
											En JS	5×10^4	LS (1.30 ± 0.65)/ RGR (93.19%)/ ODR (84.63%)/ACI (180.96)	
											Em JS	10×10^4	LS (1.57 ± 0.62)/ RGR (84.18%)/ ODR (79.69%)/ACI (170.18)	
Et-TA4	ChIL-2	pVAX1	14	25	2	7	IgY(G)	—	—	28	Et JS	5×10^4	LS (1.63 ± 0.50)/ RGR (108.87%)/ ODR (88.27%)/ACI (191.57)	Zhang et al.[1888]
Et-MZ5-7	ChIL-17	pcDNA4.0	14	100	2	7	—	—	IL-2 IFN-γ	28	Et JS	5×10^4	LS (1.18 ± 0.54)/ BWG/ODR (65.99%)/ACI (190)	Zhang et al.[1888]

(Continued)

Table 16.5 (Continued) DNA Vaccines: Antigens, Adjuvants, Experimental Designs, and Efficacy

Antigen(s)	Adjuvants	Vector	Immune Scheme[a]				Immune Responses			Challenge Information			Protection Criteria	Reference
			Age (d)	Dosage (ug)	Times	Interval (d)	Humoral	CMI	Effector	Age (d)	Species	Dosage		
Ea-GADPH	—	pVAX1	14	100	2	7	IgY(G)	CD4+ CD8+	IL-2/IFN-γ/ IL-4/IL-17/ TGF-β4/ TNF SF15	28	Et JS	5 × 10⁴	LS (0.53 ± 0.53)/ RGR (79.54%)/ ODR (85.98%)/ACI (169.24)	Zhang et al.[1888]
											Ea JS	10 × 10⁴	LS (1.35 ± 0.67)/ RGR (79.57%)/ ODR (58.59%)/ACI (165.07)	
											Em JS	10 × 10⁴	LS (1.162 ± 0.75)/ RGR (82.37%)/ ODR (44.14%)/ACI (165.17)	
											Mixed	Mixed	LS (0.47 ± 0.61)/ RGR (74.38%)/ ODR (47.75%)/ACI (164.88)	
Em-GAPDH											Et JS	5 × 10⁴	LS (0.67 ± 0.72)/ RGR (80.24%)/ ODR (82.28%)/ACI (168.54)	
											Ea JS	10 × 10⁴	LS (1.46 ± 0.86)/ RGR (87.07%)/ ODR (55.21%)/ACI (171.47)	
											Em JS	10 × 10⁴	LS (1.32 ± 0.81)/ RGR (85.01%)/ ODR (54.48%)/ACI (170.81)	
											Mixed	Mixed	LS (0.75 ± 0.54)/ RGR (79.80%)/ ODR (56.18%)/ACI (171.1)	
Et-SIR2A	—	pCAGGS	7	100	2	7	—	—	—	21	Et SH	1 × 10⁴	LS (1.09 ± 0.67)/ BWG/ODR (62.96%)	Dong et al.[381]

(Continued)

Table 16.5 (Continued)   DNA Vaccines: Antigens, Adjuvants, Experimental Designs, and Efficacy

Antigen(s)	Adjuvants	Vector	Immune Scheme[a]				Immune Responses			Challenge Information			Protection Criteria	Reference
			Age (d)	Dosage (ug)	Times	Interval (d)	Humoral	CMI	Effector	Age (d)	Species	Dosage		
Et-pEtK2	ChIL-2	pcDNA4.0(c)	14	50	2	7	—	—	—	28	Et JS	5×10^4	LS (0.97 ± 0.08)/ RGR (97.17%)/ ODR (91.02%)[b]/ ACI (186.50)	Zhang et al.[1888]
											Em YZ	5×10^4	LS (1.40 ± 0.09)/ RGR (81.85%)/ ODR (39.13%)[b]/ ACI (147.85)	
											Ea YZ	5×10^4	LS (1.50 ± 0.14)/ RGR (77.71%)/ ODR (38.78%)[b]/ ACI (142.71)	
											En GD	5×10^4	LS (1.67 ± 0.11)/ RGR (71.49%)/ ODR (91.11%)[b]/ACI (153.82)	
Et-5401	ChIFN-γ / ChIL-2	pVAX1	14	100	2	7	—	—	—	28	Et JS	5×10^4	LS (1.30 ± 0.47)/ RGR (94.01%)/ ODR (88.40%)/ACI (180.01)	Tang et al.[1669]
													LS (1.37 ± 0.61)/ RGR (91.94%)/ ODR (87.44%)/ACI (177.24)	
Em-Gam56	—	pcDNA3.1(zeo)+	7	100	2	7	IgY(G)	T-lymphocyte proliferation	—	21	Em NT	5×10^4	RGR (89.7%)/ODR (53.7%)	Zhang et al.[1888]
Ea-Hsp90	—	pVAX1	14	100	2	7	—	—	—	28	Ea	1×10^5	LS (1.56)/RGR (82.77%)/OI (1)/ ACI (166.17)	Feng et al.[523]
Ea-LDH	ChIL-2 / ChIFN-γ	pVAX1	14	100	2	7	—	CD4+ CD8+	—	28	Ea JS	1.2×10^5	LS (1.93 ± 0.63)/ BWG/ODR (57.59%)[b]/ACI (168.78)	Tang et al.[1669]
													LS (2.07 ± 0.57)/ BWG/ODR (56.82%)[b]/ACI (166.68)	
Et-rhomboid	—	pVAX1	7	100	3	7/14	IgY(G)	CD4+ CD8+	IL-2 IFN-γ	42	Et XJ	3×10^4	LS (1.29 ± 0.35)/ BWG/ODR (75.8%)[b]	Zhang et al.[1888]
Em14-3-3	—	pVAX1	14	100	2	7	IgY(G)	CD4+ CD8+	IL-4/IFN-γ/ IL-17/ TGF-β	28	Em JS	1×10^5	LS (1.18 ± 0.16)/ BWG/ODR (76.58%)[b]/ACI (170.80)	Liu et al.[1069]

(Continued)

Table 16.5 (Continued)   DNA Vaccines: Antigens, Adjuvants, Experimental Designs, and Efficacy

Antigen(s)	Adjuvants	Vector	Immune Scheme[a] Age (d)	Dosage (µg)	Times	Interval (d)	Immune Responses Humoral	CMI	Effector	Challenge Information Age (d)	Species	Dosage	Protection Criteria	Reference
Em-SAG	—	pVAX1	14	100	2	7	IgY(G)	CD4+ CD8+	IL-4/IL-17/ IFN-γ/ TGF-β1	28	Em JS	1 × 10⁵	LS (1.13 ± 0.16)/ BWG/ODR (76.64)/ ACI (175.88)	Zhang et al.[1888]
Et-SO7	ChIL-2	pVAX1	14	100	2	7	—	—	—	28	Et JS	5 × 10⁴	LS (0.50 ± 0.62)/ RGR (96.2%)/ODR (23.33%)[b]/ACI (190)	Zhang et al.[1888]
Et-SO7 / MZ5-7	ChIL-2	pVAX1	14	100	2	7	—	—	—	28	Et JS	5 × 10⁴	LS (1.10 ± 0.80)/ BWG/ODR (65.74%)/ACI (187.98)	Zhang et al.[1888]
	ChIFN-γ												LS (1.03 ± 0.56)/ BWG/ODR (68.93%)/ACI (189.92)	

Abbreviations: ACI, anticoccidial index; BWG, body weight gain; Ea, *Eimeria acervuline*; Em, *Eimeria maxima*; En, *Eimeria necatrix*; Et, *Eimeria tenella*; LS, lesion score; ODR, oocyst decrease rate; OI, oocyst index; RGR, relative growth rate.

[a] DNA vaccine is immunized through intramuscular injection (I.m.)

[b] ODR = (the number of oocysts per gram feces or content from control birds – the number of oocysts per gram feces or content from vaccinated birds)/the number of oocysts per gram feces or content from control birds × 100%.

[c] Multivalent epitope DNA vaccines consisted of En-NA4-1, Et-TA4-1, Ea-LDH-2, and Em-EMCDPK-1.

Table 16.6 Vectored Vaccines: Vector, Antigen, Experimental Designs, and Efficacy

Vector	Antigen(s)	Promoter or Expression Vector	Immunization schedule			Immunity		Challenge infection		Protection Rate/%[b]	Reference
			First Immunization Dosage (Route)	Interval (Weeks)	Second Immunization Dosage (Route)	Humoral	Cellular	Date[a]	Species (Oocysts/Bird)		
Fowlpox virus	Rhomboid	API-P7.5 × 20	$10^2/10^3/10^4$ PFU (-)	2	$10^2/10^3/10^4$ PFU (-)	—	CD4+, CD8+	14	Et F2c (5×10^4)	67.5/71.1/71.2	Zhang et al.[1888]
Mycobacterium bovis BCG	Rhomboid	pMV261[d]	10^6 CFU (i.n.)	2	10^6 CFU (i.n.)	IgY(G)	CD4+, CD8+	14	Et F2c (3×10^4)	56.04	Wang et al.,[1778]
	Rhomboid	pMV361[e]	10^6 CFU (i.n.)	2	10^6 CFU (i.n.)	IgY(G)	CD4+, CD8+	14	Et F2c (3×10^4)	51.08	Zhang et al.[1888]
	Rhomboid-chIL-2	pMV361	10^7 CFU (i.n./s.c.)	1	10^7 CFU (i.n./s.c.)	—	CD4+, CD8+	14	Et F2c (3×10^4)	64.1/56.2	Zhang et al.[1888]
	AMA1[f]	pMV261	10^7 CFU (p.o./i.n./s.c.)	1	10^7 CFU (p.o./i.n./s.c.)	IgY(G)	CD4+, CD8+	7	Em (5×10^4)	22.9/33.6/42.2	Li et al.[994]
		pMV361	10^7 CFU (p.o./i.n./s.c.)	1	10^7 CFU (p.o./i.n./s.c.)	IgY(G)	CD4+, CD8+	7	Em (5×10^4)	17.1/26.6/29.9	
	ADF	pMV261	10^7 CFU (p.o./i.n./s.c.), for three times with 1-week interval			—	—	7	Et XJ (1×10^4)	152.7/161.5/149.4[9]	Zhang et al.[1888]
		pMV361	10^7 CFU (p.o./i.n./s.c.), for three times with 1-week interval			—	—	7	Et XJ (1×10^4)	156.7/169.2/153.3[9]	
Escherichia coli	SO7	pMG36t	10^6 CFU (p.o.)	2	10^6 CFU (p.o.)	IgY(G)	CD4+, CD8+	14	Et BJ (5×10^4)	67.7	Yang et al.[1847]
Bacillus subtilis	3-1E	pBE2	10^8 CFU/kg of diet for 17 days			—	—	1	Et ZJ (5×10^4)	63.7	Zhang et al.[1888]
Lactococcus lactis	3-1E	PnisA	10^{10} CFU (p.o.), for three times and each for 3 days with 1-week interval			—	—	1	Et (5×10^4)	21.4	Ma et al.[1107]
	AMA1	PnisA	5×10^9 CFU (p.o.), AMA1/SP-AMA1/SP-AMA1-CWA[h], for three times and each for 3 days with 11-day interval			IgY(G)	T-lymphocyte proliferation	10	Et (4×10^4)	27.7/25.4/33.3	Zhang et al.[1888]
Salmonella typhimurium	5401	pcDNA3	10^8 CFU (p.o.)	2	10^8 CFU (p.o.)	IgY(G)	Blood lymphocyte proliferation	14	Et ZJ (6×10^4)	164.98[9]	Du et al.[407]
Saccharomyces cerevisiae	Mic1[i]	pCT	10^7 yeast cells (p.o.), for 27 days			IgY(G)	CD4+, CD8+	1	Et SD-01 (6×10^3)	74.4/75.7/79.0	Chen et al.[255]
	Mic2	pYSD	10^9 yeast cells (p.o.), for 20 days			sIgA	Blood lymphocyte proliferation	21	Et SD-01 (3×10^3)	76.56	Sun et al.[1643]

(Continued)

Table 16.6 (Continued) Vectored Vaccines: Vector, Antigen, Experimental Designs, and Efficacy

Vector	Antigen(s)	Promoter or Expression Vector	Immunization schedule			Immunity		Challenge infection		Protection Rate/%[b]	Reference
			First Immunization Dosage (Route)	Interval (Weeks)	Second Immunization Dosage (Route)	Humoral	Cellular	Date[a]	Species (Oocysts/Bird)		
Lactobacillus plantarum	SO7-DCpep	pSIP409	2×10^9 CFU (p.o.), for 2 weeks			IgY (G) sIgA	—	14	Et BJ (5×10^4)	75.1	Yang et al.[1848]
Eimeria tenella	IMP1[e]	SAG13	Single oral immunization with 200 oocysts, floor-reared			IgY(G)	Blood lymphocyte proliferation	14/28	Em BJ (50)	53.7/74.9	Tang et al.[1671]

Abbreviations: Em, *Eimeria maxima*; Et, *Eimeria tenella.*

a Days post the last immunization.
b Protection rate = (the number of oocysts from control birds − the number of oocysts from vaccinated birds)/the number of oocysts from control birds × 100%.
c *Eimeria tenella* F2 hybrid strain was cultivated from three parental strains isolated from Guangzhou, Baoding, and Changchun in China.
d pMV261 is an extrachromosomal vector.
e pMV361 is an integrative vector.
f These antigens are from *E. maxima*, otherwise, the antigens are from *E. tenella.*
g The authors used the anticoccidial index (ACI) to show the protection.
h The authors constructed three vectors, AMA1 (with fragment encoding 3-1E protein), SP-AMA1 (with fragment encoding signal peptide of secretion protein Usp45 [SP] and 3-1E protein) and SP-AMA1-CWA (with fragment encoding signal peptide of secretion protein Usp45 [SP], 3-1E protein and cell-wall anchor [CWA]) in this study.
i The authors constructed three yeast cell lines with different EtMic1 protein domain.

of parasites. The findings that most transgenic *Eimeria* populations have reduced fecundity and unchanged immunogenicity to their wild-type parents strongly indicate that a transgenic parasite expressing protective antigens could be a promising eukaryotic vaccine vector, especially for delivering *Eimeria* antigens.[754,1842]

One of two essential questions for establishing transgenic *Eimeria* as a vaccine vector is how much expression of the exogenous antigen is sufficient to elicit adequate protective immune responses.[1836] Solutions include, but are not limited to, the use of strong regulatory sequences, the insertion of multiple copies by techniques such as PiggyBac,[1635] and P2A,[1670] and optimizing codon usage . The most difficult task is the manipulation or adaptation of *Eimeria* to tolerate high-level expression of one or several exogenous proteins. Of course, a related question is whether the dynamics of expression controlled by stage-specific regulatory sequences will influence immune responses. Proteomics and immune-proteomics may help resolve this issue.[1836]

The second essential question is the location or compartmentalization of exogenous antigens.[1836] It was found that antigen compartmentalization affects the magnitude of the immune response. Microneme-targeted EYFP stimulates a higher IgA response as well as Ag-specific lymphocyte proliferation than cytoplasm-targeted EYFP .[754] More work to be done in this aspect includes studies on the effect of antigen compartmentalization on the magnitude of humoral, cellular, and mucosal protective immunity.[1836]

Eimeria as a vaccine vector expressing heterogeneous antigens to elicit protective immunity has been proven feasible.[1671,1674] Surface antigen 1 of *T. gondii* (TgSAG1) expressed on the cell surface of *E. tenella* sporozoites regulated by its signal peptide and GPI-anchor protects chickens from challenge with *T. gondii* RH strain tachyzoites.[1674] Transgenic *E. tenella* expressing immune mapped protein 1 of *E. maxima* (Et-EmIMP1) provides partial protection of chickens against *E. maxima* infection.[1671]

16.7 DRUGS

16.7.1 Drug Development

A new triazine compound, *N*-(4-(4-(3,5-dioxo-4,5-dihydro-1,2,4-triazine-2-(3H)-yl)-2-methylphenoxy) phenyl) acetamide (ethanamizuril [EZL], CAS:1560840-75-6), was developed using systematic analysis of the structure-activity relationship and rational design strategies.[258,1669,1903] Broilers given EZL at a dosage of 9 mg/kg have improved body weight gain and feed conversion rate and reduced mortality and intestinal lesions compared with those given diclazuril at the commercially recommended dosage of 1 mg/kg. ACIs of EZL-treated groups at 10 mg/kg are 197, 188, 194, and 190 in chickens challenged with *E. tenella, E. necatrix, E. acervulina,* and *E. maxima*, respectively.[1669] EZL treatment disturbs the process of schizont division into merozoites and results in abnormal schizonts. Overall, EZL may exert its effects during the entire endogenous stage of the parasites, but the schizogony stages are intrinsically more vulnerable.[1061]

A further study showed that a single dose of 5 mg/kg EZL by oral gavage at 4 days after inoculation significantly reduced mRNA expression of enolase, an essential enzyme that catalyzes the reversible conversion of 2-phosphoglycerate into phosphoenolpyruvate.[1065,1669] At a higher dose of 15 mg/kg EZL, differentiation of second-generation schizonts and microgamonts was inhibited, and merozoites, gametes, and zygotes became irregular in shape by electron microscopic examination.[1065,1669]

EZL has low acute oral toxicity in mice and rats. The LD_{50} in mice and rats are 5776 and 4743 mg/kg of body weight, respectively. In a subchronic toxicity study in rats dosed with 5–120 mg EZL/kg body weight for 30 days, treatment-related clinical signs of depilation on back and neck were observed in some males and females of the high-dose groups from the third week of treatment. Slight renal tubule protein casts in kidneys and alveolar wall thickening in lungs were also observed in the highest dose group of both genders. No teratogenicity or reproduction/developmental toxicity was observed in rats.[1669] On environmental assessment, the toxicities of EZL to earthworms, birds, plants, fish, algae, and daphnia were low to each nontarget organism, per the risk classification system for pesticides. In addition, the mobility of EZL in gray alluvial soil, yellow-brown soil, and red soil was very slow.[1889]

16.7.2 Mechanism of Action

The modes of action of anticoccidial drugs are diverse, and the primary targets have not been identified. Monensin, an ionophore, alters membrane fluidity and membrane-bound Na+ -K+ -ATPase activity of *E. tenella* sporozoites.[1783,1784] Genes involved in monensin resistance are those related to cytoskeletal rearrangements and energy metabolism.[745] Another ionophore, maduramicin changes ultrastructures of *Eimeria* parasites,[40,121] and the genes involved in maduramicin resistance are invasion and cytoskeletal genes as well as glycometabolism-related and potential transporter genes.[745]

Diclazuril, as a benzene acetonitrile broad-spectrum anticoccidial agent, is effective against asexual and sexual reproduction cycles of *E. tenella*. A pronounced effect of diclazuril treatment is apoptosis in second-generation merozoites of *E. tenella,* including morphological changes, loss of mitochondrial membrane potential, and increased apoptosis ratio.[1906] Treatment with diclazuril downregulates serine/threonine protein phosphatase type 5 (PP5) of second-generation *E. tenella* merozoites, reducing PP5 mRNA expression by 51.4%. PP5 downregulation increases activation of ASK1-induced apoptosis by ASK1 hypo-phosphorylation and subsequently induces apoptosis in second-generation merozoites of *E. tenella*.[1910] Another study showed that nuclear translocation and accumulation of glyceraldehyde-3-phosphate dehydrogenase is involved in diclazuril-induced apoptosis in *E. tenella*, a process accompanied by the activation of the intrinsic caspase-9 pathway.[1771]

Diclazuril also downregulates invasion-related genes. Expression levels of EtMic1 in second-generation merozoites of *E. tenella* are downregulated by 65.63%, EtMic2 by 64.12%, EtMIC3 by 56.82%, EtMic4 by 73.48%, and EtMic5 by 78.17%, leading to inhibition of binding of host cell-surface proteins as well as invasion of host cells by merozoites.[1908] Downregulation of the receptor for activated C kinase of merozoites is believed to trigger the dysfunction of downstream proteins, suppressing the signal transduction that directs the invasion-related, secreted protein expression.[1907] Further, diclazuril downregulates expression of the actin depolymerizing factor, interfering with filament turnover and inhibiting merozoite invasion into host cells, cytoskeleton remolding of the parasites, and reduces the number of second-generation merozoites.[1908,1909]

Artemisinin (ART) is a sesquiterpene lactone isolated from *Artemesia annua* and is well-known for its antimalarial effect. Beyond antimalarial, ART is also known to be effective in the control of poultry coccidiosis.[816,1194] Commercial artemisinin administered at 100 mg/kg or 5% dried leaves of *A. annua* in food can significantly reduce oocyst output and lesion scores in *E. tenella*–infected chickens.[816,1194] In addition, ART treatment effectively decreases the number of second-generation merozoites in chickens infected with *E. tenella*. Flow cytometry showed a decrease in mitochondrial membrane potential and an increase in apoptotic rate in second-generation merozoites.[1194] These findings suggest that ART treatment can directly reduce the parasite burden of chickens. *E. tenella* infection promotes the expression of antiapoptotic protein Bcl-2 while it inhibiting the expression of proapoptotic proteins Bax and cleaved caspase-3 in infected ceca at 60 hpi.[816] However, the expression trends of Bcl-2, Bax, and caspase-3 are reversed at 120 and 192 HPI, where ART treatment significantly abrogates Bcl-2 expression and increases the levels of Bax and cleaved caspase-3.[816] These results indicate that *E. tenella* can prevent apoptosis of infected cells for parasites' reproduction and survival during the early stage of infection, but ART treatment can induce apoptosis in both infected host cells and second-generation merozoites. Derivatives from ART and its parent plant *A. annua* leaves may be a potential drug effective against poultry coccidiosis

16.7.3 Drug Resistance

Drug resistance is widespread and recognized as a major cause of failure of drugs to control coccidiosis. In a large-scale study over a 5-year period, the relationship between the prevalence of coccidiosis and maduramicin resistance was studied with isolates from 525 farms across nine

geographic regions including Beijing, Sichuan, Zhejiang, Shandong, Guangdong, Fujian and Liaoning Provinces, and Inner Mongolia and Xinjiang Uyghur Autonomous Regions.[1879] Oocysts from 6.6% to 16% farms have developed high resistance. Higher resistance rates were reported in another study; 90% (18/20) of *Eimeria* field isolates from farms in Shandong, Hebei, Jiangsu, Henan, and Guangdong provinces were resistant to maduramicin.[643]

An isolate from Quzhou of the Zhejiang province developed high resistance to multiple agents, sulfachloropyrazine, toltrazuril, sulfamonomethoxine/trimethoprim, amprolium, and sulfaquinoxaline/sulfadimethoxine, in addition to light resistance to diclazuril. An isolate from Huzhou of Zhejiang Province developed light resistance to sulfaquinoxaline/ sulfadimethoxine and halofuginone, moderate resistance to nicarbazin, and severe resistance to sulfachloropyrazine, toltrazuril, diclazuril, sulfamonomethoxine/trimethoprim, and amprolium.[121]

Tests on one isolate of *E. tenella* from each of northern, eastern, southern, and middle regions of Hubei province showed that all the isolates had developed resistance to maduramicin (ACI below 160), those from northern, southern, and middle Hubei was also resistant to decoquinate, and the isolate from eastern Hubei is still susceptible to decoquinate and diclazuril.[1664]

Molecular screening, with random mRNA differential display to analyze differential expression of genes from merozoites of maduramicin sensitive and resistant strains of *E. tenella* revealed that two genes, including microneme 5 and soluble *N*-ethylmaleimide sensitive attachment protein receptor (SNARE)–like gene are upregulated in resistant strains, while 3 genes, including *E. tenella* surface antigen-17, 16 genes and one hypothetical gene are specifically expressed in sensitive strains.[121] Among the two specifically expressed in resistant strains, the SNARE-like gene was further confirmed expressing specifically in one resistant field strain and not in three sensitive field ones.[40] Linkage group selection combined with whole genome sequencing will be a high-throughput approach to identify primary target genes of anticoccidial drugs, leading to deciphering mechanisms of drug resistance.

16.7.4 Natural Compounds

Natural compounds such as plant extracts, fungal extracts, and probiotics are used or evaluated as diet supplements to alleviate the negative effects of coccidiosis (Table 16.7). Anticoccidial outcomes are often indirectly assessed by survival rates, improved growth performance, feed conversion, intestinal lesions, and bloody diarrhea in the case of *E. tenella* and *E. necatrix* challenge, rather than oocyst outputs. Trials showed that *Brucea javanica* extract, added at 2.5–10 g/kg feed, significantly reduced bloody diarrhea and lesion scores[940]; while *Dichroa febrifuga* extract, 20 mg/kg feed, significantly increased

Table 16.7 Efficacy of Single-Herb Prescription for Prevention and Treatment of Chicken Coccidiosis

| Herb | Species (Infection Dose) | Number of Chickens (Age/day) | Dose (Administration) | Time Period(day) | Criteria[a] | | | | | Reference |
					% Survival Rate ([a])	Lesion Index	Oocyst Index	Relative Weight Gain Rate	ACI	
Dichroa febrifuga vs (Toltrazuril)	Et(7 × 10⁴)	10(14)	15 mL/L (drinking)	7	90 (90)	34 (38.5)	10 (10)	95.8 (83.3)	141.8 (124.8)	Bi et al.[121]
Uncaria tomentosa vs (Diclazuril)	Et(5 × 10⁴)	10(14)	1.5mL/chicken (drinking)	10	100 (100)	2 (4)	5 (5)	95.5 (94.4)	188.5 (185.4)	Bi et al.[121]
Ophiocordyceps sinensis vs (Robenidine)	Et(6 × 10⁴)	12(28)	1 mg/chicken (drinking)	7	91.6 (100)	2.1 (1.5)	0 (1)	84.4 (78.6)	174.0 (176.2)	Bi et al.[121]

Abbreviation: Et, *Eimeria tenella*.
[a] Numbers within parentheses are those from control drug groups, on the first row, from the toltrazuril control group; on the second row, from the diclazuril control group; on the third row, from the robenidine group.

body weight gains and reduced bloody diarrhea, lesion score, and oocyst excretion.[1876] Proposed mechanisms include immune stimulation, anti-inflammatory, antioxidant activities, and beneficial effects on the gastrointestinal microbiota.

16.8 CONTROL

16.8.1 Dietary Modulation

Dietary modulation of poultry coccidiosis using "nutritious additives" is promising as various natural nutrients have functions alleviating deleterious effects of coccidiosis. Methionine supplement at 0.56% and 0.68% in the narasin-medicated diet increased chicken resistance to *E. tenella* infection, as indicated by improved immune functions and decreased cecal lesions, and fecal oocyst counts.[935] Betaine supplement in a maduramycin-medicated diet had a 19% increase in relative body weight gain.[1669] Coated sodium butyrate supplement in the diet prevents cecal microflora imbalance caused by *E. tenella* infection.[1915] *E. tenella*–infected chickens exhibited an increase in Firmicutes (mainly Ruminococcaceae, Lachnospiraceae, and vadin BB60) and Proteobacteria (mainly Enterobacteriaceae) and a decrease in Bacteroidetes (predominantly Bacteroidaceae). This imbalance of microflora was prevented by adding coated sodium butyrate to the diet of chickens.[1915] Diets supplemented with chicken oils (saturated fatty acids) aggravated mortality and decreased the levels of cecal *E. tenella* antigen-specific secretory IgA or serum IgG in chickens infected with *E. tenella*, whereas diets supplemented with fish or corn oil (unsaturated fatty acids) resulted in higher body weight gain, enhanced secretory IgA in the cecum, and lower levels of plasma carotenoids and elevated serum interleukin-6 levels in chickens infected with *E. tenella*.[1851] Dietary zinc amino acid complex prevented the reduction of

serum carotenoids and pigmentation of Three-Yellow chickens infected with *E. tenella*, but not after infection with *E. acervulina*.[1901] Plant-origin carotenoids like curcumin and lutein reduced lipid and protein oxidation and improved color stability and quality of breast meat in infected chickens.[1385] These natural products improved the chicken's resistance to coccidiosis probably through combined effects, like balanced metabolism, balanced gut microbiota, and immune modulation.

16.9 TOOLS AND REAGENTS

16.9.1 Enzyme-Linked Immunosorbent Spot Assay

The enzyme-linked immunosorbent spot (ELISPOT) assay is a sensitive and easy-to-use tool quantifying the number of cytokine-secreting T cells and offers a viable alternative for the quantitative measurement of T-cell functions in *Eimeria*-infected chickens.[1859] The assay is based on the principle of the sandwich ELISA assay and detects antigen-induced secretion of cytokines.. In *Eimeria*-immunized birds, as few as 50–100 *Eimeria* antigen-specific IFN-γ secreting cells can be detected among PBMCs using ELISpot.[1671,1674,1859] In addition, fewer than 10 IFN-γ secreting cells specific to a single antigen expressed by recombinant *Eimeria* can also be efficiently detected using this method.[1671] This sensitive and easy-to-use tool can be applied broadly to antigen discovery and vaccine evaluation of *Eimeria* and other pathogens.

16.9.2 Antibody Phage Display Technique

Phage display has become a powerful technique to produce recombinant antibodies. This technique involves the creation of combinatorial libraries of variable light and heavy chains of antibodies and their expression on the phage surface. Through the established "phage-antibody technique," a scFv sequence of 741 bp was obtained by library construction and selection of phage display antibodies derived from *E. acervulina* merozoite-immunized mice. The encoded scFv antibody specifically stains the surface protein(s) of *E. acervulina* merozoites.[1904] This high-throughput technique can help set up antibody repertoires of *Eimeria* parasites facilitating basic research and discovery of drug and vaccine targets.

16.9.3 Miscellaneous Tools and Reagents

Many tools have been developed for studying *Eimeria*, for example, the rapid and simple method for purifying merozoites through enzyme/chemical digestion and filtration[1830]; a platform for analyzing drug resistance[906,1669]; single-oocyst and -sporocyst isolation for propagating pure species or strains[39,1026,1849]; optimized DNA extraction by incubating oocysts in sodium hypochlorite followed by treatment with a saturated salt solution[1668]; a sequencing-based tool for analysis of immune repertoires[1407]; molecular analysis of a single oocyst of *Eimeria* by whole genome amplification (WGA)–based nested PCR[1781]; and transgenic *Eimeria* as a platform to test antigen immunogenicity.[754,1671] Some reagents developed for *Eimeria* research are also available including monoclonal antibodies that recognize *E. tenella* microneme proteins 1 and 2[1066] through the conventional hybridoma technique and a constitutively Cas9 expression transgenic *E. tenella* line (Hu and Suo, unpublished data). These tools and reagents have had a significant impact on the advancement of *Eimeria* research by supplying basic tools or reagents and by facilitating genetic manipulation of coccidia.

ACKNOWLEDGMENTS

I would like to thank Jin Zhu for editorial help; Xianyong Liu, Xinming Tang, Si Wang, Chunhui Duan, Jie Liu, Ying Yu, and Xia Cheng for preparing the references; Feifei Bi, Hui Dong, Chao Li, Xinming Tang, and Sixin Zhang for preparing the tables; Jian An, Jianping Cai, Xiaozhen Cui, Aifang Du, Chenzhong Fei, Hongyu Han, Dandan Hu, Bing Huang, Jingui Li, Guoqing Li, Peiguo Li, Xiangrui Li, Guohua Liu, Lili Liu, Yunyu Liu, Jianhua Qin, Tuanyuan Shi, Xiaokai Song, Mingfei Sun, Xinming Tang, Jianping Tao, Pu Wang, Feiqun Xue, Guangwen Yin, Keyu Zhang, Xichen Zhang, Junlong Zhao, Xiaomin Zhao, Mingxue Zheng, Bianhua Zhou, Yanqin Zhou, and Xingquan Zhu for supplying their selective publications and discussing their work with me. There are about 4000 publications on poultry coccidia and coccidiosis by Chinese scientists, but I cannot cite all of them. I would like to express my apology for not citing their work or only indirectly citing their work.

I am indebted to Profs. Fiona Tomley and Damer Brake for advice.

REFERENCES

39, 40, 121, 162, 232, 255, 257, 258, 284, 308, 310, 373, 374, 380–382, 406–409, 523, 579, 602, 641–643, 668–670, 673, 724, 725, 745, 749, 751, 753, 754, 814, 816, 906, 935, 940, 985, 987, 989–991, 993, 994, 996, 997, 1023, 1026–1028, 1055, 1056, 1059, 1061, 1063, 1065–1067, 1069–1071, 1101, 1106, 1107, 1194, 1370, 1371, 1373–1377, 1385, 1407, 1537, 1550, 1556, 1597, 1635–1637, 1643, 1645–1650, 1664, 1668–1674, 1712, 1771, 1778–1784, 1824, 1830, 1835, 1836, 1842, 1844–1849, 1851, 1858–1860, 1865, 1876, 1878, 1879, 1881–1883, 1888, 1889, 1891–1897, 1901–1913, 1915–1920, 1922

CHAPTER 17

Coccidiosis in Turkeys (*Meleagris gallopavo*)

T. Rathinam and U. Gadde

CONTENTS

17.1 INTRODUCTION AND HISTORY

Coccidiosis in turkeys is a disease of great economic importance to the poultry industry and ranks among the top 10 disease concerns for turkey veterinarians. Coccidiosis in turkeys is caused only by species of the genus *Eimeria*. During the late 1800s and the early decades of the twentieth century, turkey coccidiosis was inadvertently confused with histomoniasis.[283,1584] In 1923, it was proposed that coccidia in turkeys may be different from the species inflicting chickens.[833] Ernest Tyzzer of Harvard University, who also pioneered research on avian coccidiosis, later described the first two species of turkey *Eimeria*, *E. meleagridis* and *E. meleagrimitis*, along with several other newly described species infecting other avian hosts.[1717] As part of an extensive study, Tyzzer and Jones performed various cross-host experiments and showed that *E. dispersa*, a species originally isolated from Bobwhite quail, can develop in turkeys. Thus, *E. dispersa* was the third "turkey" *Eimeria* to be described.[1717] In

1950, Philip Hawkins at Michigan State University[687] published his doctoral thesis on turkey coccidiosis, extensively studying the two species described by Tyzzer[1717] and identifying a new species *E. gallopavonis*. An abbreviated version of this work was later published after his death in 1951.[688] Moore and Brown from Cornell University, New York, received several samples from the state of New York, and upon examination they found some samples that interested them "to investigate the possibility that an undescribed species might be present."[1201] They also inherited the parasite collection of Philip Hawkins. They described three species: *E. adenoeides*,[1201] *E. innocua*,[1202] and *E. subrotunda*.[1203]

17.2 MORPHOLOGY, ENDOGENOUS DEVELOPMENT, AND PATHOGENICITY

There are seven described species of *Eimeria* in turkeys (Table 17.1). Sporulation is necessary to morphologically

Table.17.1 Prepatent Period, Sporulation Time, and Oocyst Dimensions and Characteristics of Seven *Eimeria* Infecting Turkeys

Species	Prepatent Period (HPI)	Minimum Sporulation Time (hours)	Sporulated Oocyst				Sporocyst Size (L × W, mean, μm)
			Shape	Size (L × W, Mean, μm)	Shape Index (L/W)	Refractile Body	
E. adenoeides Moore and Brown, 1951	114	24	Oval	18.7 × 14.3	1.3	One	9.7 × 5.9
E. dispersa Tyzzer, 1929	114–120	48	Subspherical	26 × 21	1.2	None	14 × 8
E. gallopavonis Hawkins, 1952	144	48	Ellipsoid	27 × 19	1.4	Multiple (up to 4)	12 × 8
E. innocua Moore and Brown, 1952	114	48	Subspherical	22.4 × 20.8	1.07	None	No data
E. meleagridis Tyzzer, 1927	120	24	Ellipsoid	26.3 × 16.9	1.55	One	11 × 6
E. meleagrimitis Tyzzer, 1929	114–120	48	Subspherical	19 × 16	1.2	One	10.9 × 6.1
E. subrotunda Moore, Brown, and Carter, 1954	95	48	Subspherical	21.8 × 19.8	1.0–1.3	None	No data

Abbreviations: HPI, hours postinoculation; L × W, length and width ratio.

identify turkey *Eimeria*. The species of *Eimeria* causing turkey coccidiosis of economic importance to the industry are *E. adenoeides*, *E. gallopavonis*, *E. meleagrimitis*, and to a lesser extent *E. meleagridis*, *E. dispersa*, and *E. innocua*. *Eimeria subrotunda* is considered nonpathogenic.

The life cycle and endogenous development of *Eimeria* in the turkeys is typical of the genus' development in the chicken and is described in Chapters 1 and 15. In brief, sporulated oocysts, the infective stage, are ingested by the turkeys. The sporocysts are exposed in the crop and enter the intestines where excystation of sporozoites occur. The sporozoites invade the enterocytes to initiate a series of schizogonies followed by gametogony and production of oocysts.

17.2.1 *Eimeria adenoeides*

The species was originally described by Moore and Brown[1201] from turkey fecal samples collected in the state of New York. The life cycle has been described by Clarkson[279] and El-Sherry et al.[480] Oocyst characteristics and sporulation time are presented in Table 17.1 and Figure 17.1.

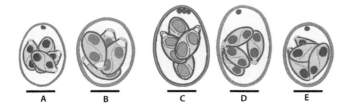

Figure 17.1 Sporulated oocysts of (A) *Eimeria adenoeides* (18.7 × 14.3 μm), (B) *E. dispersa* (26 × 21 μm), (C) *E. gallopavonis* (27 × 19 μm), (D) *E. meleagridis* (26.3 × 16.9 μm), and (E) *E. meleagrimitis* (19 × 16 μm). Scale bar 10 μm. (Redrawn from El-Sherry, S. et al. 2015. *Poult. Sci.* 94, 262–272.)

The parasite localizes in the lower ileum, ceca, and rectum. First-generation schizonts (12.9 × 10.3 μm, and contain 45–50 merozoites) can be seen as early as 32 hours postinoculation (HPI) in the lower ileum and cecal neck. The second-generation schizonts, localized in the cecal pouches, cecal neck, lower ileum, and rectum, are seen at 48 HPI, measuring 9.1 × 7.3 μm, and contains 12–16 merozoites. A third asexual generation occurs as early as 64 HPI in the same region as that of the second generation with schizonts measuring 8 × 7 μm containing six to eight merozoites. The third-generation schizonts are also seen along the sides and tips of the villi as well as in the deep glands. Gametogony occurs 104 HPI in the cecal neck, cecum, and rectum and to a lesser extent in the ileum. Macrogamonts measure 13 × 11 μm, and microgamonts measure 11.7 × 10 μm. The location of endogenous development in the intestine is diagrammatically represented in Figure 17.2, and the endogenous developmental stages are summarized in Table 17.2. The prepatent period is 114 HPI.

E. adenoeides is pathogenic to turkeys. The lesions occur primarily in the cecum and include necrosis, edema, epithelial sloughing, and formation of characteristic white caseous cores (containing cell debris, gamonts, and oocysts). Clarkson[279] reported that the pathological changes are inconsistent and may vary from individual birds that show normal ceca to those with ceca containing yellow casts with degrees of variation in between, even though they had received the same number of oocysts.[279]

17.2.2 *Eimeria dispersa*

This species was originally isolated from Bobwhite quail[1717] and was shown to produce an infection in turkeys, an unusual example in *Eimeria* species of a lack of host specificity. Oocysts obtained from quails and from

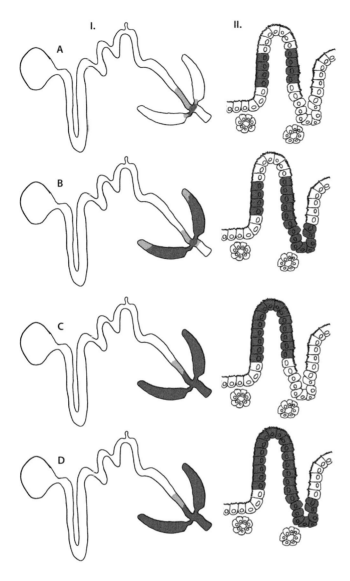

Figure 17.2 Site of development of various reproductive stages of *Eimeria adenoeides* in the intestinal tract of an infected turkey (I) and localization of developmental stages in the villi (II). (A) First asexual generation, (B) second asexual generation, (C) third asexual generation, and (D) sexual generation. In column I, the lighter intensity in shading refers to fewer parasite stages seen in that region. In column II, the general regions of the cells are grouped into tips of villi, sides of villi, base of villi, crypts, and gland cells.

pheasants have been reported to be of different size. The location where the organism parasitizes among various hosts is also not the same. These reasons and the differing immunological response to this parasite led Pellérdy[1343] to call *E. dispersa* a *species incerta*. The descriptions and development provided later are based on *E. dispersa* isolated from turkeys. The life cycle and pathogenicity of this species has been described by Hawkins,[688] Doran,[391] Long and Millard,[1083] Vrba and Pakandl,[1756] and El-Sherry et al.[482]

Oocysts' characteristics and sporulation time are provided in Table 17.1 and Figure 17.1.

Its asexual and sexual stages develop in the duodenum, jejunum, and ileum. The first-generation schizonts (21.7 × 16.8 μm with 30–35 merozoites) are first seen at 32 HPI in the duodenum and upper jejunum. Second-generation schizonts are seen at 40 HPI in the same region. Mature second-generation schizonts measure 7.5 × 6.3 μm and contain six to eight merozoites. Third-generation schizonts are present along the villi tips in the duodenum, jejunum, and after Meckel's diverticulum. They are seen at 80 HPI, measure 7.3 × 6.8 μm, and contain 14–16 merozoites. Fourth asexual generation occurs at 88 HPI at the tips of villi in the duodenum, jejunum, and ileum. Mature fourth-generation schizonts measure 9 × 8.5 μm and contain 14–18 merozoites. Gamonts are detected as early as 104 HPI in the same region as the fourth asexual generation, and in addition, the cecal neck. Mature microgamonts measure 13.3 × 10.5 μm, and the macrogamonts measure 14.7 × 12.6 μm. The location of endogenous development in the intestine is diagrammatically represented in Figure 17.3, and the endogenous developmental stages are summarized in Table 17.2. The prepatent period is 114–120 HPI.

E. dispersa is mildly pathogenic. Pathological changes include dilatation and pallor of duodenum and jejunum. Upon opening the intestine, a whitish-green mucoid fluid can be seen. Congestion, edema, and scattered petechiae may also be observed in this region.

17.2.3 *Eimeria gallopavonis*

The original description of the species was provided by Hawkins.[688] The endogenous development of *E. gallopavonis* and its pathogenicity has also been described by Farr et al.,[516] Farr,[514] Vrba and Pakandl,[1756] and El-Sherry et al.[483] Oocysts' characteristics and sporulation time can be found in Table 17.1 and Figure 17.1.

E. gallopavonis primarily infects the ileum, cecal neck, and rectum, and to some extent the jejunum. First-generation schizonts primarily develop in the neck of the ceca and rectum along the villi. Schizonts can be seen as early as 48 HPI, measure 21 × 15 μm, and contain 20–400 merozoites. The second asexual generation occurs along the villi and villi tips in the ileum, cecum, and rectum, and the second-generation schizonts measure 7 × 5 μm and usually contain six to eight merozoites. The third generation of schizonts can be observed at 88 HPI and measure 10 × 8 μm with 6–16 merozoites. They are observed in the jejunum, ileum, cecal neck, and rectum developing in the deep crypts and glands along villi and tips. Gamonts are numerous at 133 HPI along villi, deep glands, and tips in the jejunum, ileum, cecal neck, and cecum. Macrogamonts measure 15.3 × 12 μm, and microgamonts measure 17 × 12 μm. The location of endogenous development in the intestine is diagrammatically represented in Figure 17.4,

Table 17.2 Endogenous Stages, Site of Infection, and Prepatent Period of *Eimeria* spp. in Turkeys

Eimeria spp.	Location	Prepatent Period (hours)	Number of Asexual Generations	Schizont Size, μm (Number of Merozoites)	Gamonts Size, μm
E. adenoeides	Lower ileum, ceca, rectum	114	3	1G: 12.9 × 10.3 (45–50) 2G: 9.1 × 7.3 (12–16) 3G: 8 × 7 (6–8)	Macro: 13 × 11 Micro: 11.7 × 10
E. dispersa	Duodenum, jejunum, ileum	114–120	4	1G: 21.7 × 16.8 (30–35) 2G: 7.5 × 6.3 (6–8) 3G: 7.3 × 6.8 (14–16) 4G: 9 × 8.5 (14–18)	Macro: 14.7 × 12.6 Micro: 13.3 × 10.5
E. gallopavonis	Ileum, cecum, rectum	144	3	1G: 21 × 15 (20–400) 2G: 7 × 5 (6–8) 3G: 10 × 8 (6–16)	Macro: 15.3 × 12 Micro: 17 × 12
E. innocua	Anterior small intestine	114	3	Small (10–18)	Macro: 13 × 11 Micro: 11.7 × 10
E. meleagridis	Ceca, also midjejunum	108–120	4	1G: NS (50–100) 2G: NS (10–14) 3G: 8 × 7 (6–12) 4G: Small (NS)	Macro: 15 × 10 Micro: 15 × 11
E. meleagrimitis	All regions of the intestine	114–120	3	1G: 13 × 10 (45–60) 2G: 5 × 5 (12) 3G: 6 × 6 (10–12)	Macro: 15 × 12 Micro: 14 × 11
E. subrotunda	Anterior small intestine	95	NS	NS	NS

Source: Data are compiled and adapted from El-Sherry, S. et al. 2014. *Parasitol. Res.* 113, 3993–4004; El-Sherry, S. et al. 2014. *Parasitol. Res.* 113, 1135–1146; Vrba, V., Pakandl, M. 2014. *Int. J. Parasitol.* 44, 985–1000; El-Sherry, S. et al. 2017. *Parasitol. Res.* 116, 2661–2670; El-Sherry, S. et al. 2019. *Parasitol. Res.* 118, 583–598.
Abbreviations: 1G, first-generation schizonts; 2G, second-generation schizonts; 3G, third-generation schizonts; 4G, fourth-generation schizonts; macro, macrogamont; micro, macrogamont; NS, not stated.

and the endogenous developmental stages are summarized in Table 17.2. The prepatent period is 144 HPI.

E. gallopavonis is a pathogenic species capable of causing severe mortality. Farr et al.[516] have observed up to 100% mortality in heavy experimental infections. Birds infected with *E. gallopavonis* usually appear normal until day 5 postinfection when they become anorexic, lose weight, show severe diarrhea, and possibly succumb to the disease. The ileocecal junction and rectum show sloughing of epithelia and caseation necrosis. The affected regions (ileum, rectum) are filled with soft cheesy material that, if found in the cecal pouch, is usually present up to the midceca.

17.2.4 *Eimeria innocua*

The species was first described by Moore and Brown[1202] and was recently studied by Vrba and Pakandl.[1756] Oocysts' characteristics and sporulation time are provided in Table 17.1.

The primary location of development is the anterior small intestine up to Meckel's diverticulum. The schizonts develop exclusively in the tips of villi. Possibly three asexual generations, each consisting of small schizonts with 10–18 merozoites, are followed by the sexual generation that occurs at 96 HPI. Gamonts are seen in the ileum in addition to duodenum and jejunum. The location of endogenous development in the intestine is diagrammatically represented in Figure 17.5, and the endogenous developmental

stages are summarized in Table 17.2. The prepatent period is 114 HPI.

E. innocua was originally described as nonpathogenic. Vrba and Pakandl[1756] have observed white to yellow mucus in the duodenum with suppression of body weights when given a high dose. The authors conclude that the pathogenicity could be like that of *E. dispersa*.

17.2.5 *Eimeria meleagridis*

The species was first mentioned by Tyzzer[1716] and later fully described.[1717] The endogenous development in the turkey and its pathogenicity have also been reported by Hawkins,[688] Clarkson,[280] Matsler and Chapman,[1146] Vrba and Pakandl,[1756] and El-Sherry et al.[483] Vrba and Pakandl[1756] have proposed that there may be up to four distinct strains of *E. meleagridis*. Oocysts' characteristics and sporulation time are provided in Table 17.1 and Figure 17.1.

E. meleagridis is one species of turkey *Eimeria* where descriptions of endogenous development vary considerably among different researchers. *E. meleagridis* primarily develops in the ceca. The first asexual generation is detected at 48 HPI and contains 50–100 merozoites. The schizonts are present along the villi and tips in the midjejunum and ileum. Second-generation schizonts are small and contain 10–14 merozoites and are observed in the cecal pouch as early as 64 HPI. Third-generation schizonts develop in the cecal pouch (under the brush border but not in the deep glands) and measure 8 × 7 μm and contain 6–12 merozoites.

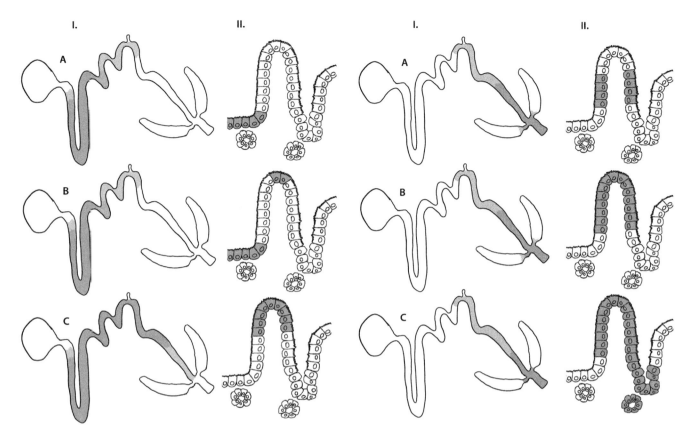

Figure 17.3 Site of development of various reproductive stages of *Emeria dispersa* in the intestinal tract of an infected turkey (I) and localization of developmental stages in the villi (II). (A) First asexual generation, (B) second asexual generation, and (C) third and fourth asexual generation and sexual generation. In column I, the lighter intensity in shading refers to fewer parasite stages seen in that region. In column II, the general regions of the cells are grouped into tips of villi, sides of villi, base of villi, crypts, and gland cells.

Figure 17.4 Site of development of various reproductive stages of *Eimeria gallopavonis* in the intestinal tract of an infected turkey (I) and localization of developmental stages in the villi (II). (A) First asexual generation, (B) second asexual generation, and (C) third asexual generation and sexual generation. In column I, the lighter intensity in shading refers to fewer parasite stages seen in that region. In column II, the general regions of the cells are grouped into tips of villi, sides of villi, base of villi, crypts, and gland cells.

A fourth generation consisting of small schizonts is detected at 108 HPI in the ceca. The gamonts are found in ileum, cecal neck, cecal pouch, and rectum, mostly in the villi, and are observed as early as 112 HPI. The macrogamonts measure 15×10 μm, and microgamonts measure 15×11 μm. The location of endogenous development in the intestine is diagrammatically represented in Figure 17.6, and the endogenous developmental stages are summarized in Table 17.2. The prepatent period is 120 HPI but may be as early as 108–112 HPI.

There are uncertainties concerning its pathogenicity. Several early studies of this species have reported that it is nonpathogenic.[280,688,1201] More recent investigations have shown that the species is mildly pathogenic. The pathogenicity is comparable to *E. acervulina* or *E. praecox* or *E. mitis* where high doses can cause weight suppression under experimental conditions.[1146] The pathology is confined to the ceca, which are swollen with thickened walls. Sometimes rows of petechial hemorrhage on the cecal

mucosa may be seen. In heavy infections, creamy-colored caseous material with cheesy consistency may also be found.

17.2.6 *Eimeria meleagrimitis*

This species was first described by Tyzzer,[1717] where he mentions that the organism "agrees very closely in morphology as well as in its distribution in the intestinal epithelium with *Eimeria mitis*" (p. 321). Several studies on endogenous development and pathogenicity have been conducted presumably due to its abundance and high pathogenicity.[281,484,688,1457,1756] Oocysts' characteristics and sporulation time are given in Table 17.1 and Figure 17.1.

E. meleagrimitis development occurs throughout the intestinal tract. The first-generation schizonts (13×10 μm, containing 45–60 merozoites) are observed at 40 HPI in the crypt cells below the cell nucleus, in the jejunum and duodenum. The second-generation schizonts (5 μm in diameter

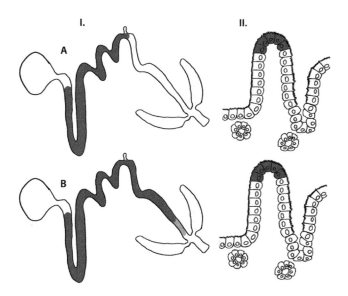

Figure 17.5 Site of development of various reproductive stages of *Eimeria innocua* in the intestinal tract of an infected turkey (I) and localization of developmental stages in the villi (II). (A) Asexual generations and (B) sexual generation. In column I, the lighter intensity in shading refers to fewer parasite stages seen in that region. In column II, the general regions of the cells are grouped into tips of villi, sides of villi, base of villi, crypts, and gland cells.

and contain 12 merozoites each) are seen at 56 HPI in the same intestinal location in the deep glands. The third asexual generation is observed around 96 HPI in the jejunum and all other parts of the intestinal tract except the ceca, along the sides and tips of the villi. The third-generation schizonts measure 6 μm in diameter and contain 10–12 merozoites. Gametogony occurs at 112 HPI in the same region and location as the third asexual generation. The macrogamonts are 15 × 12 μm, and microgamonts are 14 × 11 μm. There may be as many as six generations, starting with the first generation at 24 HPI and sixth generation developing simultaneously with gametogony at 96 HPI.[1085] The endogenous development is diagrammatically represented in Figure 17.7, and the endogenous developmental stages are summarized in Table 17.2. The prepatent period is 114–120 HPI.

E. meleagrimitis is a pathogenic species of turkey *Eimeria* causing catarrhal enteritis and mortality in severe cases. The characteristic pathogenic manifestation of this species is the excessive fluid seen in the duodenum and jejunum, which can be greenish orange with mucoid casts. This species can cause severe weight loss, and a dose-dependent severity has also been observed by El-Sherry et al.[484] They reported an inverse dose-dependent severity in the expected region of gross lesions when given an extremely high dose, which resulted in decreased pathology in duodenum and jejunum, but pathological changes were visible in the lower ileum and cecal neck.[484] This is consistent with observations by Ruff et al.[1457] who showed that the lower regions

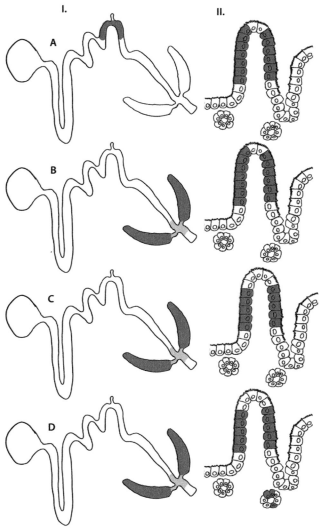

Figure 17.6 Site of development of various reproductive stages of *Eimeria meleagridis* in the intestinal tract of an infected turkey (I) and localization of developmental stages in the villi (II). (A) First asexual generation, (B) second asexual generation, (C) third asexual generation, and (D) fourth asexual and sexual generation. In column I, the lighter intensity in shading refers to fewer parasite stages seen in that region. In column II, the general regions of the cells are grouped into tips of villi, sides of villi, base of villi, crypts, and gland cells.

of intestine became infected more heavily and rapidly with increasing doses of inoculum size.

17.2.7 *Eimeria subrotunda*

This species was described by Moore et al.[1203] The description is limited in the original report, and the species has hardly been studied and has not been seen in the field except for a few brief reports without supporting evidence.[467] Oocysts' characteristics and sporulation time are presented in Table 17.1.

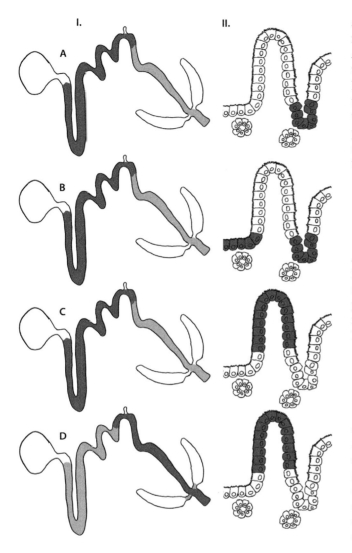

Figure 17.7 Site of development of various reproductive stages of *Eimeria meleagrimitis* in the intestinal tract of an infected turkey (I) and localization of developmental stages in the villi (II). (A) First asexual generation, (B) second asexual generation, (C) third asexual generation, and (D) sexual generation. In column I, the lighter intensity in shading refers to fewer parasite stages seen in that region. In column II, the general regions of the cells are grouped into tips of villi, sides of villi, base of villi, crypts, and gland cells.

E. subrotunda is said to develop in the upper portion of the intestine but is not seen posterior to yolk stalk or in the ceca. Asexual stages are present in the tips of villi, and some are seen in the lower two-thirds of the villi but not in crypts and deep glands. The prepatent period is 95 HPI.

Its pathogenicity is unknown.

17.3 HOST SPECIFICITY

Eimeria species are known to exhibit a marked degree of host specificity: for example, species that infect the chicken are not infective to turkeys and vice versa. Several experiments were conducted to test for the cross-infectivity of *Eimeria* species in both these hosts. Tyzzer[1717] was unable to infect chickens with *E. meleagridis* from turkeys and turkeys with *E. acervulina* from chickens. Patterson[1329] failed to infect turkeys with *E. tenella* from chickens. Several unsuccessful attempts have been made to infect chickens, pheasants, guinea-fowls, and Japanese quail with *E. adenoeides* of turkeys.[1201] *E. dispersa* and *E. innocua* isolated from turkeys develop in more than one host.[1717,1756]

17.4 PREVALENCE AND DISTRIBUTION

All species of turkey *Eimeria* described thus far, except *E. innocua* and *E. subrotunda,* have been widely reported from the field. The most common species are *E. meleagrimitis, E. adenoeides,* and *E. gallopavonis.* Prevalence studies performed in the United States and Canada show the cosmopolitan occurrence of the various species.[467,468,765,1136,1393] No such studies have been performed in Europe.

17.5 CLINICAL SIGNS

Coccidiosis in turkeys is usually seen in young poults, often 8 weeks of age or younger. However, older turkeys may also be susceptible.[62,66,185] In general, infected birds begin to consume less feed usually within 2–3 days of infection. This is followed by exhibition of ruffled feathers, huddling, closed eyes, droopy wings, and cheeping. Diarrhea with mucus, an excessive amount of urates, and in some cases, blood may be observed. In severe cases, mortality may occur around 5–7 days postinfection.

17.6 MOLECULAR TAXONOMY

Recent years have seen the application of molecular biology techniques, including development of polymerase chain reaction (PCR) assays, for the detection of turkey *Eimeria.*[290] To clarify conflicting reports, and to ascertain evolutionary relationships of turkey *Eimeria* with those of other gallinaceous birds, researchers undertook to reevaluate and redescribe known species.[480,482–484,1756] The taxonomic classification of turkey *Eimeria* and the relationship to other avian *Eimeria* have been described in recent years.[481,654,1189,1756] Based on sequence analysis of 18s rDNA, ITS rDNA, and mtCOI genes, phylogenetic trees have been generated, and the derived sequences have also been used to distinguish the different species genetically. It was reported that *E. necatrix* of chicken was more closely related to turkey *Eimeria* than other chicken *Eimeria.*[1189] The species of *Eimeria* originally isolated from turkeys were more closely related to each other than to *E. dispersa.*[481,1756] Vrba and Pakandl[1756] propose that two of the cecal species, *E. adenoeides* and *E. meleagri-dis*, are possibly synonymous. Other studies, however, have shown genetic and morphological differences between the two species.[481,483] The wide range of size and shape indexes seen in earlier reports have unfortunately not been resolved, especially for the cecal species of turkey *Eimeria*.

17.7 IMMUNITY

Eimeria species are known to induce a state of long-lasting protective immunity in the host in response to repeated infections, although this may vary depending on the particular species involved (see Chapter 3). As seen with chicken *Eimeria*, immunity to turkey *Eimeria* is species-specific, and poults immunized with one species are not protected from challenge with another species.[229,765] Turkey poults inoculated with mixed cultures of *E. adenoeides* and *E. meleagrimitis* either as a large single inoculum or multiple small inoculums over a period developed immunity and showed protection against a heavy challenge.[47] A single infection with 12.5×10^3 oocysts of *E. adenoeides* to 20-day-old turkey poults was shown to confer protection against challenge.[570] Very little information exists in the relative immunogenicity of individual turkey species and the host immune responses that occur during immunity. Gadde et al.[569,570,571] reported the immune responses occurring in turkey poults following infection with *E. adenoeides*. The infection resulted in an increase in subsets of T lymphocytes and alterations in cytokine profiles in the ceca of turkey poults.

17.8 DIAGNOSIS

As with coccidiosis in chickens, fecal examination, lesions, and molecular techniques are helpful in the diagnosis of coccidiosis in turkeys. While diagnosis of coccidiosis in chickens is based on the characteristic pathological signs presented by each species and the presence of visible lesions in the intestinal tract, in the case of turkey *Eimeria*, this is difficult as such readily identifiable lesions may not be present. Demonstration of developmental stages (schizonts, gamonts) and large numbers of immature oocysts in intestinal scrapings are aids to diagnosis. Differential diagnosis between various species depends on the morphological characteristics of the oocysts, pathogenicity, and location of lesions and developmental stages within the host. Several other criteria, such as the prepatent period, gross and microscopic lesions, and the absence of cross-protection between species should also be considered.

17.9 PREVENTION AND CONTROL

The prevention and control of coccidiosis in turkeys are accomplished principally using anticoccidial drugs but sometimes by vaccination. Anticoccidials against avian *Eimeria* are described in Chapter 6.

Ionophores are the most extensively used drugs for in-feed prophylaxis, and the approved ionophores for use in turkey production in the United States include monensin and lasalocid. Chemical anticoccidials approved for use in the United States for turkeys include amprolium, diclazuril, halofuginone, zoalene, and a combination of sulfadimethoxine and ormetoprim.

Live anticoccidial vaccines containing small numbers of sporulated oocysts of multiple *Eimeria* species have also been employed for the control of turkey coccidiosis (see Chapter 4). The first anticoccidial vaccine for turkeys, Coccivac-T was introduced in 1984[1805] and contained oocysts from wild-type strains of *E. meleagrimitis*, *E. adenoeides*, *E. dispersa*, and *E. gallopavonis*. Another vaccine, Immucox-T was introduced later and contains wild-type strains of *E. meleagrimitis* and *E. adenoeides*. Commercial vaccines containing attenuated strains of *Eimeria* are not available for turkey. In the chicken, anticoccidial vaccines have been shown to restore sensitivity to anticoccidial drugs through replacement of drug-resistant strains with drug-sensitive vaccine strains. This may also occur in the turkey. Sustainable control of coccidiosis in turkey production can be achieved by the efficient use of available drugs and vaccines. The use of shuttle and rotation programs helps reduce the development of resistance to commonly used anticoccidial drugs. The adoption of rotation programs where the use of vaccines and drugs are alternated in successive flocks results in restoration of sensitivity.

ACKNOWLEDGMENTS

The authors are grateful to Dr. H. David Chapman for his expert advice and for reviewing the manuscript.

REFERENCES

47, 62, 66, 185, 229, 279–281, 283, 290, 391, 467, 468, 480–484, 514, 516, 569–571, 654, 687, 688, 765, 833, 1083, 1085, 1136, 1146, 1189, 1201–1203, 1329, 1343, 1393, 1457, 1584, 1716, 1717, 1756, 1805

CHAPTER 18

Coccidiosis in Ducks (*Anas* spp.)

S. Wang and X. Suo

CONTENTS

18.1 INTRODUCTION

Ducks (domestic and wild) are incredibly diverse and distributed worldwide. In the past 4000 years, ducks have been a good source of meat, eggs, and feathers for human beings, especially for Asians. Asia alone accounts for 82.6% of the total duck production in the world.[10] Coccidiosis is one of the most common and economically important diseases of ducks. Duck coccidia belong to four genera, *Eimeria*, *Isospora*, *Tyzzeria*, and *Wenyonella*.

In general, the term **duck** used here is vague and includes the common domestic duck (*Anas platyrhynchos domesticus*), Pekin ducks (*Anas platyrhynchos*), Muscovy ducks (*Cairina moschata*), Mule ducks (*Anas platyrhynchos* × *Cairina moschata* hybrids), and Ferruginous duck (Aythya or *Anas nyroca*). In several instances, the ducks studied were not identified.

18.1.1 Morphology and Life Cycle

Currently 23 species of coccidia, including 14 *Eimeria* spp., 4 *Wenyonella* spp., 4 *Tyzzeria* spp., and 1 *Isospora* sp. have been identified in ducks (Figures 18.1[443,565,574,767,1762] and 18.2,[117,208,574] Table 18.1). Most species were established based on the morphology of the sporulated oocysts. The genera are classified per the number of sporocysts within

the oocyst and the number of sporozoites within the sporocysts as explained in Chapter 1. Polymerase chain reaction (PCR)–based detection and differentiation of duck coccidia have been limited to a 422 bp portion of the 18S rDNA from *Wenyonella philiplevinei*.[1825]

Information on endogenous development is limited to a few species: *Tyzzeria perniciosa*, *W. philiplevinei*, *E. mulardi*, *E. danailovi* and *E. saitamae*. One fascinating feature is the development of *E. mulardi* in the host cell nucleus.

Endogenous development of *T. perniciosa* is summarized in Table 18.2. There is some uncertainty concerning the number of asexual generations. One study reported three generations of schizonts,[27] while others reported only two generations.[1741,1861] First- and second-generation schizonts could be morphologically distinguished. First-generation schizonts were in the cytoplasm above the nuclei of villar epithelial cells. They are smaller in size and produce fewer merozoites than the second-generation schizonts, which parasitize the cytoplasm below the nuclei of mesenchymal cells. In addition, the appearance of the sexual stages shortly after the disappearance of the second-generation schizonts provides more evidence for the second-generation schizogony theory.

Three generations of schizogony are found in the life cycle of *W. philiplevinei*.[967,1862] There is no significant difference in the size of each generation schizonts (Table 18.3).

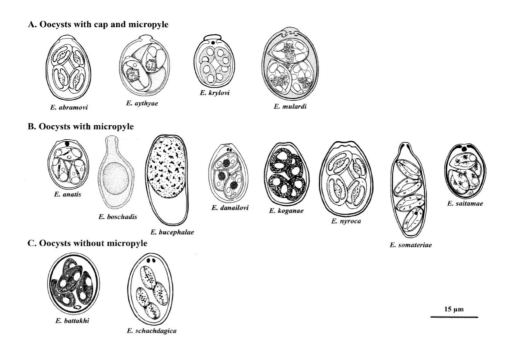

Figure 18.1 Oocysts of duck coccidia of the genus *Eimeria*: *E. abramovi*; *E. aythyae*; *E. krylovi*; *E. mulardi*; *E. anatis*; *E. boschadis*; *E. bucephalae*; *E. danailovi*; *E. koganae*; *E. nyroca*; *E. somateriae*; *E. saitamae*; *E. battakhi*; *E. schachdagica*. (From Gajadhar, A.A. et al. 1983. *Can. J. Zool.* 61, 1–24; Farr, M.M. 1965. *Proc. Helminthol. Soc. Wash.* 32, 236–238; Chauve, C.M. et al. 1994. *Parasite* 1, 15–22; Scholtyseck. 1955. *Arch. Protistenkd.* 100, 431–434; Waldén, H.W. 1961. *Arkiv för Zoologi* 15, 97–104; Christiansen, M., Madsen, H. 1948. *Dan. Rev. Game Biol.* 1, 62–73; Pecka, Z. 1992. *Folia Parasitol.* [Praha] 39, 13–18; Inoue, I., 1967. *Jpn. J. Vet. Sci.* 29, 209–215; Dubey, J.P., Pande, B.P. 1963. *Curr. Sci.* 32, 273–274 Fu, A.Q., Wu, Q.F. 1989. *China Poultry.* 1, 32–35 [in Chinese].)

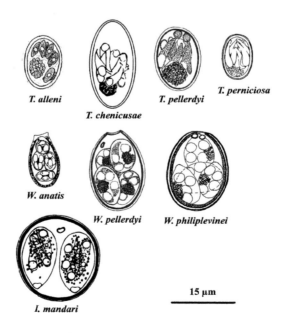

Figure 18.2 Oocysts of duck coccidia of the genera *Isospora, Tyzzeria,* and *Wenyonella*: *T. alleni*; *T. chenicusae*; *T. pellerdyi*; *T. perniciosa*; *W. anatis*; *W. pellerdyi*; *W. philiplevinei*; *I. mandari*. (From Chakravarty, M., Basu, S.P. 1947. *Sci. Cult.* 12, 106; Ray, H.N., Sarkar, A. 1967. *J. Protozool.* 14, 27; Bhatia, B.B., Pande, B.P. 1966. *Acta Vet. Acad. Sci. Hung.* 16, 335–340; Allen, E.A. 1936. *Arch. Protistenkd.* 87, 262–267; Gajadhar, A.A. et al. 1983. *Can. J. Zool.* 61, 1–24; Leibovitz, L. 1968. *Avian Dis.* 12, 670–681; Bhatia, B.B. et al. 1972. *Indian J. Anim. Sci.* 42, 625–628.)

Table 18.1 Oocyst Morphology of Duck Coccidia

Species	*Eimeria abramovi* Svanbaev and Rakhmatullina, 1967	*Eimeria anatis* Scholtyseck, 1955	*Eimeria aythyae* Farr, 1965	*Eimeria battakhi* Dubey and Pande, 1963
Range (μm)	16.1–23.4 × 10.1–13.3	14.4–19.2 × 10.8 – 15.6	14.8–23.6 × 10.5–18.2	16–21 × 19–24
Average (μm)	19.3 × 11.6	16.8 × 14.1	20.1 × 15.5	18 × 21
Oocyst shape	Ovoid to ellipsoidal	Ovoid	A shouldered round-bottomed urn to broadly elliptical	Nearly subspherical to somewhat ovoid
Oocyst wall	Bilayer, smooth, light green	Bilayer, colorless, smooth	Bilayer, pale yellow to colorless, smooth or lightly sculptured	Bilayer, pale yellow to orange outer wall, dark green inner wall
Micropyle	+	−	+	−
Oocyst residuum	−	−	−	−
Sporocyst residuum	+	+	+	+
Stieda body	−	−	+	+
Polar granule	Absent	One	Absent	One, big
Sporocyst	4	4	4	4
Sporozoite	4 × 2	4 × 2	4 × 2	4 × 2
Remarks	A 2-μm-high cap on top	A plug-like body closes the micropyle; one sporozoite is larger than the other	Oocyst wall slightly expands to form a uniformly thickened cap around the micropyle	No micropyle, one big polar granule, and a small Stieda body
Host	Mallard (*Anas platyrhynchos*), domestic duck (*Anas platyrhynchos domesticus*)	Mallard (*A. platyrhynchos*)	Lesser scaup (*Aythya affinis*)	Domestic duck (*A. platyrhynchos domesticus*)
Reference	Gajadhar et al.[574], Zuo et al.[1923]	Scholtyseck[1514], Zuo et al.[1923]	Farr[515], Zuo et al.[1923]	Dubey and Pande[443], Zuo et al.[1923], Fu and Wu[565]

Species	*Eimeria boschadis* Walden, 1961	*Eimeria bucephalae* Christiansen and Madsen, 1948	*Eimeria danailovi* Gräfner, Graubmann, and Betke, 1965	*Eimeria koganae* Svanbaev and Rakhmatullina, 1967	*Eimeria krylovi* Svanbaev and Rakhmatullina, 1967
Range (μm)	13.3–26.5 × 11.8–13.3	13–20 × 25–39	12.0–16.0 × 16.8–22.9	21–25 × 12.6–21	Varies among hosts
Average (μm)	23.9 × 12.7	15.6 × 30.3	14.0 × 20.0	21.5 × 16.1	17.8 × 14.8
Oocyst shape	Bottle-like	Ovoid to ellipsoidal	Ovoid	Ovoid or ellipsoidal	Subspherical
Oocyst wall	Colorless, finely granulated	Bilayer, light brown	Bilayer, yellowish-green or green	Bilayer, colorless	Bilayer, smooth
Micropyle	+	+	+	+	+
Oocyst residuum	−	−	−	−	−
Sporocyst residuum	−	−	+	+	−
Stieda body	+	−	+	−	−
Polar granule	Absent	Absent	One to two	Absent	One
Sporocyst	4	4	4	4	4
Sporozoite	4 × 2	4 × 2	4 × 2	4 × 2	4 × 2
Remarks	Kidney loci; bottle-like shape	Oocyst has two straight sides or one side indented	Two corpuscles on the opposite side of the micropyle	Oocyst wall often forms a collar around the micropyle	Oocyst wall forms a 1-μm-thick collar-like projection around the micropyle; both the sporocysts and the sporozoites are either ovoid or spherical
Host	Mallard (*A. platyrhynchos*), domestic duck (*A. platyrhynchos domesticus*)	Goldeneye (*Bucephala*), Domestic duck (*A. platyrhynchos domesticus*)	Domestic duck (*A. platyrhynchos domesticus*)	Pintail (*Anas acuta*), garganey (*Anas querquedula*), and gadwall or *Spatula* (*Anas strepera*)	Green-winged teal (*Anas carolinensis*), Northern shoveler (*Spatula clypeata*), garganey (*A. querquedula*), widgeon (*Mareca americana*), and gadwall (*A. strepera*)
Reference	Walden[1762], Wobeser[1812], Nation and Wobeser[1234], Fu and Wu[565]	Christiansen and Madsen[269], Fu and Wu[565]	Pecka[1333], Zuo et al.[1923]	Gajadhar et al.[574]	Gajadhar et al.[574]

(*Continued*)

Table 18.1 (*Continued*)   Oocyst Morphology of Duck Coccidia

Species	*Eimeria mulardi* Chauve, Reynaud, and Gounel, 1994	*Eimeria nyroca* Svanbaev and Rakhmatullina, 1967	*Eimeria saitamae* Inoue, 1967	*Eimeria schachdagica* Musaev, Surkova, Jelchiev, and Alieva, 1966	*Eimeria somateriae* Christiansen, 1952
Range (µm)	21.4–24.5 × 13.3–16.3	21–39.3 × 16.8–18.9	17–21 × 13–15	16–26 × 12–20	21.2–41.3 × 10.6–19.2
Average (µm)	22.6 × 14.5	25.4 × 17.7	18.6 × 13.2	22.0 × 16.0	31.9 × 13.6
Oocyst shape	Ovoid	Ovoid or ellipsoidal	Ovoid	Ovoid	Ellipsoid, asymmetric
Oocyst wall	Bilayer, smooth	Bilayer, pale green	Bilayer, colorless, smooth	Bilayer, colorless	Smooth, thin, colorless
Micropyle	+	+	+	−	+
Oocyst residuum	−	−	+	−	−
Sporocyst residuum	+	+	+	+	−
Stieda body	+	−	−	−	+
Polar granule	One	Absent	One	One to two	Absent
Sporocyst	4	4	4	4	4
Sporozoite	4 × 2	4 × 2	4 × 2	4 × 2	4 × 2
Remarks	Only infect mule duck	Micropyle is surrounded by two collars formed by the wall	Obvious micropyle	There are refractile granules at the narrow end of the oocysts, but no residuum	Kidney loci; the micropyle end is elongate, similar to a bottle neck
Host	Mule duck	Ferruginous duck (*Aythya nyroca*)	Domestic duck (*A. platyrhynchos domesticus*)	Domestic duck (*A. platyrhynchos domesticus*)	Common eider (*Somateria mollissima*), greater scaup (*Aythya marila*), Long-tailed duck (*Clangula hyemalis*) and domestic duck (*A. platyrhynchos domesticus*)
Reference	Chauve et al.[252]	Gajadhar et al.[574]	Inoue [767], Fu and Wu[565]	Fu and Wu[565]	Penner[1346], Walden[1762], Franson and Derksen[553], Fu and Wu[565]

Species	*Isospora mandari* Bhatia, Chauhan, Arora, and Agrawal, 1972	*Tyzzeria perniciosa* Allen, 1936	*Tyzzeria alleni* Chakravarty and Basu, 1946	*Tyzzeria pellerdyi* Bhatia and Pande, 1966	*Tyzzeria chenicusae* Ray and Sarkar, 1967
Range (µm)	19.5–23.4 × 18.2–22.2	9.9–13.8 × 7.8–12.3	14.5–17.3 × 9.6–11.5	11–16 × 8–11	20.4–27.6 × 14.4–20.4
Average (µm)	21.4 × 20.5	12.4 × 10.2		13.0 × 10.0	24.84 × 16.8
Oocyst shape	Spherical to subspherical	Ellipsoidal	Ovoid	Subspherical to ovoid	Broadly cylindrical
Oocyst wall	Bilayer, an outer transparent, straw-colored layer and an inner light brownish-blue layer	Bilayer, a thin outer layer and a thicker, transparent inner layer	Bilayer, colorless, smooth	Smooth, colorless	An outer thick dark layer and a thin inner layer
Micropyle	−	−	−	−	−
Oocyst residuum	−	+	+	+	+
Sporocyst residuum	+	−	−	−	−
Stieda body	+	−	−	−	−
Polar granule	One, big	Absent	Absent	Absent	Absent
Sporocyst	2	0	0	0	0
Sporozoite	2 × 4	8	8	8	8
Remarks	Dark granules dispersed around the sporozoites represent the sporocyst residuum	A large oocyst residuum composed of various-sized granules	A coarsely granular polar residuum of the oocyst, a central nucleus of the sporozoite	Sporozoite has a centrally located nucleus and a prominent globule at the broader end	A large compact residuum; a vacuole at the broader end of the club-shaped sporozoite
Host	Mandarin duck (*Aix galericulata*)	Domestic duck (*A. platyrhynchos domesticus*)	Cotton teal (*Chenicus coromandelianus*)	Gadwall (*A. strepera*) and Ferruginous duck (*A. nyroca*)	Cotton teal (*C. coromandelianus*)
Reference	Bhatia et al.[117]	Allen[27], Yin et al.[1864]	Chakravarty and Basu[208]	Bhatia and Pande[118]	Ray and Sarkar[1398]

(*Continued*)

Table 18.1 (*Continued*)   Oocyst Morphology of Duck Coccidia

Species	*Wenyonella anatis* Pande, Bhatia, and Srivastava, 1965	*Wenyonella gagari* Sarkar and Ray, 1968	*Wenyonella pellerdyi* Bhatia and Pande, 1966	*Wenyonella philiplevinei* Leibovitz, 1968
Range (μm)	11–17 × 7–10	23–26 × 17–19	13.3–19.3 × 10.0–13.3	15.5–21 × 12.5–16
Average (μm)		24 × 18.5	17.6 × 12.7	18.7 × 14.4
Oocyst shape	Ovoid	Pitcher-shaped	Ellipsoidal or ovoid	Ovoid
Oocyst wall	Bilayer, punctate, colorless	Bilayer, punctate, colorless	Bilayer, punctate, colorless	Three layers, punctate, bluish-green
Micropyle	+	+	+	+
Micropyle width (μm)	4.5–6	4.8	2–2.5	2
Oocyst residuum	–	–	–	–
Sporocyst resicuum	+	+	+	+
Stieda body	–	+	–	+
Polar granule	1	1	1	1 or 2
Sporocyst	4	4	4	4
Sporozoite	4 × 4	4 × 4	4 × 4	4 × 4
Remarks	A neck-shaped and flattened micropylar end	16 sporozoites, each sporozoite has a distinct globule at the broader end	16 sporozoites, each ovoid sporozoite has a distinct globule at the broader end	16 sporozoites, each sporozoite has large pale refractile globules
Host	Domestic duck (*A. platyrhynchos domesticus*)	Domestic duck (*A. platyrhynchos domesticus*)	Blue-winged teal (*Anas discors*)	Domestic duck (*A. platyrhynchos domesticus*)
Reference	Gajadhar et al.[574]	Sarkar and Ray[1498]	Bhatia and Pande[118]	Leibovitz[967]

Table 18.2   Endogenous Development of *Tyzzeria perniciosa* in Pekin Ducks

Reference	Oocyst Dose (×10⁴)	First-Generation Schizont					Second-Generation Schizont				Gamonts (HPI)	Oocysts (HPI)
		Detected Time (HPI)	Average Size (μm)	Merozoite Number	Localization		Detected Time (HPI)	Average Size (μm)	Merozoite Number	Localization		
Allen[27]	Nm	24	11.6 × 8.3	Nm	Nm		Nm	Nm	Nm	Nm	48	120-NS
Versényi[1741]	5	48	11.8 × 5.8	8–10	Lamina epithelialis		72–84	16 × 20	20–25	Mesenchymal cells	96	120–132
Yin et al.[1861]	216–816	48	6.4–8.8 × 5.6–8.8	6–10	Epithelial cells		96–120	11.36 × 9.87	12–24	Epithelial and glandular cells, lamina propria	96	104–120

Abbreviations: HPI, hours postinfection; Nm, not measured; NS = not stated.

Table 18.3   Endogenous Development of *Wenyonella philiplevinei* in Pekin Ducks

Detected Time (HPI)	Leibovitz[967]				Yin et al.[1862]			
	Detected Time (HPI)	Average Size (μm)	Merozoite Number	Average Merozoite Size (μm)	Detected Time (HPI)	Average Size (μm)	Merozoite Number	Average Merozoite Size (μm)
First-generation schizont	24	17 × 15	6	8.0 × 2.6	36–48	6.46 × 6.0	4–8	5.6 × 1.4
Second-generation schizont	49	14 × 10	8	8.8 × 2.4	54–72	7.95 × 6.63	4–10	8.79 × 1.73
Third-generation schizont	74	15 × 13	12	10.6 × 2.9	78–108	8.7 × 7.22	6–18	8.6 × 1.9
Macrogamont	93	12 × 10			91–120	10.58 × 8.57		
Microgamont	93	20 × 11			91–120	10.84 × 8.2		

Abbreviation: HFI, hours postinoculation.

The third-generation schizogony and gametogenesis are responsible for the pathogenicity of *W. philiplevinei*.[967,1862]

A large schizont (277×203 μm) was reported in the lamina propria of small intestine of a duck in India[444]; whether it belonged to *E. battakhi* was not certain.

Unlike other duck coccidia, *E. mulardi* develops in the nucleus rather than in the cytoplasm of the cell. The lamina propria and intestinal glands from jejunum to rectum are parasitized by *E. mulardi*.[252] At least two generations of schizogony were observed based on the size of the schizonts, the number of the merozoites, and the appearance of gamonts (Tables 18.4 and 18.5).

E. danailovi and *E. saitamae* have two generations of schizogony.[769,1333] Unlike the deep localization of *T. perniciosa* (mesenchymal cells) and *E. mulardi* (lamina propria and intestinal glands), all endogenous stages of *W. philiplevinei*, *E. danailovi*, and *E. saitamae* localize in the cytoplasm of intestinal epithelial cells. This may in part explain why *W. philiplevinei*, *E. danailovi*, and *E. saitamae* are less pathogenic than *T. perniciosa* and *E. mulardi*.

18.2 NATURAL INFECTIONS

18.2.1 Prevalence

Both domestic and wild ducks are commonly infected with coccidia (Table 18.6). Prevalence varies from 3.7% to 96.4%. In general, duck coccidia are more abundant and prevalent in domestic ducks in China, probably due to the abundance of ducks in this country. China has over 600 million domestic ducks, accounting for at least 50% of the global duck production (Food and Agriculture Organization of the United Nations [FAO]: http://kids.fao.org/glipha). The extensive animal husbandry mode and the international trade of waterfowl products increase the prevalence of duck coccidia in China.[1118] At least 11 *Eimeria* spp., 4 *Tyzzeria* spp., 4 *Wenyonella* spp., and 1 *Isospora* sp. are prevalent in China, with *T. perniciosa* and *W. philiplevinei* the most prevalent species (Table 18.6). The overall prevalence of coccidia in wild ducks is largely unknown. Special attention was given to renal coccidia in wild ducks: in a 3-year survey, renal coccidia were detected in 151 of 336 individuals of 11 species of wild ducks.[573] In other surveys, the prevalences of renal coccidia in wild ducks were relatively low, which may be due to the renal tissue not being entirely examined.[1234,1812]

18.2.2 Clinical Infections

Clinical infections of duck coccidia have been reported in the United States,[27,269,515] Denmark,[269] England,[334] Japan,[768,1514] India,[118] Canada,[1234] Iceland,[1582] and China (Table 18.7). Most of these reports confirmed duck coccidian infection by finding endogenous stages (schizonts, gamonts, and oocysts) in histological sections (Table 18.7).

Table 18.4 Size of Schizonts of *Eimeria mulardi* Chauve et al.[252] in Mule Ducks

Days postinoculation	Size Range (μm)	Mean (μm)	Merozoite Number
1	$2.5–4.9 \times 1.6–3.3$	4.0×2.6	Nm
2.5	$3.3–5.7 \times 2.0–4.9$	4.8×3.6	7–10[a]
3	$1.6–3.7 \times 1.6–2.5$	2.6×1.9	Nm
3.5	$3.3–6.6 \times 2.5–4.9$	4.5×3.0	Nm
4	$1.6–4.1 \times 1.6–3.7$	2.7×3.3	Nm
4.5	$2.5–8.2 \times 2.5–6.6$	6.0×4.4	9–16[b]
5	$4.1–9.8 \times 3.3–6.6$	7.1×5.2	12–17[b]

Abbreviation: Nm, not measured.
[a] First-generation schizont.
[b] Second-generation schizont.

Table 18.5 Size of Gamonts of *Eimeria mulardi* Chauve et al.[252] in Mule Ducks

Days postinoculation	Immature Gamonts (μm)		Macrogamonts (μm)		Microgamonts (μm)	
	Size Range	Mean	Size Range	Mean	Size Range	Mean
4.5	$1.2–1.6 \times 1.2–1.6$	1.5×1.5	Nm	Nm	Nm	Nm
5	$1.2–4.1 \times 1.2–4.1$	2.5×2.4	Nm	Nm	Nm	Nm
5.5	$2.5–10.7 \times 2.5–9.4$	6.6×5.7	Nm	Nm	Nm	Nm
6			$11.8–14.4 \times 8.4–11.8$	13.2×10.8	$13.5–18.6 \times 6.8–15.2$	16.3×11.4

Abbreviation: Nm, not measured.

Table 18.6 Prevalence of Duck Coccidiosis

Country/Region	Hosts	Number Tested	Number Positive (%)	Coccidia Species Found	Reference
Canada	Wild duck	261	64 (24.5%)	*E. boschadis*	Nation and Wobeser[1234]
Saskatchewan	11 species of wild ducks	336	151 (44.9%)	Renal coccidia	Gajadhar et al.[573]
China					
Chaohu	Domestic duck (*A. platyrhynchos domesticus*)	32 flocks (6050 ducks)	30 flocks (93.8%)	*E. abramovi* (12.5%), *E. battakhi* (50%), *E. krylovi* (3.1%), *E. nyroca* (40.6%), *E. saitamae* (28.1%), *E. schachdagica* (21.9%), *E. somateriae* (9.4%), *I. mandari* (28.6%), *T. alleni* (15.6%), *T. pellerdyi* (12.5%), *T. perniciosa* (25.0%), *W. pellerdyi* (18.6%), *W. philiplevinei* (68.8%)	Lu[1096]
Fujian	Domestic duck (*A. platyrhynchos domesticus*)	1558	106 (6.8%)	*W. philiplevinei*, *T. perniciosa*, *I. mandari*	Wu et al.[1828]
Fuzhou	Domestic duck (*A. platyrhynchos domesticus*)	6750 samples	1237 samples (18.3%)	*T. perniciosa* (16.7%), *W. philiplevinei* (14.4%), *W. pellerdyi* (3.3%), *I. mandari* (17.8%), *E. battakhi* (5.6%)	Wu et al.[1827]
Hunan	Domestic duck (*A. platyrhynchos domesticus*)	1800	258 (14.3%)	*W. philiplevinei*	Wu[1825]
Henan	Domestic duck (*A. platyrhynchos domesticus*)	28 flocks (38,000 ducks)	27 flocks (96.4%)	*T. perniciosa* (55.6%), *W. philiplevinei* (11.1%), *W. anatis* (14.8%), *E. abramovi* (7.4%), *E. battakhi* (7.4%)	Zhang et al.[1884]
Keshi	Domestic duck (*A. platyrhynchos domesticus*)	37 flocks	27 flocks (72.97%)	*W. philiplevinei* (59.4%), *T. perniciosa* (32.4%), *E. anatis* (29.7%), *E. abramovi* (21.6%), *W. anatis* (10.8%)	Zhao et al.[1899]
Kuerle	Domestic duck (*A. platyrhynchos domesticus*)	34 flocks	25 flocks (73.53%)	*W. philiplevinei* (61.8%), *T. perniciosa* (32.4%), *E. anatis* (29.4%), *E. abramovi* (20.6%), *W. anatis* (8.8%)	Jing et al.[817]
Shanghai	Domestic duck (*A. platyrhynchos domesticus*)	457 samples	278 samples (61%)	*E. anatis*, *E. abramovi*, *E. danailovi*, *E. schachdagica*, *E. battakhi*, *W. philiplevinei*, *W. pellerdyi*, *W. anatis*, *I. mandari*	Yao et al.[1853]
Yangzhou	Domestic duck (*A. platyrhynchos domesticus*)	22 flocks (about 7000 ducks)	20 flocks (90.9%)	*E. battakhi* (45.5%), *E. krylovi* (18.2%), *E. nyroca* (4.5%), *E. saitamae* (22.7%), *E. somateriae* (9.1%), *E. schachdagica* (13.6%), *W. philiplevinei* (72.7%), *W. gagari* (18.2%), *W. pellerdyi* (13.6%), *T. perniciosa* (9.1%), *T. chenicusae* (4.5%), *I. mandari* (4.5%)	Fu and Wu[565]
Yunnan	Domestic duck (*A. platyrhynchos domesticus*)	505	151 (60%)	*E. anatis* (6.3%), *E. battakhi* (4.0%), *E. aythyae* (17.6%), *E. abramovi* (3.6%), *W. philiplevinei* (36.4%), *W. anatis* (1.8%), *T. perniciosa* (38.8%)	Zuo et al.[1923]

(Continued)

Table 18.6 (Continued) Prevalence of Duck Coccidiosis

Country/Region	Hosts	Number Tested	Number Positive (%)	Coccidia Species Found	Reference
Zhanjiang	Domestic duck (*A. platyrhynchos domesticus*)	12 duck Farms	11 duck farms (91.7%)	*W. philiplevinei, E. abramovi, E. bucephalae*	Lin et al.[1022]
France					
Southwest region	Mallard (*A. platyrhynchos*)	157 Samples	40 samples (25.5%)	*T. perniciosa, T. pellerdyi, E. aythyae, E. nyroca, E. danailovi*	Chauve et al.[249]
India					
Calcutta	Mallard (*A. platyrhynchos*),	12	3 (25%)	*W. gagari*	Sarkar and Ray[1498]
Gorakhpur	Blue-winged teal (*A. discors*)	4	2 (50%)	*W. pellerdyi*	Bhatia and Pande[118]
Gorakhpur	Gadwall (*A. strepera*), common white-eye pochard (*Aythya nyroca*)	2,41	1 (50%)	*T. pellerdyi*	Bhatia and Pande[118]
Iran					
		4	2 (50%)		
Ahvaz	Domestic duck (*A. platyrhynchos domesticus*)		14 (58.33%)	*Tyzzeria* spp. (7.14%), *W. philiplevinei* (64.28%) and *I. mandari* (28.57%)	Larki et al.[944]
Sweden					
Norrkoping	Mallard (*A. platyrhynchos*), Long-tailed	27	1 (3.7%)	*E. boschadis*	Walden[1762]
Ostergotland	Duck (*C. hyemalis*)	4	1 (25%)	*E. somateriae*	Walden[1762]

Table 18.7 Histologically Confirmed Duck Coccidiosis

Country/Region	Species	Host	Signs	Lesion	Stages Found	Location of Stages	Remarks	References
Canada								
Saskatchewan	Not identified	Mallard (*A. platyrhynchos*), Pintail (*A. acuta*)	Not stated	1 to 2 mm, white foci throughout the renal parenchyma, slight urinary epithelial hyperplasia	Oocysts, gametocytes	Kidney	Oocysts are like *E. truncata* but larger	Wobeser[1812]
Saskatchewan	*E. boschadis*	Wild duck	No sign		Gametocytes, oocysts	Kidney	24.5% wild migratory ducks were infected	Nation and Wobeser[1234]
China								
Anxin	Not stated	Pekin duck	Anorexic, diarrhea, or dead	Acute hemorrhagic enteritis, distended intestine, caseous exudate	Merozoites, schizonts	Small intestines	1100 birds were sick. Anticoccidia treatment rescued most of the birds, only 160 birds died	Liu[1060]
Beijing	*T. Perniciosa, W. philiplevinei*	Pekin duck	Anorexic, emaciated, or dead	Acute hemorrhagic enteritis	Merozoites	Small intestines	First report of duck coccidiosis in China. Morbidity rates: 25%–30%; mortality rates: 5%–15.7%	Lin et al.[1024]
Changling	Not stated	Pekin Duck	Anorexic, emaciated, diarrhea, dead	Hemorrhagic or catarrhal enteritis, distended intestine, numerous punctate hemorrhaging on the mucosa	Oocysts	Small intestines	In April, 20,000 ducklings were sick, anti-enteritis drug treatment was unsuccessful	Cui et al.[311]
Fenghua	*T. perniciosa, W. philiplevinei*	Muscovy duck (*Cairina moschata*)	Anorexic, diarrhea, dead	Hemorrhagic enteritis, distended intestine, caseous exudate, numerous punctate hemorrhaging on the mucosa	Oocysts, merozoites, schizonts	Small intestines	200 day-old ducks, morbidity: 20%–70%; mortality: 10%–30%	Bao et al.[71]
Fenghua	Not stated	Muscovy duck (*C. moschata*)	Diarrhea, dead	Numerous white foci on the small intestine, caseous exudate in the lumen	Oocysts, merozoites, schizonts	Small intestines	In September, 65 sick ducks died after antibiotic treatment	Mao and Wang[1122]
Fuzhou	*T. perniciosa*	Muscovy duck (*C. moschata*)	Anorexic, diarrhea	Numerous white or red foci on the small intestine, caseous exudate in the lumen	Oocysts, merozoites, schizonts	Small intestines	One-third of the 2000 birds were infected	Lin[1029]
Fuzhou	Not stated	Muscovy duck (*C. moschata*)	Anorexic, diarrhea, dead	Distended intestine, caseous exudate, numerous punctate hemorrhaging on the mucosa	Merozoites, oocysts	Small intestines	In April, 1200 of the 1500 birds were sick, and 173 birds died 4 days later	Wu et al.[1826]
Guangdong	Not stated	Pekin duck	Anorexic, diarrhea, dead	Hemorrhagic or catarrhal enteritis	Oocysts, merozoites, schizonts, macrogametes, microgametes	Small intestines	In May, 113 ducklings died within 1 hour. After antibiotic treatment, another 80 birds died	Zhang et al.[1877]

(Continued)

Table 18.7 (Continued) Histologically Confirmed Duck Coccidiosis

Country/Region	Species	Host	Signs	Lesion	Stages Found	Location of Stages	Remarks	References
Ganzhou	Not stated	Pekin duck	Anorexic, emaciated, weak, paralysed, crying continuously, diarrhea	Distended intestine, numerous punctate hemorrhaging on the mucosa	Merozoites	Small intestines	In April, 43 of the 420 ducklings suddenly died. Terramycin treatment was unsuccessful, and another 136 birds died	Liu[1064]
Hejian	Not stated	Pekin duck	Anorexic, weak, emaciated, diarrhea, dead	Distended intestine, numerous punctate hemorrhages on the mucosa	Merozoites, schizonts, gametocytes	Small intestine	246 of the 1500 ducklings were sick and 46 died	Ji et al.[810]
Jiangjin	T. perniciosa	Pekin duck	Anorexic, emaciated, diarrhea, dead	Hemorrhagic enteritis, distended intestine, caseous exudate, sloughing of the mucosa	Oocysts, merozoites, schizonts, macrogametes, microgametes	Small intestine	In September, coccidiosis occurred among 2500 ducklings. 1868 ducks were sick, and 618 ducks died	Hu and Su[747]
Keshan	Not stated	Pekin duck	Anorexic, diarrhea, dead	Distended intestine, numerous punctate	Oocysts, merozoites	Small intestine	In June, 100 ducklings were sick, 25 of which died	Han and Sun[671]
Laibin	Not stated	Muscovy duck (C. moschata)	Anorexic, emaciated, diarrhea, dead	Distended intestine, punctate hemorrhaging, sloughing of the mucosa	Oocysts, merozoites, schizonts	Small intestines, cecum, rectum	In April, 67 of the 2500 ducklings died. Antibiotic treatment was unsuccessful	Li et al.[986]
Longyan	Not stated	Pekin duck	Anorexic, diarrhea, dead	Distended intestine, numerous white or red foci on the intestinal wall, caseous exudate, and sloughing of the mucosa	Merozoites, oocysts	Small intestines	16 birds died even after antibiotic treatment, mainly 24 day-old ducklings	Zhang[1886]
Mingxi	Not stated	Pekin duck	Anorexic, weak, diarrhea, or dead	Acute catarrhal enteritis, distended intestine	Oocysts, merozoites, schizonts	Small intestines	15% birds died in this outbreak of coccidia	Feng[524]
Nanning	Not stated	Pekin duck	Anorexic, weak, diarrhea, dead	Hemorrhagic or catarrhal enteritis, caseous exudate	Oocysts	Small intestines	In April, coccidiosis occurred on two duck farms. Mortality was 20% or 40%	Li et al.[988]
Qiqihaer	Not stated	Pekin duck	Anorexic, weak, diarrhea, dead	Distended intestine, numerous punctate hemorrhaging on the mucosa	Oocysts	Small intestines	30 ducklings died	Xu et al.[1833]

(Continued)

Table 18.7 (*Continued*) Histologically Confirmed Duck Coccidiosis

Country/Region	Species	Host	Signs	Lesion	Stages Found	Location of Stages	Remarks	References
Shanghai	Not stated	Muscovy duck (*C. moschata*)	Anorexic, weak, diarrhea, or dead	Distended intestine, destruction and sloughing of the mucosa, foamy red mucus	Oocysts, merozoites	Small intestines	Vaccination stress induced the occurrence of coccidiosis	Lu et al.[1097]
Shanghang	Not stated	Pekin duck	Anorexic, diarrhea	Hemorrhagic enteritis, distended intestine, caseous exudate, sloughing of the mucosa	Oocysts, gametocytes, merozoites	Small intestines	1200 ducklings became sick after transferred to the ground	Chen et al.[253]
Shanghang	Not stated	Muscovy duck (*C. moschata*)	Anorexic, diarrhea, dead	Hemorrhagic enteritis, distended intestine, numerous white or red foci on the intestinal wall, caseous exudate	Merozoites, oocysts	Small intestines	In June, 26 (5%) ducks died	Zhang[1885]
Shantou	Not stated	Pekin duck	Anorexic, diarrhea, dead	Hemorrhagic or catarrhal enteritis, distended intestine, caseous exudate	Oocysts, merozoites, schizonts	Small intestines	In May, 60% of the 440 ducks were sick and 10% died	Tan et al.[1663]
Shuangliao	Not stated	Mallard (*A. platyrhynchos*)	Anorexic, diarrhea, dead	Hemorrhagic or catarrhal enteritis, distended intestine, caseous exudate, sloughing of the mucosa	Oocysts, merozoites, schizonts	Small intestines	During the wet and hot summer, over 120 ducklings died within 8 days	Jia et al.[811]
Suiping	Not stated	Pekin duck	Anorexic, diarrhea, emaciated, dead	Intestinal mucosa was diffuse with punctate hemorrhages, caseous exudate	Oocysts	Small intestines	200 ducklings were sick, 50 of which died four days later	Xu et al.[1834]
Wendeng	Not stated	Pekin duck	Anorexic, emaciated	Distended intestine, caseous exudate	Merozoites, schizonts	Small intestines	15% of the adult ducks died	Kong[907]
Yongan	*T. perniciosa, W. philiplevinei*	Pekin duck	Anorexic, emaciated, diarrhea, or dead	Acute hemorrhagic enteritis, distended intestine, mucosa was diffuse with punctate hemorrhages	Merozoites, schizonts	Small intestines	10 to 20 birds died per day; antibacterial treatment was not successful	Xie[1831]
Zhangping	Not stated	Muscovy duck (*C. moschata*)	Anorexic, emaciated, dead	Hemorrhagic or catarrhal enteritis, distended intestine, caseous exudate	Merozoites, schizonts	Small intestines	In July, 238 (24%) ducklings died	Lu et al.[1097]

(*Continued*)

Table 18.7 (Continued)   Histologically Confirmed Duck Coccidiosis

Country/Region	Species	Host	Signs	Lesion	Stages Found	Location of Stages	Remarks	References
Denmark								
Halkaer bredning	E. bucephalae	Goldeneye (Bucephala)	Dead	Largely detached epithelium, increased interglandular tissue, and marked inflammatory infiltration	Oocysts	Small intestines	A new species found in wild duck	Christiansen and Madsen[269]
Iceland								
Bildudalur	E. somateriae	Eider duckling (Somateria mollissima)	Dead	Greatly enlarged kidneys variegated with white or yellowish nodules	Micro- and macrogamonts, oocysts	Kidney	E. somateriae caused significant renal dysfunction	Skirnisson[1582]
India								
Gorakhpur	W. pellerdyi	Blue-winged teal (A. discors)	No sign	No gross lesion	Macrogametes, oocysts	Middle intestine	A new species found in wild duck	Bhatia and Pande[118]
Japan								
Saitama	E. saitamae	Pekin duck	Dead	Acute catarrhal enteritis	Gametocytes and schizonts	Duodenum and the free portion of the small intestine epithelium	A new species found in domestic duck	Inoue et al.[768]
Sweden								
Norrkoping	E. boschadis	Mallard (A. platyrhynchos)	No sign	No gross lesion	Oocysts	Kidney	A new species found in wild duck	Walden[1762]
United States								
Alaska	E. somateriae	Oldsquaw (C. hyemalis)	No sign	1–2 mm white foci on kidney	Oocysts	Kidney	No serious renal impairment	Farr[515]
Iowa	E. aythyae	Lesser scaup (A. affinis)	Dead, greatly emaciated	Distended intestine, destruction and sloughing of the mucosa	Macrogametes, oocysts	Anterior small intestines	E. aythyae was responsible for die-off	Penner[1346]
Long Island Sound	E. somateriae	Greater scaup (A. marila)	No sign	No gross lesion	Oocysts, Gametocytes	Kidney	No serious renal impairment	Windingstad et al.[1810]
Nebraska	E. aytheae	Lesser scaup (A. affinis)	Dead	Epithelial destruction, sloughing of the mucosa, and hemorrhaging	Schizont, merozoites, gametocytes	Intestine	Recurrent outbreaks of coccidiosis	

Histological examination also revealed lesions caused by the localization and propagation of the parasites. In general, *E. aythyae* is the most pathogenic coccidia in lesser scaup, causing destruction and sloughing of intestinal mucosa and associated hemorrhaging.[515,1810] Heavily infected birds become greatly emaciated, and *E. aythyae* is responsible for the mortality.[515,1810] *T. perniciosa* is the most pathogenic coccidia in domestic ducks (Table 18.7). The small intestines of ducks infected with *T. perniciosa* are often distended and filled with blood and caseous exudate (Table 18.7). *T. perniciosa* induced mortality spikes to 30%, and recovered ducks are usually associated with slow weight gain, demonstrating *T. perniciosa* as a great restraint to the duck industry.[1864]

There is confusion concerning the pathogenicity of renal coccidia. *E. somateriae* is responsible for high mortality in eider ducklings: histologically, renal tubules are filled with gamonts and oocysts of *E. somateriae*, resulting in severe destruction of renal tissue.[1582] In contrast, the microscopic lesions in scaup and oldsquaw appear insufficient to cause serious renal impairment, and all infected birds are in good condition and show no overt signs of illness.[553,1234]

18.3 EXPERIMENTAL INFECTIONS

18.3.1 Cross-Transmission

Cross-transmission experiments were performed only on a few species of duck coccidia. Two *Isospora* spp. are isolated from mule ducks,[250] one of which closely resembles the goose coccidium *I. anseris*. This *Isospora* sp. is infective to mallards, Pekin ducks, Muscovy ducks, Mule ducks, and domestic geese, but not to chickens.[251] Most cross-transmission experiments with *Eimeria* spp. have failed, except *E. danailovi* and *E. mulardi*. Oocysts of *E. danailovi* from domestic ducks were successfully transmitted to domestic geese.[1398] Likewise, oocysts of *E. mulardi* from mule ducks successfully infected Muscovy ducks and domestic ducks.[1533] Mule duck is a hybrid of Muscovy duck and domestic duck, which may explain why *E. mulardi* develops in these three species of ducks.

18.4 DIAGNOSIS

Detection of duck coccidia oocysts in feces or ureteral contents confirms diagnosis. The finding of endogenous stages of the parasite in histological sections reinforces diagnosis. Routine monitoring of oocyst shedding of 2-to 6-week-old ducklings is important to prevent losses.

18.5 TREATMENT

Several drugs are effective in treating duck coccidiosis. Sulfadimethoxine (SMM, 100 mg/kg), sulfamethoxazole (SMZ, 100 mg/kg), and the combination of SMZ and trimethoprim (SMZ-TMP, 200 mg/kg) are the most effective drugs in treating duck coccidiosis.[1098,1863] Prophylactic treatment should be considered when ducklings are transferred from the net to ground. Either of the previous drugs may be added to feed for 4–5 days.

The efficacy of five polyether antibiotics (monensin, salinomycin, maduramycin, lasalocid, and naracin) against duck coccidiosis had been tested.[813,992,1025] Both maduramycin (5 mg/kg) and lasalocid (90 mg/kg) have a good anticoccidial effect when administered 2 days before infection. A single dose of toltrazuril (7 mg/kg) administered at the beginning of the life cycle of *E. mulardi* is enough to protect mallards.[1414] There is no report on the effect of toltrazuril on treating *T. perniciosa* in other species of ducks.

ACKNOWLEDGMENTS

We would like to thank Si Wang, Guangping Huang, and Lijun Yu for preparing the composite line drawings.

REFERENCES

10, 27, 71, 117, 118, 208, 249–253, 269, 311, 334, 443, 444, 515, 524, 553, 565, 573, 574, 575, 671, 747, 767–769, 810, 811, 813, 817, 907, 944, 967, 986, 988, 992, 1022, 1024, 1025, 1029, 1060, 1064, 1096, 1097, 1098, 1118, 1122, 1234, 1333, 1346, 1398, 1414, 1498, 1514, 1533, 1582, 1663, 1741, 1762, 1810, 1812, 1825–1828, 1831, 1833, 1834, 1853, 1861–1864, 1877, 1884–1886, 1899, 1923

CHAPTER 19

Coccidiosis in Horses and Other Equids

C. Bauer and J. P. Dubey

CONTENTS

19.1 INTRODUCTION AND HISTORY

Although equine coccidiosis was first recognized in 1883,[543] there are still uncertainties concerning the taxonomic status and endogenous life-cycle stages. We recently reviewed in detail its history, biology, and life cycle, and provided a comprehensive bibliography.[430] Here, we summarize essential information and add citations missed earlier.

19.2 MORPHOLOGY AND LIFE CYCLE

Eimeria leuckarti (Flesch, 1883) Reichenow, 1940, is the only valid species of *Eimeria* in equids. Two other *Eimeria* species, *E. solipedium* and *E. uniungulati*, had been described in a fecal survey on horses and donkeys[607] and were also mentioned in a few other studies; however, they are considered as spurious parasites resulting from the ingestion of oocyst-contaminated feed.[430] Endogenous stages of a protozoon found in the lungs of a horse had been ascribed to another species, *E. utinensis*[1530]; however, based on the description and illustrations, this is clearly not an *Eimeria* species. Therefore, these three species are considered as nonvalid species.

Horse (*Equus caballus*),[543] donkey (*Equus asinus*),[1403] mule (*Equus mulus*),[1363] Asian wild ass (*Equus hemionus*), Mountain zebra (*Equus zebra*), and Grant's zebra (*Equus quagga*),[1709] and probably also Przewalski's horses (*Equus ferus przewalskii*) are its hosts.

Its life-cycle stages are not fully known. Unsporulated oocysts excreted in the feces vary from 60 to 96 μm in length and 48 to 67 μm in width (Table 19.1). They are ovoid or piriform, have an up to 9 μm thick wall and a micropyle without polar cap at the narrow pole (Figure 19.1A). The oocyst wall is bilayered: the slightly roughened outer layer wall is dark brown and 6–8.6 μm thick, the smooth inner layer wall is colorless and 1 μm thick based on removal of the outer layer (Figure 19.1B).[89,451,930] A bulge of the inner layer wall is present at the pole opposite the micropyle.[163,930,1612] Sporulated oocysts have no residual body. Sporocysts are elongate, 26–45 × 9–14 μm and have an indistinct Stieda body and residual body. Sporozoites are the longest of any coccidian, up to 35 μm long (Table 19.1). The sporulation time is usually 14–21 days at temperatures of 20°C–26°C (Table 19.1).

The endogenous development of *E. leuckarti* is not fully known. Several authors had described schizonts in small intestines (Table 19.2)[102,836,898]; however, based on their descriptions and illustrations, microgamonts were most likely misidentified as schizonts. Two intraepithelial schizonts had been found in smears of the ileum 6 days after experimental infection of a pony,[89] but this finding needs confirmation. Thus, schizonts of *E. leuckarti* have not yet been unequivocally identified.

The only endogenous stages known are gamonts and oocysts occurring in the jejunum and more in the ileum (Figures 19.1C and D; Table 19.2).[74,377] They are in enterocytes that have been displaced into the lamina propria toward the luminal part of the villi, but some occur throughout the villi.[104,701,721] The host cell nucleus is hypertrophied

Table 19.1   Morphology of *Eimeria leuckarti* Oocysts Isolated from Feces of Horses or Donkeys and Sporulation Time

Size (μm) of Unsporulated Oocysts					
Range	Average	Number Tested	Remarks (Measurements in μm)	Sporulation Time	Reference
80–87 × 55–59	NS	NS	Ovoid, outer layer of wall dark brown and 6.5–7 thick, micropyle at narrow pole, inner layer of wall 1.0 and clear. Sporocysts 39–42 × 13–14, Stieda body and residual bodies present. Sporozoites 34–35 × 5	21 days at 20°C–22°C, approximately 2 weeks at 26°C	Reichenow (1940)
NS	84 × 56	NS	Oval, outer layer of wall brown and 5–7 thick, distinct micropyle without polar cap, inner layer of wall thin and transparent. Sporocysts 30 × 12, no oocyst residual body. Spindle-shaped sporozoites, 20 × 5, with residual body	15 days on "hot days"	Hiregaudar (1956)
74–78 × 48–54	77 × 52	6	Dark brown, thick-walled, prominent micropyle	NS	Benbrook and Sloss (1962)
68–94 × 49–79	81 × 57	154	Ovoid, width-length ratio 0.6–0.8, outer layer of wall dark brown and 7.7–11.2 thick, micropyle at narrow pole	21 days at 22°C, 14 days at 26°C	Dolenc (1966)
79–89 × 53–64	NS	NS	Ovoid, outer layer wall dark brown and 6–8.6 thick, micropyle at the narrow pole and 3.3–7.3 wide, inner layer wall 1 and clear. A bulge of the inner layer wall at the pole opposite the micropyle. Spindle-shaped sporocysts 38–43 × 12.5–14.7, Stieda body and residual body present, no oocyst residual body	41 days at 15°C, 19 days at 25°C, 15 days at 30°C (low sporulation rate)	Kutzer (1969)
71–85 × 51–63	77 × 55	44	Sporocyst mean length 42.7 (*n* = 24)	NS	Dunlap (1970)
73–84 × 53–67	78 × 56	NS	Oval, outer layer wall dark brown, 4.7–7.7 thick, micropyle 4.7–6.2 wide, inner layer wall thin and colorless	NS	Oğuz (1971)
80 × 47	NS	NS	Dark brown outer wall and 5–7 thick, distinct micropyle. Sporocysts 30 × 10, sporozoites 18 × 5	16 days at room temperature	Achuthan and Alwar (1972)
70–90 × 49–69	81 × 57	100	Piriform, outer wall dark brown and 7.3 thick, micropyle, inner layer of wall 1.2 and clear, length-width ratio 1.42. Sporocysts 39 × 17, Stieda body and residual bodies present	15 days at 27°C (30% sporulation rate)	Canestri-Trotti and Restani (1972)
77–84 × 51–64	80 × 57	10	NS	NS	Kistner et al. (1972)
62–85 × 46–54	76 × 50	75	Dark brown outer layer wall with distinct micropyle, lighter inner layer wall	35 days at 21°C–22°C	McQueary et al. (1977)
70–80 × 55–57	NS	NS	NS	NS	**Cotteleer and Famereé**[299]
73–76 × 51–62	74 × 55	NS	Pyriform, dark brown, trilayered 11 thick wall	NS	Wei and Wang (1986)
76–84 × 55–60	79.5 × 55.6	NS	Oval, length-width ratio 1.42, dark brown, wall 6 thick, distinct micropyle at narrow pole. Sporocysts 30 × 16, sporozoites 20 × 9	18 days at 30°C–34°C	Gatne et al. (1992)
67–90 × 49–64	79 × 54	105	Sporulated oocysts 71–94 × 50–64 (*n* = 100), length-width ratio 1.30–1.64. Sporocysts 26–45 × 9–14 (*n* = 100)	19 days at 26°C, 3 months for complete sporulation	Battelli et al. (1995)
60–68 × 50–55	NS	NS	NS	30 days at room temperature	Mandal et al. (1995)
72–85 × 47–57	81 × 56	NS	Oval, one end more flattened than the other, deep brown, oocyst wall 6.7 thick, distinct micropyle without polar cap	NS	Sharma et al. (1998)
66–96 × 49–65	80 × 56	30	Sporulated oocysts measured. Length-width ratio 1.2–1.5. Sporocysts 24–46 × 8–14, length-width ratio 2.7–3.6 (*n* = 30)	NS	de Souza et al. (2009)

(Continued)

Table 19.1 (Continued)   Morphology of *Eimeria leuckarti* Oocysts Isolated from Feces of Horses or Donkeys and Sporulation Time

Size (μm) of Unsporulated Oocysts					
Range	Average	Number Tested	Remarks (Measurements in μm)	Sporulation Time	Reference
63–85 × 46–60	NS	NS	Ovoid or ellipsoidal, brown, thick outer layer wall, micropyle at the narrow pole, 3–5 in width, thin inner layer wall	NS	Sinyakov and Mironenko (2011)
77–90 × 50–55	79 × 53	NS	Ovoidal, length-width ratio 1.4–1.6, oocyst wall bilayered, 7.3 thick. Projection/enlargement of the inner layer wall at the pole opposite the micropyle	No sporulation at 23°C–28°C	Spitz dos Santos et al. (2014)
77–91 × 53–59	82 × 56	NS	Ovoid, outer layer wall dark brown and 6–9 thick, micropyle at narrow pole, inner layer wall 1.0 and transparent, characteristic fossa on the inner layer wall at the pole opposite the micropyle	>1 month at 25°C	Bundina and Khrustalev (2016)
75–89 × 50–58	80 × 54	NS	Ovoidal, wall bilayered	NS	Buono et al. (2016)

Source: Modified from Dubey, J.P., Bauer, C. 2018. *Vet. Parasitol.* 256, 58–70.
Note: In bold is addition to Dubey and Bauer.
Abbreviation: NS, not stated.

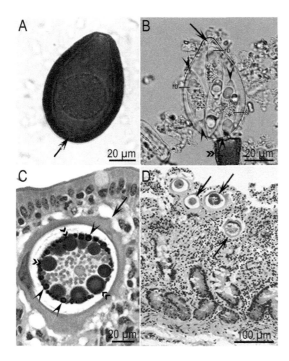

Figure 19.1 *E. leuckarti* stages. (A) Unsporulated oocyst with a central sporont. Note a bulge of the inner layer wall (arrow). Unstained. (B) Sporulated oocysts. The inner layer of oocyst has been mechanically squeezed from the outer layers; part of the broken wall (double arrowheads) is still attached to the inner layer. Note thin, colorless inner layer containing four sporocysts that are about 40 μm long (opposing arrowheads). Also, note the polar granule (arrow) in the oocyst, sporocystic residuum (sr), and two refractile bodies (rb) in each sporocyst. The outlines of sporozoites are not clear. (C and D) Stages in sections of small intestine of naturally infected horses. Hematoxylin and eosin stain. (C) Note a macrogamont (arrow) with two types of wall-forming bodies (type 1 double arrowheads, type 2 single arrowheads) in the lamina propria. (D) Several gamonts (arrows) in luminal parts of villi.

and indented. The parasite stages are enclosed in a thick parasitophorous vacuole that is thicker for macrogamonts than for microgamonts (Figures 19.1C and D).

Per experimental infections of ponies, the gametogony proceeds as follows.[74] At 14 days post-inoculation (DPI), the gamonts are 4–7 μm in size and still undifferentiated. At 23 DPI, microgamonts (29–68 μm in diameter) can be differentiated from macrogamonts by the presence of nuclei. At 28 DPI, the size of microgamonts has increased up to 81 μm in diameter. At 36–39 DPI, the microgamonts have matured, are grossly visible as white spots being up to 243 μm in diameter, and contain hundreds of 3–5 μm long microgametes each with two flagella of 8–12 μm length. Up to 300 μm sized microgamonts have been found in naturally infected equids.[925] Macrogamonts can be identified 23 DPI by the presence of wall-forming bodies. The youngest macrogamonts are 13.6 × 23.8 μm in diameter, and their parasitophorous vacuoles are 30.6–47.6 μm in diameter. At 28 DPI, macrogamonts have increased to 40.8–57.8 μm in diameter and two types of wall-forming bodies (see Figure 19.1C). Oocysts can be seen in histological sections beginning at 36 DPI, at a time they are also detected in feces. In developing oocysts, the wall-forming bodies are 12–15 μm in diameter. The size of oocysts in sections is 50–68 × 35–38 μm,[1653] 75–78 × 50–55 μm,[925] 80–88 × 55–59 μm,[701] or 89–90 × 64–69 μm.[543]

The prepatent period is 30–37 days.[74,89,377,1169] The patency usually lasts 3–18 days after experimental single infection[74,89,377,1169] and may last 4 months in naturally infected foals.[88]

Horses can become immune after primary infection. In ponies reinfected with 80,000 *E. leuckarti* oocysts 82 days after initial dosing, the number of oocysts excreted after challenge was significantly lower than after primary infection.[89] Under natural conditions, infections are much more

Table 19.2 Histologically Confirmed *Eimeria leuckarti* Infection in Equids

Country	Number	Age	Breed	Signs	Lesion	Stages Found	Location of Stages	Reference
Australia								
Tasmania	1	4–5 mo	NS	Diarrhea	Hepatic necrosis, necrosis area in large intestine	Oocysts	Small intestine, lamina propria of villi	Mason and King (1971)
New South Wales	1	8 wk	Arab-cross	Pneumonia	Severe bronchopneumonia, multifocal hepatic abscesses, ulcerative colitis, no enteritis	Gamonts	Small intestine with exception of duodenum, lamina propria of villi	Reppas and Collins (1995)
	1	6 wk	Standardbred	Short diarrhea	Ulcerative rhinitis, multifocal abscesses in large intestine	Micro- and macrogamonts, oocysts	Duodenum, lamina propria at tip of villi	
	1	6 mo	Quarter horse	Chronic diarrhea	Multiple gastric ulcers	Gamonts	Jejunum, lamina propria of villi	
Belgium	3	2 mo	NS	Chronic diarrhea, bronchopneumonia	NS	Micro- and macrogamonts	Small intestine	Navez (1925)
Brazil	1	6 mo		Chronic diarrhea	Ceco-colic intussusception	Gamonts, oocysts	NS	Figueiredo et al. (1993)
France	3	NS	NS	NS	NS	NS	NS	Brumpt, E. (1913) personal communication to Neveu-Lemaire (1943)
Germany	1	1 yr	(Warmblood)	Sudden death, grayish-white plaques in jejunum and ileum	Fist-sized aneurysm of mesentery artery, mucosa of small intestine as strewn with sand grains	Micro- and macrogamonts, oocysts	Small intestine, lamina propria at tip of villi	Hobmaier (1922), Kupke (1923)
	1	Adult	Warmblood (military horse)	Weakness	Gastric rupture	Micro- and macrogamonts, oocysts	Small intestine, subepithelial at tip of villi	Hemmert-Halswick (1943)
	1	8 mo	Zebra	Fracture of leg	NS	"*E. leuckarti*"	NS	Seitz (1961)
	1	8 wk	NS	Diarrhea	NS	Microgamonts, mature oocysts	Ileum, lamina propria	Bauer and Bürger (1984)
Ireland	1	2 mo	Thoroughbred	Acute illness, sudden death	Diffuse hemorrhages in small and large intestines	Micro- and macrogamonts	Small intestine, lamina propria at tip of villi	Sheahan (1976)
Japan	7	2–7 mo	Thoroughbred, Anglo-Arabian	NS	NS	Micro- and macrogamonts, oocysts	Jejunum and ileum, lamina propria at tip of villi	Sutoh et al. (1976)
	5	Foals	Thoroughbred	Mycotic guttural pouch, gastric ulcer, obscure diarrhea	NS	Micro- and macrogamonts, oocysts	Jejunum and ileum, lamina propria at tip of villi	Hirayama et al. (2002)

(Continued)

Table 19.2 (Continued) Histologically Confirmed *Eimeria leuckarti* Infection in Equids

Country	Number	Age	Breed	Signs	Lesion	Stages Found	Location of Stages	Reference
Kenya	2	Adult	Donkey	No symptoms	NS	Micro- and macrogamonts, oocysts	Ileum, lamina propria of villi	Karanja et al. (1994)
New Zealand	1	7 mo	Thoroughbred	Colic	Peritonitis, perforated large intestines	Gamonts, "schizonts"[a]	Jejunum and ileum, lamina propria of villi	Johnstone et al. (1982)
Nigeria	1	2 yr	Donkey	No symptoms	Numerous grayish-white plaques in jejunum and ileum	Micro- and macrogamonts	Jejunum and ileum, lamina propria of villi	Chineme et al. (1979)
	1	1.5 yr	Donkey	Unthrifty, anemic, mild diarrhea	Numerous grayish-white plaques in jejunum and ileum, catarrhal enteritis	Micro- and macrogamonts	Jejunum and ileum, lamina propria of villi	
Serbia	1	4 yr	Thoroughbred	Colic and diarrhea	Diffuse hemorrhagic-necrotic jejunoileitis, focal colitis, peritonitis	Microgamonts	Jejunum and ileum, epithelial cells	Marinković et al. (2013)
Sudan	Several	NS	NS	NS	NS	NS	NS	Bennett (1923) cited by Neveu-Lemaire (1943)
Switzerland	1	Adult	NS	NS	NS	Micro- and macrogamonts, oocysts	Small intestines with exception of duodenum, lamina propria at tip of villi	Flesch (1883, 1884)
United Kingdom								
Scotland	1	3 yr	Welsh pony	Chronic diarrhea	Enteritis	Micro- and macrogamonts	Small intestines, subepithelial at tip of villi	Wheeldon and Greig (1977)
England	1	17 yr	Horse	No diarrhea	NS	Micro- and macrogamonts, oocysts	Small intestines, subepithelial at tip of villi	Roberts and Cotchin (1973)
	1	7 mo	Thoroughbred	No enteritis	NS	Micro- and macrogamonts, oocysts	Small intestines, subepithelial at tip of villi	
	1	10 mo	Welsh mountain pony	Nervous condition	NS	Micro- and macrogamonts, oocysts	Small intestines, subepithelial at tip of villi	
United States								
Arizona or Mexico	1	NS	Donkey	NS	NS	Gamonts, oocysts	Small intestines subepithelial in villi	Benbrook and Sloss (1962)

(Continued)

Table 19.2 (Continued) Histologically Confirmed *Eimeria leuckarti* Infection in Equids

Country	Number	Age	Breed	Signs	Lesion	Stages Found	Location of Stages	Reference
Georgia	1	6 mo	Quarter horse	Acute abdominal pain, diarrhea	Ceco-colic intussusception, peritonitis, numerous mature *Parascaris equorum*	Microgamonts, oocysts	Distal ileum, within villi	White et al. (1988)
Indiana	1	5 mo	Quarter horse	Pneumonia, umbilical hernia	*Corynebacterium* abscess in lung, focal hepatic necrosis, mild enteritis	Micro- and macrogamonts, "schizonts"[a]	Small intestines, lamina propria, also within crypts	Kitchen and Gaafar (1974)
Minnesota	1	3 mo	Arabian	NS	Hemorrhagic enteritis	Micro- and macrogamonts, oocysts, "schizonts"[a]	Small intestines, lamina propria of villi	Bemrick et al. (1979)
	1	7 wk	Arabian	NS	Shortening of villi	Gamonts, oocysts	Small intestines, at tips of villi	
	1	7 mo	Standardbred	NS	Infarction	Macrogamonts	Small intestines, lamina propria	
	1	3 yr	Thoroughbred	Peritonitis	Perforation of small intestine	Gamonts, "schizonts"[a]	NS	
	1	8 mo	Quarter horse	Mucoid chronic diarrhea	NS	Macrogamonts	Small intestines, villi	
Texas	1	6 mo	Miniature horse	Acute diarrhea, sudden death	Colitis, spleen necrosis	"numerous coccidiae"	Small intestine, "embedded in mucosa"	Eugster and Jones (1985)

Source: From Dubey, J.P., Bauer, C. 2018. *Vet. Parasitol.* 256, 58–70.
Abbreviations: Mo, months; NS, not stated; wk, weeks; yr, years.
[a] "Schizonts" = misidentification of microgamonts.

Table 19.3 *Eimeria leuckarti* Prevalence in Equids Using Fecal Examinations

Country	Host	Number Tested	Number Positive (%)	Method Used	Remarks	Reference
Albania	Horse	68	2 (3)	Telemann's sedimentation		Postoli et al. (2010)
	Donkeys, mules	268	11 (4.1)	sedimentation		
Australia	Horses	>2000	1 (0.05)	Sedimentation		Palmer[1317]
Austria	Horses (7 farms)	646	6 (0.9)	Sedimentation-flotation	Positive horses in two of seven farms	Rehbein et al. (2002)
Belarus	Horses	3066	9 (0.3)	NS	From livestock farms	Sinyakov and Mironenko (2011)
		66 foals (6–18 months)	6 (9)			
Belgium	Horses	5065	4 (0.08)	NaCl-ZnCl₂ flotation		Cotteleer and Famerée (1981)
Brazil						
Rio de Janeiro state	Horses	396	2 (0.5)	Centrifugation	Aged <3 years 1 of 58 positive, aged <4 years 1 of 338 positive	De Souza et al. (2009)
Rio de Janeiro state	Horses	57	10 (18)	Sugar flotation (sp. gr. 1.24) and sedimentation	Foals	Spitz dos Santos et al. (2014)
Pernambuco state	Horses	49	1	Sugar flotation		Cintra Ferreira et al.[272]
Canada						
Quebec	Horses	11	2	NS	1 of 10 foals and a 3-year-old horse positive	Fréchette and Marcoux (1974)
China (Taiwan)	Horses (one stud farm)	63	1 (2)	NS		Tsai Yujen et al. (1998)
China (PRC)						
Inner Mongolia Ergunyou banner	Horses and donkey	66	2 (3)	Potassium carbonate flotation	62 foals 1–2 months old, 3 adult horses, 1 donkey	Wei and Wang (1986)
Inner Mongolia Ewenki banner and Hailar	Horses	85	85 (100)	Potassium carbonate flotation	Adult horses	
Hu Meng	Horses	151	2 (1.3)	Potassium carbonate flotation		
Chifeng	Horses	32	32 (100)	Potassium carbonate flotation		
Czech Republic	Thoroughbred (one stud farm)	36–69	Positive, % not clear	Breza solution (sp. gr. 1.3) flotation	Repeated examinations for >1 year, sucklings 0.6% positive Weaners 0.4% positive, horses aged <2 years 0.8% positive, mean OPG 4–14	Langrová (2000)
	Coldblooded horses	431	3 (0.6)	NS		Nápravník et al. (1992)

(Continued)

Table 19.3 (Continued) *Eimeria leuckarti* Prevalence in Equids Using Fecal Examinations

Country	Host	Number Tested	Number Positive (%)	Method Used	Remarks	Reference
	Horses	98	4 (4)	Sedimentation (MIFC)	Repeated examinations, positivity in foals (3–6 months) and yearlings only	Wagnerová (2011)
Finland	Horses	139	8 (5.8)	Magnesium sulfate flotation	Foals and young horses	**Aromaa et al.**[43a]
Germany						
Holstein	Horses	100	4 (4.0)	Benedek's sedimentation		Nebel (1976)
Bavaria	Horses	2824	21 (0.7)	Potassium acetate flotation (sp. gr. 1.35)		Brem (1977)
Hesse	Donkeys	106	1 (0.9)	Benedek's sedimentation		Gothe and Heil (1984)
Northwest Germany	Horses (mostly from boarding stables)	2314	23 (1.0)	Benedek's sedimentation	Samples from 1977 to 1983	Bauer and Stoye (1984)
Northwest Germany	Horses (mostly from boarding stables)	9192	55 (0.6)	Benedek's sedimentation	Samples from 1984 to 1991	Epe et al. (1993)
Northwest Germany	Horses (mostly from boarding stables)	3103	11 (0.4)	Benedek's sedimentation	Samples from 1993 to 1997	Epe et al. (1998)
Northwest Germany	Horses (mostly from boarding stables)	4399	2 (0.05)	Benedek's sedimentation	Samples from 1998 to 2002	Epe et al. (2004)
Northwest Germany	Horses (mostly from boarding stables)	3475	3 (0.1)	Benedek's sedimentation	Samples from 2003 to 2012	Raue et al. (2017)
Lower Saxony	Thoroughbred (one stud farm)	14 foals and their dams	14 foals (100) 0 mares	Benedek's sedimentation	Repeated examinations, 0.1–33 OPG	Bauer (1988)
Bavaria	Horses	30 foals and their dams	24 foals (80) 1 mare (3)	Benedek's sedimentation	Repeated examinations, 0.2–189 OPG	Beelitz et al. (1994)
Bavaria	Horses	37 foals and their dams	24 foals (65) 1 mare (3)	Benedek's sedimentation	Repeated examinations, positive foals aged 28–32 weeks	Beelitz et al. (1996a)
Bavaria	Horses (10 farms) Donkeys	23 37	1 1	Benedek's sedimentation	Repeated examinations on 10 farms, positivity in foals <1 year only	Beelitz et al. (1996b)
Bavaria, Saxonia, Thuringia, Mecklenburg-Western Pomerania	Horses (49 farms)	2034	2 (0.1)	Sedimentation-flotation	Positive horses in 2 of 49 farms	Rehbein et al. (2002)

(Continued)

Table 19.3 (Continued) *Eimeria leuckarti* Prevalence in Equids Using Fecal Examinations

Country	Host	Number Tested	Number Positive (%)	Method Used	Remarks	Reference
Greece						
Skyros Island	Ponies	63	2 (3)	NS		Kinis et al. (1985)
Macedonia, Thessalia	Horses	226	6 (2.7)	Telemann's sedimentation		Sotiraki et al. (1997)
	Donkeys	37	3 (8)			
Central and northern	Horses (6 farms)	223	9 (4.0)	Telemann's sedimentation		Papazahariadou et al. (2009)
Hungary	Horses	846	2 (0.2)	Breza solution (sp. gr. 1.3) flotation		Széll et al. (1999)
India						
Maharashtra state	Horses	Approximately 750	3 (0.4)	NS		Gatne et al. (1992)
Madhya Pradesh state	Horses	8	5	NS		Mandal et al. (1995)
Uttar Pradesh state	Donkeys	30	1 (3)	Sugar flotation (sp. gr. 1.26)	250 OPG	Sharma et al. (1998)
Haryana	Horses, donkeys, mules	141	2 (1.4)	NS	Mean OPG 100	Sengupta and Yadav (1998)
Gujarat state	Horses	502	13 (2.6)	Sedimentation	5 of 43 foals, 5 of 187 yearlings, but only 3 of 272 old horses positive	Mavadiya (2009)
Gujarat state	Donkeys	1794	117 (6.5)	Sedimentation-flotation		Parsani et al. (2013)
Gujarat state	Donkeys	354	23 (6.5)	Sedimentation		Prajapati (2016)
Rajasthan state	Horses	100	1 (1.0)	Sedimentation		Khan (2012)
Rajasthan state	Donkeys	100	1 (1.0)	Sedimentation		Kumar (2012)
Tamil Nadu state	Donkeys	30	1 (3)	Sedimentation-flotation		Sowmiya et al. (2017)
Iran						
Urmia	Working horses	221	1 (0.5)	Sedimentation		Tavassoli et al. (2010)
Southwest	Working horses	26	2	ZnSO$_4$ flotation		Karimighahfarrokhi et al. (2014)
	Donkeys	26	2			
Italy						
Emilia, Marche, Toscana, Abruzzo	Horses	150	9 (6.0)	Flotation (sp. gr. 1.3)		Canestri-Trotti and Restani (1972)
	Donkeys	10	1			
Emilia	Donkey (one farm)	72	1 (1)	NS	1.4 OPG	**Trentini et al.**[1704]
Udine	Horses	73	9 (12)	NS	6 of 51 young and 3 of 22 old horses from stud farms were positive	Battelli et al. (1995)
11 regions	Donkeys (77 farms)	1775	17 (1.0)	Sugar flotation (sp. gr. 1.25)	Positive donkeys on 10 of 77 farms	Buono et al. (2016)
Mexico	Horses	90	61 (68)	NaCl flotation	Horses aged 3–7 years	Güiris et al. (2010)

(Continued)

Table 19.3 (Continued) *Eimeria leuckarti* Prevalence in Equids Using Fecal Examinations

Country	Host	Number Tested	Number Positive (%)	Method Used	Remarks	Reference
Mongolia						
Gobi Desert	Domestic horses	29	2	Benedek's sedimentation		Painer et al. (2011)
	Asiatic wild asses	31	0			
	Przewalski's horses	40	0			
Netherlands	Horses	3791	12 (0.3)	Centrifugation-flotation		Mirck (1978)
Poland						
Lublin district	Horses	899	60 (6.7)	Sedimentation-flotation		Gundlach et al. (2004)
Lublin district	Horses	207 foals	19 (9.2)	Sedimentation-flotation	Foals aged 6–12 months, 50–1100 OPG	Studzińska et al. (2008)
	Thoroughbred, Arabian (from stud farms)	516 foals	12 (2.3)	Sugar flotation (sp. gr. 1.28)	Aged 1–3 months 6 of 37 positive, aged 4–6 months 3 of 106 positive, aged 7–9 months 3 of 316 positive, aged 10–12 months 0 of 57 positive	Kornaś et al. (2011)
Romania	Horses	158	3 (1.9)	NaCl flotation		Ioniţă et al. (2013)
	Horses (from stud farms and recreational establishments)	112	14 (12.5)	NaCl flotation		Buzatu et al. (2016)
	Working horses	121	19 (15.7)			
Saudi Arabia						
Eastern province	Horses	302	1 (0.3)	Sedimentation	99 OPG	Al-Qudari et al. (2015)
Switzerland	Horses	4158	3 (0.1)	Sedimentation-flotation (sp. gr. 1.3)	Samples from 1968 to 1975	Eckert (personal communication to CB, 1984)
Turkey						
Kars province	Horses	184	7 (3.8)	Benedek's sedimentation		Arslan and Umur (1998)
	Donkeys	82	8 (2)			
Gemlik	Horses (from a military center)	85	5 (6)	Benedek's sedimentation		Bakirci et al. (2004)
Konya province	Horses	111	5 (4.5)	Benedek's sedimentation		Uslu and Guçlu (2007)
	Donkeys	81	3 (4)			
Different cities	Horses	620	20 (3.2)	Benedek's sedimentation		Soykan and Öge (2012)
Northwest	Sport horses (21 farms)	549	16 (2.9)	Sugar flotation (sp. gr. 1.28)	9 of 21 farms with positive horses, aged <1 years 4 of 26 positive, aged 1–2 years 5 of 233 positive, aged 3–5 years 4 of 125 positive, aged >5 years 3 of 165 positive	Gülegen et al. (2016)

(Continued)

Table 19.3 (Continued) *Eimeria leuckarti* Prevalence in Equids Using Fecal Examinations

Country	Host	Number Tested	Number Positive (%)	Method Used	Remarks	Reference
Uganda	Donkeys	26	1	Sedimentation-flotation		Nakayima et al. (2017)
United Kingdom	Horses	1836	6 (0.3)	NS	Quarterly surveillance reports 2016, reported as "coccidia"	Anonymous (2016a,b, 2017a,b)
	Horses	2274	22 (1.0)	NS	Quarterly surveillance reports 2017, reported as "coccidia"	Anonymous (2017c,d,e, 2018)
United States						
Montana	Horses	22	13	Sugar flotation (sp. gr. 1.25)	Repeated examinations, 25–400 OPG	McQueary et al. (1977)
Kentucky	Thoroughbred (13 farms)	164 foals	67 (40.9)	Sugar flotation (sp. gr. 1.28)	Repeated examinations in 1986, positive foals aged 38–85 days, positive foals on 11 of 13 farms	Lyons et al. (1988)
Kentucky	Thoroughbred (14 farms)	733 foals	305 (41.6)	Sugar flotation (sp. gr. 1.28)	Repeated examinations in 2003, positive foals aged 29–191 days, positive foals on all 14 farms	Lyons and Tolliver (2004)
Kentucky	Thoroughbred (7 farms)	349 foals	96 (28)	Sugar flotation (sp. gr. 1.28)	Repeated examinations in 2004, positive foals aged 28–301 days, positive foals on six of seven farms	Lyons et al. (2006)
Kentucky	Thoroughbred (3 farms)	79 foals	36 (47)	Sugar flotation (sp. gr. 1.28)	Repeated examinations in 2004, positive foals aged 81–300 days, positive foals on all three farms	Lyons et al. (2007)
Former Yugoslavia						
Slovenia	Rural horses / Horses (5 stud farms) / Lipizzan (Lipica stud farm)	2634 / 460 / 107	24 (0.9) / 12 (2.6) / 39 (36.4)	Flotation (sp. gr. 1.53)	Aged <1 years 75% positive, aged 1–3 years 26% positive, aged >3 years 0.5% positive	Dolenc (1966)
Serbia	Horses	62	10 (16)	NS		Vujić et al. (1983)

Source: For full citations, see Dubey, J.P., Bauer, C. 2018. *Vet. Parasitol.* 256, 58–70.
Note: In bold are additions to Dubey and Bauer.
Abbreviations: NS, not stated; OPG, oocysts per gram of feces; Sp. gr., specific gravity.

Table 19.4 *Eimeria leuckarti* Single/Isolated Reports in Equids Using Fecal Examinations

Country	Host	Number Tested	Remarks	References
Austria	Horse, pony	3	Adults	Kutzer (1969)
Denmark	Horse	1	Imported horse	Henriksen (1975)
Germany	Donkey	1		Reichenow (1940)
	Horse, donkey, Asian wild ass, zebra	NS	Living in zoological garden; Przewalski's horses were negative	Tscherner (1978)
Iceland	Horse	NS		**Eydal**[509a]
India				
Mumbai	Horse	1		Hiregaudar (1956)
Chennai	Race horse	1		Achuthan and Alwar (1972)
Russia	Horse	1	11 years old	Bundina and Khrustalev (2016)
Turkey	Horse	7	Foals	Oğuz (1971)
United States				
Nebraska	Donkey	1	9-month-old foal	Benbrook and Sloss (1962)
Washington	Thoroughbred	7	1- to 6-month-old foals	Dunlap (1970)
Georgia	Horse	1	11-month-old foal	Kistner et al. (1972)
Texas	Miniature horse	1	6-month-old foal with "acute" diarrhea	Eugster and Jones (1985)

Source: For full citations, see Dubey, J.P., Bauer, C. 2018. *Vet. Parasitol.* 256, 58–70.
Note: In bold is addition to Dubey and Bauer.
Abbreviation: NS, not stated.

common in foals than in adult equids (Tables 19.2 through 19.4). Both findings indicate that an immunity against *E. leuckarti* infection is acquired.

19.3 PREVALENCE AND EPIDEMIOLOGY

E. leuckarti infections occur worldwide and have been reported from many countries (Tables 19.2 through 19.4). In general, the prevalence of fecal oocyst excretion is low but much higher in foals than in adult animals (Table 19.3). In stud farms, 75%–100% of the foals can be positive as observed in longitudinal studies.[88,95,377,942,1102–1105] The monthly prevalence of oocyst excretion may vary from 1.8% to 5.4%.[942]

E. leuckarti is a parasite occurring mainly in stud farms (Table 19.3). In studies where foals and their dams had been repeatedly tested, mostly foals excreted oocysts.[88,93–95] Foals can acquire the infection on the day of birth,[95,377,1102,1103–1105] probably rather from the contaminated environment than from oocysts excreted by their mares because of the long sporulation time. Under field conditions, oocysts were found in foals as young as 28 days.[1102–1105] The finding of oocysts in feces of a 15-day-old foal was considered passive excretion of unsporulated oocysts ingested from the environment.[1102] The oocyst excretion can start soon after turnout onto pasture in early spring,[88,95,377,942] suggesting oocysts overwintered on the pasture after sporulation during the previous grazing period. This is also because unsporulated *E. leuckarti* oocysts are killed even by brief freezing.[89] An oocyst excretion can be observed in most months but is mainly found in spring and autumn.[88,377,942] The individual oocyst

output is usually very low (<100 oocysts per gram feces) (Table 19.3).

19.4 PATHOGENICITY, PATHOLOGY, AND CLINICAL SIGNS

E. leuckarti is considered only mildly pathogenic. Its endogenous stages were found in histological sections of intestines of approximately 50 equids from several countries (Table 19.2). In most instances, there are only minor lesions. Parasitized villi may be atrophied without erosions or ulcers.[721] An eosinophilic infiltration is often present, but it is uncertain if the response was to *E. leuckarti* or to concurrent helminth infections. Lesions characterized by hemorrhage and mild or severe mononuclear cell infiltration have also been described.[1653] In most of these reports, infections were considered incidental. However, in a few cases, *E. leuckarti* was considered as the cause of or contributing to enteritis in foals.[102,1548,1793] There is only one report on a foal with acute diarrhea excreting *E. leuckarti* oocyst, but other infectious agents were not excluded.[508] In all successful experimental *E. leuckarti* infections, the equids fed oocysts remained asymptomatic.[73,74,89,377,1169]

19.5 DIAGNOSIS

In vivo, an *E. leuckarti* infection is diagnosed by the detection of oocysts in feces (Figure 19.1A, Table 19.1). For this, it is important to use a sedimentation technique or flotation methods using solutions with a specific gravity of 1.25 or higher (e.g., Sheather's sugar flotation) because the oocysts are large and heavy; saturated sodium chloride solution is unsuitable.[89,930,1403] Postmortem, the diagnosis is made by histological sections in which the presence of thick and large parasitophorous vacuoles in the lamina propria of jejunum and ileum are diagnostic, because occasionally the contained parasite stages fall out of the section (Table 19.2).[74,377] Mature microgamonts are macroscopically visible as small white spots and are characterized by the presence of microgametes or numerous nuclei. Macrogamonts can be distinguished by the presence of large (up to 15 μm wide) eosinophilic wall-forming bodies (Figure 19.1C). Oocysts are easily recognizable by their dark brown wall and, in longitudinal sections, the ovoid shape.

19.6 CONTROL

There is no information on therapeutic or preventive measurements to control *E. leuckarti* infection, probably because of its very low pathogenicity.

REFERENCES

43a, 73, 74, 88, 89, 93, 94, 95, 102, 104, 163, 272, 299, 377, 430, 451, 508, 509a, 543, 607, 701, 721, 836, 898, 925, 930, 942, 1102–1105, 1169, 1317, 1363, 1403, 1530, 1548, 1612, 1653, 1704, 1709, 1793

CHAPTER 20

Coccidiosis in Dogs (*Canis familiaris*)

J. P. Dubey and D. S. Lindsay

CONTENTS

20.1 INTRODUCTION AND HISTORY

Although coccidian parasites have been known in dog feces for more than a century, until 1960 little was known regarding their life cycles.[438] We previously reviewed in detail the history and biology of coccidial infections in dogs.[438] Here, we present essential information of coccidiosis in dogs.

There are no valid species of *Eimeria* infecting dogs; they are considered pseudoparasites resulting from ingestion of viscera on feces of rodents or other animals.

20.2 *CYSTOISOSPORA* INFECTIONS

Currently, there are four species of *Cystoisospora* considered to be valid in dogs, *C. canis*, *C. ohioensis*, *C. burrowsi*, and *C. neorivolta* (Table 20.1). Of these, *C. canis* is distinctive because of its large-sized oocysts, whereas the latter three are grouped as *C. ohioensis*–like because their oocysts overlap in size.[438] Extraintestinal stages of

C. canis, *C. neorivolta*, and *C. burrowsi* in tissues of dogs are unknown; however, biological evidence indicated that *C. ohioensis* invaded the spleens and mesenteric lymph nodes of dogs fed oocysts; dogs fed individual extraintestinal tissues excreted oocysts.[414] Monozoic tissue cysts are present in mice infected with oocysts of *C. ohioensis* or *C. canis* and tissues containing these monozoic cysts produce patent infections in dogs and coyotes.[417]

20.2.1 *Cystoisospora canis* (Neméséri, 1959) Frenkel, 1977

Information on life-cycle stages is summarized in Table 20.1. *C. canis* oocysts are the largest among canine coccidia, measuring 34–40 × 28–32 μm. *C. canis* multiplies asexually and sexually in the lamina propria of both small and large intestines (Table 20.1). Dogs excreted *C. canis* oocysts after being fed tissues from sheep, camels, donkeys, pigs, and water buffalos, demonstrating that these animal species can serve as paratenic hosts for *C. canis*.[717,718,1874] The ultrastructure of the monozoic tissue cysts of *C. canis* has been described from the mesenteric lymph nodes of experimentally infected mice,[1126] and coyotes that ingested tissues of mice orally inoculated with *C. canis* oocysts excreted *C. canis* oocysts with an appropriate prepatent period.[417]

C. canis can be pathogenic.[438] Some of the dogs experimentally infected with 10,000 or more oocysts became ill and developed diarrhea.[34,160,971,1191,1237,1406] Lesions included villous atrophy, rare foci of inflammation, and desquamation of villar contents into the lumen.[438]

Dogs experimentally infected with *C. canis* developed immunity to reexcretion of *C. canis* oocysts.[971] However, there was no cross-protection between *C. canis* and *C. ohioensis*.[744]

20.2.2 *Cystoisospora ohioensis* (Dubey, 1975) Frenkel, 1977

C. ohioensis oocysts are smaller than *C. canis* and measure 18–27 × 16–25 µm (Table 20.1). Its asexual and sexual development occurs in surface epithelium of intestines only, irrespective of the ingestion of oocysts or tissue cysts (Table 20.1).

Mice, sheep, camel, donkey, pigs, and water buffalo can be paratenic hosts for *C. ohioensis*. Tissue cysts were identified in mesenteric lymph nodes of mice fed *C. ohioensis* oocysts.[441] Dogs fed tissues of experimentally infected mice excreted *C. ohioensis* oocysts.[414] Dogs fed tissues of naturally exposed tissues of camel,[717,718] sheep,[718] swine, donkey, and water buffalo[1874] excreted *C. ohioensis* oocysts; there was no microscopic confirmation of monozoic tissue cysts in these reports. However, in another study, monozoic tissue cysts could be found by excysting using pepsin digestion.[743,1272]

In two studies, experimentally infected young pups developed coccidiosis after infection with *C. ohioensis*.[160,415] The inoculated pups developed diarrhea. Histologically, stunted villi, necrosis, and desquamation of villar tips were found.[415] Weaned pups inoculated with *C. ohioensis* became immune as judged by lack of clinical disease and excretion of oocysts after challenge.[415]

C. ohioensis–associated coccidiosis with vomiting, anorexia, diarrhea, and dehydration was reported in a naturally infected 3-month-old female Maltese puppy.[962]

20.2.3 *Cystoisospora neorivolta* (Dubey and Mahrt, 1978) Frenkel, 1977

The measurements and structure of oocysts or tissue cysts of *C. neorivolta* are unknown.[440] It develops both asexually

Table 20.1 Comparison of *Cystoisospora* spp. Infections in Dogs

Character	C. canis (Neméséri, 1959)	C. ohioensis (Dubey, 1975)	C. neorivolta (Dubey and Mahrt,1978)	C. burrowsi (Trayser and Todd, 1978)	C. ohioensis–like
Location of endogenous stages	Small and large intestines	Entire length of small intestines	Distal one-half of small intestines	Distal three-fifths of small intestines	Distal one-half of small intestines
Villus[a]	LP	Epi	LP + Epi	LP + Epi	LP + Epi
Number of asexual generations	Three or more	Four or more	Four or more	Two	Two or more
Schizonts	Present	Present	Present	Not reported	Present
Multinucleated zoites					
Microgamonts Sections	20–38 × 14–26[b] (27 × 18)	13–17 × 8–15 (15.3 × 11.4)	10–22 × 7–18 (14.2 × 10.1)	13–27 × 10–21 (19.8 × 14.1)	7–12 × 5–10 (9.6 × 7)
Smears	No data	24–30 × 15–24 (21.7 × 17.6)	No data	No data	15–25 × 9–19 (19.5 × 15.6)
Macrogamonts Sections	22–29 × 14–23 (25 × 18)	13–17 × 11–12 (14.5 × 12.8)	11–15 × 9–13 (12.6 × 10.8)	11–25 × 8–18 (17.1 × 11.5)	10–16 × 9–13 (12.5 × 10.8)
Smears	No data	21–26 × 17–25 (21.7 × 17.6)	No data	No data	12–24 × 12–21 (18–1 × 15.7)
Prepatent period	9–12 days	4–5 days	6 days	7–11 days	Unknown
Oocysts Sections	No data	15–19 × 13–16 (16.5 × 14.6)	13–15 × 11–13 (12.6 × 11.4)	No data	12–17 × 10–13 (13 × 11.5)
Smears	34–40 × 28–32 (36 × 30)	18–27 × 16–25 (22.3 × 20.6)	No data	16–23 × 14–22 (21 × 18)	16–23 × 14–20 (19 × 16.4)
Sporocysts	18–21 × 15–18 (20 × 16)	15–19 × 10–13 (17 × 12)	No data	12–16 × 8–11 (14.4 × 9.7)	
Sporozoites	No data	9–13 × 2.5–5.0			
References	Lepp and Todd [971]; Dubey and Lindsay[438,438a,439]	Dubey[410,414,415]	Dubey and Mahrt[440]	Trayser and Todd[1703]; Rommel and Zielasko[1434]	Dubey et al.[448]; Dubey[428]

[a] Epithelium (Epi), lamina propria (LP).
[b] Range in µm followed by (mean) in µm.

and sexually in host cells located within the lamina propria of the small and large intestines and occasionally epithelial cells on villi.[440,1116] The dogs experimentally infected with *C. neorivolta* by Mahrt[1116] remained asymptomatic.

20.2.4 *Cystoisospora burrowsi* (Trayser and Todd, 1978) Frenkel, 1977

C. burrowsi oocysts are 16–23 × 14–22 μm. Its developmental stages are in epithelial cells and in the lamina propria near the tips of villi in the posterior three-fifths of the small intestine and cecum. There are two generations of schizonts. Dogs experimentally infected with *C. burrowsi* remained asymptomatic (Table 20.1). Mice and rats were shown to be paratenic hosts based on feeding tissues to naïve dogs. The prepatent period was 7–11 days, irrespective of the stage of the parasite ingested.

20.2.5 *Cystoisospora ohioensis* Complex

It is not certain whether *C. burrowsi* is different from *C. neorivolta*. There are no archived specimens of *C. burrowsi*. Therefore, the real identity of these species will remain unknown. Therefore, for diagnostic purposes, this group of parasites is called *C. ohioensis*–like.

Dubey et al.[448] reported clinical coccidiosis in a naturally infected dog in association with a *C. ohioensis*–like organism. It differed structurally and biologically from *C. ohioensis* (Table 20.1).

20.2.6 Transmission of *Cystoisospora* spp.–Like Oocysts from Wild Canids to Domestic Dogs

Wild canids are thought to share *C. canis* and *C. ohioensis*–like oocysts, but little is known of their cross-transmission to the domestic dog. *C. canis* isolated from a domestic dog was transmitted successfully to coyote (*Canis latrans*) via paratenic host.[417]

Bledsoe[138] transmitted *Cystoisospora vulpina* (Nieschulz and Bos, 1933) Frenkel, 1977, from silver foxes (*Vulpes vulpes*) to the domestic dog; *C. vulpina* oocysts are morphologically *C. canis*–like. Five coccidia-free dogs fed oocysts from the fox excreted *C. vulpina* oocysts with a prepatent period of 6 or 7 days; one control dog did not excrete oocysts. These studies indicate that these parasites might not be strictly host specific.

20.3 CLINICAL COCCIDIOSIS

Before the recognition of enteric viral pathogens of dogs and effective immunization against distemper virus infection in the 1960s, coccidiosis was considered a common disease affecting as many as 50% of dogs (reviewed in Dubey and Lindsay[438]). In the last 20 years, there have been only a few reports of clinical coccidiosis in dogs.[296,438,575,852,1275] Depression, weakness, loss of appetite, diarrhea, and dehydration were the common clinical signs. Blood can sometimes be present, but there is not extensive hemorrhagic diarrhea.

By far the most striking case with a definitive diagnosis of clinical coccidiosis was due to a *C. ohioensis*–like organism in a 10-week-old Chihuahua pup with a history of weight loss. The pup had yellow pasty feces and died despite sulfaguanidine therapy for 2 days.[448] Severe enteritis was associated with asexual and sexual stages of the *C. ohioensis*–like organism.

20.4 PREVALENCE AND EPIDEMIOLOGY

Coccidia are prevalent in dogs worldwide (Table 20.2). The ingestion of food and water contaminated with oocysts is the major mode of transmission of *Cystoisospora* infections in dogs. Although *Cystoisospora* stages occur in extraintestinal organs, there is no evidence for lactogenic or congenital transmission. The role of paratenic hosts in the natural epidemiology of coccidial transmission is unknown. Experimentally, newborn puppies are susceptible to infection. Coccidiosis is a disease of young dogs, and most become infected by 4 months of age.[160]

During a detailed epidemiological investigation in a commercial kennel in South Africa, oocysts were detected in pups starting at 3 weeks, and by week 5 oocysts were seen in 15 of 16 litters.[1347] The oocyst excretion peaked at 5 weeks reaching 139,600 oocysts per gram of feces (OPG), and there was no pattern of association between oocyst excretion in pups and bitches. The authors concluded that the most likely source of infection in pups was the oocysts excreted by their dams.[1347] Similar results were reported from Germany[332] and Austria.[160] In another study from Austria, 3-week-old puppies were already excreting oocysts; as many as 95,250 OPG were detected in some pups.[1395]

These findings obtained on dogs from breeding establishments were corroborated by Barutzki and Schaper[82] in a very large sample of pet dogs. Among the 24,677 feces of dogs submitted to a commercial diagnostic laboratory,[81] data from 2319 dogs up to 1 year of age were analyzed with respect to enteropathogens. *Cystoisospora* spp. oocysts were first seen at the beginning of 4 weeks of age. Peaks of infection were at week 6 for *C. ohioensis*–like organisms, and week 15 for *C. canis*. Coinfections of *Toxocara canis*, *Giardia* sp. were seen starting in the sixth week.

In a study of families of dogs in Germany, *Cystoisospora* spp. oocysts were detected in feces of 41 of 50 litters and in 25 of 37 bitches[605,606]; the prevalence of *C. canis* (16 litters) was much lower than that of *C. ohioensis*–like (41 litters) parasites.

Table 20.2   Prevalence of Cystoisospora in Feces of Dogs

Country	Region	Number of Dogs	C. canis	C. ohioensis–like	C. sp.	Remarks Source, Others	Reference[a]
			Number of Positives (%)				
Albania	Tirana	111	19 (17.1)	35 (31.5)		Intestinal tracts of stray dogs	Xhaxhiu et al. (2011)
Argentina	Buenos Aires	2,193	66 (3.0)	264 (12.0)		Pets	Fontanarrosa et al. (2006)
Australia	Victoria	690	20 (2.9)	110 (15.9)		Shelter	Blake and Overend (1982)
Australia	Sydney	110		6 (5.5)		Clinics	Collins et al. (1983)
Australia	Southern Victoria	493		39 (7.9)		Pets, veterinary, kennel, stray dogs, and fecal samples from public areas	Johnston and Gasser (1993)
Australia	Kimberley	182		4 (2.2)		Aboriginal communities	Meloni et al. (1993)
Australia	Perth	421	29 (6.9)	19 (4.5)		Refuges, pet shops, vet clinics, exercise areas, breeding kennels	Bugg et al. (1999)
Australia	Not specified	1,400	15 (1.1)	49 (3.5)		Pets	Palmer et al. (2008)
Austria	Carinthia	220		11 (5.0)		Clinics. Stated only coccidia, no genus	Krebitz (1982)
Austria	Vienna	1,246	83 (6.7)	122 (9.8)		Shelter, pets	Supperer and Hinaidy (1986)
Austria	Vienna	3,106		155 (5.0)		Includes all coccidia	Arnold et al. (2004)
Austria	Vienna	3,590	89 (2.5)	168 (4.7)	314 (8.7);17.8% had both C canis and C. ohioensis–like	Diagnostic center	Buehl et al. (2006)
Austria	Vienna and surrounding	1,486	13 (0.9)			Species not distinguished	Hinney et al. (2017)
Belgium	Brussels	2,432	32 (1.3)	61 (2.5)	5 (0.2)	Brussels dogs	Cotteleer and Famerée (1980)
Belgium	Brussels	52			2 (3.8)	Necropsied dogs	Gerin et al. (1980)
Belgium	Several regions	2,324	85 (3.7)			Stray	Vanparijs et al. (1991)
Brazil	Guanabara	251	13 (5.2)	19 (7.5)		Not stated	Lage et al. (1974)
Brazil	Rio de Janeiro	197	6 (3.0)	43 (21.8)		Stray	Franken et al. (1975)
Brazil	São Paulo	167	5 (3.0)	2 (1.2)		Not stated	Ogassawara et al. (1978)
Brazil	São Paulo	271		23 (8.5)		Pets and stray	Oliveira-Sequeira et al. (2002)
Brazil	Santa Catarina	158		10 (6.3)		Stray	Blazius et al. (2005)
Brazil	Paraná	280		21 (7.5)		Clinics	Tesserolli et al. (2005)
Brazil	Ribeirão Preto	331		11 (3.3)		Feces pools from recreational areas	Capuano and Rocha (2006)
Brazil	Santa Maria	109		20 (18.3)		Pet shops and breeding kennels	da Silva et al. (2008)
Brazil	Botucatu	254		9 (3.5)		Pets and stray	Katagiri and Oliveira-Sequeira (2008, 2010)
Brazil	Botucatu	872 feces		75 (8.6)		Clinic	Torrico et al. (2008)
Brazil	Minas Gerais	141		2 (1.4)		Feces from 42 squares in the city of Belo Horizonte	Ribeiro et al. (2013)
Brazil	São Paulo	278		33 (11.9)		Urban and rural pets	Oliveira-Arbex et al. (2017)
Bulgaria	Stara Zagora	20		2 (10.0)		Stray	Georgieva et al. (1999)
Cambodia	Preah Vihear	94	13 (13.8)			Pets	Schär et al. (2014)

(Continued)

Table 20.2 (*Continued*) Prevalence of *Cystoisospora* in Feces of Dogs

Country	Region	Number of Dogs	C. canis	C. ohioensis–like	C. sp.	Remarks Source, Others	Reference[a]
Canada	Several regions, northwest	959		85 (8.9)		Pets	Unrih et al. (1973)
Canada	Montréal	239	4 (1.7)	83 (34.7)		Stray	Seah et al. (1975)
Canada	Prince Edward Island	209			Pet store 49% of 69, 13% of 78 from clinic, 6% of 62 from shelter	Various sources. Only dogs <1 year of age were included	Uehlinger et al. (2013)
Canada	Several regions	1,086			113 (10.4)	Shelter	Villeneuve et al. (2015)
Chile	San Miguel	480	9 (1.9)	18 (3.8)		Urban areas	Gorman et al. (1989)
Chile	Santiago	972			89 (9.2)	Pets	López et al. (2006)
Colombia	Medellín, Antioquia	68	3 (4.4)			Stray	**Sierra-Cifuentes et al.**[1574]
Cuba	Havana	293			27 (9.2)	Pets and stray	**Luis Enrique et al.**[1099]
Czech Republic	Prague	500	16 (3.2)	6 (1.2)		Feces from 10 Prague housing developments	Valkounová (1982)
Czech Republic	Brno	663	2 (0.3)	14 (2.1)		Clinic	Svobodová et al. (1984)
Czech Republic	South Moravia	699	51 (7.3)	26 (3.7)		Farm dogs	Borkovcová (2003)
Czech Republic	Prague	4,320 feces			449 (10.4)	Fecal samples from public areas, animal shelter, rural areas	Dubná et al. (2007)
Denmark	Zealand	31			7 (22.6)	*Coccidia* spp. in hunted dogs	Tonsberg et al. (2004)
Ecuador	Galapagos Islands	97	4 (4.0)			Pets	Gingrich et al. (2010)
Egypt	Dakahlia Governorate	125	122 (97.6)	49 (39.2)		Stray. Oocysts measured	Abdel Magied et al. (1982)
Egypt	Ismailia	500	23 (4.6)	65 (13.0)	88 (17.6)	Feces from the roadsides and public places	Abou-Eisha and Abdel-Aal (1995)
France	Paris	500			25 (5.0)		Petithory and Ardoin (1990)
France	Paris	93			8 (8.6)	Clinic	Beugnet et al. (2000)
France	St. Pierre	57	5 (8.8)			Pets, shelter	Bridger and Whitney (2009)
Germany	Not stated	512			37 (7.2)	Data includes all coccidia	Brahm (1974)
Germany	Hamburg, Hannover	565	13 (2.3)	13 (2.3)		Shelter, clinics	Potters (1978); Boch et al. (1981)
Germany	South Germany	500	4 (0.8)	20 (4.0)		Pets; *C. burrowsi*: 9 (1.8%)	Böhm (1979); Boch et al. (1979, 1981)
Germany	Rhineland-Palatinate	725			51 (7.1)	Stated only coccidia, no genus	Jonas (1981)
Germany	Northwest Germany	3,029		130 (4.3)		Rural and urban	Bauer and Stoye (1984)
Germany	Munich	554			32 (5.8)	Stated only coccidia, no genus	Deumer (1984)
Germany	Hannover	92	1 (1.0)	4 (4.3)		Shelter	Schwennicke (1985)
Germany	Berlin	141			10 (7.0)		Jungmann et al. (1986)

(*Continued*)

Table 20.2 (Continued) Prevalence of Cystoisospora in Feces of Dogs

Country	Region	Number of Dogs	Number of Positives (%)			Remarks Source, Others	Reference[a]
			C. canis	C. ohioensis–like	C. sp.		
Germany	Wuppertal	1,246			140 (11.2)	Mentioned coccidia, no genus	Emde (1988)
Germany	Southern Germany	50 litters and 37 bitches	8 (16.0) litters and 4 (10.8) bitches	18 (36.0) litters and 9 (24.3) bitches		Kennel (see text)	Gothe and Reichler (1990a,b)
Germany	Northern Germany	3,329			140 (4.2)	Pets, clinics from 1984 to 1991	Epe et al. (1993)
Germany	Rostock	1,555			31 (2.0)		Dibbert and Methling (1995)
Germany	Northern Germany	2,289			49 (2.1)	Pets, clinics from 1993 to 1997	Epe et al. (1998)
Germany	Not specified	8,438	219 (2.6)	464 (5.5)	499 (5.9)	Clinic	Barutzki and Schaper (2003)
Germany	Central Germany	270	5 (2.0)	24 (9.0)		Shelter	Cirak and Bauer (2004)
Germany	Northern Germany	1,281			30 (2.3)	Pets, clinics from 1998 to 2002	Epe et al. (2004)
Germany	Halle	340	2 (0.6)	4 (1.1)		Clinics, shelter	Gottschalk and Prange (2004)
Germany		141			5 (3.5)		Beck (2006)
Germany	Several regions	24,677	588 (2.4)	973 (3.9)	1,391 (5.6)	Pets (see text)	Barutzki and Schaper (2011)
Germany	Lower Saxony	445			11 (2.5)	Stray and foster	Becker et al. (2012)
Germany	Several regions	2,319	See text	See text		Pets, <1 year old (see text)	Barutzki and Schaper (2013)
Germany	Several regions	2,731			154 (5.6)	Clinics	Raue et al. (2017)
Ghana	Greater Accra region	380			33 (8.7)	Pets and hunting	Johnson et al. (2015)
Greece	Thessaloniki	232		9 (3.9)		Pets and hunting	Haralabidis et al. (1988)
Greece	Serres	281			11 (3.9)	Shepherd and hunting	Papazahariadou et al. (2007)
Greece	Several regions	1,036			129 (12.4)	Clinic, shelter	Symeonidou et al. (2017)
Hungary	Eastern and Northern Hungary	220	18 (8.2)				Nemeseri (1960)
Hungary		490			17 (3.5)	Pets, animal ambulance service, and shelter	Fok et al. (2001)
India	Maharashtra	385	18 (4.6)	6 (1.5)	9 (2.3)	Stray	Shastri (1989)
India	Assam	101			2 (2.0)	Pets	Traub et al. (2002)
Iran	Teheran	255		10 (4.0)		Pets	Mirzayans et al. (1972)
Iran	Kerman	100	1 (1.0)			Pets	Mirzaei and Fooladi (2013)
Iran	Hamadan	1,500			41 (2.7)	Pets and stray	Sardarian et al. (2015)
Iran	Meta-analysis	1,539			5 (0.3)	Pets and stray	**Sarvi et al.**[1499]
Ireland	Dublin	612	20 (3.2)			Unwanted	**Garcia-Campos et al.**[581]
Iraq	Basra Province	93	6 (6.5)			Clinics	Al-Jassim et al. (2017)
Italy	Rome	100		14.0		Not stated	Pellegrino et al. (1953)
Italy	North	52			0		Petithory and Ardoin (1990)
Italy	Naples	6,288				395 (6.2%), Only coccidia mentioned	Sanna et al. (1993)
Italy	Naples	415	17 (4.1)			Feces collected from public sites	Rinaldi et al. (2006)
Italy	Veneto and Abruzzi	406			85 (21.0)	Pets, kennel, and stray	Capelli et al. (2006)

(Continued)

Table 20.2 (*Continued*)　Prevalence of Cystoisospora in Feces of Dogs

Country	Region	Number of Dogs	Number of Positives (%)			Remarks Source, Others	Reference[a]
			C. canis	C. ohioensis–like	C. sp.		
Italy	Tuscany	239			18 (7.5)	Pets	Riggio et al. (2013)
Japan	Iochigi City	1979 y (262); 1991 y (260)			6 (5.5); 10 (11.6)	Pets	Asano et al. (1992)
Japan	Hachinohe	1,105			81 (7.3)	Pets	Itoh et al. (2009)
Japan	Saitama	906	5 (0.6)	19 (2.1)		Shelter	Yamamoto et al. (2009)
Korea	Chonbuck	412		66 (16)			Baek et al. (1993)
Mexico	Northwest	380			17 (4.4%)	Stray	**Trasvina-Muñoz et al.[1702]**
Morocco	Rabat	57	2 (3.5)			Stray	Pandey et al. (1987)
Netherlands		224	3 (1.3)	3 (1.3)		Shelter	le Nobel et al. (2004)
Nigeria	Ibadan	203			29 (14.3)	Feces from streets	Ayinmode et al. (2016)
New Zealand	North Island	481	19 (4.0)	44 (9.2)			McKenna and Charleston (1980)
Philippines	Cebu	200			15 (7.5)	Pets and stray	Urgel et al. (2019)
Poland	Several regions	831			4 (0.5)	Asylums and clinics	Balicka-Ramisz et al. (2004)
Poland		135			10 (7.4)	Cystoisospora spp.	Michalczyk and Sokól (2008)
Poland	Chelmno	339			37 (10.9)	Feces collected from seven sites from accessible public areas	Felsmann et al. (2017)
Portugal	Évora	126			7 (5.5)	Shelter, clinics	Ferreira et al. (2011)
Portugal	Cantanhede	301			12 (4.0)	Rural	Cardoso et al. (2014)
Portugal	Ponte de Lima	592			56 (9.5)	Hunting, farm dogs, and feces from environment	Mateus et al. (2014)
Romania	Several regions	52	4 (7.7)	12 (23.1)		Shelter, kennels, shepherd, and household	Mircean et al. (2012)
Russia	Voronezh	587	9 (1.5)			2008–2010	**Menyaylova and Gaponov[1178]**
Russia	Moscow	2,652	59 (2.2)	129 (4.9)		2004–2009	**Kurnosova[926]**
Russia	Vladivostok	94			5 (5.3)	2014	**Moskvina and Zheleznova[1210]**
Russia	Moscow region; cities of Kirov, Astrakhan and Novosibirsk	430	7 (1.6)	0		Shelters; 2010–2016	**Yastreb and Shaytanov[1856]**
Russia	Perm	505			32 (6.3)	2014	**Sivkova and Sogrina[1580]**
Russia	Moscow	1,752	18 (1)		36 (2)	2012–2017, pets	**Kurnosova et al.[927]**
Slovakia	Bratislava	457			19 (4.1)	Feces from public sites	Totková et al. (2006)
Slovakia	Several regions	752			78 (10.4)	Pets, guard dogs, hunting dogs, shelter and center for import/export of animals	Szabová et al. (2007)
South Africa	Durban and Coast	240			3 (1.3)	Stray	Mukaratirwa and Singh (2010)
Spain	Zaragoza	81			8 (9.9)	Pets and stray	Causapé et al. (1996)

(*Continued*)

Table 20.2 (Continued)　Prevalence of Cystoisospora in Feces of Dogs

Country	Region	Number of Dogs	Number of Positives (%)			Remarks Source, Others	Reference[a]
			C. canis	C. ohioensis–like	C. sp.		
Spain	Barcelona	505			3 (0.6)	Pets, stray. Stated only coccidia, no genus	Gracenea et al. (2009)
Spain	Murcia	265	27 (10.2)			Pets, shelter, stray	Martínez-Carrasco et al. (2007)
Spain	Córdoba	1,800	396 (22.0)		184 (10.2)	Homeless or housed	Martínez-Moreno et al. (2007)
Spain	Madrid	1,562			47 (3.0)	Shelter	Miró et al. (2007)
Spain	Barcelona	544			45 (8.2)	Shelters	**Ortuno and Castella**[1289]
Switzerland		662			30 (4.5)		Seiler et al. (1983)
Switzerland	Lugano	371			11 (3.0)	Shelter	Deplazes et al. (1995)
Switzerland	Bern	505			19 (3.7)	Clinics, pets, and farm dogs	Sager et al. (2006)
Switzerland	Zurich	402			8 (2.0)	Samples from 14 grassland areas, disposal units for dog waste bags	Hauser et al. (2015)
Taiwan		376	28 (7.5)			Feces from imported dogs	Ho et al. (2006)
Thailand	Bangkok	229			23 (10.0)	Pets	Inpankaew et al. (2007)
Thailand	Nakhon Nayok	500			0	Shelter	Rojekittikhun et al. (2014)
United Kingdom	Not specified	608			11 (1.8)	Hearing dogs. Stated only coccidia, no genus	Guest et al. (2007)
United States	Ohio	113	4 (3.5)	5 (4.4)		Clinics	Catcott (1946)
United States	Illinois	139	22 (15.9)	25 (18.0)		Pets, stray, and breeding kennels dogs; morphology described	Levine and Ivens (1965)
United States	New Jersey	660	90 (13.6)	70 (11.0)		Stray	Burrows and Lillis (1967)
United States	Chicago	846			14 (1.6)	Urban	Jaskoski (1971)
United States	Ohio	500	9 (1.8)	18 (3.6)		Stray	Streitel and Dubey (1976)
United States	Missouri	2,093			398 (19.0)	Pets	Becker et al. (1977)
United States	Atlanta	143			13 (9.1)	Pets and kennels	Stehr-Green et al. (1987)
United States	Pennsylvania	6,555	80 (1.2)	129 (2.0)		Clinic	Gates and Nolan (2009)
Venezuela	Maracaibo	614			50 (8.1)	Pets	Ramírez-Barrios et al. (2004)
Zambia	Several regions	540			31 (5.7)	Pets	Nonaka et al. (2011)

Source: Modified from Dubey, J.P., Lindsay, D.S. 2019. *Vet. Parasitol.* 266, 34–55.

[a] For references, see Dubey and Lindsay; additional references missed in Dubey and Lindsay are in bold.

20.5 DIAGNOSIS

Cystoisospora infection in dogs can be diagnosed by identification of the unsporulated oocysts with any of the fecal flotation methods commonly used to diagnose parasitic infections. In dogs, only *C. canis* can be identified with certainty by oocyst size and shape (Figure 20.1). The oocysts of the other three species of *Cystoisospora*, namely, *C. ohioensis, C. burrowsi,* and *C. neorivolta,* may overlap in size, and their distinction is not clinically important. Rarely, epithelial casts may be found in feces; schizonts, merozoites, and partially formed oocysts can be found in smears made in normal saline (not water). Unsporulated oocysts measuring 10–14 μm should be either *Hammondia/Toxoplasma/Neospora,* and bioassay or specific polymerase chain reaction assays are needed for definitive identification.[1508] Unlike other coccidia, *Sarcocystis* species oocysts/sporocysts are excreted sporulated. They would not be seen in dogs who were not fed meat or in puppies.

Molecular data using the 18S rRNA and internal transcribed spacer (ITS)-1 genes indicates close phylogenetic similarity between dog and cat *Cystoisospora* species,[80,690,177,1148,1480] and this information may be useful in differential diagnosis of *C. ohioensis*–like parasites.[962]

20.6 TREATMENT

The presence of underlying disease or host immunosuppression should be suspected when coccidial infections persist for extended periods in older animals or when associated with chronic diarrhea. Treatment is often indicated in bitches and their newborn puppies because of the severity of clinical signs at this age. If diarrhea or dehydration is severe, parenteral fluid therapy must be considered as a supportive measure. Blood transfusion may be required when severe intestinal hemorrhage results in anemia.[434] Specific therapy involves the use of drugs that are coccidiostatic rather than curative (Table 20.3).

Sulfonamides have long been the drugs of choice for the treatment of canine coccidiosis.[943] Rapid-acting sulfonamides, such as sulfadimethoxine or sulfaguanidine, can be given alone or in combination with other antifolate drugs such as trimethoprim. Trimethoprim-sulfonamide offers the advantages of being readily available and being less toxic than other drugs. It should be considered a drug of first choice; however, to reduce the chance of toxicity, dosage rates vary per the body weight (Table 20.3). Amprolium is considered an effective preventive and treatment for coccidiosis in kenneled puppies. Although it is not approved for use in dogs, it can be administered as an undiluted liquid and a paste, but it is unpalatable in these forms.[434]

Currently, toltrazuril and ponazuril are most commonly used (Table 20.3); medication with these compounds reduced or stopped oocyst excretion both in naturally exposed and experimentally infected dogs (reviewed in Dubey and Lindsay[438]). Dosages of 10 mg/kg are effective in reducing oocysts and clinical signs.[332] Toltrazuril is relatively nontoxic even at the dose of 250 mg/kg.[246] Supportive therapy is needed to prevent dehydration.

20.7 PREVENTION

Coccidiosis tends to be a problem in unsanitary environments; however, once a "clean" kennel becomes contaminated with oocysts from an incoming pet, they are very difficult to eliminate. The fecal excretion of large numbers of environmentally resistant oocysts makes infection likely under such conditions. Animals should be housed in a way that does not allow contamination of food and water bowls by oocyst-laden soil or infected feces. Feces should be removed daily and incinerated. Oocysts survive freezing temperatures. Runs, cages, food utensils, and other implements should be disinfected by steam cleaning or immersion in boiling water or by a 10% ammonia solution. Animals should have limited access to intermediate hosts and should not be fed uncooked meat. Insect control is essential in animal quarters and food storage areas because cockroaches and flies may serve as mechanical vectors of oocysts. Coccidiostatic drugs can be given to infected bitches before or soon after whelping to control the spread of infection to puppies. Treatment of equipment with a steam cleaner or hot water (>70°C) is more effective in killing or damaging unsporulated oocysts than sporulated oocysts. Attempts should be made to minimize stress during the transport of puppies.

REFERENCES

34, 80–82, 138, 160, 177, 246, 296, 332, 410, 414, 415, 417, 428, 434, 438, 438a, 439–441, 448, 575, 581, 605, 606, 690, 717, 718, 743, 744, 852, 926, 927, 943, 962, 971, 1099, 1116, 1126, 1148, 1178, 1191, 1210, 1237, 1272, 1275, 1289, 1347, 1395, 1406, 1434, 1480, 1499, 1508, 1574, 1580, 1702, 1703, 1856, 1874

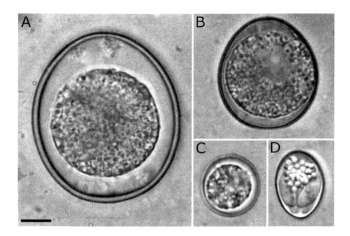

Figure 20.1 Unsporulated oocysts of canine coccidia. (A) *Cystoisospora canis,* (B) *C. ohioensis,* (C) *Hammondia heydorni,* and (D) *Sarcocystis* sp. All canid coccidia, except *Sarcocystis,* are excreted in feces unsporulated. Bar = 5 μm.

Table 20.3   Anticoccidial Drugs for Dogs

Drug[a]	Dose (mg/kg)[b]	Interval (Hours)	Duration (Days)
Sulfamethoxine[c]	50–60	24	5–20
Sulfaguanidine	100–200	8	5
Trimethoprim-sulfonamide*	30–60[d]	24	5
	15–30[e]	12–24	5
Ormetoprim-sulfadimethoxine*	66[f]	24	7–23
Furazolidone[g]	8–20	12–24	5
Amprolium	300–400 (total)[h]	24	5
	110–200 (total)[i]	24	7–12
Quinacrine	10	24	5
Toltrazuril	15–30	24	1–6[j]
Ponazuril	30–50[k]	24	1–7

Source: Reprinted from *Infectious Diseases of the Dog and Cat,* 4, Dubey, J.P., Greene, C.E., Greene, Copyright 2012, with permission from Elsevier.

[a]   Drugs given orally; * can also be given subcutaneously.
[b]   Dose per administration at specified interval.
[c]   Other sulfonamides, such as sulfadimidine and sulfaguanadine, can be used, but sulfaquinoxaline should not be used because it interferes with vitamin K synthesis and may result in hemorrhagic complications.
[d]   Greater than 4 kg body weight.
[e]   Less than 4 kg body weight.
[f]   11 mg ormetoprim and 55 mg of sulfadimethoxine.
[g]   When furazolidone is combined with sulfonamides, 50% of this dose is used. Not available in some countries.
[h]   Total dose per day. Lower dose recommended for puppies, with a maximum of 300 mg total per day. Has been added to drinking water at 1.5 tablespoon (23 mL) per gallon (3.8 L) water as a sole water source, with a duration not to exceed 10 days.
[i]   Total dose per day. Combine 150 mg amprolium and 25 mg sulfadimethoxine per kilogram per day for 14 days.
[j]   Doses of 30 mg/kg have been used for 1 day; however, treatment at half that dose for at least 3 days, repeating if needed, has been more effective in treatment of pups with coccidiosis without relapses.
[k]   Dose based on efficacy studies in pups.

CHAPTER 21

Coccidiosis in Cats (*Felis catus*)

J. P. Dubey

CONTENTS

21.1 INTRODUCTION AND HISTORY

Although *Isospora*-like coccidian parasites have been known in cat feces for more than a century, until 1970 they were considered not host specific and to have a direct fecal-oral transmission cycle confined to the feline intestine. In the 1970s, extraintestinal stages of *Isospora felis* and *I. rivolta* were found,[433,560] and they were reclassified under the genus *Cystoisospora*.[559]

Recently, the history, taxonomy, biology, and epidemiology of feline coccidiosis was reviewed in detail and a complete bibliography was provided.[424] Here, essential information is summarized, and citations missed in the review were included. There are no species of *Eimeria* in cats; they are considered pseudoparasites resulting from the ingestion of viscera of rodents or other animals. There are two species of *Cystoisospora* in cats, *C. felis* and *C. rivolta*.

21.2 *CYSTOISOSPORA FELIS* (WENYON, 1923) FRENKEL, 1977

21.2.1 Morphology and Life Cycle

Its oocysts are the largest in size among the feline coccidia. Unsporulated oocysts in feline species are ovoid, up to 53 μm long and up to 43 μm wide with a smooth wall, 1.3 μm thick. Measurements of sporulated oocysts, sporocysts, and sporozoites based on a clone culture of oocysts are shown in Table 21.1. Variability in its oocyst size was discussed recently.[424]

Information on *C. felis* biology is summarized in Table 21.1. The endogenous stages of *C. felis* occur in villar enterocytes of the small intestine (Figure 21.1). Ultrastructurally, development of *C. felis* in feline intestine is like other coccidians.[526–528] Extraintestinal stages of *C. felis* in cats are illustrated in Figure 1.9A–C, Chapter 1. Monozoic tissue cysts of *C. felis* are illustrated in Figure 1.9D–G, Chapter 1.

Mice and several other hosts can act as paratenic or transport hosts.[421,490,560,1048,1172] Bioassay studies revealed that rodents,[560] dog,[409] cattle,[518,1813] pigs,[1175,1176] camels,[717] albino mice,[556–558,698] and rabbit[297,313,314] can act as paratenic hosts. There are no ill effects of *C. felis* infection in paratenic hosts. Dung beetles and other arthropods can act as transport hosts for the oocysts.[1477]

C. felis is transmitted very efficiently by oral uptake of oocysts, and this is the main mode of transmission. However, some aspects of its transmission are a mystery because cats kept even in meticulous hygienic conditions can become infected.[1278] It is likely that adult cats may excrete low numbers of oocysts that are sources of infection

Table 21.1 Comparison of Two Species of *Cystoisospora* Infections in Cats

Character	*C. felis* (Wenyon, 1923) Frenkel, 1977	*C. rivolta* (Grassi, 1879) Frenkel, 1977
Location of endogenous stages in small intestine	Villi	Villi and glands of Lieberkühn
Number of asexual generations	Three or more	Three or more
Schizonts/types with multinucleated zoites	Present	Present
Microgamonts in sections	18–32 × 46 × 26 (46 × 26)[a]	9–15 × 6–9 (11.3 × 8.0)
Number of microgametes	>200	≤70
Macrogamonts		
Sections	16–22 × 8–13 (18 × 10)	11–18 × 5–13 (13.3 × 12.8)
Smears	ND	(18 × 16)
Prepatent period (days)	7–8 (ingestion of oocysts) 5–9 (ingestion of tissues)	6–7 (ingestion of oocysts or tissue cysts)
Oocysts		
Sections	ND	10–15 × 15–16 (16.5 × 14.6)
Smears	ND	17–24 × 17–23 (19.8 × 18.0)
In feces		
Unsporulated	ND	18–25 × 16–23 (22.3 × 19.7)
Sporulated	38–51 × 27–39 (42 × 31)	23–29 × 20–26 (25.4 × 23.4)
Sporocysts	20–26 × 17–22 (23 × 18)	13–21 × 10–15 (17.2 × 15.0)
Sporozoites	12–16 × 3–4 (13 × 3)	10–14 × 2.5–3.0 (12.4 × 2.8)
References	Dubey,[421] Shah[1535]	Dubey[416]

Abbreviation: ND, not done.

[a] Range (average), measurements in micrometers (μm).

for newborn kittens. Lactogenic and transplacental transmission from chronically infected queens has been suggested for *C. felis*.[1278] However, this mode of infection is unlikely. *C. felis* and *C. rivolta* oocysts were not found in feces of 48 kittens up to 106 days of age; the kittens were born to eight queens that were experimentally infected with *C. felis* and *C. rivolta* before pregnancy.[412] In summary, the postnatal ingestion of parasite from the environment (by ingestion of oocysts or infected tissues) is the only proven mode of transmission.

21.2.2 Immunosuppression Induced by *C. felis* and Reexcretion of *Toxoplasma* Oocysts

C. felis is biologically important with respect to certain other protozoan infections. It can modify *Toxoplasma gondii* oocyst excretion, and these oocysts are key in the transmission of the parasite to humans and other hosts. Cats excrete *T. gondii* oocysts for 1–2 weeks after eating infected tissues and seldom reexcrete oocysts. However, infection of cats with *C. felis* induces reexcretion of *T. gondii* oocysts in the absence of any clinical signs.[259,411,1278] The *C. felis*–induced relapse is specific because *C. rivolta* does not induce relapse of *T. gondii* infection, and the effect can be blocked by immunization of cats with *C. felis* before *T. gondii* infection.[411,413] Both *C. felis* and *T. gondii* can be acquired simultaneously if the intermediate hosts are infected with these coccidian parasites. Cats chronically infected with *T. gondii* can reexcrete *T. gondii* oocysts, not only after experimental infection with *C. felis* but also by spontaneous *C. felis* infection.[413] The mechanism of interaction of *C. felis* and *T. gondii* is not known, but these organisms share some antigens.[1277,1279]

21.3 *CYSTOISOSPORA RIVOLTA* (GRASSI, 1879) FRENKEL, 1977

Life-cycle stages are summarized in Figure 1.11, Chapter 1 and in Table 21.1. Unsporulated oocysts of *C. rivolta* are approximately two-thirds of the size of *C. felis* oocysts. Data on sizes of its oocysts, sporocysts, and sporozoites are summarized in Table 21.1. Asexual and sexual development of *C. rivolta* occurs throughout the small intestine, in epithelial cells of the villi and glands of Lieberkühn (Figure 21.2), both after the ingestion of oocysts or tissue cysts.[416]

Rodents can act as paratenic hosts for *C. rivolta*.[560,1151] The prepatent period was 4–7 days, and patent periods ranged from 2 to several weeks.[416,1898]

C. rivolta was pathogenic for newborn but not for weaned cats. Newborn cats fed 100,000 sporocysts or infected mice usually developed diarrhea 3–4 days post-inoculation (DPI). Microscopically, desquamation of the tips of the villi, and cryptitis were seen in the ilium and cecum in association with meronts and gamonts.

21.4 PREVALENCE OF *C. FELIS* AND *C. RIVOLTA* IN CATS

Worldwide reports are summarized in Table 21.2. In general, *C. felis* was more common than *C. rivolta*, and infections were more common in kittens versus adults.[81,82] Kittens were excreting *Cystoisospora* spp. oocysts by the third week of age and had peaked by the 15th week when as many as 33% were excreting *C. felis*.[82] An unusually high prevalence of *C. rivolta* was reported from Portugal.[1759]

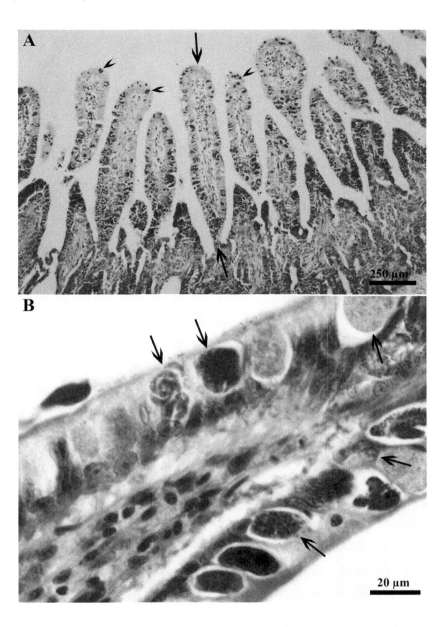

Figure 21.1 Endogenous stages of *Cystoisospora felis* in the ileum of cats. (A) Severe parasitization of the villi (arrow), 120 hours post-inoculation with tissue stages. Giemsa stain. The parasites are confined in surface epithelium (arrowheads). (B) Asexual and sexual stages (arrow) of *C. felis*, 7 days after feeding oocysts. Hematoxylin and eosin stain. (From Dubey, J.P., 2014. *J. Eukaryot. Microbiol.* 61, 637–643; Dubey, J.P., 2018. *Vet. Parasitol.*, 263, 34–48.)

In addition to data in Table 21.2, coccidia (species not specified) were found in 148 (3.2%) of 1519 cats in one survey[113] and 129 (6.5%) of 1990 cats in another report.[592] Both studies were from cats in European countries (Austria, Belgium, Bulgaria, France, Greece, Hungary, Italy, Portugal, Romania, Spain, Switzerland, and the United Kingdom).

21.5 CLINICAL COCCIDIOSIS IN CATS INFECTED WITH *C. FELIS* AND *C. RIVOLTA*

There are conflicting reports concerning the pathogenicity of *C. felis* infection in cats. In some reports, especially before prophylaxis for enteric viruses was available, severe diarrhea was observed in cats infected with *C. felis*. The author considers *C. felis* to not be important clinically as a primary pathogen because experimentally infected cats remained asymptomatic while excreting thousands of oocysts.[424]

Diarrhea was reported in cats naturally infected with *C. felis* in Canada, New Caledonia, and the United Kingdom[114,1256,1355]; positive response to anticoccidial drugs was considered in etiology.

As mentioned earlier, *C. rivolta* was more pathogenic than *C. felis*, perhaps related to the location of development; *C. felis* multiplies in surface epithelial enterocytes (fast

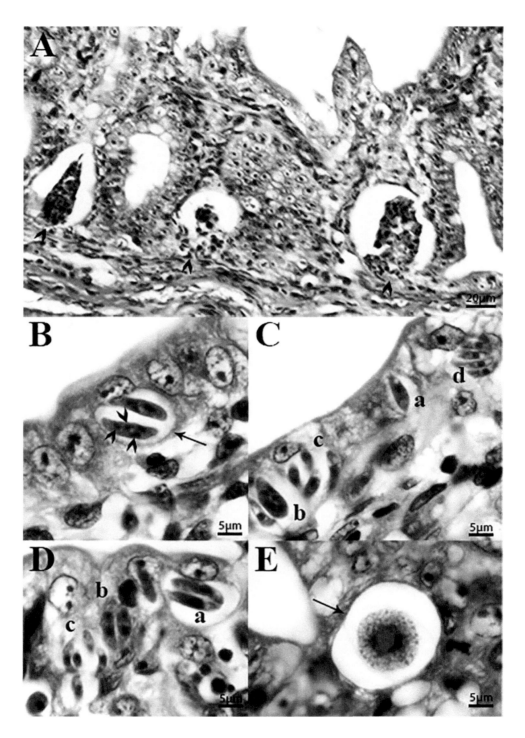

Figure 21.2 Endogenous stages of *Cystoisospora rivolta* in the small intestine of experimentally infected kittens. Iron-hematoxylin stain. Bar in A = 20 μm, bar in B–E = 5 μm. (A) Inflammatory exudate in the lumen of three glands of Lieberkühn (arrowheads). *C. rivolta* stages are present but not visible at this magnification. (B) Two multinucleated (arrowheads) schizonts in a parasitophorous vacuole (arrow). (C) A schizont with one nucleus (a), meront with five or more nuclei (b), meront with four large merozoites (c), and a group with four small merozoites (d). (D) Schizont with two merozoites/meronts each with one nucleus (a), meront with two merozoites/meront each with two nuclei (b), and meront with merozoites (c). (E) An oocyst (arrow) with crumpled wall. (From Dubey, J.P., 1979, *J. Protozool.*, 26, 433–443.)

Table 21.2 Prevalence of *Cystoisospora* spp. Oocysts in Feces of Cats

Country	Region	Number of Cats	C. felis (%)	C. rivolta (%)	Cystoisospora sp. (%)	Remarks	Reference
Albania	Tirana	18	1 (5.6)	2 (11.1)		Suburban areas cats from 2008 to 2009	Knaus et al. (2011)
Argentina	Buenos Aires	271			55 (20.3)	Feces (spaces surrounding the buildings of public hospitals)	Sommerfelt et al. (2006)
Australia	Tasmania	55	7 (12.7)	3 (5.4)		Feral cats trapped	Gregory and Munday (1976)
Australia	Victoria, New South Wales	300	12 (4.0)	9 (3.0)		Feral cats trapped	Coman et al. (1981)
Australia	Brisbane	400	42 (10.5)	8 (2.0)		Pets	Wilson-Hanson and Prescott (1982)
Australia	Sydney	71	2 (2.8)	1 (1.4)		Clinic	Collins et al. (1983)
Australia	Perth	89	8 (7.2)	6 (5.3)		Higher in urban versus rural cats	Shaw et al. (1983)
Australia	Western Australia	33	6 (18.2)	3 (9.1)		Aboriginal community	Meloni et al. (1993)
Australia	Perth	418	19 (4.5)	6 (1.4)		Pets, pet shops, shelter. Pet shops had 31.4% of C. felis	McGlade et al. (2003)
Australia	National	1063	59 (5.6)	28 (2.7)		Higher prevalence in refuge (n = 491) versus clinic cats (n = 572); C. felis 10.2% refuge versus 1.7% clinic and for C. rivolta 5.5% refuge versus 0.3% clinic	Palmer et al. (2008)
Australia	Several regions	64			7 (10.9)	Catteries	Bissett et al. (2009)
		41			4 (9.8)	Shelter	
Austria	Carinthia	95			12 (12.6)		Krebitz (1982)
Austria	Vienna	1228	380 (25.2)	345 (28.1)			Kral (1986)
Austria	NS	421	48 (11.4)	42 (10.0)		Urban and rural	Supperer and Hinaidy (1986)
Belgium	Several areas	500			193 (38.6)	Stray	Vanparijs and Thienpont (1973)
Belgium		30	6 (20.0)	3 (10.0)		Stray	Vanparijs et al. (1991)
Brazil	Guanabara, Rio de Janeiro	125	26 (24.0)	18 (14.4)		Pets	Nery-Guimarães and Lage (1973)
Brazil	Goiás	50	38 (76.0)	15 (30.0)		Pets; oocysts measured	Barbosa et al. (1973)
Brazil	São Paulo	103	12 (11.7)	3 (2.9)	1 (1.0)	Pets	Ogassawara et al. (1980)
Brazil	Paraná	30			3 (10.0)	Pets	Tesserolli et al. (2005)
Brazil	São Paulo	140			30 (21.4)	Clinic	Torrico et al. (2008)

(Continued)

Table 21.2 (Continued) Prevalence of Cystoisospora spp. Oocysts in Feces of Cats

Country	Region	Number of Cats	C. felis (%)	C. rivolta (%)	Cystoisospora sp. (%)	Remarks	Reference
Brazil	São Paulo	51			22 (43.1)	Cats euthanized at Zoonosis Control Center	Coelho et al. (2009)
Canada	Western	635			24 (3.8)	Commercial lab samples	Hoopes et al. (2013)
Canada	National	636			89 (14.0)	Pets, feral, shelter	Villeneuve et al. (2015)
Chile	Santiago	230			28 (12.2)	Cats with diarrhea	López et al. (2006)
China	Kunming	85	15 (17.6)	28 (33.0)		Pets	Meng and Hu (2011)
China	Kunming	100			28 (28.0)	Pets	Chen et al. (2012)
China	Henan and Beijing	360	61 (13.4)	41 (11.4)		Stray, pet, market, tissue cysts found in bioassayed mice	Yang and Liang (2015)
Egypt	Nile Delta region	113			2 (1.9)	Stray	Khalafalla (2011)
Finland	NS	411	3 (0.7)			Pets	Näreaho et al. (2012)
France	Paris	34			1 (2.9)	1998–1999	Beugnet et al. (2000)
Germany	Southern	694	20 (2.9)	35 (0.5)		Pets	Walter (1979); Boch et al. (1981)
Germany	Brandenburg	369	10 (2.7)	5 (1.4)		Stray	Hansel and Rusher (1980)
Germany	Northwest Germany	910			49 (5.4)	1974–1983	Bauer and Stoye (1984)
Germany	Berlin	13			1 (7.7)		Jungmann et al. (1986)
Germany	North	170	7 (4.1)			Urban and rural	Hiepe et al. (1988)
Germany	Wuppertal	264			23 (8.7)	1984–1986	Knaus and Fehler (1989)
Germany		821			23 (2.8)	1983–1986	Emde (1991)
Germany	Lubeck	704	61 (8.7)	31 (4.4)		1989–1990	Unbehauen (1991)
Germany	Southern	70	47 (67.0)	34 (49.0)		Catteries- litters-outdoors	Beelitz et al. (1992)
Germany	NS	30	14 (47.0)	10 (34.0)		Catteries- litters-indoors	
Germany	North	1562			72 (4.6)	Pets, clinic from 1984 to 1991	Epe et al. (1993)
Germany	Gera, Jena, Leipzig	111	19 (17.1)	14 (12.6)		1990–1992	Raschka et al. (1994)
Germany	Eastern Brandenburg	155			17 (11.0)	1993–1995	Schuster et al. (1997)
Germany	North	1496		34 (2.3)		Pets, clinic from 1993 to 1997	Epe et al. (1998)
Germany	Hannover	932	18 (1.9)	19 (2.0)		1996–1997	Mundhenke and Daugschies (1999)

(Continued)

Table 21.2 (Continued)   Prevalence of *Cystoisospora* spp. Oocysts in Feces of Cats

Country	Region	Number of Cats	C. felis (%)	C. rivolta (%)	Cystoisospora sp. (%)	Remarks	Reference
Germany	Monchengladbach	293	15 (5.1)	4 (1.4)		1998	Hecking-Veltmann et al. (2001)
Germany	NS	3167	484 (15.3)	250 (7.9)		Veterinary Laboratory, Freiburg from 1999 to 2002	Barutzki and Schaper (2003)
Germany	Central	100	7 (7.0)	10 (10.0)		Shelters	Cirak and Bauer (2004)
Germany	Deutschland	20,914	610 (2.9)	200 (1.0)		2004–2006	Vrhovec (2006)
Germany	North	441			48 (10.7)	Pets, clinics from 1998 to 2002	Epe et al. (2004)
Germany	Mecklenburg	100	2 (2.0)				Dieffenbacher (2006)
Germany	NS	8560	376 (4.4)	188 (2.2)	513 (6.0)	Pets, commercial lab samples. Most prevalent in August	Barutzki and Schaper (2011)
Germany	NS	1206	401 (33.3)	124 (10.3)	401 (33.3)	Pets. Commercial lab samples, age-related prevalence	Barutzki and Schaper (2013)
Germany	Several areas	903			22 (2.4)	Clinic	Raue et al. (2017)
Hungary	Western	235	7 (3.0)	3 (1.3)		Clinically normal house cats	Capári et al. (2013)
India	Maharashtra	9	1 (11.0)	1 (11.0)		Pets	Shastri and Ratnaparkhi (1992)
Iran	Kashan	113	6 (5.3)	6 (5.3)		Stray cats trapped	Arbabi and Hooshyar (2009)
Iran	Zanjan	100	70 (70.0)	80 (80.0)		Stray	**Esmaeilzadeh et al.**[505]
Iran	Mashhad	52	12 (23.7)			Residential areas from 2009 to 2010	Borji et al. (2011)
Iran	Meshkin	103			6 (5.8)	Stray	**Mohebali et al.**[1198]
Iran	Meta-analysis	682			75 (10.9)	Pets and stray	**Sarvi et al.**[1499]
Ireland	Dublin	271	10 (3.7)			Unwanted	**Garcia-Campos et al.**[581]
Italy	Rome	50	12 (24.0)			Pets	Pellegrino et al. (1953)
Italy	Naples	515			36 (7.0)	Pets	Sanna et al. (1993)
Italy	Sardina	160	17 (10.6)	1 (0.6)		Pets	Porqueddu et al. (2004)
Italy	Tuscany (Florence, Siena, Pisa, Pistoia, Lucca)	273	8 (2.9)	5 (1.8)		Indoor/outdoor, from 2008 to 2010	Mugnaini et al. (2012)
Italy	Milan	139			6 (4.3)	Stray	Spada et al. (2013)
Italy	Central	81	4 (4.9)	1 (1.2)		Total four positive cats	Riggio et al (2013)

(Continued)

Table 21.2 (Continued)   Prevalence of *Cystoisospora* spp. Oocysts in Feces of Cats

Country	Region	Number of Cats	C. felis (%)	C. rivolta (%)	Cystoisospora sp. (%)	Remarks	Reference
Japan	Osaka	200	19 (9.5)	3 (1.5)		Five cats infected with both species	Tomimura (1957)
Japan	Saitama	1079	48 (4.5)	24 (2.2)		Humane shelter	Yamamoto et al. (2009)
Kenya	Thika	103			45 (43.7)	Indoor/outdoor	Njuguna et al. (2017)
Korea	Seoul	41			4 (9.8)	Purchased from market	Huh et al. (1993)
Malaysia	Selangor	100	19 (19.0)	11 (11.0)		Stray	Amin-Babjee (1978)
New Zealand	North Island	508	89 (17.5)	11 (2.2)		Pets	McKenna and Charleston (1980)
Netherlands	NS	305	59 (19.3)	43 (14.1)		22 shelters	Robben et al. (2004)
Poland	Olsztyn	35			2 (7.7)	Shelter, pets	Michalczyk and Sokół (2008)
Poland	Szczecin	128			1 (0.7)	Shelter	Ladczuk and Balicka-Ramissz et al (2010)
Portugal	Lisbon	74	4 (5.4)			Pets	Duarte et al. (2010)
Portugal	Évora	22	0	0	1 (4.5)	Shelter	Ferreira et al. (2011)
Portugal	Lisbon	162	23 (14.2)	75 (46.0)		Stray	Waap et al. (2014)
Quatar	Doha, Al-Saad, Al-matar	824	4 (0.5)			Public grounds	Abu-Madi et al. (2007)
Romania	Transylvania Region	414	22 (5.3)	37 (8.9)		Pets	Mircean et al. (2010)
Russia	Voronezh	420	11 (2.6)			2008–2010	**Menyaylova and Gaponov**[1178]
Russia	Moscow	1448	42 (2.9)	25 (1.7)		2004–2009	**Kurnosova**[926]
Russia	Moscow region, cities of Kirov and Krasnodar	119	7 (5.9)	1 (0.8)		Shelters; 2014–2016	**Yastreb and Shaytanov**[1856]
Russia	Vladivostok	51			7 (13.7)	2014	**Moskvina and Zheleznova**[1210]
Russia	Perm	637			30 (4.7)		**Sivkova and Sogrina**[1580]
Russia	Moscow	1261	32 (5.0)	11 (0.8)		2012–2017, pets	**Kurnosova et al.**[927]
Switzerland		94	5 (5.3)	5 (5.3)			Seiler et al. (1983)
Taiwan	NS	96	3 (3.1)	5 (5.2)		Breeder, clinic	Lin et al. (1990)

(Continued)

Table 21.2 (Continued) Prevalence of *Cystoisospora* spp. Oocysts in Feces of Cats

Country	Region	Number of Cats	C. felis (%)	C. rivolta (%)	Cystoisospora sp. (%)	Remarks	Reference
Thailand	Nakhon Nayok	300			17 (5.7)	Shelter	Rojekittikhun et al. (2014)
Turkey	Nigde	72			9 (12.5)	Stray	Karatepe et al. (2008)
Turkey	Kirikkale	100			66 (65.9)	Stray	Korkmaz et al. (2016)
United Kingdom	NS	58			49 (84.4)	Cat colony. Treatment with sulfonamides	Wilkinson (1977)
United Kingdom	England	69	3 (4.3)			Feral	Nichol et al. (1981)
United Kingdom	NS	1355	46 (3.0)			Pets with clinical signs of gastrointestinal disease	Tzannes et al. (2008)
United Kingdom	NS	57	4 (7.0)			Pets	Gow et al. (2009)
United Arab Emirates	Dubai	240	31 (12.9)	22 (9.2)		Feral cats. 2004–2008	Schuster et al. (2009)
United States	Kansas City	516	89 (17.2)	50 (9.6)		Pets, stray, highest prevalence in recently weaned kittens	Dubey (1973)
United States	Ohio	1000	62 (6.2)	32 (3.2)		Shelter, Columbus	Christie et al. (1976)
United States	Illinois	217	49 (23.0)	52 (24.0)		Pets and stray	Guterbock and Levine (1977)
United States	Pennsylvania	1566	43 (3.7)	19 (2.1)		Clinic	Gates and Nolan (2009)
United States	New York	1322			278 (21.0)	Two shelters and affiliated foster homes from 2006–2010	Lucio-Forster et al. (2011)

Note: References in bold are from additional information not included in Dubey.
Source: For references, see Dubey, J.P. 2018. *Vet. Parasitol.* 263, 34–48.
Abbreviation: NS, not stated.

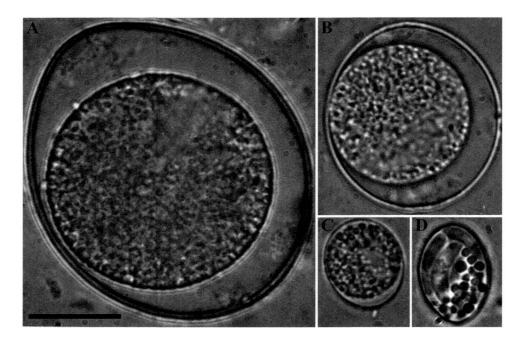

Figure 21.3 Unsporulated oocysts of *Cystoisospora felis* (A), *C. rivolta* (B), and *Toxoplasma gondii* (C) compared with sporulated sporocysts of *Sarcocystis muris* (D). All feline coccidia, except *Sarcocystis*, are shed unsporulated. Scale bar = 10 μm and applies to all figures. (From Dubey, J.P., 2018. *Vet. Parasitol.* 263, 34–48.)

turnover rate) compared to *C. rivolta* that can multiply in enterocytes in glands of Lieberkühn (germinal cells affecting reproduction of enterocytes).

21.6 *C. FELIS* AND *C. RIVOLTA*–LIKE PARASITES IN WILD FELIDAE

C. felis and *C. rivolta*–like oocysts have been reported in wild Felidae, including Indian jungle cat, lion, tiger, bobcat, and mountain lion.[424] Transmission of *C. felis* from a wild felid (bobcat, *Lynx rufus*) to domestic cat (*Felis catus*) was reported using paratenic hosts.[436] The parasite from bobcat was transmissible to domestic cats. Schizonts, gamonts, and oocysts, morphologically like *C. felis,* were detected in histological sections of domestic cats but differed in location; the bobcat-derived parasites were clearly in the lamina propria, whereas *C. felis* of the domestic cat is in the surface epithelium. Limited DNA characterization of DNA isolated from *C. felis* oocysts from the donor bobcat revealed that

Table 21.3   Anticoccidial drugs for cats

Drug[a]	Dose (mg/kg)[b]	Interval (hours)	Duration (days)
Sulfamethoxine[c]	50–60	24	5–20
Sulfaguanidine	100–200	8	5
Trimethoprim-sulfonamide*	15–30[d]	12–24	5
Amprolium	60–100 (total)	24	7
Furazolidone[e]	8-20	12-24	5
Quinacrine	10	24	5
Clindamycin	10	12	7-28
Diclazuril	25	24	1
Ponazuril	15[f]	24	7

Source: From Dubey, J.P., Greene, C.E., 2012. *Infectious Diseases of the Dog and Cat.* 828–839.
[a] Drugs given orally; * can also be given subcutaneously.
[b] Dose per administration at specified interval.
[c] Other sulfonamides, such as sulfadimidine and sulfaguanadine, can be used, but sulfaquinoxaline should not be used because it interferes with vitamin K synthesis and may result in hemorrhagic complications.
[d] Less than 4 kg body weight.
[e] When furazolidone is combined with sulfonamides, 50% of this dose is used. Not available in some countries.
[f] A loading dose of 50 mg/kg PO can be given every 24 hours for 4 days.

sequences of the internal transcribed spacer (ITS)-1 region was 87% like the ITS1 region of *C. felis* from domestic cats. It was concluded that the *C. felis* from bobcat was different than *C. felis* of domestic cat.

21.7 DIAGNOSIS

The detection of oocysts in feces aids diagnosis. Any of the flotation methods can be used to detect feline coccidia; their specific gravity is lower than 1.18. Oocysts of several species of coccidia (*Toxoplasma*, *Hammondia*, *Besnoitia*, and *Sarcocystis*) can be present in cats. Among these, oocysts of *C. felis* are the largest, and oocysts of *C. rivolta* are of medium size (Figure 21.3). Merozoites might be present in smears of intestines with acute diarrhea.[424] Molecular data using the 18S rRNA and ITS1 genes may be useful to differentiate *Cystoisospora* species in cats.[177,1148,1480]

Differential diagnosis of unsporulated oocysts measuring less than 16 μm in diameter is difficult and requires PCR or bioassay to distinguish *Toxoplasma* and *Hammondia*[1509] from *Besnoitia* spp.[450,1739] Oocysts/sporocysts of numerous species of *Sarcocystis* are present in cat feces, but these are usually excreted in the sporulated stage.[431]

21.8 TREATMENT AND PREVENTION

Several anticoccidial drugs (amprolium, furazolidone, ponazuril, diclazuril, toltrazuril, sulfadimethoxine, and trimethoprim-sulfonamides) have been used to treat *Cystoisospora* infections in cats.[424] The number of oocysts excreted is reduced markedly by administration of toltrazuril to cats during the prepatent period.[1354]

Doses are summarized in Table 21.3.[434] Although *Cystoisospora* infections may be self-limiting, anticoccidial therapy can speed up resolution of clinical signs and may lessen environmental contamination.[943] These drugs cannot kill or eliminate oocysts. Symptomatic treatment is necessary in clinical cases, including electrolyte replacement.

Prophylaxis should include daily cleaning of cat litter boxes, disinfection of litter boxes using hot water (>70°C), and general disinfection. Raw meat should never be fed to cats. Cats should be kept indoors to prevent hunting.

REFERENCES

81, 82, 113, 114, 177, 259, 297, 313, 314, 409, 411–413, 416, 421, 424, 431, 433, 434, 436, 450, 490, 505, 518, 526–528, 556–560, 581, 592, 698, 717, 926, 927, 943, 1048, 1148, 1151, 1172, 1175, 1176, 1178, 1198, 1210, 1256, 1277–1279, 1354, 1355, 1477, 1480, 1499, 1509, 1535, 1580, 1739, 1759, 1813, 1856, 1898

CHAPTER 22

Coccidiosis in Humans

S. Almeria, H. N. Cinar, and J. P. Dubey

CONTENTS

Cyclospora and *Cystoisospora* are the only genera discussed here. There are no valid *Eimeria* species infecting humans.[427]

I. *CYCLOSPORA CAYETANENSIS*

22.1 INTRODUCTION

Cyclospora cayetanensis is the only species of the genus *Cyclospora* known to infect humans. *C. cayetanensis* was first described and named 25 years ago.[1282,1288] Earlier, there were reports of organisms initially known as *Cyanobacterium*-like bodies or coccidian-like bodies, blue-green algae, large *Cryptosporidium* or small *Isospora*-like organisms associated with diarrhea in humans, which in retrospect were probably *C. cayetanensis*.[1285] Some other species of the genus *Cyclospora* have been described in nonhuman primates and other animals, but *C. cayetanensis* is host specific.[589]

22.2 MORPHOLOGY AND LIFE CYCLE

C. cayetanensis has a one-host fecal-oral transmission cycle (Figure 22.1). Unsporulated oocysts are excreted in freshly passed feces. They are spheroidal, 8–10 μm in diameter, with little or no size variation. Sporulation occurs outside the host. The oocyst wall is colorless, thin (<1 μm), and bilayered. Polar body and oocyst residuum are present.[1282] Sporocysts are ovoidal, ~4 × 6 μm, and contain both Stieda and substieda bodies, and a large residuum. A sporulated oocyst contains two sporocysts, each with two sporozoites. The sporozoites are elongated, ~1 × 9 μm.[1288] Sporozoites apparently lack crystalloid or refractile bodies.

The life cycle of *C. cayetanensis* has not been fully described. The oocyst is the only stage definitively identified. After the ingestion of sporulated oocysts in contaminated food, water, or soil by a host, sporozoites excyst in the gut lumen and invade the enterocytes of the epithelium of small intestine (Figure 22.1), there the sporozoites round up and subsequently form two types of schizonts. Type I schizonts (size unknown) contain 8–12 small (3–4 μm long) merozoites. Type II schizonts contain four long (12–15 μm long) merozoites.[1283] The type II merozoites form gamonts. The dimensions of gamonts are unknown. In the sexual multiplication, the microgamont fertilize the macrogamont to form the zygote; the flagella have not yet been identified. Oocysts are formed in enterocytes and excreted unsporulated in feces (Figure 22.2). The prepatent period is thought to be around 1 week.[1283]

Unsporulated oocysts have been reported in human sputum.[367,757] Cholecystitis and biliary involvement have been confirmed histologically in HIV-infected patients.[343,1575] Oocysts sporulate outside the host within 1–2 weeks, depending on the temperature.[1500,1591]

22.3 TRANSMISSION AND EPIDEMIOLOGY

The modes of transmission of *C. cayetanensis* are still not completely documented, although fecal-oral transmission is the major route.[1287] Direct person-to-person transmission is unlikely. Indirect transmission can occur if an infected person contaminates the environment, the oocysts sporulate under the right conditions, and then contaminated food and water are ingested. The role of soil in transmission has also been proposed.[201] The relative importance of these various modes of transmission and sources of infection is not known.

C. cayetanensis infection has been reported worldwide, in both developed and developing countries, but it is most common in tropical and subtropical areas.[589] Initially identified endemic areas were Haiti, Guatemala, Peru, and Nepal, where the first outbreaks were reported. Currently, endemic areas are Central and South America, several countries in Middle East (Egypt, Turkey), the Indian subcontinent with Nepal, and South East Asia including Indonesia.[170,589]

In the 1990s, studies in susceptible populations in endemic areas showed prevalence levels around or higher than 10%. In 2010, a review of previous studies on endemic areas from 22 countries (Mexico, Guatemala, Honduras, Brazil, Peru, Venezuela, Cuba, Turkey, Jordan, Saudi Arabia, China, Nepal, Bangladesh, Lao PDR, Thailand, Indonesia, Egypt, Nigeria, Uganda, Kenya, Tanzania, and Mozambique) reported that the infection rates in those countries ranged from 0% to 13% in 47,642 people.[202] Based on the same review, rates from matched asymptomatic controls varied from 0% to 4.2% (average 0.4%). In the same metadata analysis, higher prevalence rates were observed in immunocompromised persons; among 3340 immunocompromised persons, mostly HIV/AIDS patients with diarrhea, prevalence ranged from 0% to 36% (average 4.5%).[202] A recent review gives detailed information on prevalence and geographical distribution of *C. cayetannesis* worldwide.[589]

22.3.1 Seasonality

C. cayetanensis infection is remarkably seasonal worldwide.[110,111,458,589,656] This seasonality varies by regions, most likely due to human activities, environmental contamination, and the optimal sporulation conditions in each area. The reasons for the apparent absence of symptomatic human infection for prolonged periods in environments where the parasite is present, and which biological conditions are needed for the survival of the parasites during these prolonged periods are unknown.[1284]

Factors such as rainfall, temperature, humidity, and perhaps photoperiod could affect the seasonality, which clearly cannot be related to rainfall alone, as there is a marked seasonal variation in very dry environments.[110] The incidence of *C. cayetanensis* infection increases in warm periods of maximal rainfall in countries such as Guatemala, Honduras,

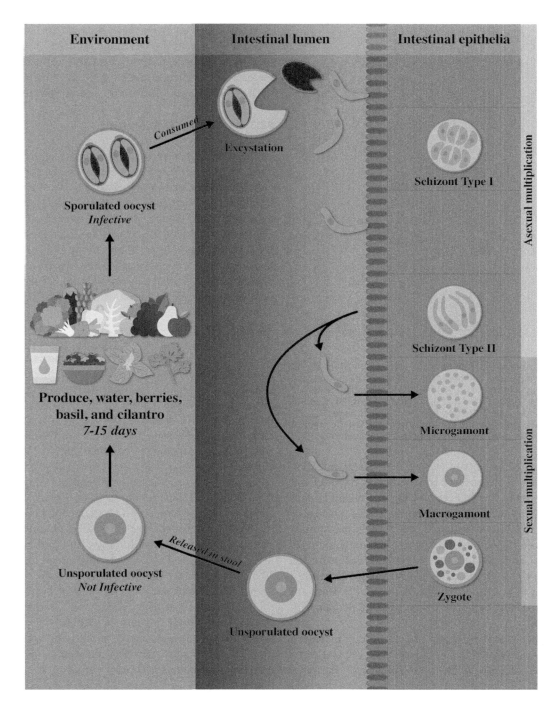

Figure 22.1 Life cycle of *Cyclospora cayetanensis*. If a susceptible human ingests sporulated oocysts in contaminated food or water, the sporozoites inside the sporocysts excyst in the gut lumen and invade enterocytes of the epithelium of duodenum and jejunum where the sporozoites transform into trophozoites. Trophozoites subsequently form two types of schizonts (asexual multiplication). Type I schizonts contain 8–12 merozoites. Type II schizonts contain four merozoites. Then, type II merozoites form gamonts (sexual multiplication). There are two types of gamonts: microgamonts and macrogamonts. Microgamonts fertilize macrogamonts to form the zygote. Oocysts then are formed in enterocytes and are excreted unsporulated in the feces. The prepatent period is thought to be around 1 week. Unsporulated oocysts are not infectious; they need to sporulate to became infective for a host. Under laboratory conditions, at 22°C and 30°C, sporulation will take around 7–14 days to occur outside the host. A sporulated oocyst contains two sporocysts, each with two sporozoites.

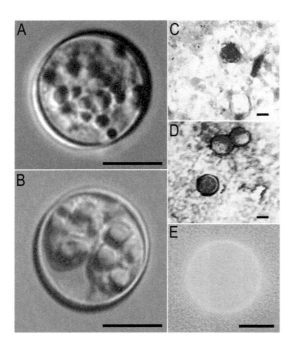

Figure 22.2 *Cyclospora cayetanensis* oocysts. (A and B) Unstained, differential interference contrast, (C) acid-fast stain, (D) hot-safranin stain, (E) ultraviolet fluorescence microscopy. Oocyst in (B) is sporulated. Bars in (A) through (E) = 5 μm. (Images [C], [D], and [E] were public images from DPDx CDC: https://www.cdc.gov/dpdx/cyclosporiasis/index.html.)

Mexico, Jordan, Nepal, or China.[110,111,730] However, infection is more prevalent in the absence of rain, during the drier and hotter months of the year in Peru and Turkey. In Haiti, infections occur during the driest and coolest time of the year or at the cooler wet season in Indonesia.[458] In India, clinical cases were more frequent in the summer before the rainfall. Therefore, it is difficult to explain a common factor for the differences observed in seasonality. It should be considered that temperatures at the cooler time of the year in Haiti are closer to the warmest months of the year in Guatemala City and Kathmandu.[458]

In Vietnam, contamination of produce increased before the rainy season,[1701] and in Guatemala clinical cases increased in April through June, coinciding with the raspberry harvest.[111] Furthermore, the seasonal pattern observed in endemic areas such as Mexico[1281] coincides with maximal clinical prevalence in the United States.[655,656]

22.3.2 Risk Factors

In general, children, foreigners, and immunocompromised patients in endemic developing countries will be the most vulnerable to *C. cayetanensis* infection. The main risk factors for cyclosporiasis in industrialized countries include international travel to cyclosporiasis-endemic areas and domestic consumption of contaminated food, mainly fresh produce imported from these regions. In most developed countries, the disease has been primarily associated with foodborne outbreaks. There are likely to be unknown risk factors, particularly in endemic areas, where studies have been skewed toward those with clinical symptoms.

22.3.2.1 Contact with Animals

Several studies showed that contact with animals (e.g., dogs, chickens, ducks) was a risk factor for infection in endemic countries and increased the risk for human infection with *Cyclospora*.[110,111,202,1553] However, this was not the case in Haiti[1089] where key risk factors for infection with *Cyclospora* included using water from an artesian well, having a shallow, porous well, and living in a stick and adobe house rather than a cement house. In that study, eating uncooked foods and having animals did not show any statistically significant correlation with infection.[1089]

22.3.2.2 Age

In the developed world, cyclosporiasis has been observed in the general population regardless of age.[655,656] In endemic areas, on the other hand, young children are most affected by the disease.[111,202,729,1552] Prevalence in children varied with region as well as in the studies within each region.[202] Prevalence ranged from 0% in Bangladesh, Kenya, Mozambique, or Tanzania to 33% (123/386) positive children in a cohort study in a community of Peru.[110] More recent studies (since 2010) have reported prevalence levels from 0.1% to 5.3% in children from Turkey, Kenya, India, Egypt, Mexico, Morocco, and Nepal. High prevalence (5.3% of 150 children tested) was observed in children in an intensive care hospital unit in Turkey.[127] In Egypt, higher prevalence was observed in immunosuppressed children (7.8%, 13 of 166 children) compared to the immunocompetent children tested in the same study (2.1%, 3 of 142).[5]

The highest risk of infection and diarrhea in children occurs in the first 5 years of life.[110,202,205,729] Infections in children younger than 18 months of age are uncommon,[728] which may partially be due to protection via maternal antibodies. In older children (>11 years) and adults, clinical symptoms are not always present.[204,206] The causes for this age distribution pattern are not clear but may be related to predominant modes of exposure, shared foods, and water from which very young children are relatively protected.[110] After an initial episode of cyclosporiasis, the likelihood of diarrhea and duration of symptoms decreases significantly with each subsequent infection.[110] High percentages of asymptomatic carriers have been noted in endemic areas,[202] suggesting that persistent contact with oocysts during the first years of age induces protective immunity against disease that will last into adulthood in endemic areas.

22.3.2.3 Gender

Gender does not have a significant effect on the *Cyclospora* infection rate in different geographical areas.

22.3.2.4 Socioeconomic Status

The epidemiology of *C. cayetanensis* infections is affected by socioeconomic status. Poverty and low socioeconomic status are considered as risk factors for infection.[204,1287]

Cyclosporiasis is common in impoverished endemic areas where water and food sanitation are poor or nonexistent, particularly affecting children.[110,1288] A correlation between socioeconomic status and infection was observed in Venezuela.[204] In this country, most cases of cyclosporiasis were clustered in areas of extreme poverty where residences were without a latrine or toilet; contact with fecal-contaminated soil was also strongly associated with infection.[204] Higher prevalences associated with deficient sanitary facilities were also observed in other endemic regions.[1089,1777,1914] Even in developed countries such as Germany, workers without proper toilet facilities were believed to be the source of an outbreak.[378] Studies in low socioeconomic areas have shown high prevalence, such as in Chennai, India (22.2% in 256 samples collected),[365] and in an indigenous Karina community in Venezuela (10% of 141 fecal samples collected).[599]

Socioeconomic status also influences the age pattern of infection by *C. cayetanensis*. In very poor areas of Peru, *C. cayetanensis* prevalence was highest in young children (aged 2–4 years); the infection was almost never detected after 11 years of age, and adults usually did not have any clinical infection. In contrast, in middle- to upper-class families who lived in dwellings with suitable sanitation, children rarely appeared to become infected, and infections occurred mainly in adults.[1287]

22.3.2.5 Immunocompromised Hosts

C. cayetanensis affects both immunocompetent and immunocompromised persons. However, it is more severe in immunocompromised hosts, particularly HIV-infected patients for whom it is an important cause of diarrhea.[202,1321] Clinical illness due to *C. cayetanensis* in immunocompromised patients is prolonged and severe and associated with a high rate of recurrence that can be attenuated with long-term suppressive therapy.[1321,1575,1735] The average duration of diarrhea for HIV-infected patients is longer than that for HIV-negative patients, and other manifestations, such as acalculous cholecystitis, have been reported in HIV-positive patients.[1575]

Since the 1990s, there have been many reports on *C. cayetanensis* infection in immunocompromised patients worldwide, mainly in AIDS/HIV-infected people, but also in immunosuppressed persons, including those undergoing cancer treatments.[202,710] In HIV-positive patients with chronic diarrhea, very different prevalence levels are reported in different parts of the world, with marked geographical variations.[589]

High prevalence is generally observed in patients immunosuppressed with pathologies such as Hodgkin's lymphoma and acute lymphoblastic leukemia.[700] In a study in cancer patients receiving chemotherapy in Saudi Arabia, very high prevalence was observed (52% of 54 patients), and particularly high *C. cayetanensis* prevalence was observed in patients with lymphomas.[1483]

22.3.2.6 Resident Foreigners, Expatriates, and Traveler's Diarrhea

Resident foreigners and travelers to endemic areas are at high risk of infection with clinical disease and are more susceptible to the disease than the indigenous population, including children. Between 1997 and 2008, 33.5% of laboratory confirmed cases of infection in the United States were related to travel.[655] In Canada, 71% of reported cyclosporiasis cases between 2000 and 2010 were in travelers.[1696] The remainder were domestically acquired, presumably foodborne.

Most cases of cyclosporiasis reported in Europe and Australia have been acquired by visitors in regions where the parasite is endemic.[1285] There have been several outbreaks in expatriates living in developing countries such as Nepal and Indonesia and in foreign visitors to endemic countries.[589,1285]

22.3.2.7 Consumption of Contaminated Food

C. cayetanensis contamination has been reported in fresh produce surveillance studies in several countries, mainly in endemic areas (Table 22.1).[29] To date, no surveillance studies have been published in the United States. The cases identified in the United States prior to 1995 were all thought to be linked to imported food or were associated with people who had traveled to areas where the disease was endemic. During the period of 2004–2009, 37.8% (70/185) of the cases were classified as domestically acquired.[656]

Recent studies have shown *C. cayetanensis* contamination in ready-to-eat and prepackaged/bulk vegetable products in Canada and Europe.[591] The contamination of ready-to-eat and prepackaged/bulk vegetables is an indication that the current sanitation processes do not guarantee food safety when dealing with certain parasites of fecal origin.[173] Global trade of foods may play a significant role in the transmission of *C. cayetanensis* in developed countries, such as the United States, considering that some of the outbreak cases have been traced back to fresh produce imported from developing regions.[30]

Table 22.1 Positive Reports and Surveillance Studies of *Cyclospora cayetanensis* Detection of Oocysts in Fresh Produce Worldwide

Location	% (Number Positive/ Total Samples Analyzed)	Food Type	Reference
Cambodia	8.3 (3/36)	Water spinach	Anh et al. (2007)
Costa Rica	8.0 (2/25)	Lettuce	Calvo et al. (2004)
Canada	1.7 (9/544)	Precut salads and leafy greens	Dixon et al. (2013)
Canada	0.5 (6/1171)	Arugula/baby arugula, baby spinach and spring mix	Lalonde and Gajadhar (2016a)
Egypt	16 (4/25)	Lettuce heads	Abou el Naga (1999)
Egypt	21.3 (64/300)	Rocket, lettuce, parsley, leek, green onion	El Said Said (2012)
Egypt	25.7 (9/35)	Fresh strawberry juice	Mossallam (2010)
Ethiopia	6.9 (25/360)	Vegetables and raw fruits (avocado, lettuce, cabbage, carrot, tomato, banana and mango)[a]	Bekele et al. (2017)
Ghana	5.1 (20/395)	Cabbage, green pepper, onion, tomato, lettuce	Duedu et al. (2014)
Italy	12.2 (6/49)	Fennel, cucumber, celery, tomato	Giangaspero et al. (2015a)
Italy	1.3 (8/648)	Ready-to-eat/prepackaged salads	Caradonna et al. (2017)
Korea	1.2 (5/404)	Winter grown cabbage, sprouts, blueberries, and cherry tomatoes	Sim et al. (2017)
Nepal	Number not indicated	Cabbage, lettuce, mustard leaves	Sherchand et al. (1999)
Nepal	Number not indicated	Lettuce, spinach, mustard and basil leaves	Sherchan et al. (2010)
Peru	Two surveys: 1.8 (2/110) and 1.6 (1/62)	Lettuce, mint, black mint	Ortega et al. (1997b)
Venezuela	5.9% (6/102)	Lettuce	Devera et al. (2006)
Vietnam	8.4 (24/287)	Herbs (basil, coriander sativum and coriander, Vietnamese mint, marjoram, persicaria) and lettuce	Tram et al. (2008)

Source: Almeria S. et al. 2019. *Cyclospora cayetanensis* and cyclosporiasis: An update. *Microorganisms*. vol. 7, 317.
[a] Unclear which commodity was contaminated by *Cyclospora*.

Produce commodities implicated in numerous food-borne *C. cayetanensis* outbreaks worldwide, include raspberries, blackberries, mesclun (mixture of varieties of lettuce), bagged mixed greens, snow and snap peas, cilantro, and basil (Table 22.2).

Historically, cilantro and raspberries have been two of the main food matrices linked to cyclosporiasis outbreaks in North America.[710] Contaminated Guatemalan raspberries were responsible for high-profile foodborne outbreaks in the United States and Canada in the 1990s.[710] Recently, the main cause of outbreaks in both the United States and Canada has been consumption of contaminated cilantro.

Basil is another leafy green that has been linked to outbreaks in the USA and Canada. The most recent outbreaks associated with basil were two clusters of eight confirmed cases identified in two states in the USA in 2018 and one multistate outbreak in 2019, with 205 lab-confirmed cases from 11 states linked to fresh basil imported from Mexico (as of August 28th, 2019) (Table 22.2).

Salad greens, such as lettuce, were linked to outbreaks in the United States and Europe,[710,378] and romaine-carrot mixes were linked to a recent outbreak in 2018 due to the consumption of domestic salads from a fast-food restaurant chain in the United States. Lettuce contaminated

with *C. cayetanensis* oocysts has been found in many countries (Canada, Costa Rica, Egypt, Ethiopia, Ghana, Italy, Nepal, Peru, Venezuela, and Vietnam) (Table 22.2). Contaminated snow peas were linked to an outbreak in the United States,[189] and Guatemalan imported snap peas were linked to two separate outbreaks in Europe and Canada (Table 22.2).[29]

In 2016, a small outbreak in the United States was linked to coleslaw (cabbage and carrot mix with dressing).[30] In 2018, in the most recent outbreak in the United States, prepackaged vegetable trays containing carrots, broccoli, cauliflower, and dill dip were the cause of infection.

For many outbreaks, the contaminated food source has not been identified. The identification of food items that serve as vehicles in cyclosporiasis outbreaks represents a major challenge. The unknown incubation period for *C. cayetanensis* infection, the short shelf-life of implicated commodities (i.e., fresh produce), and the complex epidemiological investigations required to identify the contaminated produce item present in a dish with multiple ingredients, are among the factors that hamper these investigations.[30] Fresh produce is often consumed raw and with little or no washing and may become contaminated by food handlers or through crop irrigation with untreated water. Factors including poor

Table 22.2 Summary of Outbreaks Associated with *C. cayetanensis* by Country and Year of Occurrence and Possible Sources of Exposure

Country	Year	Disease Cases (If Laboratory Confirmed: Number of Cases)	Source of Exposure Suspected or Known	Origin/Notes	Reference
Australia (cruise)	2010	266 (73)	Lettuce (suspected)	Two consecutive voyages	Gibss et al. (2013)
Brazil	1999–2002	132 (16)	Not indicated	Not available	Zini et al. (2004)
Canada (two provinces) **and United States (20 states)**	1996	1465 (978)	Raspberries	Guatemala	Dixon *et al.* (2011); Herwaldt et al. (1997); Manuel et al. (2000)
Canada (Ontario) **and United States (14 states)**	1997	1012 (422)	Raspberries	Guatemala	Dixon et al. (2011); Herwaldt et al. (1999)
Canada (Ontario)	1998	315	Raspberries	Guatemala	Herwaldt (2000); Dixon et al. (2011)
Canada (Ontario)	1999	104	Dessert berries (blackberries suspected)	Blackberries (Guatemala), strawberries (United States), frozen raspberries (Chile)	Herwaldt (2000); Dixon et al. (2011)
Canada (BC[a])	1999	15	Undetermined	Undetermined	Dixon et al. (2011)
Canada (BC)	2001	30 (17)	Thai basil	Imported from Thailand (supplier in United States). Not confirmed	Hoang et al. (2005)
Canada (BC)	2003	11	Cilantro	Undetermined, community	Kozak et al. (2013)
Canada (BC)	2004	17 (9)	Mango or basil (suspected)	Not confirmed, community	Kozak et al. (2013)
Canada (BC)	2004	8	Cilantro suspected	Undetermined, community	Kozak et al. (2013)
Canada (Quebec)	2005	250 (142)	Fresh basil	Mexico, workers who ate in a restaurant	Milord et al. (2012)
Canada (Ontario)	2005	44 (16)	Basil (suspected)	Retreat. Pasta salad with basil, origin not confirmed (shipment from Peru and Costa Rica)	Kozak et al. (2013)
Canada (BC)	2006	28	Basil or garlic	Undetermined	Kozak et al. (2013)
Canada (BC)	2007	29 (14)	Organic basil	Mexico	Shah et al. (2009)
Canada (Sarnia)	2010	210	Basil, pesto	Fundraiser event	Ortega and Sherchand (2015)
Canada	2013	25	Leafy greens suspected	Undetermined	Dixon et al. (2016)
Canada (multiple provinces)	2015	97	Undetermined, multistate (BC: 5, Alberta: 1, Ontario: 84, Quebec: 7)	Travelers from Mexico	Nichols et al. (2015); CFIA-PHAC (2017)
Canada (multiple provinces)	2016	87	Undetermined	BC 2, Alberta 2, Ontario 75, Quebec 8	CFIA-PHAC (2017)
Canada (multiple provinces)	2017	164	Undetermined	BC (17), Ontario (143), Quebec (3), Nova Scotia (1)	CFIA-PHAC (2017)
Colombia	2002	56 (31)	Salad, juices	University employees	Botero-Garces et al. (2006)
Germany	2000	34	Salad, green leafy herbs	France, Italy, Germany	Doller et al. (2002)
Nepal	1989	535 (55)	Drinking water suspected	Foreigners, Travelers from United Kingdom	Shlim et al. (1991)
Nepal	1989	14 (12)	Drinking water suspected	Foreigners	Rabold et al. (1994)
Nepal	1992	964 (108)	Drinking water suspected	Foreigners	Hoge et al. (1993)
Mexico	2001	97 (55/70 fecal samples analyzed)	Watercress (salad berros)	Party attendees at wedding and christening	Ayala-Gaytan et al. (2004)

(Continued)

Table 22.2 (Continued)   Summary of Outbreaks Associated with C. cayetanensis by Country and Year of Occurrence and Possible Sources of Exposure

Country	Year	Disease Cases (If Laboratory Confirmed: Number of Cases)	Source of Exposure Suspected or Known	Origin/Notes	Reference
Peru	2004	127/274 people with diarrhea, 24/77 positive by microscopy	Undetermined (salsa sauces suspected)	Recruits	Torres-Slimming et al. (2006)
Peru	2005	52 recruits (37 positive, 15 control) 20/35 positive by PCR	Undetermined (food, water)	Recruits	Mundaca et al. (2008)
Poland	2013	3	Drinking water suspected	Travelers from Indonesia	Bednarska et al. (2015)
Spain	2003	13 (7)	Raspberry juice suspected	Travelers from Guatemala	Puente et al. (2006)
Sweden	2009	18 (12)	Snap peas	Guatemala	Insulander et al. (2010)
The Netherlands	2001	29 (14)	Could not investigate potential food sources	Dutch participants at a scientific meeting in Bogor, Indonesia	Blans et al. (2005)
Turkey	2005	35	Drinking water suspected, coinfection with *Cryptosporidium*	Undetermined	Aksoy et al. (2007)
Turkey	2007	505 stools (14/17 positive by PCR)	Undetermined, suspected to be related to lack of rain and use of contaminated water	Unwashed green salad suspected	Ozdamar et al. (2010)
United Kingdom	2015	79	Undetermined	Travelers from Mexico	Nichols et al. (2015)
United States (Illinois)	1990	21	Tap water or food	Not completely clarified	Huang et al. (1995)
United States (Florida)	1995	38	Raspberries suspected, risk factor soil contact	(Guatemala as possible source)	Koumans et al. (1998)
United States (New York)	1995	32	Fruit suspected	Undetermined	Herwaldt (2000)
United States (Massachusetts)	1996	57 (12)	Berries	Wedding, strawberries (California), blueberries (Florida), blackberries (Guatemala), raspberries (Guatemala/Chile)	Fleming et al. (1998)
United States (Florida)	1996	86	Raspberries (suspected)	Guatemala	Katz et al. (1999)
United States (Charleston, South Carolina)	1996	38	Raspberries	Guatemala	Caceres et al. (1998)
United States (20 states) **and Canada (2 provinces)**	1996	1465 (978)	Raspberries	Guatemala	Dixon et al. (2011); Herwaldt et al. (1997); Manuel et al. (2000)
United States (Florida)	1997	220 (including people in cruise ship that departed from Florida)	Mesclun	Peru or United States (if related to 12 cases from Florida above, then mesclun from Peru most probable source)	Herwaldt (2000)
United States (14 states) **and Canada (Ontario)**	1997	1012 (422)	Raspberries	Guatemala	Dixon et al. (2011); Herwaldt et al. (1999)
United States (Northern Virginia, Washington DC-Baltimore metropolitan area)	1997	341 (48)	Basil	Multiple possible sources, may be local contamination	Herwaldt (2000)
United States (Virginia)	1997	21	Fruit plate	Undetermined	Herwaldt (2000)

(Continued)

Table 22.2 (*Continued*) Summary of Outbreaks Associated with *C. cayetanensis* by Country and Year of Occurrence and Possible Sources of Exposure

Country	Year	Disease Cases (If Laboratory Confirmed: Number of Cases)	Source of Exposure Suspected or Known	Origin/Notes	Reference
United States (Georgia)	1998	17	Probable fruit salad	Undetermined	Herwaldt (2000)
United States (Florida)	1999	94	Berries likely	Undetermined	Herwaldt (2000)
United States (Missouri)	1999	62	Basil in chicken pasta and tomato basil salad	Mexico or United States, two events	Lopez et al. (2001)
United States (Georgia)	2000	19	Raspberries and/or blackberries (suspected)	Suspected to be from Guatemala	CDC (2017)
United States (Pennsylvania)	2000	54	Raspberry, wedding cake	Guatemala	Ho et al. (2002)
United States (Florida)	2001	39	Undetermined	Undetermined	CDC (2017)
United States (New York City)	2001	3	Undetermined	Undetermined	CDC (2017)
United States (Vermont)	December 2001–January 2002	22	Raspberry (likely)	Suspected to be from Chile	CDC (2017)
United States (Massachusetts)	2002	8	Undetermined	Undetermined	CDC (2017)
United States (New York)	2002	14	Undetermined	Undetermined	CDC (2017)
United States (Texas, Illinois)	2004	95 (38 in Texas, 57 in Illinois)	Undetermined	Undetermined, basil likely	Ortega and Sanchez (2010); CDC (2017)
United States (Tennessee)	2004	12	Undetermined	Undetermined	CDC (2017)
United States (Pennsylvania)	2004	96	Snow peas	Guatemala	CDC (2004)
United States (Florida)	2005	582	Basil, restaurants	Peru	Ortega and Sherchand (2015); CDC (2017)
United States (South Carolina)	2005	6	Undetermined	Undetermined	CDC (2017)
United States (Massachusetts)	2005	74	Two different outbreaks (58 and 16 cases)	Undetermined	CDC (2017)
United States (Connecticut)	2005	30	Basil suspected	Undetermined	CDC (2017)
United States (Minnesota)	2006	14	Undetermined	Undetermined	CDC (2017)
United States (New York)	2006	20	Undetermined	Undetermined	CDC (2017)
United States (Georgia)	2006	3	Undetermined	Undetermined	CDC (2017)
United States (Wisconsin)	2008	4	Sugar snap peas (likely)	Guatemala not confirmed	CDC (2017)
United States (California)	2008	45	Raspberries and/or blackberries (likely)	Undetermined	CDC (2017)
United States (District of Columbia)	2009	34	Blackberries and raspberries	Undetermined	CDC (2017)
United States (Connecticut)	2009	8			CDC (2017)
United States (Florida)	2011	12	Undetermined	Undetermined	CDC (2017)
United States (Georgia)	2011	88[b]	Undetermined	Undetermined	CDC (2017)
United States (Texas)	2012	16	Undetermined	Undetermined	CDC (2017)
United States (Iowa and Nebraska and neighboring states)	2013	162	Bagged salad mix	Mexico	CDC (2017)
United States (Texas)	2013	270 (38)	Cilantro	Mexico, multistate	Abanyie et al. (2013)

(*Continued*)

Table 22.2 (Continued)   Summary of Outbreaks Associated with C. cayetanensis by Country and Year of Occurrence and Possible Sources of Exposure

Country	Year	Disease Cases (If Laboratory Confirmed: Number of Cases)	Source of Exposure Suspected or Known	Origin/Notes	Reference
United States (Wisconsin)	2013	8	Berry salad (suspected)	Undetermined	CDC (2017)
United States (Michigan)	2014	14	Undetermined	Undetermined	CDC (2017)
United States (Iowa, Nebraska)	2014	227 (161)	Lettuce (imported romaine lettuce)	Mexico	Buss et al. (2016a,b)
United States (Texas)	2014	304 (26)	Cilantro	Mexico	CDC (2017)
United States (South Carolina)	2014	13	Cilantro (suspected)	Mexico	CDC (2017)
United States (31 states)	2015	546 (90 cases in Georgia, Texas and Wisconsin)	Cilantro (suspected)	Mexico	CDC (2017)
United States (Texas)	2016	6[c]	Carrots or green cabbage in coleslaw (suspected)	Undetermined	CDC (2017); Fox (2017)
United States (40 states)	2017 (summary)	1065	Undetermined	Undetermined	CDC (2017)
United States (Florida)	2017	6	Berries (suspected)	Undetermined	CDC (2017)
United States (Texas)	2017	38[d]	Scallions (i.e., green onions)	Undetermined	CDC (2017)
United States (Michigan)	2017	29	Undetermined	Undetermined	CDC (2017)
United States (Tennessee)	2017	4[e]	Undetermined	Undetermined	CDC (2017)
United States (Connecticut)	2017	3	Undetermined	Undetermined	CDC (2017)
United States (Florida)	2017	3[f]	Undetermined	Undetermined	CDC (2017)
United States (33 states)	2018 (summary)	2299 total cases (partial data indicated in a, b, c, and d)	Many cases not directly linked, rest indicated in a, b, c, and d cases	Undetermined	CDC (2018a); Casillas et al. (2018)
United States (4 states)[b]	2018	250 (250)	Vegetable trays with broccoli, cauliflower, carrots, and dill dip	Bought in supermarket. It was not possible to determine if an individual component of the vegetable trays was the likely vehicle of infection	CDC (2018b)
United States (15 states and New York)[c]	2018	511 (511)	Romaine lettuce and carrot mix	Salads purchased from a fast-food restaurant chain	CDC (2018c)
United States (2 states)[d]	2018	8 (8)	Basil	Undetermined	CDC (2018a)
United States (Midwest, 3 clusters)[e]	2018	53 (53)	Cilantro	Mexican-style restaurants	CDC (2018a)
USA (30 states)	2019	580 (580)	Basil (205)	Mexico	CDC (2019)[g]

Source: Almeria S. et al. 2019. *Cyclospora cayetanensis* and cyclosporiasis: An update. *Microorganisms 7*, 317.

Note: In bold: Outbreaks in two countries at the same time. In 2018, a, b, c and d show cases directly linked to specific food produce. & As of August 28, 2019.

Abbreviations: CDC, Centers for Disease Control and Prevention; PCR, polymerase chain reaction.

a   British Columbia.

b   An additional 10 probable cases associated with this outbreak, according to CDC (2017), were not included in the total.

c   Additional nine suspected cases were identified in persons associated with this outbreak but were not counted in the table because of reporting issues (e.g., insufficient case data) according to CDC (2017).

d   An additional three probable cases were identified in persons associated with this outbreak but were not counted in the table because of reporting issues (e.g., insufficient case data).

e   An additional two probable cases were identified in persons associated with this outbreak but were not counted in the table because of reporting issues (e.g., insufficient case data).

f   One additional probable case was identified in a person associated with this outbreak but was not counted in the table because of a reporting issue.

g   As of July 2019.

worker hygiene practices, contaminated soil, and contaminated agricultural water could play a role in contamination. In many instances, the fresh produce linked to outbreaks may be a component of complex dishes with many produce ingredients, which makes detection and determining the contaminated ingredient more difficult.[30,1284]

22.3.2.8 Waterborne Infection of *Cyclospora cayetanensis*

Water contaminated with fecal matter may act as a vehicle of transmission for *C. cayetanensis* infection. The source of drinking water has been determined as a risk factor for cyclosporiasis in endemic areas.[1089] More importantly, *C. cayetanensis* oocysts have been detected in several types of water (Table 22.3),[29] including chlorinated water, and wastewater in endemic areas and in nonendemic areas, which suggests the potential spread of the parasite via drinking

and recreational water. *C. cayetanensis* oocysts have been detected in different sources of water in many endemic countries such as Guatemala, Haiti, Ghana, Vietnam, and Egypt, among others (Table 22.3).

C. cayetanensis contaminated water and the potential for the oocysts to be transmitted by waste water contamination of drinking or irrigation water has also been found in developed countries.[897] In Italy, treated wastewater, tap water, and well water were found, by molecular methods, to be contaminated by *C. cayetanensis*.[590]

Some *C. cayetanensis* outbreaks are waterborne, but the source of contamination has not been established, and other sources have not been ruled out.[710] In countries where *C. cayetanensis* is endemic and water and sewage treatment systems are insufficient, waterborne oocysts are a likely source of infection. Oocysts can pass through physical barriers and are not affected by chlorine and other water disinfectants. Cyclosporiasis was associated with consumption

Table 22.3 Water Sources Contaminated by *Cyclospora cayetanensis* in Different Countries

Country	Type of Water	Percentage (Positive/Total Analyzed)	Reference
Egypt	Household water tanks in Alexandria	9.0 (9/100)	Khalifa et al. (2001)
Egypt	Finished piped water, irrigation canals, shallow underground water and drain water	Positive detection from five residential areas. No number indicated	El-Karamany et al. (2005)
Egypt	Treated potable water from tanks	0.2 (2/840)	Elshazly et al. (2007)
Egypt	River Nile, water works, water pumps, water tank, pond and canals	5.9 (20/336)	Khalifa et al. (2014)
Ghana	Sachet drinking water	59.3 (16/27)	Kwakye-Nuako et al. (2007)
Guatemala	Rivers	6.7 (2/30)	Bern et al. (1999)
Guatemala	Drinking water sources	41.7 (5/12)[a]	Dowd et al. (2003)
Italy	Tap water	30.0 (3/10)[a]	Giangaspero et al. (2015a)
Italy	Treated wastewater	21.3 (20/94)[a]	Giangaspero et al. (2015b)
Italy	Well water	6.2 (1/16)[a]	Giangaspero et al. (2015b)
Malaysia	(1) Drinking water treatment plants and (2) recreational water (man-made lake)	(1) 8.3 (2/24) and (2) 16.7 (2/12)	Bilung et al. (2017)
Nepal	Chlorinated water	Presence of oocysts	Rabold et al. (1994)
Nepal	Sewage contamination	22.2 (4/18); 41.7 (5/12)	Sherchand et al. (1999); Sherchand and Cross (2001)
Nepal	Irrigation water, pond water, tap water, and tube wells water	2 of 8 irrigation canals, 1 of 12 pond water samples (none in tap water or tube wells)	Sherchan et al. (2010)
Peru	Wastewater	72.7 (8/11)	Sturbaum et al. (1998)
Spain	DWTP[b], WWTP[c], rivers	9.0 (20/223)	Galván et al. (2013)
Tunisia	Wastewater	0.4 (1/232)[a]	Ben Ayed et al. (2012)
Turkey	(1) Streams and (2) drinking water	Total: 24.6 (56/228) (1) 31.1 (56/180), (2) 0.0 (0/48)	Karaman et al. (2017)
United States	WWTP[b] (1) influent and (2) effluent	(1) 25.0 (6/24) (2) 12.5 (3/24)[a]	Kitajima et al. (2014)
Vietnam	Lakes and rivers	63.6 (84/132)[a]	Miegeville et al. (2003)
Vietnam	Water samples from markets and farms	12.6 (12/95)	Tram et al. (2008)

Source: Almeria S. et al. 2019. *Cyclospora cayetanensis* and cyclosporiasis: An update. *Microorganisms.* vol. 7, 317.
[a] PCR methods.
[b] Drinking water treatment plants.
[c] Wastewater.

of unchlorinated water and drinking water that was inadequately filtered. Oocysts also seem to be able to survive treatment protocols used in wastewater treatment plants (WWTPs), since both influent and effluent treated water showed similar frequencies of *Cyclospora* spp. in these plants (Table 22.3).

C. cayetanensis can contaminate plant crops via different pathways including black water (waste water from toilets) used for irrigation or spraying of crops, contact with contaminated soil, infected food handlers, or hands that have been in contact with contaminated soil. Irrigation of crops using untreated or poorly treated water is a likely source of contamination for fruits and vegetables. Contaminated water used for applying fertilizers and for washing and processing foods are also likely sources of foodborne transmission. In addition, recreational exposure to water contaminated with *C. cayetanensis* oocysts may also be a source of infection.[126]

A few studies evaluated the role of shellfish in the transmission of *Cyclospora*. The Asian freshwater clam (*Corbicula fluminea*) could be used as a biological indicator for recovery of *C. cayetanensis* oocysts from water.[610] *C. cayetanensis* oocysts have been found in bivalves, gandofli (*Caelatura Iaronia pruneri*) in Alexandria, Egypt,[1236] and *C. cayetanensis* DNA was also detected by real-time polymerase chain reaction (PCR) with high-resolution melting analysis in mussels (*Mytilus galloprovincialis*) (26.4% of 53) collected at the Aegean coast of Turkey.[18] Using mollusk bivalves as biological sentinels, *C. cayetanensis* oocysts were also recently observed in Tunisian coastal waters. The presence of *C. cayetanensis* in shellfish could indicate that freshwater runoff from land could carry oocysts into the marine ecosystem.[203]

22.3.2.9 Soil as Source of Infection and/ or Transmission for *Cyclospora cayetanensis* Oocysts

Soil is a potential and possibly important mode of transmission and source of infection for *C. cayetanensis*.[204,201] Contamination of soils by inadequate defecation disposal might be a significant determinant for infection. Some studies have included contact with soil as a risk factor for *C. cayetanensis* infections in both developing and developed countries.[204] In Venezuela, most cases of *C. cayetanensis* were clustered in the areas of extreme poverty, where living in a hut, not having a toilet, and having contact with soil contaminated with human feces were strongly associated with infection.[204] *C. cayetanensis* was more prevalent where agricultural work and lack of handwashing were present.[1665] More recently, soil was found to be positive for oocysts in Italy (11.8% positive samples, 6/51).[590] Higher rates of infection have been noted in additional areas where risk factors such as deficient sanitary facilities, poor personal hygiene, and soil contaminated with human feces were present.[1089,1777]

22.4 *CYCLOSPORA CAYETANENSIS* OUTBREAKS

Table 22.2 presents a summary of the outbreaks associated with *C. cayetanensis* worldwide with possible routes of transmission.

Most outbreaks due to *C. cayetanensis* described to date have been related to fresh produce consumption. *Cyclospora cayetanensis* outbreaks have been mostly reported in North America, probably due to better detection methods and disease surveillance that have helped in tracking outbreaks.

In the mid-1990s, *C. cayetanensis* was recognized as the causative agent of multistate outbreaks of diarrheal illness in the United States and Canada. The outbreak that brought cyclosporiasis to importance in North America, affecting the population in both the United States and Canada, occurred in the spring of 1996; it was due to consumption of fresh raspberries imported from Guatemala. A total of 1465 cases were reported by 20 states and the District of Columbia in the United States and in two Canadian provinces.[711] Infections were linked to fresh produce, mostly berries and leafy vegetables imported from Mexico and Central America into the United States and Canada (Table 22.2). Between 1990 and 2000, nearly all reported outbreaks in the United States and Canada were associated with food and mostly related to Guatemalan raspberries. Since 2000, at least 31 outbreaks have been reported worldwide, 18 of those in North America.[203] The 2013 multistate outbreaks in the United States with 631 laboratory-confirmed cases contributed to the largest annual number of cases of cyclosporiasis in the United States since 1997.[2] The 2014 and 2015 multistate outbreaks in this country involved 304 and 546 confirmed cases in 19 and 31 states, respectively. In 2016, a restaurant-associated subcluster of cyclosporiasis in Texas was epidemiologically linked to consumption of coleslaw containing shredded carrots and cabbage.[30] In 2017, although many cases (1065) were diagnosed in the United States, only a few of them were clustered as outbreaks and linked to a specific commodity, e.g., 38 cases in Texas linked to consumption of scallions (i.e., green onions) and 6 cases in Florida suspected of being caused by consumption of berries (Table 22.2). In 2018, the incidence of *C. cayetanensis* infections increased markedly, in part related to large outbreaks associated with produce. Two main outbreaks and several smaller ones took place in 2018 in the United States. An outbreak in four states, with 250 laboratory-confirmed cases of *Cyclospora* infection, was linked to consumption of prepackaged vegetable trays containing broccoli, cauliflower, carrots, and dill dip from supermarkets. Eight people were hospitalized. No deaths were reported. It was not possible to determine if an individual component of the vegetable trays was the likely vehicle of infection. A separate outbreak involved 511 laboratory-confirmed cases of *Cyclospora* infections in people from 16 states who reported consuming a variety of salads from fast-food restaurants in the Midwest. Twenty-four people were hospitalized; no deaths were reported. Epidemiologic and traceback evidence indicated that salads purchased from fast-food restaurants were one likely source of this outbreak.[180]

In 2018, from the total of 2299-confirmed cases, as of October 2018, approximately 35% ill people were associated with either of the two outbreaks indicated: vegetable trays and salads.[180] In addition, two basil-associated clusters of 8 confirmed cases in two states and multiple cilantro-associated clusters in Mexican-style restaurants including 53 confirmed cases associated to three clusters in the Midwest, took place. Many cases of cyclosporiasis could not be directly linked to any outbreak.[180]

In 2019, as of August 28, 2019, 1,696 laboratory-confirmed cases of cyclosporiasis were reported to CDC by 33 states, District of Columbia and New York City in people who became ill since May 1, 2019 and who had no history of international travel during the 14-day period before illness onset. At least 92 people were hospitalized.

Waterborne outbreaks have been suspected (see Section 22.2.8). In one outbreak reported in the United States,[752] repair of a water pump and refilling storage tanks in a penthouse area of the dormitory of a physician was thought to be the cause and this would have been the first described waterborne outbreak in the United States. However, examination of water samples did not reveal *Cyclospora* oocysts, and the mean time of incubation was inconsistent.[710] Some outbreaks related to cruises have been documented. The most important outbreak was related to two consecutive voyage cruises departing from Australia in 2010 in which 266 people were affected (73 were laboratory confirmed), and lettuce was suspected as the cause of the outbreak.

Several outbreaks have been reported in expatriates or visitors to developing countries.[589] For example, after a scientific meeting of a group of Dutch people in Bogor, Indonesia, 14 of 29 were positive for *C. cayetanensis*, and in another instance, Spaniard workers who traveled for international aid–related purposes to Guatemala were affected. A small outbreak was reported in three Polish businessmen who traveled to Indonesia.[589] Interestingly, cyclosporiasis outbreaks have also been reported in local populations of developing areas.[589]

22.5 CLINICAL SYMPTOMS AND PATHOGENESIS

The main symptoms of *C. cayetanensis* infection are voluminous watery diarrhea, abdominal cramps, nausea, low-grade fever, fatigue, and weight loss.[1285] Although the disease is self-limiting in most of the immunocompetent patients, it may present as a severe, protracted, or chronic diarrhea in immunocompromised patients.[1285]

The clinical presentation in endemic settings shows differences by age, with elderly persons and young children having more severe clinical symptoms, while infections are milder in older children and adults. In addition, asymptomatic infections are frequent in endemic areas.[599,759] The

severity and duration of infection tend to become milder after repeated episodes.[1285] The median incubation period is around 7 days.[711] The average duration of diarrhea is longer in HIV-positive patients than in HIV-negative patients (199 days and 57.2 days, respectively).[1285,1575] Another clinical manifestation of *C. cayetanensis* infection in HIV-positive patients is biliary disease, acalculous cholecystitis, and cholangitis in AIDS patients.[343,1575,1873] The pathogenesis of biliary infections is unknown. Presumably, some sporozoites from intestinal lumen travel to bile ducts and initiate the development of *Cyclospora* there; extrabiliary infections have not been reported.

The pathogenesis underlying these symptoms has not been defined. Jejunal biopsies have shown mucosal alterations in intestinal villi, diffuse edema and infiltration by inflammatory cells, reactive hyperemia, vascular dilation, and congestion of capillaries in the presence of the parasite, which are compatible with inflammation of the upper intestinal tract.[1283]

22.6 DIAGNOSIS

22.6.1 Serological Studies

Currently, no serological assays are commercially available. In a study, specific IgG and IgM antibodies in individuals with oocysts were tested by enzyme-linked immunosorbent assay (ELISA).[1777]

22.6.2 Oocyst Detection in Clinical Samples

22.6.2.1 Oocyst Testing

Multiple stool samples should be examined to rule out a *C. cayetanensis* infection. Three stool specimens collected on alternate days within a 10-day period should be examined to achieve a greater than 95% detection rate.[580] Wet smears, with or without iodine, may be used to detect *C. cayetanensis* oocysts. Commercial concentration devices are available to ensure consistent performance of the technique in the detection of a small number of *Cyclospora* oocysts in stool samples. Due to the small size (8–10 μm) and round shape of the oocysts, they can be confused with amoebae or inflammatory cells, and alternative microscopic methods are required to achieve a higher detection sensitivity.[580]

22.6.2.2 Modified Acid-Fast Staining

Cyclospora, Cryptosporidium, and *Cystoisospora* oocyst walls contain acid-fast lipids,[580] which is a common property and makes acid-fast staining relevant for the screening of these three parasites in a single test. Although modified acid-fast staining can be used to identify these organisms, in *Cyclospora,* variable levels of dye uptake may result in ghost cells, or poorly stained cells, along with well-stained ones.[580,1285] There have been minor variations in modified acid-fast stains to improve *Cyclospora* detection. One of the favored modifications is the use of 1% H_2SO_4 as a decolorizer without alcohol.[580] Another variation is the addition of dimethyl sulfoxide (DMSO) to the phenol-basic fuchsine and the incorporation of acetic acid with malachite green as a combined decolorizer-counterstain to achieve better penetration for the visualization of the internal structures of the oocysts.[580]

22.6.2.3 Heated Safranin Staining

This staining was initially used for *Cryptosporidium* identification. A modified heated safranin stain was reported to uniformly stain *Cyclospora* oocysts a brilliant reddish-orange color.[1749] Safranin staining showed agreement in sensitivity and specificity with the Ziehl Nielsen acid-fast staining technique.[578]

22.6.2.4 Autofluorescence

The oocysts of *Cyclospora*, *Cystoisospora*, and *Cryptosporidium* have autofluorescence properties.[122] Strong autofluorescence of *Cyclospora* oocysts is a useful microscopic test for identification.[1073] *Cyclospora* appears blue when exposed to 365 nm ultraviolet (UV) light[1730] and looks green under 450–490 nm excitation.[1286]

22.6.3 Molecular Detection and Characterization

Molecular methods have various strengths for the diagnosis of cyclosporiasis. Methods with the ability to simultaneously detect several pathogens using multiplex platforms, rapid assessment, and high sensitivity that have been developed over the years,[1733,1743,938,1675] but until recently, no commercially available molecular diagnostic test was available for use in clinical laboratory settings. The BioFire FilmArray gastrointestinal (GI) panel (BioMerieux) is the only commercially available molecular diagnostic product capable of detecting *C. cayetanensis*. This fully automated system can detect 12 enteric bacterial pathogens, five groups of viruses, and the protozoan parasites *C. cayetanensis*, *Cryptosporidium*, *Giardia*, and *Entamoeba histolytica*. After a simple sample loading process, fully automated cell lysis, nucleic acid purification, and high-order multiplex PCR reactions occur in a pouch that contains all the reagents in microfluidics chambers where the FilmArray reactions and analysis occur. The multicenter evaluation of the BioFire FilmArray GI panel was performed on 1556 clinical stool samples. Performance of the FilmArray was compared with traditional and molecular assays to determine the sensitivities and specificities of the four protozoans in the GI panel. This study showed that both sensitivity and specificity for the *C. cayetanensis* assay were 100% in the FilmArray GI panel.[165] Recently, in a clinical practice setting, results using

the BioFire FilmArray GI panel were found to be reproducible (34/35, 97%).[722]

Whole genome sequencing of the parasite[1380] and mitochondrial and apicoplast genome sequencing were recently achieved.[75,270,271,604] They will be extremely useful in the development of new diagnostic assays for *C. cayetanensis*, including genotype analysis of the parasite. A multilocus sequence typing (MLST) method based on five microsatellite markers amplified by nested PCR was described.[644–646] This method was evaluated in *C. cayetanensis*–positive stool specimens from 54 patients, including 51 from the United States.[727] Poor discriminatory power was found, and many specimens had what appeared to be a mixture of sequence types at one of the loci. The authors suggested that an alternative approach to MLST could be to perform next-generation sequencing (NGS).[727]

Detection of *C. cayetanensis* in produce is a challenge. Usually low numbers of oocysts are detected in naturally contaminated produce, and the methods used for clinical samples are not always extrapolatable for detection in produce. One very important step is an efficient recovery of oocysts from fresh produce after careful washing. For the recovery of oocysts, different washing solutions have been used. Of those, a commercial laboratory detergent (Alconox) showed improved recovery compared to other solutions.[1558] The use of lectin-coated paramagnetic beads for isolation of *Cyclospora* oocysts from fruits and vegetables was described, but no significant differences in recovery efficiencies could be detected with or without this procedure. The isolation and concentration of *C. cayetanensis* oocysts using antibody-specific coated beads, as used for the detection of *Cryptosporidium parvum*, will likely improve efficiency, but antibodies are not yet commercially available. In recent years, several molecular techniques, including quantitative PCR (qPCR) have been developed for detection in fresh produce.[938,939,1225,1345] As few as 3 oocysts per gram (OPG) of fruit, or 5 OPG of herbs or green onions were reliably detected by qPCR melting curve analyses.[939] Furthermore, as low as five oocysts in raspberries, cilantro, parsley, basil, and carrots, in 25 g for leafy greens and carrots, and 50 g for raspberries, were detected by qPCR using a U.S. Food and Drug Administration (FDA) validated technique.[30,1224,1225]

A validated wash protocol for the recovery of *C. cayetanensis* oocysts from fresh produce, together with DNA extraction and a specific real-time PCR for detection of *C. cayetanensis* DNA published in 2017 in the Bacteriological Analytical Manual (Chapter 19) of the FDA.[1223] The wash protocol for fresh produce is performed in a filter bag (BagPage+) by adding 0.1% Alconox detergent as wash solution. Bags containing leafy greens or sturdy vegetables (but not those containing fragile matrices such as berries) are massaged gently with fingertips a few times to remove most of the air. Bags containing berries should be sealed without massaging and without removing air. Once sealed, the bags containing leafy greens are laid flat in a tray on a rocker platform for 30 minutes at 85 rpm at room temperature, inverting the bags after 15 minutes; bags containing berries are placed upright in the tray and slowly rocked on a rocker platform for 30 minutes at a lower speed. Afterwards, the supernatant from the filtrate side of each filter bag is transferred to individual centrifuge tubes, and sequential centrifugations are performed to recover, pool, and concentrate the wash debris. The wash debris pellets may then be stored at 4°C for up to 24 hours or frozen at −20°C for longer periods prior to DNA isolation.[1223]

22.7 TREATMENT

Trimetoprim-sulfamethoxazole (TMP-SMX) is the antibiotic of choice used for the treatment of cyclosporiasis.[589,729,1321,1735] Ciprofloxacin can be used as an alternative therapy in patients with sulfonamide allergies, although it is not considered as effective as TMP-SMX.[1735]

22.8 CONTROL AND PREVENTION

Infection of *C. cayetanensis* could be prevented by improved personal hygiene and sanitary conditions to prevent possible fecal-oral transmission from contaminated food, water, and possible environmental samples in endemic areas. Infection could also be eliminated by avoiding consumption of raw fresh produce, particularly in endemic areas.

There are some exploratory methods to remove or inactivate oocysts in fresh fruits and raw vegetables. Studies conducted on other coccidia may shed light on the control and prevention of *C. cayetanensis*. Using the chicken coccidian, *Eimeria acervulina*, γ-irradiation, at 1.0 KGy and higher was effective in decontamination of raspberries.[956] Using the same surrogate, hydrostatic pressure (HPP) (550 MPa at 40°C for 2 minutes) in raspberries and basil appeared to be effective since broiler chickens that were fed the contaminated produce with treated oocysts were asymptomatic and did not excrete oocysts.[902] Sodium dichloroisocyanurate (NaDCC) has been used in disinfection studies against common intestinal protozoa, including *C. cayetanensis,* where raw vegetables and fruits were dipped into NaDCC solution (1 g/L), and parasite numbers were reduced.[473] Treatment of *C. cayetanensis* oocysts with magnesium oxide nanoparticles showed significant reductions in sporulation rates compared to untreated oocysts and could be used safely as a preventive agent in food and water disinfectant treatments.[758] Water used for drinking, food preparation, and washing of fresh produce to be eaten raw, should be boiled or filtered. As indicated earlier, *C. cayetanensis*, and coccidia in general, are highly resistant to sanitizers and disinfectants.

Controlling sources of contamination in the field, in packing houses, and from farm workers is the key to prevent *C. cayetanensis* infection, particularly in endemic areas.

Access to toilet facilities, thorough handwashing, and proper disposal and treatment of human sewage are essential. Workers having any symptoms of gastroenteritis should not be allowed contact with vegetables or food. Other aspects of control and prevention used for other coccidian infections may also be applicable to *C. cayetanensis*. There is no vaccine to protect humans against this coccidian infection.

II. *CYSTOISOSPORA BELLI* (WENYON, 1923) FRENKEL, 1977

22.9 HISTORY

Isospora-like intestinal coccidia have been known for more than 100 years to parasitize humans, but there was uncertainty of the species involved.[429] Wenyon[1791] proposed the name *Isospora belli* for the large, bell-shaped 25–30 × 12–15 μm oocysts in human feces. Despite the characteristic shape of its oocysts, *I. belli* continued to be misdiagnosed as *Isospora hominis*.[554,784] Until the 1970s, *Isospora* species were considered non-host-specific and to have a direct fecal-oral transmission cycle. When the life cycle of *Sarcocystis* was discovered in 1972, it became clear that the parasite *I. hominis* was a mixture of more than two species of *Sarcocystis* with an obligatory two-host cycle involving cattle and pigs as intermediate hosts and humans as definitive hosts.[431] Additionally, *Isospora* spp. of cats were found to have a tissue cyst stage in extraintestinal organs of paratenic hosts,[560] leading to the creation of a new genus, *Cystoisospora*,[559] for *Isospora* species with a tissue cyst stage. In 1987, the tissue cyst stage of *I. belli* was discovered.[1411] Based on morphological and phylogenetic relationships with feline and canine *Isospora*, *I. belli* was transferred to the genus *Cystoisospoira*.[80] Thus, the correct designation for *I. belli* is *Cystoisospora belli* (Wenyon, 1923) Frenkel, 1977.

22.10 MORPHOLOGY AND LIFE CYCLE

Oocysts are excreted intermittently or continuously up to 50 days.[796] In freshly passed human feces, the oocysts are excreted in an unsporulated stage. Oocysts are 17–37 × 8–21 μm, colorless, and the oocyst wall is very thin and smooth. The oocysts are not always bell shaped and have one, both, or no pointed ends (Figures 22.3 and 22.4). The length-to-width ratio is greater than 1.2 (usually 2.1). Usually the sporulated oocysts contain two sporocysts and four sporozoites in each sporocyst, but occasionally, *Caryospora*-like oocysts (oocysts with one sporocyst containing eight sporozoites) are present.[839,1043] A micropyle and polar granule are present in some oocysts. The sporocysts are 9–14 × 7–12 μm, spherical to ellipsoidal, and without a Stieda body (Figure 22.3). Sporulation occurs in the environment, but apparently, in some cases, oocysts sporulate in the gut lumen[151]; also partially and fully sporulated oocysts have been seen in freshly

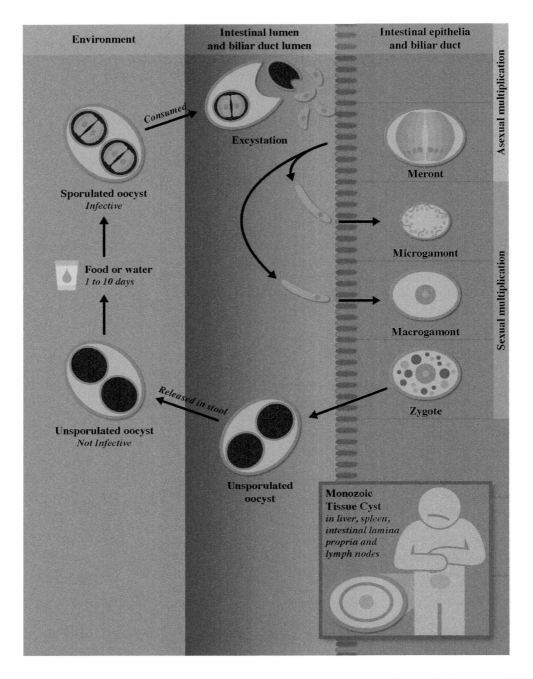

Figure 22.3 Life cycle of *Cystoisospora belli*. *Cystoisospora belli* has a direct fecal-oral transmission cycle. If a susceptible human ingests sporulated oocysts in contaminated food or water, the sporozoites inside the sporocysts excyst in the gut lumen and invade epithelial cells of the intestine, bile ducts and gallbladder where the parasite multiplies asexually and sexually within parasitophorous vacuole (pv) of host. In the asexual reproduction, shizogony takes place and merozoites are formed. After unknown numbers of schizogonies, merozoites form gamonts (sexual multiplication). There are two types of gamonts: microgamonts and macrogamonts. After a microgamete fertilize a macrogamont, oocyst wall is formed around the zygote and unsporulated oocyst is excreted in feces. Some sporozoites encyst in extra-intestinal organs (spleen, liver, mediastinal, trachea-bronchial, and mesenteric lymph nodes) and in intestinal lamina propria and produce monozoic tissue cysts. Oocysts sporulate in the environment and can survive in soil and water for months. All stages of the parasite are microscopic (<50 μm in maximum dimension).

excreted feces. Sporulation time varies depending on the environmental conditions from 24 hours to 10 days.

Monozoic tissue cysts (MTCs) are present in extraintestinal organs of immunosuppressed humans, but a paratenic host has not been demonstrated. Tissue cysts were found in the spleen, liver, mediastinal, trachea-bronchial, and mesenteric lymph nodes, and in the intestinal lamina propria (Table 22.4). The MTC wall is up to 4.0 μm thick.[1045] The zoites are 10.0–14.0 × 1.5–4.0 μm and mostly crescent shaped. A pale eosinophilic area was present distal to nucleus.

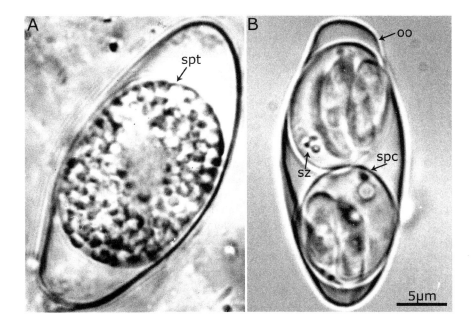

Figure 22.4 Oocysts of *Cystoisospora belli*. (A) Unsporulated with a central sporont (spt). (B) Sporulated oocyst. Note thin oocyst wall (oo), two sporocysts (spc), each with four sporozoites (sz). (Courtesy of Dr. Donald Duszynski.)

Ultrastructurally, MTC consists of a parasitophorous vacuolar membrane enclosing the thick granular cyst wall, and intravacuolar tubules (Figure 22.5). The zoite inside the cyst has the structure of coccidian sporozoite, including numerous micronemes, a few rhoptries, dense granules, polysaccharide granules, and a crystalloid body (Figure 22.6). Occasionally two tissue cysts were seen in one vacuole.

Like *C. cayetanensis*, *C. belli* is specific to humans. Attempts to infect nonhuman primates, livestock, rodents, and other animals with *C. belli* were unsuccessful.[796] Experimental

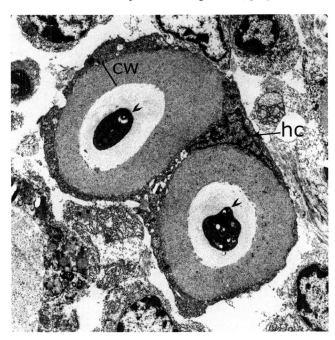

Figure 22.5 Transmission electron microscopy of two monozoic tissue cysts of *Cystoisospora belli* within one host cell (hc) in mesenteric lymph node of an AIDS patient. Note thick cyst wall (cw) enclosing zoites within a vacuole. (From Lindsay et al. 1997. *Clin. Microbiol. Reviews.* 10, 19–34.)

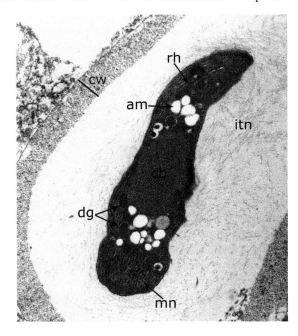

Figure 22.6 Transmission electron microscopy of a monozoic tissue cyst of *Cystoisospora belli* from the same patient as in Figure 22.5. Note longitudinal section of the sporozoite. Note, rhoptry (rh), numerous micronemes (mn), a crystalloid body (cb), dense granules (dg), and amylopectin (am). (From Lindsay et al., 1997. *Clin. Microbiol. Reviews.* 10, 19–34.)

infections in human volunteers[530,1147] confirmed the direct fecal-oral transmission cycle of *C. belli*. Human volunteers who ingested sporulated oocysts became infected and excreted unsporulated *C. belli* oocysts 9–17 days later. The incubation period (first day of symptoms) was 7–10 days. Symptoms recorded in some of these volunteers included: fever, nausea, vomiting and headache, asthenia, abdominal pain, meteorism (excess gas), fetid flatus, diarrhea, and voluminous stool.

Asexual and sexual stages of *C. belli* are confined to the intestines, bile ducts, and gallbladder epithelium (Table 22.4). Schizonts, gamonts, and unsporulated oocysts are present in enterocytes of the small intestine and in the biliary epithelium (Figure 22.1). Schizonts are often crescent shaped, up to 25×18 μm, and contain up to 10 merozoites that are $10–11 \times 3–4$ μm. The macrogamonts are elongated. The microgamonts contain as many as 30 nuclei and one to three residual bodies. The microgametes were about 4 μm long[432] and had flagella. The life cycle of *C. belli* is illustrated in Figure 22.3.

Partial development of schizonts containing two to four merozoites was seen in human cell lines seeded with *C. belli* sporozoites *in vitro*.[1274,1579]

22.11 DISTRIBUTION AND PREVALENCE

C. belli is globally distributed, but infections are found mainly in tropical and subtropical areas of the world such as the Caribbean, Central and South America, Africa, and Southeast Asia (Tables 22.4–22.7). There are more reports of *C. belli* infections from India than other countries, and these are summarized in Table 22.7.

Most *C. belli* infections have been reported in the last century. A report summarized more than 1500 cases from the Western Hemisphere.[517] Most of these reports were based on finding *C. belli* oocysts in feces (Tables 22.5 and 22.6). Many studies were reported after the emergence of HIV, and currently, the prevalence of *C. belli* is being reported worldwide (Table 22.6). Reports confirmed by autopsy or biopsy are summarized in Table 22.4. Epidemic outbreaks of cystoisosporiasis were reported in the 1960s and in the late 1970s in some countries. Oocysts of *C. belli* were found in an industrial water treatment plant, which may have been used to water and contaminate vegetables.[1475] The epidemic reported in Brazil occurred in a children orphanage.[171]

Prevalence rates vary even in endemic areas. Consistently high prevalence of *C. belli* infection (12%–15%) was observed in several studies in Haiti.[354,1322,1735] In Africa, prevalence levels vary greatly among the different countries, ranging from 0.3% to 28% (Table 22.6). In nonendemic areas, such as Europe, the United States, and Australia, prevalences of *C. belli* are low (Table 22.6). Cases initially reported in Europe, the United States, and Australia were mostly people who came from endemic areas or who had traveled to tropical and subtropical countries, such as Haiti, South America,

India, or Africa (Tables 22.5 and 22.6). In fact, in the United States, one of the risk factors for infection was immigration from or travel to Latin America.[1598] Clinical cases related to traveler's diarrhea have been reported in several countries (Tables 22.5 and 22.6). Since the 1990s, many studies have been reported on *C. belli* infection in immunocompromised patients worldwide. The prevalence of *C. belli* infection is significantly higher in HIV-infected patients compared to HIV-negative patients in different geographical areas (Table 22.6).

C. belli oocysts have been found in vegetables and fruits[98] as well as in surface and recreational water[126,489] in endemic areas. Eleven (3.1%) of 360 fruit and vegetable samples (avocado, lettuce, cabbage, carrot, tomato, banana, and mango) collected in Southern Ethiopia markets were positive for the presence of this parasite,[98] although it is unclear which individual commodities were contaminated. *C. belli* oocysts were also found in 4 of 12 water samples used for recreational activities in Malaysia,[126] and in Egypt 0.47% positive samples of 840 treated potable water samples tested positive for the presence of *C. belli*.[489]

22.12 PATHOGENESIS

C. belli is an intracellular parasite. It multiplies in enterocytes that are replaced every few days during the normal host cycle. Judging from the reports of examination of biopsy specimens from patients, the severity of symptoms does not seem to correlate with parasite density. In a typical coccidian parasite, such as *Eimeria* infections in livestock, coccidiosis is self-limiting. *C. belli* infections, however, can persist for months.[1705] One hypothesis for persistency of infection is that oocysts can sporulate in the host and cause reinfection. Another hypothesis is that tissue cysts formed by *C. belli* in extraintestinal organs or in the lamina propria of the intestine can initiate relapse. However, there is no report of histological evidence for tissue cyst rupture. It remains uncertain that the high prevalence of *C. belli* in immunosuppressed patients is due to relapse of subclinical infections or recently acquired infections. There are no data pertaining to the infectious dose of *C. belli*. The occasional findings of schizonts and gamonts with associated disease in the bile duct and gallbladder are probably due to the spread of intestinal infection by reverse peristalsis.

22.13 CLINICAL SYMPTOMS

Common symptoms of *C. belli* infection are profuse diarrhea (chronic or intermittent), abdominal discomfort, fever, nausea, anorexia, and considerable weight loss. In a study of 57 patients sampled for 8 years,[784] the author noted intense watery diarrhea in 98.2%, eosinophilia in 53.6%, fever in 75%, weight loss in 86.3%, asthenia in 88.2%, anorexia in 71.4%, and colic pain in 61% of patients. Fatty stools and

Table 22.4 Summary of Reports of Cystoisospora belli Infections in Humans with Histologic Findings Presented in Chronological Order, Including Stages Found, Treatments, and Outcome

Patient Data	Country	Symptoms	Immunocompromised (Yes, No) Type	Method of Diagnosis	Endogenous Stages Found	Treatment (which) Successful or not	Outcome of Patient	Reference
3 cases, no personal data on patients	Chile	Diarrhea, fever, abdominal pain and eosinophilia	Unknown	Feces, biopsy of small intestine	SC;	ND		Niedmann (1963)
6 cases, Case 1: F, 42 yr Puerto Rican; Case 2: M, 30 yr Cuban with Hodgkin's disease Case 3: M, 48 yr, had visited Syria; Case 4: F, 55 yr; Case 5: 12-month-old infant who died; Case 6: no data on sex, age	United States, California	Intense, chronic diarrhea and steatorrhea	Yes, in case 2 patient with Hodgkin's disease (involving liver, lymph nodes, and spleen but not intestine)	Oocysts in feces of cases 1–3, not in 4–6 Small intestine biopsies from 6 patients (total 19 biopsies)	Oo in feces of 2, SC, GA, Oo in sections of intestine, Oo in duodenal contents of 1 but no Oo in feces	Case 3 improved without treatment, nitrofurantonin for Giardia	3 patients died from pulmonary edema or pulmonary embolism (case 1, case 4, and case 5) Case 3 recovered	Brandborg et al. (1970)
1 case, M, 23 yr	Italy, Sardinia	Diarrhea, weight loss, malabsorption for 6 years	IC, but α-chain disease	TEM of jejunal biopsy	Unidentified zoites	ND		Henry et al. (1974)
1 case, M, 58 yr	United States, Massachusetts. After military service in Italy and North Africa	Chronic diarrhea for more than 20 years. Eosinophilia and probable malabsorption for more than 7 years	No, IC	Feces, histology, and TEM. Multiple biopsies of duodeno-jejunal junction	SC, GA, Oo in biopsy, oocysts in feces	Pyrimethamine and sulfadiazine combined	Prompt disappearance of symptoms and intestinal coccidia. Asymptomatic and no intestinal coccidial reinfestation for 3 years	Trier et al. (1974)
1 case, F, 24 yr	United States, Oklahoma	Acute lymphoblastic leukemia. Severe chronic diarrhea for 30 months, weight loss	Yes, chemotherapy for acute lymphoblastic leukemia	Feces, duodenal aspirate	No Oo in feces but present in 7 of 10 duodenal aspirates	TMP-SMX	Successful, diarrhea subsided in 48 hours, negative 3-month follow-up	Westerman and Christensen (1979)
1 case, M, 6 months	United States, California	Severe diarrhea and vomiting for 1.5 weeks. Perforation of sigmoid colon. Laparotomy at necropsy	No	TEM of biopsy of ileum	Yes, not specific diagnosis "coccidia" poor images of no diagnostic value	30 weeks of continuous total parental nutrition	Died	Liebman et al. (1980)
1 case, M, 65 yr	Spain	Diarrhea and weight loss for 3.5 years. Lost 23 kg 3 months before admission to hospital and got to be 38 kg and cachectic	No	Feces. Small bowel biopsy	Oo in feces. No parasites in biopsy	Pyrimethamine-sulfadoxine	After treatment diarrhea subsided and patient started to gain weight progressively	Guisantes et al. (1982)

(Continued)

Table 22.4 (Continued) Summary of Reports of Cystoisospora belli Infections in Humans with Histologic Findings Presented in Chronological Order, Including Stages Found, Treatments, and Outcome

Patient Data	Country	Symptoms	Immunocompromised (Yes, No) Type	Method of Diagnosis	Endogenous Stages Found	Treatment (which) Successful or not	Outcome of Patient	Reference
1 case, M, 35 yr	Israel, Tel Aviv	Diarrhea for more than 5 years. Malabsorption syndrome. Combined humoral and cellular immunodeficiency	Yes, combined humoral and cellular immunodeficiency	Feces. Duodneal biopsy. Diagnosis uncertain whether C. belli or other coccidians	Oo in feces, no parasites in biopsy of duodenum	Metronidazole (2 g/day for 30 days and 1 g/day for 100 days) initially induced clinical remission that lasted for 6 months	Died after 6 months suffering from acute lymphoproliferative disease	Hallak et al. (1982)
1 case, M, 37 yr	The Netherlands	Gonorrhea, syphilis, Condylomata acuminata, and hepatitis B, severe diarrhea and weight loss	Yes, AIDS	Feces, biopsy of small intestine	Oo in feces. Unidentified stage in biopsy	Pyrimethamine and sulfadiazine (discontinued due to pancytopenia) Spiramycin and nivaquina (stopped) Amprolium (patient consent)	Spiramycin and nivaquina (only partially successful) Amprolium successful. When stopped recurrency, treatment again successful. She died from other infection	Veldhuyzen van Zanten et al. (1984)
1 case, M, 38 yr	Chile	Chronic diarrhea, Kaposi's sarcoma, steatorrhea, weight loss, fever	Yes, AIDS	Feces, biopsy in duodenum and colon	Oo in stools. Merozoites and schizonts in enterocytes in duodenum **and also in epithelial cells in large intestine (colon)**	TMP-SMX	Treatment suspended because of neutropenia. Died of sepsis after 16 months	Figueroa et al. (1985)
1 case, M, 32 yr	United States, Pennsylvania, patient originally from Haiti, emigrated 5 yr prior	Diarrhea and weight loss. History of malaria, syphilis, hepatitis B, and toxoplasmosis	Yes, inversion T helper–suppressor cells. It is not indicated if AIDS but could be	Feces, biopsy of jejunum. Duodenal washing	Oo in feces. Biopsy inconclusive	Previous TMP-SMX intermittent, cyclic diarrhea. Also tretracycline, furazolidone, spiramycin	Intermittent cyclic diarrhea after all treatments	Gaska et al. (1985)
1 case, M, 30 yr	Republic of Cabo Verde	Diarrhea, weight loss. Developed typhoid fever.	Yes, AIDS	Feces, jejunal fluid examination, duodenal-jejunal and ileal biopsies. TEM	Oo in feces and in biopsy fluid. ME in TEM	Transiently cured by pyrimethamine-sulfadiazine. Recurrent diarrhea, treated again	Successful response after treatment of recurrence	Modigliani et al. (1985)
1 case, F, 11 yr	Chile, Temuco	Intense diarrhea, malabsorption, eosinophilia	IC	Stool examination, Biopsy small intestine	Oo in stool, SC with ME in biopsy	TMP-SMX	Numerous relapses, when treatments were stopped	Gamboa et al. (1986)

(Continued)

Table 22.4 (Continued) Summary of Reports of Cystoisospora belli infections in Humans with Histologic Findings Presented in Chronological Order, Including Stages Found, Treatments, and Outcome

Patient Data	Country	Symptoms	Immunocompromised (Yes, No) Type	Method of Diagnosis	Endogenous Stages Found	Treatment (which) Successful or not	Outcome of Patient	Reference
3 cases, No individual sex or age data	Uganda	Diarrhea	Yes, AIDS	Stool examination. Duodenal biopsies	Of 3 patients positive[l] in stools, one showed SC inside enterocytes	Not indicated	N/A[m]	Sewankambo et al. (1987)
1 case, M, 38 yr	United States, Maryland (NIH, Bethesda)	History of cystoisosporiasis and AIDS, found infected with cytomegalovirus at necropsy	Yes, AIDS, homosexual	Necropsy. Light microscopy and TEM in intestinal (small and large intestine) and extraintestinal tissues	Oo in feces, SC in biopsy, and **TC in extraintestinal tissues (lamina propria of small and large intestine, mesenteric and trachea-bronchial lymph nodes)**	TMP-SMX	Died. Studies at necropsy	Restrepo et al. (1987)
5 cases (12%) of 42 patients	Zaire, Kinshasa	Diarrhea	Yes, AIDS	Stool examination. Duodenal biopsy and TEM	Positive stools in 5 patients. In one patient C. belli detected in duodenal biopsy. TEM	ND	N/A	Colebunders et al. (1988)
1 case, M, 34 yr	Belgium, Antwerp, African patient	Chronic diarrhea (2 yrs), anorectal pain, hemorrhage, weight loss (10 kg in 2 months). Surgery for hemorrhoidal thrombosis	Yes, AIDS	Feces. Duodenal and jejunal biopsies	Oo in feces, biopsy negative	Resistant to TMP-SMX, pyrimethamine and folinic acid needed to be stopped for decreasing white blood cells. Roxithromycin	Diarrhea intermittent and less severe after treatment. No *I. belli* observed after 10 days of treatment Four months after treatment had no diarrhea in the last 2 months	Musey et al. (1988)
1 case, F, 42 yr	Taiwan	Hodgkin's disease with chronic watery diarrhea for 6 months HTLV-1 positive, delayed hypersensitivity	Yes, Immunocompromised by chemotherapy for Hodgkin's disease HTLV-1 positive	Feces, biopsy	Oo in feces. SC in terminal ileum	TMP-SMX. Recurrence treated again with same therapy	Remained in maintenance therapy with TMP-SMX at publication	Peng and Tsai (1991)
1 case, F, 30 yr	Italy	Chronic watery diarrhea and fever	Yes, AIDS, (heroin drug addict)	Biopsy of duodenojejunal junction. TEM	**SC, ME in enterocytes. Zoites in the lamina propria and within lymphatic vessels**	TMP-SMX	Resolution of diarrhea within 48 hours	Comin and Santucci (1994)
1 case, M, 39 yr	United States, Washington, DC	Diarrhea, nausea, vomiting, abdominal pain, weight loss. Acalculous cholecystitis.	Yes, AIDS (drug use, homosexual)	Feces. Biopsy of intestine and bile ducts. HE-stained sections at postmortem	No oocysts in feces, no parasites in duodenal biopsy. SC and GA in bile duct epithelium and epithelial cells of gallbladder			Benator et al. (1994)

(Continued)

Table 22.4 (Continued) Summary of Reports of *Cystoisospora belli* Infections in Humans with Histologic Findings Presented in Chronological Order, Including Stages Found, Treatments, and Outcome

Patient Data	Country	Symptoms	Immunocompromised (Yes, No) Type	Method of Diagnosis	Endogenous Stages Found	Treatment (which) Successful or not	Outcome of Patient	Reference
1 case, M, 22 yr	France	Diarrhea, travel history	Yes, AIDS	Feces negative, biopsy ileum	*C. belli*-like stages	ND	N/A	Alfandari et al. (1995)
1 case, F, 30 yr	France, originally from Burkina Faso	Chronic diarrhea, vomiting, weight loss. Malabsorption syndrome	Yes, HIV-1 positive, AIDS	Light microscopy and TEM after necropsy	SC, GA in enterocytes, **TC in liver, spleen, and lymph nodes.** Epithelial stages: ME, GA, and Oo within enterocytes	Several TMP -SMX treatments followed by prophylaxis with same drugs	TMP-SMP did not improve conditions	Michiels et al. (1994); Bernard et al. (1997); Lindsay et al. (1997b)
1 case, M, 26 yr	Two episodes of self-limiting diarrhea and vomiting	United Kingdom	Yes, AIDS	Feces. Duodenal biopsy, TEM	SC in enterocytes	Low-dose co-trimoxazole gradually built up to 960 mg 4 times a day for 10 days, had to be discontinued due to skin rash. Then, treated with pyrimethamine	Patient compliance was poor	Hamour et al. (1997)
8 cases, no age or sex data	Argentina	Chronic diarrhea	Yes, AIDS	Feces, endoscopy, duodenal biopsy (TEM and light microscopy)	**TC in 2 patients in duodenal lamina propria** with no oocysts in feces. Negative stools	TMP-SMX (4 times daily for 14 days)	2 patients no resolution of diarrhea, 6 temporary resolution but relapses	Velásquez et al. (2001); Velásquez et al. (2011)
1 case, M, 60 yr	Germany, emigrant from Greece	Malabsorption. Severe diarrhea, loss of weight. Cholecystectomy. Damaged biliary tree	No	Duodenal aspirates and bile	Oo in duodenal aspirates and bile	Failed treatment TMP-SMX and nitazoxanide. Stopped Oot excretion with IV TMP-SMX in 5 days	IV TMP-SMX: patient discharged. Asymptomatic for the next 3 months under observation	Bialek et al. (2001)
1 case, M, 54 yr	Bangkok	Chronic diarrhea. Intestinal malabsorption	No. Homozygous hemoglobin E. hemoglobinopathy	Feces. Biopsy of jejunal mucosa	SC, Oo in epithelium	TMP-SMX, pyrimetamine or albendazole but relapses. Pyrimetamine 25 mg/d for 20 weeks successful	Follow-up negative stools	Jongwutiwes et al. (2002)
1 case, M, 26 yr	Brazil	Patient with a long history of parasitism (15 yr) HIV-positive and hepatitis C positive at 20 yr. Last admission with fever, abdominal pain, diarrhea, and vomiting. Cause of death staphylo-coccal septicemia	Yes, HIV-positive, drug user	Histology at autopsy. Sections of esophagus, duodenum, ileum, colon, appendix, and gallbladder studied	Few GA in gallbladder epithelium. **TC in lymph nodes**	TMP-SMX in several occasions, also anti-HIV- therapy	Resistant to chemotherapy. Died	Frenkel et al. (2003)

(Continued)

Table 22.4 (Continued) Summary of Reports of Cystoisospora belli Infections in Humans with Histologic Findings Presented in Chronological Order, Including Stages Found, Treatments, and Outcome

Patient Data	Country	Symptoms	Immunocompromised (Yes, No) Type	Method of Diagnosis	Endogenous Stages Found	Treatment (which) Successful or not	Outcome of Patient	Reference
1 case, M, 44 yr	Japan	Diarrhea, appetite loss, malabsorption and body weight loss for over 10 years	No, IC	Feces, biopsy of duodenum **Immunohistochemical examination using the patient's sera**	SC, GA	TMP-SMX	Successful. Diarrhea dramatically attenuated. Patient discharged.	Sasaki et al. (2004)
28 cases. No sex or age data	France, 6827 Patients HIV-positive 1995–2003 in two hospitals in France	HIV patients from France. Eight with developed AIDS-defining events (tuberculosis [n = 3], non-Hodgkin's lymphoma [n = 2], esophageal candidiasis [n = 2] and Kaposi's sarcoma [n = 1]). All patients with cystoisosporiasis presented with diarrhea, which was severe enough to lead to hospital admission for 60% of them. Fever was uncommon (7%)	Yes, HIV- pos	Feces, duodenal and bile duct biopsy in three patients. **The prevalence of isosporiasis increased from 0.4 per 1000 patients in the pre-HAART° era (1995–1996) to 4.4 per 1000 patients in the HAART era (2001–2003)**	Oo in feces of all 28, bile duct involvement, and cholangitis in 3. Cystoisosporiasis more frequently in sub-Saharan Africa (72%) in female and heterosexual, and with patients who had a higher median CD4 count at diagnosis (142 cells/mL)	TMP-SMX. HAART. Treatment was longer (median 15 days) and at a higher dose (median daily dose of 3200 mg) than recommended, but relapses of 45% were observed	27 patients treated with TMP-SMX: Relapse occurred in six of 16 patients (38%) despite maintenance TMP-SMX therapy and HAART	Lagrange-Xélot et al. (2008)
1 case, M, 43 yr	Iran	Chronic severe debilitating watery diarrhea, intermittent fever, severe dehydration, vomiting, abdominal pain	Yes, Primary interpulmonary thymic epithelial tumor (mediastinal thymoma)	Feces, duodenal biopsies.	**TC cysts in lamina propria** of intestine	The patient was first treated by oral TMP-SMX	Recurrence, treated with cotrimoxazole. No diarrhea in the following 6 months. Patient had a thymectomy performed	Meamar et al. (2009)
1 case, M, 42 yr	United States, Connecticut	Abdominal pain, vomiting, and diarrhea. Acute diffuse biliary disease associated with isosporiasis	AIDS	Bile duct biopsy. Histology, TEM, PCR	SC, GA, Oo in histologic bile duct sections. TEM demonstrated intracellular coccidian stages, and microgametes. PCR-positive	TMP-SMX and ivermectin	Lost to follow-up	Walther and Topazian (2009); Dubey et al. (2019)
1 case, M, 23 yr	Argentina	Abdominal pain, clinical dehydration	Ultra-short bowel syndrome. Isolated **intestinal transplantation**	Feces. Endoscopic biopsies	Oo in lumen	TMP-SMX followed by prophylaxis	Highly effective, improvement within 48 hours. Histology normalization after the first week; however, abnormal endoscopic findings persisted for several weeks	Gruz et al. (2010)

(Continued)

Table 22.4 (Continued) Summary of Reports of *Cystoisospora belli* Infections in Humans with Histologic Findings Presented in Chronological Order, Including Stages Found, Treatments, and Outcome

Patient Data	Country	Symptoms	Immunocompromised (Yes, No) Type	Method of Diagnosis	Endogenous Stages Found	Treatment (which) Successful or not	Outcome of Patient	Reference
1 case, M, 44 yr	Mexico	Diarrhea	Yes, HIV	Feces. Ileum biopsy, PCR-ITS	SC, GA			Murphy et al. (2011)
8 cases, W	South Africa	Chronic diarrhea	Yes, AIDS. However, evidence of reconstitution of CD4 T-cell count and suppression of HIV replication in both cases	Feces, duodenal biopsies	Oo in feces of all and in biopsy of 7. Biopsy positive but feces negative in acute cases	TMP-SMX and other antibiotics	2 patients died after all kind of treatments, and despite immune reconstitution for AIDS	Boyles et al. (2012)
1 case, M, 70 yr	South Korea	Chronic diarrhea with a 35 kg weight loss in 2 yr	No, alcoholic	Stool examination (negative results in three different samplings). Biopsy from upper jejunum	SC, GA	TMP-SMX	Successful. Follow-up evaluation at 2.5 years later revealed marked improvement of body weight (40 kg to 68 kg)	Kim et al. (2013)
1 case, M, 50 yr	United States, Ohio	Diarrhea, abdominal pain, nausea, vomiting, peripheral eosinophilia	Yes, receiving systemic corticosteroids for eosinophilic gastroenteritis (EGE)	*C. belli* superinfection in EGE. Biopsy duodenum	SC in enterocytes	TMP-SMX	Successful. Diarrhea and peripheral eosinophilia resolved	Navaneethan et al. (2012)
1 case, M, 39 yr	Argentina	Chronic diarrhea	Yes, AIDS	Microscopic analysis of blood, stool, and duodenal biopsy samples. Blood samples were also examined with the molecular techniques for *C. belli* DNA detection	GA in epithelium. **Tissue cysts in the lamina propria. Parasitemia.** Extraintestinal	ND	N/A	Velásquez et al. (2016)
2 cases: Case 1: W, 25 yr; Case 2: M, 35 yr	Iran	Case 1: abdominal discomfort and diarrhea. Case 2: abdominal pain, vomiting, and diarrhea	Yes, (1) prolonged corticosteroid therapy. (2) AIDS. cholecystectomy due to acalculous cholecystitis several months prior to fecal examinations	Oo in feces of both. Gallbladder biopsy Case 2: PCR (+)	SC, Oo, in gallbladder mucosa	Case 1: TMP-SMX	Case 1: diarrhea ceased within 3 days of starting treatment	Agholi et al. (2016a)

(Continued)

Table 22.4 (Continued) Summary of Reports of Cystoisospora belli Infections in Humans with Histologic Findings Presented in Chronological Order, Including Stages Found, Treatments, and Outcome

Patient Data	Country	Symptoms	Immunocompromised (Yes, No) Type	Method of Diagnosis	Endogenous Stages Found	Treatment (which) Successful or not	Outcome of Patient	Reference
1 case, M, 28 yr	Australia, refugee from Myanmar	Chronic diarrhea, nausea, vomiting, abdominal pain	No, IC	Feces, colon biopsy. Molecular study	Oo in feces. Ribosomal RNA ITS locus, and mitochondrial COI locus PCR tests, and amplicon sequencing positive in DNA extracted from stored colon biopsies	TMP-SMX	Successful with 1 month of TMP-SMX	Woon et al. (2016)
1 case, M, 69 yr	Italy	Vomiting, profuse and intermittent watery diarrhea, and weight loss, lasting 7 months	Yes, **Good's syndrome**	Feces, molecular detection in duodenal biopsy	First, PCR amplification and amplicon sequencing of Apicomplexan18S rRNA: 100% identity with the 18S ribosomal RNA gene of *C. belli*. Stool examination: Eventually, *Cystoisospora* spp. were detected in the stool specimen	TMP-SMX Onset of suspected drug-induced pancytopenia, TMP/SMX terminated and instead ciprofloxacin	The patient fully recovered and gained weight. Recurrence of diarrhea never occurred during the 6-month period of follow-up	Esvan et al. (2018)
1 case, M, 23 yr	United States, Utah			Duodenal biopsy	SC, GA			Swanson et al. (2018); Dubey et al. (2019)

Source: Dubey, J.P., Almeria, S. 2019. *Cystoisospora belli* infections in humans—The past 100 years. *Parasitology* http://doi.org/10.1017/S0031182019000957.

Note: Important/rare findings are in bold.

Abbreviations: ART, active antiretroviral therapy; F, female; HAART, highly active antiretroviral therapy; IC, immunocompetent; ID, immunosuppressed, M, male; N/A, not applicable; ND, not done or no data; Oo, oocysts; SC, schizonts; TMP-SMX, trimethoprim sulfamethoxazole, cotrimoxazole; yr, age in years.

Table 22.5 Early Reports (1935–1983, Before the Emergence of AIDS) of Intestinal *Cyclospora belli* Infections in Humans Based Only on Stool Examination, Presented in Chronological Order

Patient Data	Country, Region	Symptoms	Remarks	Treatment (which) Successful or not	Outcome of Patient	Reference
10 cases (2.6%) of 384 stools tested from soldiers in World War I	Egypt, Alexandria, and Turkey, Gallipoli		Soldiers who had been in these areas were infected	N/A	N/A	Woodcock and Penfold (1916) (included in Magath, 1935)
153 cases	Multiple	Digestive disorders	Some named *Isospora hominis*	N/A	N/A	Connal (1922)
208 cases, World War I soldiers	Multiple	Digestive disorders		ND	N/A	Magath (1935)
5 cases, soldiers (19–29 yr)	Japan, Okinawa, and Saipan	Diarrhea	Soldiers stationed in Okinawa (2–16 weeks), then evacuated to Saipan. One patient excreted *C. belli* oocysts for 38 days	Atabrine, quinine, tetrachlorethylene, or carbarsone. No effect	Self-limited infection after patient moved to nonendemic area	Liebow et al. (1948)
50 cases	United States	Diarrhea	Army soldiers	ND	ND	Barksddale and Routh (1948)
1 case, M, no age indicated	Chile	Diarrhea, tuberculosis		ND	N/A	Neghme and Silva (1950)
11 cases, 9 M, 2 F, 17–52 yr	Chile	Chronic diarrhea, fever (6 of 11), slight eosinophilia, abdominal pain, frequent Charcot–Leyden crystals		Sulfonamides, terramycin, chlromicetine, penicillin, streptomycin	No effect	Balmaceda et al. (1953)
1 case, F, 17-month-old	United States, Florida	Slight fever, watery diarrhea, weakness	Oocysts in feces, malnutrition	ND	N/A	Beck et al. (1955)
12 cases (1.26%) of 955 children and 11 (0.14%) of 7621 adults	South Africa, Durban, Natal	Stool samples from hospitalized patients	Oocysts more frequently observed during **Autumn** (March to May) and in children	ND	N/A	Dodds and Elsdon-Dew (1955)
3 cases, F, 10, 31, and 77 yr	United States, Tennessee	Nausea, abdominal discomfort/pain, greenish-yellow diarrhea with mucus		No treatment was given	Spontaneous recovery in two, one died due to possible electrolyte imbalance	Webster (1957)
1 case, no data on age or sex	Chile	Diarrhea, dyspepsia, abdominal pain, eosinophilia	Stools with oocysts, **also oocysts in duodenal juice**	Sulfadiazine	Oocysts disappeared 1 week later	Orrego et al. (1959)
189 cases (3.3%) of 5763 patients (29 followed up)	Chile	Onset with fever, acute or subacute diarrhea, asthenia, anorexia, weight loss, eosinophilia, and Charcot–Leyden crystals	98% diarrhea, 88% asthenia, 86% weight loss, 75% fever,73% Charcot-Leyden 71% anorexia, 70% meteorism, 61% abdominal pain	Opiates, antibiotics, sulfonamides	Variable effect of treatment. All benign cases	Jarpa et al. (1960)
835 cases reviewed	North and South America			N/A	N/A	Faust et al. (1961)

(Continued)

Table 22.5 (Continued) Early Reports (1935–1983, Before the Emergence of AIDS) of Intestinal *Cyclospora belli* Infections in Humans Based Only on Stool Examination, Presented in Chronological Order

Patient Data	Country, Region	Symptoms	Remarks	Treatment (which) Successful or not	Outcome of Patient	Reference
12 cases, 6 yr or older	United States, Texas, Austin	Severe diarrhea, fever, chills, nausea, and considerable weight loss		Treatment with terramycin, glycobiarasol, diiodoquin, and chloroquine	No effect	Henderson et al. (1963)
1 case, M, 11 yr	Egypt, Cairo	Constipation for 1 year, no diarrhea, anemia	Malnutrition	Sulfadiazine for 1 week	Successful	Rifaat and Salem (1963)
8 cases, 5 F, 3 M, 20–40 yr	Chile	Acute diarrhea, fever, abdominal pain, asthenia, anorexia, nausea, and vomiting; eosinophilia (6)	Epidemic outbreak in summer (March–July) Charcot–Leyden crystals (4)	ND	N/A. Two needed hospitalization	Daiber et al. (1964)
1 case, M, 34 yr	Great Britain	Exacerbated tropical sprue, diarrhea, eosinophilia	Oocysts in feces	Nitrofurantoin	Partly successful	French et al. (1964)
1 case, M, 34 yr	Belgium, traveler from Congo	Diarrhea, fever		Chloroquine	Successful	Limbos et al. (1965)
1 case, M, 30 yr	Chile, Santiago de Chile	Diarrhea, abdominal colic, fever, weight loss	*C. belli* oocysts infection	Corticoid therapy (prednisone)	Improved after therapy	Sapunar et al. (1965)
38 cases (23.1%) of 164? children in a 3-month period (4 months to 3 yr)	Romania, Jassy	No morbid clinical symptoms	12 cases associated with *Giardia*. Unclear number of children analyzed	No treatment, just follow-up	Resolved without treatment	Burdea et al. (1966)
392 cases (3.2%) of 12,398 patients in 8 years from a medical center	Chile, Santiago de Chile	Intense diarrhea in 98.2%, eosinophilia in 53.6%, fever (75%), weight loss (86.3%), asthenia (88.2%), anorexia (71.4%), colic pain (61%). Fatty stools	Long-term follow-up of 57 patients	No treatment performed	N/A	Jarpa Gana (1966)
7 cases (10.2%) of 685 stools	The Netherlands	No symptoms	Samples from subjects who lived in tropical and subtropical regions	N/A	N/A	Smitskamp and Oey-Muller (1966)
1 case, f, 38 yr	United States, New York **traveler**	Dysentery, slight fever, moderate abdominal pain, mucus in stools	Diarrhea after a month in rural Argentina	Carbasone for 14 days	Recovered	Cahill and Tsai (1968)
12 cases (7.2%) of 165 children (2–6 yr) in an orphanage	Brazil, Sao Paulo	Diarrhea, abdominal pain	Epidemic in March. Good hygienic conditions	ND	N/A	Campos et al. (1969)
2 cases, F, 18 yr; M, 56 yr	United States, New York	(C1) nausea, vomiting, and diarrhea; (C2) nausea and diarrhea	Patients returned from visits to Puerto Rico and Mexico	(C1) Not treated, did not return to clinic (C2) Tetracycline	(C2) Cured	Miller et al. (1971)
2 cases, M, 35 and 37 yr	Belgium	Diarrhea, anorexia, vomiting, weight loss, intermittent abdominal pain	Traveler's diarrhea, visited tropics	(C1) Chloroquine, metronidazole (C2) chloroquine	(C1) No effect (C2) Cured	Limbos et al. (1972)
1 case, F, 23 yr	England	Violent diarrhea and abdominal pain	Traveler's diarrhea, visited West Africa	No treatment performed	Self-cured	Skinner (1972)

(Continued)

Table 22.5 (Continued) Early Reports (1935–1983, Before the Emergence of AIDS) of Intestinal Cyclospora belli Infections in Humans Based Only on Stool Examination, Presented in Chronological Order

Patient Data	Country, Region	Symptoms	Remarks	Treatment (which) Successful or not	Outcome of Patient	Reference
1 case, 8 yr, F,	United States	Diarrhea				McCracken (1972)
1 case, F, 51 yr	Israel	Intermittent diarrhea, mucoid, nausea, vomiting, malaise	Duodenal intubation (immature oocysts). Malabsorption	TMP-SMX	Recovery in a few days	Syrkis et al. (1975)
1 case, M, 47 yr	Japan, Sendai	Diarrhea, malabsorption		ND	N/A	Ohtaki et al. (1976)
1 case, M, 48 yr. Army soldier in the South Pacific, returned to United States	United States, South Carolina	**Recurrent diarrhea for 26 years**	Oocysts in stool. Jejunal biopsy but negative results	Tetracycline and dithiazanine iodide	Continued to have intermittent episodes	Ravenel et al. (1976)
90 cases in a 3-month period, 51 M, 39 F; 2–69 yr (18 cases under 14 yr)	Chile, Antofagasta	Diarrhea, meteorism, weight loss. Charcot–Leyden (95.6%), eosinophilia (76%), anorexia (50%)	**Epidemic outbreak. In 12 of the 18 pediatric cases no symptoms More frequent 30- to 40-year-olds**	Symptomatic treatment (diet, antispasmodic), tinidazol	ND	Sagua et al. (1978)
26 cases, pediatric, in 3 years, 16 M, 10 F, 2–15 yr	Chile, Antofagasta	Diarrhea, anorexia, intestinal pain, weight loss	Increased cases in autumn-winter. Good education and socioeconomic level. 15 cases asymptomatic (58%)	ND	N/A	Sagua et al. (1979)
1 case, F, 24 yr	United States, Oklahoma	Diarrhea		Co-trimoxaole	Successful	Westerman and Christensen (1979)
5 cases (0.14% of 3500 stools, M	France	Diarrhea, weight loss, eosinophilia in one case	Travelers from tropical areas (Nigeria, Togo, French Guyana, Syria)	Tinidazole	Less symptoms except one case	Deluol et al. (1980)
1 case, M, 29 yr	Australia	Watery, yellow-green (6 motions/day) diarrhea, weight loss, weakness, night sweats		Metronidazole, tinidazole	A few oocysts still present after treatment. Patient did not return for checkups	Butler and de Boer (1981)
452 cases (0.8%) of 55,421 in a **17-year observation period** (1963–1979)	Chile	56% had Charcot–Leyden crystals	Stool examination. More frequent in males. Monthly (April to June) and annual variations	ND	N/A	Jarpa et al. (1981)
1 case, M, 35 yr	Israel, Tel Aviv	Diarrhea, malabsorption	Oocysts labelled as Isospora hominis		N/A	Hallak et al. (1982)
1 case, M, 65 yr	Spain	Diarrhea, megablastic anemia				Guisantes et al. (1982)
1 case, M, 35 yr	Brazil, Salvador-Bahia	Diarrhea, anorexia. Nausea, asthenia, fever	Stool examination	Not indicated	N/A	Faria and Brust (1983)

Source: Dubey, J.P. Almeria. S. 2019. Cystoisospora belli infections in humans—The past 100 years. Parasitology http://doi.org/10.1017/S0031182019000957.
Note: Important findings are in bold.
Abbreviations: F, female; M, male; N/A, not applicable; ND, not done or no data; TMP-SMX, trimethoprim sulfamethoxazole or cotrimoxazole; yr, age in years.

Table 22.6 Summary of Positive Reports of Intestinal *C. belli* Infections in Humans after the Emergence of AIDS, Based Only on Stool Examination, Presented in Chronological Order

Patient Data	Country, Region	Symptoms	Immunocompromised (Yes, No) Type	Remarks	Treatment (which) Successful or Not	Outcome of Patient	Reference
3 cases of 20 patients selected (17 M, 3 F, 22–43 yr)	United States, Georgia. Patients from Haiti	Chronic enteritis	Yes, AIDS associated with Kaposi's sarcoma and opportunistic infections	Two patients were diagnosed by duodenal string test and one by stool examination	ND	Two patients were alive. One was dead at the end of 2-yr	Pitchenik et al. (1983)
1 case, F, 18 yr	Thailand	Diarrhea. Severe dehydration, inappetence, and weakness	No, IC		Treatment with electrolytes and TMP-SMX[f]	Diarrhea ceased within 5 days	Teschareon et al. (1983)
3 cases, M (l)	United States, California	Several months of diarrhea	Homosexual, likely AIDS	Oo[g] cysts in feces, *C. belli*–like stages in duodenal biopsy	Case (1) Metronidazole for 10 days Case (2) lost track of patient before treatment started. Case (3) TMP-SMX begun but discontinued due to increasing neutropenia. Subsequently, he received metronidazole	Case (1) resolution of symptoms with metronidazole. Case (3) Resolution of the diarrhea	Forthal and Guest (1984)
3 cases, M, 29, 36, and 41 yr	United States, New York	Watery diarrhea in 3, weight loss in 1	ND	Patient 1 had traveled to Guatemala and Mexico 3 weeks before. The other patients were homosexuals	Atabrine 7 days (patient 1), sulfa-trimethoprim (patient 2), Dose regimen not reported (patient 3)	Full recovery in all three	Ma et al. (1984)
1 case, M, 34 yr	United States, California	History of intermittent or episodic diarrhea, low-grade fever and adenopathy	Yes, AIDS. Kaposi's sarcoma	Other parasites present	TMP-STX Metronidazole and diiodohydroxyquin for *Entamoeba histolytica, Giardia lamblia*; he was treated with quinacrin	Symptomatic improvement but episodic diarrhea continued	Ng et al. (1984)
10 cases, unknown age and sex	United States, Miami (Three patients were from Haiti and lived in the United States at the time of the study)	Profuse diarrhea (8–10 stools/day) weakness, anorexia, weight loss	Yes, AIDS (Kaposi's sarcoma or multiple opportunistic infections, or both)	**Duodenal string test,** 1 patient negative stool but positive in string test	TMP-SMX prolonged course. Relapses (in 2 of the 3 patients) treated with furazolidone and pyrimetamine-sulfadiazine	Successfully re-treated with a 4-week course of TMP-SMX	Whiteside et al. (1984)

(Continued)

Table 22.6 (Continued) Summary of Positive Reports of Intestinal C. belli Infections in Humans after the Emergence of AIDS, Based Only on Stool Examination, Presented in Chronological Order

Patient Data	Country, Region	Symptoms	Immunocompromised (Yes, No) Type	Remarks	Treatment (which) Successful or Not	Outcome of Patient	Reference
1 case (0.1%) in 110 stools from children	Chile, South	ND	No, IC	Stool examination	ND	N/A[i]	Gayan and Norambuena (1985)
1, M, 37 yr	United States, Hispanic	Diarrhea, nausea, vomiting, intermittent fever, weight loss (23 pounds), not able to sleep, dehydration	Not indicated, homosexual and diarrhea	Stool examination	TMP-SMX, loperamide, compazine (for nausea)	Symptoms decreased, and patient was discharged	Kobayashi et al. (1985)
20 cases (15%) of 131 AIDs patients	Haiti	Chronic watery diarrhea and weight loss	Yes, AIDS 86% HTLV-III seropositive		TMP-SMX (160 mg and 800 mg) 4 times daily for 10 days, and then twice daily for 3 weeks	Seven had recurring cystoisosporiasis in 2–20 weeks after therapy	DeHovitz et al. (1986)
9 cases (19.5%) of 46 adults, Unknown age and sex. Initial suspicion of AIDS	Zaire	Episodic chronic diarrhea from several months to years, weight loss more than 10% body weight, fever	Yes, 37 ID, 9 IC	8 of 37 **ID, 1 of 9 IC**	ND	N/A	Henry et al. (1986)
1 case (0.4%) of 372 pooled stools from 274 patients, M, 55 yr	United States, Chicago	Diarrhea	No specified, homosexuals with diarrhea	2 (0.7%) of 372 specimens. Patient Oo in stool	Metronidazole and iodoquin	Protected of symptoms but patient died	Peters et al. (1986)
1 case, M, 34 yr	United States, Returning from a trip to India	Watery diarrhea, low-grade fever and periumbilical cramps	No, IC	Traveler's diarrhea	TMP-SMX, relapse treated with double-strength treatment	Cleared for next 15 months	Godiwala and Yaeger (1987)
1 case, M, 57 yr	Thailand, Chiang Mai	Diarrhea after prednisolone administration for the management of nephrotic syndrome	Yes, Acute lymphoblastic leukemia		No specific treatment	Recovery without specific treatment	Morakote et al. (1987)
1 case, F, 23 yr	United States, Hispanic origin	Diarrhea	Yes, HIV-positive		TMP-STX	**Oo in feces still 6 months after treatment**	Peters et al. (1987)
3 cases (5%) of 60, M	Spain, Barcelona	Watery diarrhea	Yes, AIDS, 1 drug addict. 1 Kaposi's sarcoma		TMP-SMX	Successful. One discontinued treatment and had recurrence 2 weeks later, treated successfully with same treatment	Ros et al. (1987)
2 cases (2%) of 100 patients	United States, New York	Diarrhea	Yes, AIDS	C. belli in 2 patients with diarrhea			Antony et al. (1988)

(Continued)

Table 22.6 (Continued) Summary of Positive Reports of Intestinal *C. belli* Infections in Humans after the Emergence of AIDS, Based Only on Stool Examination, Presented in Chronological Order

Patient Data	Country, Region	Symptoms	Immunocompromised (Yes, No) Type	Remarks	Treatment (which) Successful or Not	Outcome of Patient	Reference
61 cases (0.2%) of 30,032 patients	United States	Chronic enteric disease	Yes, AIDS	Haitian-born adults had 13 times higher cystoisosporiasis (1.7%) than all other AIDS patients	ND	N/A	Salik et al (1987)
11 cases (9.3%) of 118 patients	Congo, Brazzaville	Diarrhea in 75% of patients	Yes, AIDS		ND	N/A	Carme et al. (1988)
2 cases, Haitians, M, 40 yr; F 47 yr	United States	Debilitating profuse watery diarrhea in both	Yes, aggressive T-cell malignancy (ATL) adenocarcinoma		P1: TMP-SMX P2: IV TMP-SMX	P1: Recurred. P2: resolution but discontinued after 4 days, recurrence. She died	Greenberg et al. (1988)
40 cases (38 adults, 2 children)	France	Diarrhea, low-grade fever, steatorrhea in severe diarrhea cases. Hypereosinophilia	No, IC	Retrospective study. Traveler's diarrhea	TMP-SMX in 17 cases	Successful in the immunocompetent cases treated: all cured	Junod (1988)
2 cases, M, 62 yr, 43 yr	United States, New York	Diarrhea	Yes, AIDS		TMT-SMX. Treatment 2 patients with AIDS, sulfonamide allergy, pyrimethamine worked TMT-SMX	Recurrency treated successfully with pyrimethamine alone or with folinic acid	Weiss et al. (1988)
8 cases, AIDS patients. No age and sex data	Zaire	Abdominal pain, cramps, watery diarrhea	Yes, AIDS		**Diclazuril** for 7 days	Disappearance of abdominal pain and cramps in all, diarrhea stopped in 4 of 5 with watery diarrhea, no changes in 3 with semiformed stools. One recurrence	Kayembe et al. (1989)
10 cases (10.1%) of 99 HIV patients	Brazil, Rio de Janeiro	ND	Yes, HIV-positive (99 group IV), IC: 260	Only *C. belli* observed in HIV-positive patients	ND	N/A	Moura et al. (1989)
1 case, M, 40 yr	Chile	Chronic diarrhea	Yes, HIV		ND	N/A	Neira and Villalón (1989)
34 cases (12%) 291 Haitian patients	Haiti	Chronic diarrhea	Yes, AIDS		TMP-SMX (32 patients). Recurrence. Same treatment in 10 patients, sulfadoxine and pyrimetamine (12 patients) or placebo (3 patients)	Only 1 patient had *C. belli* while on treatment	Pape et al. (1989)

(Continued)

Table 22.6 (Continued) Summary of Positive Reports of Intestinal *C. belli* Infections in Humans after the Emergence of AIDS, Based Only on Stool Examination, Presented in Chronological Order

Patient Data	Country, Region	Symptoms	Immunocompromised (Yes, No)Type	Remarks	Treatment (which) Successful or Not	Outcome of Patient	Reference
1 case, M, 23 yr	Spain	Diarrhea, abdominal pain, nausea, vomiting, fever, lymphadenopathia	Yes, AIDS (drug addict), HIV-positive	Patient developed Lyell syndrome after TMP-SMX	TMP-SMX. Metronidazole	After 2 weeks TMP-SMX developed generalized rash in palms, soles, conjunctival and glans involvement. After metronidazole: improvement, neg *C. belli* at 2 months follow-up	Romeu et al. (1989)
7 case (11.1%) of 63 HIV-positive patients	Zambia	Diarrhea (70%), abdominal pain (19%), weight loss (10%). Rectal discharge (1%)	Yes, 63 HIV-positive, IC: 36 controls	7 (16%) of 44 HIV-positive with diarrhea. 0 of HIV-positive without diarrhea	ND	N/A	Conlon et al. (1990)
1 case, M, 65 yr	Japan	Watery diarrhea for 2 months	Yes, HTLV-1 positive, ATL		TMP-SMX	Effective for diarrhea	Kawano et al. (1992)
2 cases of 81 HIV patients	France	Diarrhea, malabsorption	HIV	Feces of 1 and duodenal biopsy of 1			Cotte et al. (1993)
17 cases (13%) of 131 AIDS and 0 of 81 IC patients	Brazil, reference center	Gastrointestinal manifestations	Yes, AIDS in 131		ND	N/A	Sauda et al. (1993)
1, M, 53 yr	Japan	Watery diarrhea, anorexia, progressive weight loss, leukocytosis	Yes, HTLV-1 positive, ATL	Died from leukemia	TMP-SMX	Recurrence, treated again with TMP-SMX effective	Yamane et al. (1993)
11 cases (15.3%) of 72 patients	Senegal, Dakar	Diarrhea	Yes, HIV-positive	6 (12.8%) of 47 HIV-1 positive, 5 (23.8%) of 21 in HIV-2 positive	ND	N/A	Dieng et al. (1994)
1 case, F, 57 yr	Spain	Chronic diarrhea and polyarthritis (reactive arthritis). Eosinophilia	Yes, HIV-positive		TMP- SMX and diclofenac	Arthritis improved and diarrhea abated, but patient died due to AIDS	Gonzalez-Dominguez et al. (1994)
14 cases (4.9%) of 287 patients	Zambia	Diarrhea	Yes, HIV (242). IC: 45 with diarrhea	From two different centers	ND	N/A	Khumalo-Ngwenya et al. (1994)
15 cases (4.3%) of 351 patients	Tanzania	Diarrhea	Yes, HIV-positive (112), HIV-negative[i] (239)	13 (11.6%) in HIV-positive, 2 (0.8%) in HIV-negative. Five were in HIV-positive children	ND	N/A	Gomez-Morales et al. (1995)
127 cases (1.0) of 16,351 AIDS patients between 1985 and 1992	United States, California	Chronic diarrhea	Yes, AIDS	Not indicated (diarrhea): 127 cases (1.0%)	TMP-SMX	Prevented new infection	Sorvillo et al. (1995)

(Continued)

Table 22.6 (Continued)   Summary of Positive Reports of Intestinal *C. belli* Infections in Humans after the Emergence of AIDS, Based Only on Stool Examination, Presented in Chronological Order

Patient Data	Country, Region	Symptoms	Immunocompromised (Yes, No) Type	Remarks	Treatment (which) Successful or Not	Outcome of Patient	Reference
9 cases (2.1%) 420 AIDS patients	United States, California,	Chronic diarrhea	Yes, AIDS	2 staining techniques compared	ND	N/A	Berlin et al. (1996)
2 cases, M, 28 and 36 yr	Italy	Chronic watery diarrhea	Yes, AIDS		Both patients. Albendazole and ornidazole. Patient 2 same treatment	Resolution of symptoms. **Hypersensitivity to TMP-SMX**	Dionisio et al. (1996)
2 cases: case 1, F, 38 yr; case 2, F, 31 yr	Case 1, Brazil, Case 2 Germany, Cologne	Diarrhea	Kaposi's sarcoma	Oos in aspirated duodenal juice; biopsy negative	TMP-SMX	Successful	Franzen et al. (1996)
21 cases (28%) of 77 adult patients	Zambia	Diarrhea	Yes, AIDS	Hospital study. **High prevalence**	ND	N/A	Kelly et al. (1996)
9 cases (7.2%) of 124 HIV patients	Uganda	Diarrhea (64 AIDS-positive and 31 HIV-negative), nondiarrhea (60 AIDS-positive, 100 IC)	Yes, AIDS (124, of those 64 with diarrhea), IC: 131	8 (12.5%) of 64 AIDS patients with diarrhea, 1 (1.6%) of 60 AIDS-positive without diarrhea	ND	N/A	Ravera et al. (1996)
7 cases (5.6%) of 123	Tanzania	Diarrhea	Yes, HIV-positive				Tarimo et al. (1996)
4 cases (0.9%) of 430 adults	Central Africa Republic, Bangui	Diarrhea (290), 140 no diarrhea		*C. belli* only in HIV-positive. 1 (1.3%) of 79 with acute diarrhea, 3 (2.7%) of 110 persistent diarrhea	ND	N/A	Germani et al. (1998)
4 cases (2%) of 200 HIV patients	Brazil	Diarrhea	Yes, HIV/AIDS				Cimerman et al. (1999)
1 case, M, 60 yr	Mozambique	Pulmonary tuberculosis, diarrhea, weight loss	Yes, AIDS		TMP-SMX	Diarrhea stopped	Clavero et al. (1999)
1 case (0.65%) of 154 patients	Italy, Apulia	Diarrhea (65), rest no diarrhea	Yes, HIV-positive	1.5% group with diarrhea	ND	N/A	Brandonisio et al. (1999)
1 case (1.5%) of 67 HIV patients	Cuba	**Asymptomatic**	Yes, HIV-positive (67). IC:136	Infected patient was asymptomatic	ND	N/A	Escobedo and Nunez (1999)
11 cases (32.3%) of 34 AIDS adults	Brazil	Persistent chronic diarrhea	Yes, HIV-positive		ND	N/A	Lainson and da Silva (1999)
22 cases. No age and sex data	Haiti (Port-au-Prince)	Chronic diarrhea	Yes, HIV-positive	TMP-SMX better than ciprofloxacin	Treatment of 22 patients: TMP-SMX in 10 patients; ciprofloxacin 12 patients	Ciprofloxacin: 3 of 12 persistent *I. belli* elimination, 2 with diarrhea. Treated with TMP-SMX, successful 9, only 1 persistent elimination *I. belli* (no diarrhea)	Verdier et al. (2000)

(Continued)

Table 22.6 (Continued) Summary of Positive Reports of Intestinal C. belli Infections in Humans after the Emergence of AIDS, Based Only on Stool Examination, Presented in Chronological Order

Patient Data	Country, Region	Symptoms	Immunocompromised (Yes, No) Type	Remarks	Treatment (which) Successful or Not	Outcome of Patient	Reference
9 cases (1.5%) of 594 samples	Senegal, Dakar	Diarrhea (279), nondiarrhea (315)	Yes, HIV-positive (318) HIV-negative (276)	7 (4.4%) of 158 HIV-positive with diarrhea and 2 (1.2%) of 160 HIV-positive no diarrhea	ND	N/A	Gassama et al. (2001)
4 cases (7.7%) of 52 patients	Guinea-Bissau	Chronic diarrhea	Yes, HIV-positive (37). IC (15)	1 (20%) of 5 HIV-1 positive; 3(10.7%) of 28 HIV-2 positive	ND	N/A	Lebbad et al. (2001)
3 cases (5%) of 60 patients. No age and sex data	Thailand	Diarrhea	Yes, HIV-positive	2 patients had diarrhea and one did not. The 3 had CD4 <200/uL			Wiwanitkit (2001)
56 cases (13.3%) of 422 patients	Brazil, Natal	Diarrhea	Yes, HIV-positive	Humid weather, bad sanitary conditions	ND	N/A	Da Rocha and Dos Santos (2002)
93 cases. No age and sex data	Germany	Chronic diarrhea, 1 patient with biliary cystoisosporiasis (in Bialek et al., 2001)	Yes, **bone marrow transplant recipients**, patients HIV-positive	Sensitivity of iodine staining was 48.4% (95% CI, 37.7–59.1), but a sensitivity of 95.7% (95% CI, 85.2–99.5) was calculated for autofluorescence	ND	N/A	Bialek et al. (2002)
4 cases (0.8%) of 484 stools analyzed. No age and sex data	Uganda	Diarrhea	Yes, HIV	Low prevalence in this cohort	ND	N/A	Brink et al. (2002)
55 cases (14%) of 397 HIV-infected patients	Venezuela	98% of the positive patients had acute or chronic diarrhea	Yes, HIV-positive	Epidemiological cross-sectional study	ND	N/A	Certad et al. (2003)
18 cases (7.4%) of 243 patients in hospital in Malawi:	Malawi	121 patients with diarrhea and 122 without diarrhea	Yes, All C. belli positive were HIV-positive	15 of 121 in patients with diarrhea, 3 of 122 without diarrhea	ND	N/A	Cranendonk et al. (2003)
1 case, M, 38 yr	France, The patient was from Mali living in France for 8 years	Chronic diarrhea. Severe watery diarrhea and metabolic disorders	Yes, Stage IV Non-Hodgkin's lymphoma HIV-negative		TMP-SMX	Successful	Resiere et al. (2003)
2 (3.3%) of 60 patients	South Africa	Diarrhea	Yes, HIV/AIDS (30). IC: 30	Both positive were HIV-positive and had diarrhea	ND	N/A	Oguntibeju (2006)
3 cases (1.9%) of 154 HIV adult patients	Cameroon	29% had diarrhea	Yes, HIV	Cross-sectional study	ND	N/A	Sarfati et al. (2006)

(Continued)

Table 22.6 (Continued) Summary of Positive Reports of Intestinal C. belli Infections in Humans after the Emergence of AIDS, Based Only on Stool Examination, Presented in Chronological Order

Patient Data	Country, Region	Symptoms	Immunocompromised (Yes, No) Type	Remarks	Treatment (which) Successful or Not	Outcome of Patient	Reference
1 case, M, 25 yr	Turkey	Diarrhea	Renal transplant	Oo in feces	Cotrimoxazole	Successful	Yazar et al (2006)
1 case, F, 25 yr	Turkey	Liver transplant 8 months prior. Watery diarrhea	Yes, Immunosuppressive therapy prior to transplant		TMP-SMX	Responded well	Atambay et al. (2007)
37 cases (10.3%) of 359 patients (638 fecal samples)	Brazil, Triangulo Mineiro region	252 patients with diarrhea, 107 no diarrhea	Yes, HIV/AIDS	29 (8.1%) positive with diarrhea, 8 nondiarrhea	ND	N/A	De Oliveira-Silva et al. (2007)
164 cases (0.2%) of 74,174 HIV-infected enrolled in French program 1992–2003	France	Diarrhea	Yes, HIV	Risk assessment study—higher risk in people from sub-Saharan Africa	If TMP-SMX prophylaxis lower risk of parasitism	N/A	Guiguet et al. (2007)
38 cases (33 ID, 5 IC)	Thailand	ND. Selection based on positive fecal samples to C. belli	Yes, AIDS ($n = 30$) and corticosteroid-treated patients ($n = 3$) Also, 5 IC	Morphological and molecular characterization 5.8S rRNA, ITS-1, and ITS-2	N/A	N/A	Jongwutiwes et al. (2007)
17 cases (30.4%) of 56 patients	Honduras	Diarrhea	Yes, AIDS		No treatment, no retroviral treatment either	N/A	Kaminsky et al. (2007)
1 case, M, 32 yr	Turkey, Ankara	Acute onset of abdominal cramps, watery diarrhea, low-grade fever, and nausea	Yes, Renal transplant recipient		Ciprofloxacin (two times because of recurrence, second time IV for 3 days). Then, TMP-SMX	C. belli oocysts still detected after ciprofloxacin. TMP-SMX treatment successful	Koru et al. (2007)
26 cases (12.2%) of 214 HIV-positive, 0 of 164 HIV-negative	Ethiopia	ND	Yes, 214 HIV-positive No, 164 HIV- negative	<200 CD4 cells/uL had more prevalence of infection and diarrhea	ND	N/A	Assefa et al. (2009)
28 cases (8.4%) of 334 HIV-positive and 50 (2.9%) of 1722 HIV-negative	Peru	ND	Yes, 334 (16.3%) HIV- positive No, 1722 HIV-negative	Cross-sectional study of 2056 patients			Chincha et al. (2009)
9 cases (3.1%) of 268 HIV-positive, 0 of 20 HIV-negative	Nigeria	Diarrhea	Yes, 268 HIV-positive No, 20 HIV-negative	<200 CD4 cells/uL 19.0% (4/21) 200–500 CD4/uL 2% (5/247)	ND	N/A	Olusegun et al. (2009)
1 case, M, 55 yr	France, expatriate returning from Mauritania	Traveler diarrhea	No, IC		TMP-SMX previously. In France ciprofloxacin and symptomatic	Improved, no follow-up	Agnamey et al. (2010)

(Continued)

Table 22.6 (Continued) Summary of Positive Reports of Intestinal C. belli Infections in Humans after the Emergence of AIDS, Based Only on Stool Examination, Presented in Chronological Order

Patient Data	Country, Region	Symptoms	Immunocompromised (Yes, No) Type	Remarks	Treatment (which) Successful or Not	Outcome of Patient	Reference
28 cases (7.8%) of 360 HIV-infected	Nigeria	Not indicated	Yes, HIV-positive	CD4 counts <200/uL associated with *C. belli*	ND	N/A	Akinbo et al. (2010)
2 cases, M, 30 yr and 27 yr	Chile	Diarrhea	Yes, HIV- positive	Fecal examination, PCR and sequencing	Case 1: TMP-SMX, 3 months later ciprofloxacin and prophylaxis TMP-SMX. Case 2: ND	Case 1: died. Case 2: no follow-up	Neira et al. (2010)
3 cases (1.7%) of 175 AIDS patients	Democratic Republic of Congo, Kinshasa	Diarrhea	Yes, AIDS	Stools examination	ND	N/A	Wumba et al. (2010)
35 cases (10.1%) of 346 HIV	Malaysia	Diarrhea	Yes, HIV-positive		ND	N/A	Asma et al. (2011)
6 cases (1.2%) 500 with diarrhea and 0 of 357 no diarrhea	Brazil	Diarrhea in 143 patients, nondiarrhea in 357 patients	Yes, HIV/AIDS	Retrospective study 500 HIV patients (1998–2008)	ND	N/A	Cardoso et al. (2011)
1 case, M, 32 yr	Spain, tourist returning from Senegal	Dengue infection in a traveler tourist returning from Senegal	No, IC	Traveler diarrhea	No treatment. Self-limiting	Auto-cured	Pérez-Ayala et al. (2011)
29 cases (15.4%) of 188 HIV patients	Ethiopia		Yes, HIV-positive	0 of 66 non-HIV patients			Alemu et al. (2011)
24 cases (7.8%) of 450 stools from **children**	Egypt, Minia district	Chronic diarrhea	Yes, 200 immunosuppressed (severe malnutrition, chronic diseases, corticosteroids, malignancies). IC: 250	15 Immunosuppressed (9.1%), 9 (6.3%) IC	ND	N/A	Abdel-Hafeez et al. (2012)
1 case, F, 44 yr	United States, New York	Debilitating diarrheal illness and profound weight loss, and abdominal pain	Yes, HTLV-1, diagnosed with ATL later, HIV-negative		TMP-SMX	Initial resolution of diarrhea. Recurrence, repeat TMP-SMX, with no significant improvement. Patient died a few weeks after discharge	Ud Din et al. (2012)
1 case, M, 35 yr	Turkey	Abdominal pain, malaise, and recurrent diarrhea	Yes, **liver transplant**		TMP-SMX	Recurrence	Usluca et al. (2012)
2 cases (0.6%) of 356 patients	Iran	Diarrhea	Yes, HIV-positive	**Molecular detection (ITS-2)** <200 CD4 T cells/uL	ND	N/A	Agholi et al. (2013)

(Continued)

Table 22.6 (Continued) Summary of Positive Reports of Intestinal *C. belli* Infections in Humans after the Emergence of AIDS, Based Only on Stool Examination, Presented in Chronological Order

Patient Data	Country, Region	Symptoms	Immunocompromised (Yes, No) Type	Remarks	Treatment (which) Successful or Not	Outcome of Patient	Reference
4 cases (6.7%) 59 HIV-positive	Brazil	Diarrhea	Yes, HIV-positive	CD4 T lymphocytes <200 cells/mm^3 significantly related to parasitism	ND	Lack of adherence to antiretroviral therapy more prevalence of parasitism	Assis et al (2013)
35 cases (1.7%) of 2112 children under 5 yr	Kenya, Nairobi	Diarrhea	No, IC	Poor urban environment	ND	N/A	Mbae et al. (2013)
6 cases, 5 M, 1 F, 32 yr to 55 yr (mean 38 yr)	Peru	Recurrent diarrhea	Yes, HIV/AIDS	Refractory to treatment, high number died	HIV prophylaxis with TMP-SMX, ciprofloxacine, nitaxozanide, and/or pyrimethamine	Refractory to treatment, 5 died	Montalvo et al. (2013)
9 cases (17.65%) of 56 patients	Venezuela	Diarrhea (79%), weight loss (28.6%), abdominal pain and/or colic and vomits (18%)	Yes, HIV-positive		ND	N/A	Rivero-Rodriguez et al. (2013)
1 case, 61 yr, M	Germany	Ulcerative colitis (13 yr history) Severe diarrhea, abdominal cramps, weight loss and low-grade fever	ID, long-term systemic corticosteroids and immunomodulators, azathioprine and infliximab	Oocysts in feces	Initial treatment with metronidazole and ciprofloxacin. Then treated with TMP-SMX	Successful treatment after TMP-SMX double strength	Stein et al. (2013)
2 cases (6%) of 58 patients in Latin America	From 6 Latin-American countries	Recurrent diarrhea, in a child 15-yr-old case cachexia with body index of 10.4 kg/m^2	Yes, Hyper-IgM syndrome	Review Hyper-IGM syndrome in Latin America	ND	N/A	Cabral-Marques et al. (2014)
1 case (0.3%) of 316 HIV-positive	Ethiopia, Addis Ababa	Not indicated	Yes, HIV-positive 316		ND	N/A	Taye et al. (2014)
23 cases (10.1%) of 207 HIV-positive	Cameroon	Not indicated	Yes, HIV-positive		ND	N/A	Vouking et al. (2014)
1 case, 3 yr	Iran	Diarrhea, fever	Yes, AIDS		TMP-SMX	Successful	Nateghi Rostami et al. (2014)
5 cases (1.3%) of 199 patients	Ethiopia	Diarrhea	Yes, HIV		ND	N/A	Kiros et al. (2015)
1 case, F, 13 yr	Portugal, patient born in São Tomé Island	Intermittent course of diarrhea, abdominal pain, and vomiting	Yes, immunosuppressive therapy after a cardiac transplant		Ivermectin, albendazole, praziquantel, and ciprofloxacin	Clinical and microbiological resolution	Sanches et al. (2015)
1 case (0.3%) of 291 (146 M, 145 F). 0–89 yr, (29.2 ± 20 yr)	Burkina Faso	ND	No	Hospital survey	ND	N/A	Sangare et al. (2015)

(Continued)

Table 22.6 (Continued) Summary of Positive Reports of Intestinal *C. belli* Infections in Humans after the Emergence of AIDS, Based Only on Stool Examination, Presented in Chronological Order

Patient Data	Country, Region	Symptoms	Immunocompromised (Yes, No) Type	Remarks	Treatment (which) Successful or Not	Outcome of Patient	Reference
3 cases (1.5%) of 200 children	Egypt	Mentally handicapped	No, IC	Four institutions	ND	N/A	Shehata and Hassanein (2015)
9 cases (1.2%) of 741	Iran	Diarrhea	Yes, AIDS/HIV (387), malignancy (187), transplant recipients (184), corticosteroids long term or hypogammaglobulinemia (43)	Description of *Sarcocystis cruzi* in one patient	ND	N/A	Agholi et al. (2016b)
3 cases, M, 4, 10 and 13 yr	Turkey	Abdominal pain, diarrhea, lack of appetite, weight loss, fatigue	Leukemia in 1		All three cases co-trimoxazole	Case 1 showed relapse after 2 weeks and treatment repeated with success	Cengiz et al. (2016)
13 cases (3.4%) of 300 patients	Cameroon	Not selected based on symptoms	Yes, HIV	Significantly associated with CD4 T cells below 200 cells/uL in patients on HIV prophylaxis	ND	N/A	Nsagha et al. (2016)
1 case, F, 46 yr	Iran	Debilitating diarrhea, intermittent fever, night sweat, abdominal pain, severe weight loss, malnutrition	Yes, HTLV-1	Stool positive, **DNA positive by ITS-1 PCR**	TMP-SMX	Improved diarrhea, but she died from malnutrition	Shafiei et al. (2016)
4 cases (1.1%) of 350. No age and sex data	Iran	Immunosuppressed (AIDS, malignancy, organ transplant recipients, others)	Yes, HIV/AIDS and other immunosuppressive malignancies	2 (2.5%) of 80 HIV/AIDS-positive, 1 (0.4%) of 234 with malignancy, 1 (4.7%) of 21 with other immunosuppression	ND	N/A	Salehi-Sangani et al. (2016)
1 case, M, 63 yr	Taiwan	Vietnamese	Yes, HIV/AIDS and other immunosuppressive malignancies	PCR-positive on biliary aspirate	ND	N/A	Chiu et al. (2016)
1 case (0.2%) of 517 samples from HIV-positive	Mozambique, Maputo		Yes, HIV (371 samples (71.8%) IC: 146 (28.2%)	The positive sample was in a HIV-negative patient	ND	N/A	Cerveja et al. (2017)
9 (2.8%) of 323 patients	Ethiopia	HIV, not selected based on symptoms	Yes, HIV/AIDS	Other intestinal parasites studied	ND	N/A	Gedle et al. (2017)
1 case, F, 31 yr.	United States, New Jersey, Newark. Haitian patient	Acute worsening of chronic diarrhea and weight loss of 1 yr duration	Yes, HTLV-1 positive with ATL		TMP-SMX with recurrence and repeat treatment	After recurrence, prophylactic TMP-SMX	Hasan et al. (2017)

(Continued)

Table 22.6 (Continued)   Summary of Positive Reports of Intestinal *C. belli* Infections in Humans after the Emergence of AIDS, Based Only on Stool Examination, Presented in Chronological Order

Patient Data	Country, Region	Symptoms	Immunocompromised (Yes, No) Type	Remarks	Treatment (which) Successful or Not	Outcome of Patient	Reference
7 cases (retrospective study). No age and sex data	Peru	Diarrhea and HIV-positive. 1 had concomitant hepatitis C, 1 tuberculosis, 1 with syphilis	HIV-positive		TMP-SMX forte in all (1–7 times) 5 of them with ciprofloxacin or nitazoxanide	4 had recurrent diarrhea even after treatment, 3 solved symptoms after treatment. 1 died due to complications	Silva-Diaz et al. (2017)
1 case (1.1%) of 90 HIV patients	Brazil	ND	Yes, HIV/AIDS	Epidemiological study	N/A	N/A	Barcelos et al. (2018)
27 cases (25.0%) of 108 HIV patients	Mozambique, Maputo	Diarrhea when admitted to hospital	Yes, 83 HIV-positive, whereas the HIV status of the remaining 25 patients had not been determined		ND	No	Casmo et al. (2018)
1 case, F, 71 yr	France	Fever and severe watery diarrhea	Yes, corticosteroids and immunosuppressive therapy for rheumatic arthritis, HIV-negative		TMP-SMX	Patient died	Post et al. (2018)
1 case, M, 77 yr	Spain	Chronic diarrhea, monoclonal gammopathy	Yes, monoclonal gammopathy, HIV-negative		TMP-SMX	Diarrhea ceased	Ros Die and Nogueira Coito (2018)
1, M, 56 yr	Iran	History of thymectomy, persistent recurrent diarrhea, weight loss	Yes, Good's syndrome and thymoma		TMP-SMX	Responsive, but died due to syndrome	Tavakol et al. (2018)

Source: Dubey, J.P., Almeria, S. 2019. *Cystoisospora belli* infections in humans—The past 100 years. *Parasitology*146, 1490–1527.
Note: Important/rare findings are in bold.
Abbreviations: F, female; IC, immunocompetent; ID, immunosuppressed, M, male; N/A, not applicable; ND, not done or no data; Oo, oocysts; TMP-SMX, trimethoprim sulfamethoxazole or cotrimoxazole; yr, age in years.

Table 22.7 Summary of Positive Reports of *C. belli* Infections in Humans in India, Presented in Chronological Order

Patient Data	State, City	Symptoms	Immunocompromised (Yes, No) Type	Remarks	Treatment (which) Successful or not	Outcome of Patient	Reference
1 case, M, 19 yr	Delhi	Abdominal pain, intermittent diarrhea with alternating constipation	No, IC	Initially diagnosed as amebiasis	Sulfonamides (sulfatriad)	No oocysts detected after treatment	Prakash et al. (1969)
1 case, M, 5 yr	Delhi	Fever, diarrhea, abdominal pain	No, IC		Unspecified amebic drugs. **Metronidazole**	No improvement after metronidazole.	Mirdha et al. (1993)
3 cases (12%) of 25 HIV patients	Maharastra, Karad	Diarrhea	Yes, HIV		ND	N/A	Ghorpade et al. (1996)
1 case, M, 30 yr		Fever, diarrhea	Yes, acute lymphocytic leukemia		TMP-SMX	Successful	Jayshree et al. (1996)
4 cases (5.2%) of 77 patients	Maharastra, Mumbai	Diarrhea (4), abdominal pain (3), weight loss (4), oral candidiasis (1)	Yes, AIDS		ND	N/A	Lanjewar et al. (1996)
1 case (0.1%) of 1029 cancer patients	Karanataka, Banglore	Diarrhea	Yes, cancer chemotherapy		ND	N/A	Rudrapatna et al. (1997)
1 case (1.3%) of 75 AIDS and cancer patients	Karanataka, Banglore	Diarrhea	Yes, AIDS (45 patients), cancer (30 patients)		ND	N/A	Ballal et al. (1999)
13 cases (11.8%) of 111 HIV- positive	Tamil Nadu, Vellore	Acute diarrhea (30 patients), chronic diarrhea (31 patients). No diarrhea (50 patients)	Yes, HIV-positive	3 of 30 with acute diarrhea, 8 of 31 chronic diarrhea, 2 in patients without diarrhea	TMP-SMX,	Symptoms improved	Mukhopadhya et al. (1999)
1 case, M, 28 yr	Tamil Nadu, Dharampuri	Chronic diarrhea, fever, abdominal pain, weight loss	Yes, HIV-positive		TMP-SMX	No follow-up	Parija and Bhattacharya (2000)
8 cases (**30.8%**) of 26 diarrheic patients	Uttar Pradesh, Lucknow	Diarrhea	Yes-HIV-positive		ND	N/A	Prasad et al. (2000)
14 cases (13.7%) of 102 HIV- positive with diarrhea	Tamil Nadu, Chennai	102 HIV-positive patients with diarrhea (43 acute diarrhea, 59 chronic diarrhea), weight loss (9), vomiting (7), fever (5), abdominal pain (4)	152 HIV-positive (102 HIV-positive patients with diarrhea (43 acute diarrhea, 59 chronic diarrhea) and 50 HIV-positive and no diarrhea. 50 IC		ND	N/A	Kumar et al. (2002)
11 (18.6%) of 59 of chronic diarrhea	Tamil Nadu, Chennai	*C. belli* association with diarrhea	HIV patients		ND	N/A	Satheesh Kumar et al. (2002)
16 cases (17%) of 94 AIDS patients	Maharashtra, Mumbai	Diarrhea	Yes, AIDS	Higher percentage in AIDS and chronic diarrhea (12, 12.8%) than in acute diarrhea (4, 4.2%)	ND	N/A	Joshi et al. (2002)

(Continued)

Table 22.7 (Continued)   Summary of Positive Reports of *C. belli* Infections in Humans in India, Presented in Chronological Order

Patient Data	State, City	Symptoms	Immunocompromised (Yes, No) Type	Remarks	Treatment (which) Successful or not	Outcome of Patient	Reference
7 cases (0.7%) of 10,126 children (4 month to 8 yr) over a decade study	Delhi	Diarrhea	Yes, HIV-positive (2). Oral thrush (1), nephrotic syndrome (1) HIV-negative (3)		Treated with cotrimoxazole	Successful. No recurrence in the 18-months follow-up	Mirdha et al. (2002)
3 cases (2.5%) of 120 HIV-positive	Chandigarh	Diarrhea	0 of 50 control patients		ND	N/A	Mohandas et al. (2002)
51 cases (19.8%) of 258 HIV-positive (0.5%) of 4103 HIV-negative with diarrhea	Tamil Nadu, Vellore	HIV-negative all with diarrhea	Yes, HIV-positive (258). IC	Tertiary care center. 5 yr study	ND	N/A	Banerjee et al. (2005)
1 case, 2 yr, M.	Delhi	Diarrhea	Yes, prolonged corticosteroid therapy for systemic vasculitis	Numerous *C. belli* oocysts. Unusual presence of merozoites	Dihydrofolate reductase inhibitor and TMP-SMX	Refractory to treatment	Malik et al. (2005)
4 cases (2.9%) of 120 stools	Uttar Pradesh, Varanasi	Diarrhea	Yes, HIV-positive	Low CD4 T cells	ND	N/A	Attili et al. (2006)
2 cases (2.7%) of 75	New Delhi	Diarrhea in 50, no diarrhea in 25	Yes, HIV	CD4 levels lower in HIV with diarrhea	N/A	N/A	Dwivedi et al. (2007)
64 cases (26.1%) of 245	Tamil Nadu, Chennai	Diarrhea	Yes, HIV-positive		ND	N/A	Vignesh et al. (2007)
1 case, Fh, 9 yr	Delhi	Loose stools, nausea, vomiting, weight loss	Malnourished, protein-energy malnutrition grade IV	Poor nutrition coupled with unsanitary environmental conditions	TMP-SMX	Successful	Kochhar et al. (2007)
1 case (1%) of 100, 1 case (2%) of 50 adults	Delhi		No, but malnourished	0 of 50 adults and 1 of 50 children	ND	N/A	Behera et al. (2008)
19 cases (8.6%) of 226. Positive were all HIV-positive (13% of 113) patients. 0 cases of 113 HIV- negative patients	Delhi	Chronic diarrhea in 34 HIV-positive patients and in 113 HIV-negative patients	Yes, HIV (113). IC (113)	14 (41.2%) of 34 HIV-positive patients with diarrhea, 5 (6.3%) of 79 HIV-positive without diarrhea	ND	N/A	Gupta et al. (2008)
2 cases (0.5%) of 366 HIV- positive	Uttar Pradesh, Varanasi	Diarrhea	Yes, HIV (366); IC (200)	Both cases occurred in summer and patients with CD4 less than 200 cells/uL	ND	N/A	Tuli et al. (2008)
11 cases (8.0%) of 137 HIV-positive	Masharashtra, Pune	Diarrhea	Yes, HIV		ND	N/A	Kulkarni et al. (2009)
1 case, M, 35 yr	Masharashtra, Kolhapur	Diarrhea	No, but malnutrition		TMP-SMX	Patient died	Mudholkar and Namey (2010)

(Continued)

Table 22.7 (Continued) Summary of Positive Reports of *C. belli* Infections in Humans in India, Presented in Chronological Order

Patient Data	State, City	Symptoms	Immunocompromised (Yes, No) Type	Remarks	Treatment (which) Successful or not	Outcome of Patient	Reference
14 cases (7.2%) in 194 patients	Delhi	Diarrhea	Yes, 144 HIV-positive. IC: 50	13 (9.03%) of 144 HIV-positive with diarrhea, 11 with counts lower than 200 cells/uL. 1 (2%) of 50 IC	ND	N/A	Jha et al. (2012)
2 cases: (1) 41 yr M; (2) postrenal transplant. No age, sex data		(1) Chronic watery diarrhea (8 months), (2) diabetic patient on immunosuppressive therapy. Diarrhea of 1 yr duration	(1) ND (2) Yes. Immunosuppressive therapy	Parasites in biopsy of duodenum or ileum. Feces negative	(1) TMP-SMX (2) Not treated	(1) Responded well. (2) Diarrhea subsided without any treatment	Rao et al. (2012)
29 cases (10.9%) of 266 HIV patients	Rajasthan, Jaipur	Diarrhea (100 patients acute diarrhea, 166 chronic diarrhea)	Yes, HIV (266), IC: 100	24 of 166 chronic diarrhea, 5 of 100 with acute diarrhea, 0 of 100 HIV-negative without diarrhea	ND	N/A	Vyas et al. (2012)
12 cases (6%) of 200 patients	Tamil Nadu, Chennai	Diarrhea	No, IC	Low-income adults	ND	N/A	Chopra and Dworkin (2013)
19 cases (16.5%) of 115 HIV patients	Odisha, Berhampur	Diarrhea	Yes, HIV-positive (115) HIV-negative (92)	All *C. belli*–positive patients were HIV-positive	ND	N/A	Dash et al. (2013)
21 cases (21%) of 100 HIV-positive patients	Chennai	38 acute diarrhea: 30 chronic diarrhea; 32 no diarrhea	Yes, HIV-positive	Significantly associated with chronic diarrhea in HIV patients	9 of 21 were on TMP-SMX therapy	Not stated	Janagond et al. (2013)
16 cases (10.7%) of 150 HIV patients	Delhi	Diarrhea	Yes, HIV-positive	2 (2.7%) of 75 HIV-treated, 14 (18.7%) of 75 not HIV-treated	Prophylaxis TMP-SMX given to patients with CD T cells <200 cell/mm.	Persistence of oocysts after specific therapy	Jha et al. (2013)
18 cases (28%) of 65 HIV-positive, and 1 (0.4) of 266 HIV-negative	Maharashtra, Pune	Diarrhea, weakness, abdominal pain, anorexia, fever, nausea, vomiting, blood/mucus in stools	Yes, HIV-positive		ND	N/A	Kulkarni et al. (2013)
1 case, M, 43 yr	Maharashtra, Pune	Diarrhea	HIV	No oocysts in feces. Sschizonts reported in duodenal biopsy	ND	N/A	Malik et al. (2013)
1 case, M, 50 yr	Gujrat, Vadodara	Acute-onset watery diarrhea, low-grade fever, and nausea	Yes, renal transplant		Combination TMP-SMX (Bactrim) double strength and Nitazoxanide	Responded	Marathe and Parikh (2013)

(Continued)

Table 22.7 (Continued) Summary of Positive Reports of *C. belli* Infections in Humans in India, Presented in Chronological Order

Patient Data	State, City	Symptoms	Immunocompromised (Yes, No) Type	Remarks	Treatment (which) Successful or not	Outcome of Patient	Reference
42 cases (7.7%) of 544 HIV-positive	Gujrat, Jamnagar	Of 544, 343 had prolonged diarrhea, 57 acute diarrhea, while 144 were asymptomatic	Yes, HIV	39 (17.0%) of 230 chronic diarrhea, 3 (7.5%) of 40 acute diarrhea	ND	N/A	Mathur et al. (2013)
46 cases (22%) of 250 HIV-positive patients		200 patients with diarrhea, 50 no diarrhea; CD4 cells <200 cells/uL associated with diarrhea	Yes, HIV-positive	*C. belli* in 44 (22%) of 200 with diarrhea, 2 (4%) of 50 without diarrhea	ND	N/A	Mohanty et al. (2013)
41 cases (2.4%) of 1700 stools -ID; patients. Of those 3 were children	Punjab, Hissar, Chandigarh	Diseases included: Inflammatory bowel disease, interstitial lung disease, polymyositis or post-transplant, 3 children with nephrotic syndrome and malnutrition	Yes, All ID: HIV-positive or ID due to prolonged use of steroids or other immunosuppressive drugs	30 in HIV-positive (26 had diarrhea). 11 in HIV-negative (all had diarrhea). Seasonality observed (highest May–August). Tertiary care center	HIV-negative treated with TMP-SMX	In those treated the diarrhea improved and follow-up samples were negative for *C. belli*	Gautam et al. (2014)
1 case, F, 50 yr	Maharashtra, Mumbai	*Pemphigus vulgaris.* Recurrent diarrhea, abdominal pain, loss of appetite, occasional fever	Yes, long-term (4 yr) immunosuppressants or rituximab for pemphigus vulgaris	Disease recalcitrant	TMP-SMX	Responded	Sahu et al. (2014)
22 cases (11.5%) of 192 patients	Maharashtra, Mumbai	Diarrhea	Yes, HIV-positive (142), IC: 50	22 of 142 HIV-positive with diarrhea and 0 of 50 HIV-negative with diarrhea			Ahmed and Chowdhary (2015)
3 cases (3.4%) of 88 organ transplant recipients	Delhi	38 recipients presenting with diarrhea (29 postrenal, 2 liver, and 7 bone marrow transplant recipients) and 50 recipients without diarrhea	Yes, all transplant recipients	*C. belli* in 3 of 38 with diarrhea and 0 of 50 without diarrhea	Albendazole and TMP-SMX	N/A	Yadav et al. (2016)
9 cases (20%) of 45 HIV- positive patients	Maharashtra, Pune	Diarrhea (27), no diarrhea (18)	Yes, HIV	7 (25.9%) of 27 HIV with diarrhea, 2 (11.1%) of 18 with no diarrhea	ND	N/A	Shah et al. (2016)

(Continued)

Table 22.7 (Continued)   Summary of Positive Reports of C. belli Infections in Humans in India, Presented in Chronological Order

Patient Data	State, City	Symptoms	Immunocompromised (Yes, No) Type	Remarks	Treatment (which) Successful or not	Outcome of Patient	Reference
4 cases (2%) of 200 children	Delhi	Diarrhea	Yes, C. belli–positive children were HIV-positive		N/A	N/A	Kumar et al. (2017)
1 case of 968 stool samples	Rajasthan, Jodhpur	Diarrhea and other gastrointestinal symptoms	Yes, patient positive was HIV-positive	Tertiary care center	ND	N/A	Saurabh et al. (2017)
173 cases (20.9%) of 829 HIV-positive patients	Tamil Nadu, Chennai	Diarrhea	Yes, HIV-positive	Epidemiological study. C. belli was the most common pathogen	N/A	N/A	Swathirajan et al. (2017)

Source: Dubey, J.P., Almeria, S. 2019. *Cystoisospora belli* infections in humans—The past 100 years. *Parasitology* http://doi.org/10.1017/S0031182019000957

Note: Important/rare findings are in bold.

Abbreviations: ART, active antiretroviral therapy; F, female; IC, immunocompetent; ID, immunosuppressed; M, male; N/A, not applicable; ND, not done or no data; Oo, oocysts; pos, positive; SC, schizonts; TMP-SMX, trimethoprim sulfamethoxazole, cotrimoxazole; yr, age in years.

the presence of Charcot–Leydel crystals were common and observed in more than 75% cases.[784]

Immunocompromised people can experience more severe disease with extreme diarrhea, anorexia, and weight loss.[13,16,457,639,809,934] Clinical illness due to *C. belli* infection is more severe and of longer duration in HIV-positive than in HIV-negative patients.[198] HIV-positive individuals with diarrhea have a higher prevalence of *C. belli*,[1197] and the risk for clinical disease is even higher in HIV-positive individuals with low CD4$^+$ lymphocyte counts (usually <200 cells/μL)[46,354,1197,1276,1522] In fact, some studies showed that among different parasites found in HIV-infected individuals with diarrhea, *C. belli* was the most common.[919,1501]

C. belli infections can be persistent; symptoms can last from weeks to months. The case in point is a *C. belli* infection in a 58-year-old male U.S. veteran who had intermittent episodes of diarrhea for 20 years since his discharge from the army in 1947,[1705] and a similar case in another U.S. veteran from the South Pacific with recurrent diarrhea for 26 years.[1396] Profound weight loss may be associated with chronic diarrhea. Frequently, *C. belli* infection is associated with malabsorption.[840,1181,1705] The presence of Charcot–Leydel crystals in fecal samples[784] and steatorrhea (high fat presence) are found in a high percentage of patients.[151]

Fever, mostly low grade, and peripheral eosinophilia can also be features of *C. belli* infection.[884] Infection with *C. belli* in immunosuppressed patients has been reported in association with viral infections other than HIV, with cancers such as Hodgkin's lymphoma, mediastinal thymoma, malignant lymphoma, acute leukemias, hypogammaglobulinemia, or after organ transplant.[429]

Other disorders observed in persons infected with *C. belli* include α-chain disease (disordered IgA), homozygous hemoglobin E (hemoglobinopathy)[840], ultrashort bowel syndrome with transplant, diabetes insipidus with or without immunosuppressive therapy, eosinophilic gastroenteritis (reactive arthritis, monoclonal gammopathy, Lyell syndrome (active pulmonary tuberculosis), hyper-IgM syndrome, hypogammaglobulinemia), or Good syndrome.[429]

Clinically, gallbladder and biliary tract infection, mainly in immunosuppressed HIV patients, can also accompany cystoisoporiasis.[12,103] Reports of biliary involvement associated with *C. belli* are summarized in Table 22.4. However, care must be taken when diagnosing *C. belli* in the gallbladder. A recent study analyzed eight patients in which epithelial cytoplasmic vacuoles and inclusions within the gallbladder epithelium were previously diagnosed as due to *C. belli*. None of the patients could be confirmed by subsequent molecular methods.[1656]

22.14 DIAGNOSIS

Oocysts of *C. belli* are morphologically distinctive and easy to diagnose by microscopical examination of fecal samples if large numbers are present. However, oocysts are excreted irregularly and in low numbers or are absent during acute infection. Therefore, repeated stool examinations and concentration procedures are recommended. Although *C. belli* oocysts can be detected in direct fecal smears or by Lugol wet mounts, concentration methods such as Sheather's sugar flotation or sedimentation concentration followed by light microscopy are superior.

Staining of fecal smears made from concentrated samples may improve detection. Among staining techniques, safranin, modified acid-fast staining, auramine-rhodamine, and Giemsa techniques can be used.[1238,1296,1435] Better results were found with modified Ziehl–Neelsen or safranin staining compared to auramine, which showed irregularity of fluorochrome uptake by *C. belli*.[1296]

The use of fluorescent staining using 1% Unitex 2B was compared to the modified fast stain in stools and duodenal/bile juice, and found to be a suitable method for diagnosis.[555] Epifluorescence using a 330–380 nm UV filter may also be used to detect autofluorescence of the oocysts.[122] Similar sensitivity was observed between the Kinyoun acid-fast stained smear and autofluorescence, but autofluorescence analysis was recommended because of its simple preparation.[109] Higher sensitivity was observed using autofluorescence (95.7% [95% CI, 85.2–99.5]) compared to iodine staining (48.4% [95% CI, 37.7–59.1]).[122]

Internal parasitic stages may also be identified in duodenal aspirates.[1705] However, histological examination of intestinal biopsies of infected individuals, particularly in HIV-positive patients, are best. Although rare, as indicated earlier, intracellular stages have been found in other extraintestinal locations.

There are currently several PCR methods that facilitate the identification of *C. belli*.[507,938,1211,1226,1675,1693,1815] *C. belli* oocysts were morphologically and molecularly characterized in a study based on the small subunit ribosomal RNA (rRNA), 5.8S rRNA, ITS-1, and ITS-2, which showed that *C. belli* is highly conserved. This indicates that there were no cryptic species or extensive strain as variations of the parasite.[839] However, the analysis of genetic profiles by restriction fragment length polymorphism (RFLP) showed that the same patient with extraintestinal infection may have been infected with several genotypes at the same time.[1410a]

No serological tests have been described.

22.15 TREATMENT

Several anticoccidials have been evaluated for treatment of *C. belli* infections. Among them, trimethoprim sulfamethoxazole (TMP/SMX or cotrimoxazole) is the drug of choice for cystoisosporiasis. However, it is common for immunosuppressed patients to relapse with clinical disease.[934,1322] Up to 38% relapses (6/16 patients) were observed by Walther and Topazian.[1769] When recurrence occurs, patients may need to be treated longer and/or with higher daily doses to clear infections.

Pyrimethamine and sulfanomides combination, Ciprofloxacin, nitazoxanide, diclofenac, metronidazole, albendazole and ornidazole, or diclazuril, amprolium, nitrofurantoin, and roxitrhomycin are some of the other drugs tried with varying success.[429]

22.16 CONTROL AND PREVENTION

See Section 22.8.

REFERENCES

2, 5, 12, 13, 16, 18, 29, 30, 46, 75, 80, 98, 103, 109, 110, 111, 122, 126, 127, 151, 165, 170, 171, 173, 180, 189, 198, 201–206, 270, 271, 343, 354, 365, 367, 378, 427, 429, 431, 432, 457, 458, 473, 489, 507, 517, 530, 554, 555, 559, 560, 578, 580, 589, 590, 591, 599, 604, 610, 639, 644–646, 655, 656, 700, 710, 711, 722, 727–730, 752, 757–759, 784, 796, 809, 839, 840, 884, 897, 902, 919, 934, 938, 939, 956, 1043, 1045, 1073, 1089, 1147, 1181, 1197, 1211, 1223–1226, 1236, 1238, 1274, 1276, 1281–1288, 1296, 1321, 1322, 1345, 1380, 1396, 1410a, 1411, 1435, 1475, 1483, 1500, 1501, 1552, 1553, 1558, 1575, 1579, 1591, 1598, 1656, 1665, 1675, 1693, 1696, 1701, 1705, 1730, 1733, 1735, 1743, 1749, 1769, 1777, 1791, 1815, 1873, 1914

References

C. K. Cerqueira-Cézar, F. H. A. Murata, O. C. H. Kwok, and R. Calero-Bernal

1. Aarthi S., Raj, G.D., Raman, M., Blake, D., Subramaniam, C., Tomley, F., 2011. Expressed sequence tags from *Eimeria brunetti*—Preliminary analysis and functional annotation. *Parasitol. Res.* 108, 1059–1062.

2. Abanyie, F., Harvey, R.R., Harris, J.R., Wiegand, R.E., Gaul, L., Desvignes-Kendrick, M., Irvin, K. et al., 2015. 2013 multistate outbreaks of *Cyclospora cayetanensis* infections associated with fresh produce: Focus on the Texas investigations. *Epidemiol. Infect.* 143, 3451–3458.

3. Abbas, I.E., El-Alfy, E., Al-Araby, M., Al-Kappany, Y., El-Seadawy, R., Dubey, J.P., 2019. Prevalence of *Eimeria* species in camels (*Camelus dromedarius*) from Egypt and variability in structure of *Eimeria cameli* oocysts. *J. Parasitol.* 105, 395–400.

4. Abdel-Baki, A.A.S., Al-Quraishy, S., 2013. Prevalence of coccidia (*Eimeria* spp.) infection in domestic rabbits, *Oryctolagus cuniculus*, in Riyadh, Saudi Arabia. *Pakistan J. Zool.* 45. 1329–1333.

5. Abdel-Hafeez, E.H., Ahmad, A.K., Ali, B.A., Moslam, F.A., 2012. Opportunistic parasites among immunosuppressed children in Minia District, Egypt. *Korean J. Parasitol.* 50, 57–62.

6. Abdel-Rady, A., 2014. Epidemiological studies on parasitic infestations in camels (*Camelus dromedaries*) in Egypt. *Inat. J. Agro Vet. Med. Sci.* 8, 142–149.

7. Abu-El-Ezz, N.M.T., Abdel Megeed, K.N., Mahdy, O.A., Hassan, S.E., 2012. ELISA assessment in the diagnosis of hepatic coccidiosis in experimentally infected rabbits. *Global Veterinaria* 9, 517–523.

8. Abubakr, M.I., Nayel, M.N., Fadlalla, M.E., Abdelrahman, A.O., Abuobeida, S.A., Elgabara, Y.M., 2000. Prevalence of gastrointestinal parasites in young camels in Bahrain. *Revue Élev. Méd. vét. Pays Trop.* 53, 267–271.

9. Adl, S.M., Simpson, A.G.B., Farmer, M.A., Andersen, R.A., Anderson, O.R., Barta, J.R., Bowser, S.S. et al., 2005. The new higher level classification of eukaryotes with emphasis on the taxonomy of protists. *J. Eukaryot. Microbiol.* 52, 399–451.

10. Adzitey, F., Adzitey, S.P., 2011. Duck production: Has a potential to reduce poverty among rural households in Asian communities—A review. *J. World's Poult. Res.* 1, 7–10.

11. Afonso, E., Baurand, P.E., Tournant, P., Capelli, N., 2014. First amplification of *Eimeria hessei* DNA from the lesser horseshoe bat (*Rhinolophus hipposideros*) and its phylogenetic relationships with *Eimeria* species from other bats and rodents. *Exp. Parasitol.* 139, 58–62.

12. Agholi, M., Aliabadi, E., Hatam, G.R., 2016. Cystoisosporiasis-related human acalculous cholecystitis: The need for increased awareness. *Pol. J. Pathol.* 67, 270–276.

13. Agholi, M., Hatam, G.R., Motazedian, M.H., 2013. HIV/AIDS-associated opportunistic protozoal diarrhea. *AIDS Res. Hum. Retroviruses* 29, 35–41.

14. Agtarap, A., Chamberlin, J.W., Pinkerton, M., Steinrauf, L., 1967. The structure of monensic acid, a new biologically active compound. *J. Am. Chem. Soc.* 89, 5737–5739.

15. Agyei, A.D., Odonkor, M., Osei-Somuah, A., 2004. Concurrence of *Eimeria* and helminth parasitic infections in West African Dwarf kids in Ghana. *Small Ruminant Res.* 51, 29–35.

16. Ahmed, N.H., Chowdhary, A., 2015. Pattern of co-infection by enteric pathogenic parasites among HIV seropositive individuals in a tertiary care hospital, Mumbai, India. *Indian J. Sex. Transm. Dis. AIDS* 36, 40–47.

17. Ahmed, W.M., Hassan, S.E., 2007. Applied studies on coccidiosis in growing buffalo-calves with special reference to oxidant/antioxidant status. *World J. Zool.* 2, 40–48.

18. Aksoy, U., Marangi, M., Papini, R., Ozkoc, S., Bayram Delibas, S., Giangaspero, A., 2014. Detection of *Toxoplasma gondii* and *Cyclospora cayetanensis* in *Mytilus galloprovincialis* from Izmir Province coast (Turkey) by real-time PCR/high-resolution melting analysis (HRM). *Food Microbiol.* 44, 128–135.

19. Al-Afaleq, A.I., Elamin, E.A., Fatani, A., Homeida, A.G.M., 2018. Parasitic profile of Saudi Arabian camels. *J. Camel Prac. Res.* 25, 93–97.

20. Al-Habsi, K., Yang, R., Ryan, U., Miller, D.W., Jacobson, C., 2017. Morphological and molecular characterization of three *Eimeria* species from captured rangeland goats in Western Australia. *Vet. Parasitol. Reg. Stud. Rep.* 9, 75–83.

21. Albanese, G.A., Tensa, L.R., Aston, E.J., Hilt, D.A., Jordan, B.J., 2018. Evaluation of a coccidia vaccine using spray and gel applications. *Poult. Sci.* 97, 1544–1553.

22. Alcaíno, H., Laval, E., Gorman, T., Pinochet, L., Díaz, I., 1989. Isosporosis y criptosporidiosis en cerdos de criaderos industriales de la Región Metropolitana de Chile. *Arch. Med. Vet.* 21, 131–135.

23. Alcala-Canto, Y., Ibarra-Velarde, F., 2008. Cytokine gene expression and NF-κB activation following infection of intestinal epithelial cells with *Eimeria bovis* or *Eimeria alabamensis in vitro. Parasite Immunol.* 30, 175–179.

24. Ali, N.A., Binnerts, W.T., Klimes, B., 1972. Immunization by irradiated *Eimeria acervulina. J. Protozool.* 19, 177–180.

25. Aliaga-Leyton, A., Friendship, R., Dewey, C.E., Todd, C., Peregrine, A.S., 2011. *Isospora suis* infection and its association with postweaning performance on three southwestern Ontario swine farms. *J. Swine Health Prod.* 19, 94–99.

26. Alicata, J.E., Willet, E.L., 1946. Observations on the prophylactic and curative value of sulfaguanidine in swine coccidiosis. *Am. J. Vet. Res.* 7, 94–100.

27. Allen, E.A., 1936. *Tyzzeria perniciosa* gen. et sp. nov., a coccidium from the small intestine of the Pekin duck, *Anas domesticus* L. *Arch. Protistenkd.* 87, 262–267.

28. Allen, P.C., Fetterer, R.H., 2002. Recent advances in biology and immunobiology of *Eimeria* species and in

diagnosis and control of infection with these coccidian parasites of poultry. *Clin. Microbiol. Rev.* 15, 58–65.

29. Almeria, S., Cinar, H.N., Dubey, J.P., 2019. *Cyclospora cayetanensis* and cyclosporiasis: An update. *Microorganisms.* 7, 317.

30. Almeria, S., da Silva, A.J., Blessington, T., Cloyd, T.C., Cinar, H.N., Durigan, M., Murphy, H.R., 2018. Evaluation of the U.S. Food and Drug Administration validated method for detection of *Cyclospora cayetanensis* in high-risk fresh produce matrices and a method modification for a prepared dish. *Food Microbiol.* 76, 497–503.

31. Almería, S., López-Gatius, F., 2015. Markers related to the diagnosis and to the risk of abortion in bovine neosporosis. *Res. Vet. Sci.* 100, 169–175.

32. Almería, S., Serrano, B., Yàniz, J.L., Darwich, L., López-Gatius, F., 2012. Cytokine gene expression profiles in peripheral blood mononuclear cells from *Neospora caninum* naturally infected dams throughout gestation. *Vet. Parasitol.* 183, 237–243.

33. Alnassan, A.A., Kotsch, M., Shehata, A.A., Krüger, M., Daugschies, A., Bangoura, B., 2014. Necrotic enteritis in chickens: Development of a straightforward disease model system. *Vet. Rec.* 174, 555–561.

34. Altreuther, G., Gasda, N., Schroeder, I., Joachim, A., Settje, T., Schimmel, A., Hutchens, D., Krieger, K.J., 2011. Efficacy of emodepside plus toltrazuril suspension (Procox oral suspension for dogs) against prepatent and patent infection with *Isospora canis* and *Isospora ohioensis*–complex in dogs. *Parasitol. Res.* 109 (Suppl 1), S9–S20.

35. Alyousif, M.S., Kasim, A.A., Al-Shawa, Y.R., 1992. Coccidia of the domestic goat (*Capra hircus*) in Saudi Arabia. *Int. J. Parasitol.* 22, 807–811.

36. Alzieu, J.P., Mage, C., Maes, L., de Mûelenaere, C., 1999. Economic benefits of prophylaxis with diclazuril against subclinical coccidiosis in lambs reared indoors. *Vet. Rec.* 144, 442–444.

37. Amiruddin, N., Lee, X.W., Blake, D.P., Suzuki, Y., Tay, Y.L., Lim, L.S., Tomley, F.M., et al. 2012. Characterisation of full-length cDNA sequences provides insights into the *Eimeria tenella* transcriptome. *BMC Genomics* 13, 21

38. Ammar, S.I., Watson, A.M., Craig, L.E., Cope, E.R., Schaefer, J.J., Mulliniks, J.T., Gerhold, R.W., 2019. *Eimeria gilruthi*–associated abomasitis in a group of ewes. *J. Vet. Diagn. Invest.* 31, 128–132.

39. An, J., Wang, M., Wang, L., Chen, Z., Zhao, J., Yan, Y., Zhang, Y., 2006. Establishment of single-sporocyst isolation for *Eimeria* propagation. *Chin. J. Vet. Med.* 42, 10–12 (in Chinese).

40. An, J., Wang, M., Wang, L., Sheng, S., 2007. Identification of the drug resistant strain by molecular biological technique. *Chin J Vet Sci.* 27, 340–346 (in Chinese).

41. Andrews, A.H., 2013. Some aspects of coccidiosis in sheep and goats. *Small Ruminant Res.* 110, 93–95.

42. Arakawa, A., Tanaka, Y., Baba, E., Fukata, T., 1991. Effects of clopidol on sporulation and infectivity of *Eimeria tenella* oocysts. *Vet. Parasitol.* 38, 55–60.

43. Arendt, M.K., Sand, J.M., Marcone, T.M., Cook, M.E., 2016. Interleukin-10 neutralizing antibody for detection of intestinal luminal levels and as a dietary additive in *Eimeria* challenged broiler chicks. *Poult. Sci.* 95, 430–438.

43a. Aromaa, M., Hautala, K., Oksanen, A., Sukura, A., Näreaho, A., 2018. Parasite infections and their risk factors in foals and young horses in Finland. *Vet. Parasitol. Reg. Stud. Rep.* 12, 35–38.

44. Aruna, M., Subramanian, N., Muthu, M., 2016. Survey study on gastro-intestinal parasites of buffalo in Cheyyar Taluk Thiruvannamalai District. *Int. J. Curr. Res.* 8, 42619–42628.

45. Ashton, P.D., Curwen, R.S., Wilson, R.A., 2001. Linking proteome and genome: How to identify parasite proteins. *Trends Parasitol.* 17, 198–202.

46. Assefa, S., Erko, B., Medhin, G., Assefa, Z., Shimelis, T., 2009. Intestinal parasitic infections in relation to HIV/AIDS status, diarrhea and CD4 T-cell count. *BMC Infect. Dis.* 9, 155.

47. Augustine, P.C., 1988. *Eimeria adenoeides* and *E. meleagrimitis*: Effect of poult age on susceptibility to infection and development of immunity. *Avian Dis.* 32, 798–802.

48. Augustine, P.C., Danforth, H.D., 1986. A study of the dynamics of the invasion of immunized birds by *Eimeria* sporozoites. *Avian Dis.* 30, 347–351.

49. Augustine, P.C., Denbow, D.M., 1991. Effect of coccidiosis on plasma epinephrine and norepinephrine levels in turkey poults. *Poult Sci.* 70, 785–789.

50. Augustine, P.C., Doran, D.J., 1978. Development of *Eimeria meleagrimitis* Tyzzer from sporozoites and merozoites in turkey kidney cell cultures. *J. Protozool.* 25, 82–86.

51. Augustine, P.C., Watkins, K.L., Danforth, H.D., 1992. Effect of monensin on ultrastructure and cellular invasion by the turkey coccidia *Eimeria adenoeides* and *Eimeria meleagrimitis*. *Poult Sci.* 71, 970–978.

52. Avery, S., Rothwell, L., Degen, W.D.J., Schijns, V.E.J.C., Young, J., Kaufman, J., Kaiser, P., 2004. Characterization of the first nonmammalian T2 cytokine gene cluster: The cluster contains functional single-copy genes for IL-3, IL-4, IL-13, and GM-CSF, a gene for IL-5 that appears to be a pseudogene, and a gene encoding another cytokinelike transcript, KK34. *J. Interferon Cytokine Res.* 24, 600–610.

53. Baba, E., Gaafar, S.M., 1985. Interfering effect of *Isospora suis* infection on *Salmonella typhimurium* infection in swine. *Vet. Parasitol.* 17, 271–278.

54. Bach, U., Kalthoff, V., Mundt, H.C., Popp, A., Rinke, M., Daugschies, A., Luttge, B., 2003. Parasitological and morphological findings in porcine isosporosis after treatment with symmetrical triazintriones. *Parasitol. Res.* 91, 27–33.

55. Badawy, A.I.I., Lutz, K., Taubert, A., Zahner, H., Hermosilla, C., 2010. *Eimeria bovis* meront I-carrying host cells express parasite-specific antigens on their surface membrane. *Vet. Res. Commun.* 34, 103–118.

56. Bækbo, P., Christensen, J., Henriksen, S.A., Nielsen, K., 1994. Attempts to induce colostral immunity against *Isospora suis* infections in piglets (oral vaccination of sows). *Proc. 13th IPVS Congr.*, Bangkok, Thailand, p. 244.

57. Bafundo, K.W., 1989. Protective responses produced by immunisation of day-old chicks with either *Eimeria maxima*, *E. acervulina* or *E. tenella* live oocyst vaccines. In Yvore, P. (Ed.), *Coccidia and Intestinal Coccidiomorphs*. INRA. Paris. 395–400.

58. Bahrami, S., Alborzi, A.R., 2013. Prevalence of subclinical coccidiosis in river buffalo calves of southwest of Iran. *Acta Parasitol.* 58, 527–530.

59. Baker, N.F., Walters, G.T., Fisk, R.A., 1972. Amprolium for control of coccidiosis in feedlot lambs. *Am. J. Vet. Res.* 33, 83–86.

60. Balicka-Ramisz, A., 1999. Studies on coccidiosis in goats in Poland. *Vet. Parasitol.* 81, 347–349.

61. Balicka-Ramisz, A., Ramisz, A., Vovk, S., Snitynskyj, V., 2012. Prevalence of coccidia infection in goats in Western Pomerania (Poland) and West Ukraine region. *Ann. Parasitol.* 58, 167–171.

62. Ball, S.J., 1963. The effect of sulfaquinoxaline and amprolium against *Eimeria adenoeides* and *E. meleagrimitis* in turkeys. *Res. Vet. Sci.* 4, 39–47.

63. Ball, S.J., 1966. The development of resistance to glycarbylamide and 2-chloro-4-nitrobenzamide in *Eimeria tenella* in chicks. *Parasitology* 56, 25–37.

64. Ball, S.J., Pittilo, M.R., Snow, K.R., 2014. Observations on oocyst development of *Eimeria stiedai* in rabbits. *Acta Parasitol.* 59, 544–547.

65. Ball, S.J., Pittilo, R.M., Long, P.L., 1989. Intestinal and extraintestinal life cycles of eimeriid coccidia. *Adv. Parasitol.* 28, 1–54.

66. Ball, S.J., Warren, E.W., 1963. The effect of long-term medication with sulphaquinoxaline and amprolium upon serial infections of *Eimeria adenoeides* and *E. meleagrimitis* in turkeys. *Br. Vet. J.* 119, 549–558.

67. Bangoura, B., Daugschies, A., 2007. Influence of experimental *Eimeria zuernii* infection in calves on electrolyte concentrations, acid-base balance and blood gases. *Parasitol. Res.* 101, 1637–1645.

68. Bangoura, B., Daugschies, A., 2007. Parasitological and clinical parameters of experimental *Eimeria zuernii* infection in calves and influence on weight gain and haemogram. *Parasitol. Res.* 100, 1331–1340.

69. Bangoura, B., Daugschies, A., Fuerll, M., 2007. Influence of experimental *Eimeria zuernii* infection on clinical blood chemistry in calves. *Vet. Parasitol.* 150, 46–53.

70. Bangoura, B., Mundt, H.C., Schmäschke, R., Westphal, B., Daugschies, A., 2012. Prevalence of *Eimeria bovis* and *Eimeria zuernii* in German cattle herds and factors influencing oocyst excretion. *Parasitol. Res.* 110, 875–881.

71. Bao, S.D., 2009. Diagnosis and treatment of Muscovy duck coccidiosis. *Zhejiang Anim. Sci. Vet. Med.* 34, 16 (in Chinese).

72. Barbosa, M.A., Blasi, A.C., de Oliveira, M.R., Corrêa, F.M.A., 1992. Natural parasitism of buffalo cows in Botucatu, SP, Brazil—III. Dynamics of gastro-intestinal parasitism in cows and calves. *Mem. Inst. Oswaldo Cruz* 87 (Suppl I), 37–41.

73. Barker, I.K., Remmler, O., 1970. Experimental *Eimeria leuckarti* infection in ponies. *Vet. Rec.* 86, 448–449.

74. Barker, I.K., Remmler, O., 1972. The endogenous development of *Eimeria leuckarti* in ponies. *J. Parasitol.* 58, 112–122.

75. Barratt, J.L.N., Park, S., Nascimento, F.S., Hofstetter, J., Plucinski, M., Casillas, S., Bradbury, R.S., Arrowood, M.J., Qvarnstrom, Y., Talundzic, E., 2019. Genotyping genetically heterogeneous *Cyclospora cayetanensis* infections to complement epidemiological case linkage. *Parasitology.* 146, 1275–1283.

76. Barriga, O.O., Arnoni, J.V., 1979. *Eimeria stiedae*: Weight, oocyst output, and hepatic function of rabbits with graded infections. *Exp. Parasitol.* 48, 407–414.

77. Barriga, O.O., Arnoni, J.V., 1981. Pathophysiology of hepatic coccidiosis in rabbits. *Vet. Parasitol.* 8, 201–210.

78. Barta, J.R., Coles, B.A., Schito, M.L., Fernando, M.A., Martin, A., Danforth, H.D., 1998. Analysis of infraspecific variation among five strains of *Eimeria maxima* from North America. *Int. J. Parasitol.* 28, 485–492.

79. Barta, J.R., Martin, D.S., Liberator, P.A., Dashkevicz, M., Anderson, J.W., Feighner, S.D., Elbrecht, A. et al., 1997. Phylogenetic relationships among eight *Eimeria* species infecting domestic fowl inferred using complete small subunit ribosomal DNA sequences. *J. Parasitol.* 83, 262–271.

80. Barta, J.R., Schrenzel, M.D., Carreno, R., Rideout, B.A., 2005. The genus *Atoxoplasma* (Garnham 1950) as a junior objective synonym of the genus *Isospora* (Schneider 1881) species infecting birds and resurrection of *Cystoisospora* (Frenkel 1977) as the correct genus for *Isospora* species infecting mammals. *J. Parasitol.* 91, 726–727.

81. Barutzki, D., Schaper, R., 2011. Results of parasitological examinations of faecal samples from cats and dogs in Germany between 2003 and 2010. *Parasitol. Res.* 109, S45–S60.

82. Barutzki, D., Schaper, R., 2013. Age-dependant prevalence of endoparasites in young dogs and cats up to one year of age. *Parasitol. Res.* 112, S119–S131.

83. Basso, W., Marti, H., Hilbe, M., Sydler, T., Stahel, A., Bürgi, E., Sidler, X., 2017. Clinical cystoisosporosis associated to porcine cytomegalovirus (PCMV, *Suid herpesvirus 2*) infection in fattening pigs. *Parasitol. Int.* 66, 806–809.

84. Bastianetto, E., 2010. Infecção por *Eimeria* spp. em búfalos jovens e avaliação de esquemas terapêuticos metafiláticos. Dr. Anim. Sc. thesis. Universidade Federal de Minas Gerais.

85. Bastianetto, E., Filho, E.J.F., Lana, A.M.Q., Cunha, A.P., Teixeira, L.V., Bello, A.C.P.P., Teixeira, C., Leite, R.C., 2007. Epidemiology of *Eimeria* sp. infection in buffaloes (*Bubalus bubalis*) bred in Minas Gerais, Brazil. *Ital. J. Anim. Sci.* 6, 911–914.

86. Bastianetto, E., Freitas, C.M.V., Bello, A.C.P.P., Cunha, A.P., Dalla Rosa, R.C., Leite, R.C., 2008. Primeiro diagnóstico de *Eimeria bareillyi* (Apicomplexa: Eimeridae) nas fezes de bezerros bubalinos (*Bubalus bubalis*) naturalmente infectados no estado de Minas Gerais, Brasil. *Rev. Bras. Parasitol. Vet.* 17 (Suppl 1), 234–238.

87. Bastiani, F.T., Da Silva, A.S., Dück, M.R.K., Tonin, A.A., Monteiro, S.G., 2012. Outbreak of eimeriosis and giardiasis associated to mortality of lambs in southern Brazil. *Comp. Clin. Pathol.* 21, 371–373.

88. Bauer, C., 1988. Prevalence of *Eimeria leuckarti* (Flesch, 1883) and intensity of faecal oocyst output in a herd of horses during a summer grazing season. *Vet. Parasitol.* 30, 11–15.

89. Bauer, C., Bürger, H.J., 1984. Zur Biologie von *Eimeria leuckarti* (Flesch, 1883) der Equiden. *Berl. Münch. tierärztl. Wochenschr.* 97, 367–372.

90. Beach, J.R., Corl, J.C., 1925. Studies in the control of avian coccidiosis. *Poult. Sci.* 4, 83–93.

91. Beck, H.P., Blake, D., Dardé, M.L., Felger, I., Pedraza-Díaz, S., Regidor-Cerrillo, J., Gómez-Bautista, M. et al., 2009. Molecular approaches to diversity of populations of apicomplexan parasites. *Int. J. Parasitol.* 39, 175–189.

92. Bedrnik, P., 1967. Development of sexual stages and oocysts from the 2nd generation of *Eimeria tenella* merozoites in tissue cultures. *Folia Parasitol. (Praha)* 14, 364.

93. Beelitz, P., Göbel, E., Gothe, R., 1996. Artenspektrum und Befallshäufigkeit von Endoparasiten bei Fohlen und ihren Mutterstuten aus Zuchtbetrieben mit und ohne Anthelminthika-Prophylaxe in Oberbayern. *Tierärztl. Prax.* 24, 48–54.

94. Beelitz, P., Göbel, E., Gothe, R., 1996. Endoparasiten von Eseln und Pferden bei gemeinsamer Haltung in Oberbayern: Artenspektrum und Befallshäufigkeit. *Tierärztl. Prax.* 24, 471–475.

95. Beelitz, P., Rieder, N., Gothe, R., 1994. *Eimeria-leuckarti*-Infektionen bei Fohlen und ihren Mutterstuten in Oberbayern. *Tierärztl. Prax.* 22, 377–381.

96. Behrendt, J.H., Hermosilla, C., Hardt, M., Failing, K., Zahner, H., Taubert, A., 2008. PMN-mediated immune reactions against *Eimeria bovis. Vet. Parasitol.* 151, 97–109.

97. Behrendt, J.H., Ruiz, A., Zahner, H., Taubert, A., Hermosilla, C., 2010. Neutrophil extracellular trap formation as innate immune reactions against the apicomplexan parasite *Eimeria bovis. Vet. Immunol. Immunopathol.* 133, 1–8.

98. Bekele, F., Tefera, T., Biresaw, G., Yohannes, T., 2017. Parasitic contamination of raw vegetables and fruits collected from selected local markets in Arba Minch town, Southern Ethiopia. *Infect. Dis. Poverty* 6, 19.

99. Beldomenico, P.M., Uhart, M., Bono, M.F., Marull, C., Baldi, R., Peralta, J.L., 2003. Internal parasites of free-ranging guanacos from Patagonia. *Vet. Parasitol.* 118, 71–77.

100. Belli, S.I., Smith, N.C., Ferguson, D.J.P., 2006. The coccidian oocyst: A tough nut to crack! *Trends Parasitol.* 22, 416–423.

101. Beltrán-Saavedra, L.F., Nallar-Gutiérrez, R., Ayala, G., Limachi, J.M., Gonzalez-Rojas, J.L., 2011. Estudio sanitario de vicuñas en silvestría del Área Natural de Manejo Integrado Nacional Apolobamba, Bolivia. *Ecol. Bolivia* 46, 14–27.

102. Bemrick, W.J., O'Leary, T.P., Barnes, D.M., 1979. *Eimeria leuckarti* in five Minnesota horses. *Vet. Med. Small Anim. Clin.* 74, 77–80.

103. Benator, D.A., French, A.L., Beaudet, L.M., Levy, C.S., Orenstein, J.M., 1994. *Isospora belli* infection associated with acalculous cholecystitis in a patient with AIDS. *Ann. Intern. Med.* 121, 663–664.

104. Benbrook, E.A., Sloss, M.W., 1962. Coccidial oocysts (*Eimeria leuckarti*) from North American donkeys (*Asinus asinus*). *J. Am. Vet. Med. Assoc.* 140, 817–818.

105. Bergeland, M.E., 1981. *Isospora suis* enteritis in piglets: Diagnosis and epizootiology. *Proc. Ann. Meet. Am. Assoc. Vet. Lab. Diagn.* 24, 427–435.

106. Bergeland, M.E., Henry, S.C., 1982. Infectious diarrheas of young pigs. *Vet. Clin. North Am. Large Anim. Pract.* 4, 389–399.

107. Berger, J., Rachlin, A.I., Scott, W.E., Sternbach, L.H., Goldberg, M.W., 1951. The isolation of three new crystalline antibiotics from *Streptomyces. J. Am. Chem. Soc.* 73, 5295–5298.

108. Bergstrom, R.C., Maki, L.R., 1976. Coccidiostatic action of monensin fed to lambs: Body weight gains and feed conversion efficacy. *Am. J. Vet. Res.* 37, 79–81.

109. Berlin, O.G.W., Conteas, C.N., Sowerby, T.M., 1996. Detection of *Isospora* in the stools of AIDS patients using a new rapid autofluorescence technique. *AIDS* 10, 442–443.

110. Bern, C., Arrowood, M.J., Eberhard, M., Maguire, J.H., 2002. *Cyclospora* in Guatemala: Further considerations. *J. Clin. Microbiol.* 40, 731–732.

111. Bern, C., Hernandez, B., Lopez, M.B., Arrowood, M.J., de Mejia, M.A., de Merida, A.M., Hightower, A.W., Venczel, L., Herwaldt, B.L., Klein, R.E., 1999. Epidemiologic studies of *Cyclospora cayetanensis* in Guatemala. *Emerg. Infect. Dis.* 5, 766–774.

112. Bethencourt, A.M., Quijada, J.J., Cabrera, P., Aguirre, A.M., García, M.E., Sulbarán, D.C., Vivas, I.H., 2013. Prevalencia y abundancia de huevos de estróngilos digestivos y ooquistes de *Eimeria* spp. en búfalos de agua infectados naturalmente. *Rev. Fac. Cs. Vets. UCV* 54, 17–28.

113. Beugnet, F., Bourdeau, P., Chalvet-Monfray, K., Cozma, V., Farkas, R., Guillot, J., Halos, L. et al., 2014. parasites of domestic owned cats in Europe: Co-infestations and risk factors. *Parasit. Vectors* 7, 291.

114. Beugnet, F., Chardonnet, L., 1993. Note à propos d'un cas de coccidiose digestive chez trois chatons. *Rev. El. Méd. Vét. N. -C.* 17, 21–24.

115. Bevill, R.F., 1988. Sulphonamides. In Booth, N.H. and McDonalds, L.E. (Ed.), *Veterinary Pharmacology and Therapeutics.* Iowa State University Press. Ames, IA. 6th ed., 717–727.

116. Bezerra, P.S., Driemeier, D., Loretti, A.P., Riet-Correa, F., Kamphues, J., de Barros, C.S., 1999. Monensin poisoning in Brazilian horses. *Vet. Hum. Toxicol.* 41, 383–385.

117. Bhatia, B.B., Chauhan, P.P.S., Arora, G.S., Agrawal, R.D., 1972. Observations on some coccidian infections in birds and a mammal at the Delhi Zoo. *Indian J. Anim. Sci.* 42, 625–628.

118. Bhatia, B.B., Pande, B.P., 1966. On two new species of coccidia from wild Anatidae. *Acta Vet. Acad. Sci. Hung.* 16, 335–340.

119. Bhatia, B.B., Pande, B.P., 1967. Giant eimerian schizonts in the Indian water-buffalo. *Acta Vet. Acad. Sci. Hung.* 17, 351–357.

120. Bhatia, B.B., Pande, B.P., Chauhan, P.P.S., Arora, G.S., 1968. A study on the sporulated oocysts of twelve eimerian species in Indian buffalo (*Bubalus bubalis*). *Acta Vet. Acad. Sci. Hung.* 18, 115–133.

121. Bi, F., Hao, Z., Sun, P., Yu, Y., Suo, X., Liu, X., 2018. Studies on anticoccidial drugs and drug resistance of coccidiosis in chickens. *Acta Parasitol. Med. Entomol. Sinica* 25, 242–253 (in Chinese).

122. Bialek, R., Binder, N., Dietz, K., Knobloch, J., Zelck, U.E., 2002. Comparison of autofluorescence and iodine staining for detection of *Isospora belli* in feces. *Am. J. Trop. Med. Hyg.* 67, 304–305.

123. Biester, H.E., Murray, C., 1934. Studies in infectious enteritis of swine. VIII. *Isospora suis* n. sp. in swine. *J. Am. Vet. Med. Assoc.* 85, 207–219.

124. Biester, H.E., Schwarte, L.H., 1932. Studies in infectious enteritis of swine. VI. Immunity in swine coccidiosis. *J. Am. Vet. Med. Assoc.* 81, 358–375.

125. Bila, C.G., Perreira, C.L., Gruys, E., 2001. Accidental monensin toxicosis in horses in Mozambique. *J. S. Afr. Vet. Assoc.* 72, 163–164.

126. Bilung, L.M., Tahar, A.S., Yunos, N.E., Apun, K., Lim, Y.A.L., Nillian, E., Hashim, H.F., 2017. Detection of *Cryptosporidium* and *Cyclospora* oocysts from environmental water for drinking and recreational activities in Sarawak, Malaysia. *Biomed Res. Int.* 2017, 4636420.

127. Birdal Akis, F., Beyhan, Y.E., 2018. Distribution of intestinal parasites in patients hospitalized in child intensive care unit. *Turkiye Parazitol. Derg.* 42, 113–117.

128. Biswal, G., 1948. Coccidiosis in buffalo calves. *Indian Vet. J.* 25, 37–38.

129. Blagburn, B.L., Boosinger, T.R., Powe, T.A., 1991. Experimental *Isospora suis* infections in miniature swine. *Vet. Parasitol.* 38, 343–347.

130. Blake, D.P., Alias, H., Billington, K.J., Clark, E.L., Mat-Isa, M.N., Mohamad, A.F.H., Mohd-Amin, M.R. et al., 2012. *Emax*DB: Availability of a first draft genome sequence for the apicomplexan *Eimeria maxima*. *Mol. Biochem. Parasitol.* 184, 48–51.

131. Blake, D.P., Billington, K.J., Copestake, S.L., Oakes, R.D., Quail, M.A., Wan, K.L., Shirley, M.W., Smith, A.L., 2011. Genetic mapping identifies novel highly protective antigens for an apicomplexan parasite. *PLOS Pathog.* 7, e1001279.

132. Blake, D.P., Clark, E.L., Macdonald, S.E., Thenmozhi, V., Kundu, K., Garg, R., Jatau, I.D. et al., 2015. Population, genetic, and antigenic diversity of the apicomplexan *Eimeria tenella* and their relevance to vaccine development. *Proc. Natl. Acad. Sci. U.S.A.* 112, E5343–E5350.

133. Blake, D.P., Hesketh, P., Archer, A., Carroll, F., Shirley, M.W., Smith, A.L., 2005. The influence of immunizing dose size and schedule on immunity to subsequent challenge with antigenically distinct strains of *Eimeria maxima*. *Avian Pathol.* 34, 489–494.

134. Blake, D.P., Oakes, R., Smith, A.L., 2011. A genetic linkage map for the apicomplexan protozoan parasite *Eimeria maxima* and comparison with *Eimeria tenella*. *Int. J. Parasitol.* 41, 263–270.

135. Blake, D.P., Pastor-Fernández, I., Nolan, M.J., Tomley, F.M., 2017. Recombinant anticoccidial vaccines—A cup half full? *Infect. Genet. Evol.* 55, 358–365.

136. Blake, D.P., Tomley, F.M., 2014. Securing poultry production from the ever-present *Eimeria* challenge. *Trends Parasitol.* 30, 12–19.

137. Blandino, T., Gomez, E., 1985. Evaluación del formaldehído sobre oocistos de *Eimeria zurnii* en condiciones simuladas de producción. *Rvta. Cub. Cienc. Vet.* 16, 67–72.

138. Bledsoe, B., 1976. *Isospora vulpina* Nieschulz and Bos, 1933: Description, and transmission from the fox (*Vulpes vulpes*) to the dog. *J. Protozool.* 23, 365–367.

139. Bliss, S.K., Marshall, A.J., Zhang, Y., Denkers, E.Y., 1999. Human polymorphonuclear leukocytes produce IL-12, TNF-α, and the chemokines macrophage-inflammatory protein-1α and -1β in response to *Toxoplasma gondii* antigens. *J. Immunol.* 162, 7369–7375.

140. Boch, J., Pezenburg, E., Rosenfeld, V., 1961. Ein Beitrag zur Kenntnis der Kokzidien der Schweine. *Berl. Münch. tierärztl. Wochenschr.* 74, 449–451.

141. Boch, J., Wiesenhütter, E., 1963. Beitrag zur Klärung der Pathogenität der Schweinekokzidien. *Tierärztl. Umschau* 18, 223–225.

142. Bohrmann, R., 1991. Treatment with toltrazuril in a natural outbreak of coccidiosis in calves. *Dtsch. Tierarztl. Wochenschr.* 98, 343–345.

143. Boles, J.I., Becker, E.R., 1954. The development of *Eimeria brunetti* Levine in the digestive tract of chickens. *Iowa State Coll. J. Sci.* 29, 1–26.

144. Borghi, E.D., Araoz, C., Jofré, C., Duarte, A., Mera y Sierra, R.L., 2004. Gastrointestinal parasites of guanacos (*Lama guanicoe*) of Midwest Argentina (Mendoza and San Juan). *Biocell* 28, 185.

145. Borji, H., Razmi, G., Movassaghi, A.R., Naghibi, A.G., Maleki, M., 2009. Prevalence of *Cryptosporidium* and *Eimeria* infections in dromedary (*Camelus dromedarius*) in abattoir of Mashhad, Iran. *J. Camel Prac. Res.* 16, 167–170.

146. Bornstein, S., Gluecks, I.V., Younan, M., Thebo, P., Mattsson, J.G., 2008. *Isospora orlovi* infection in suckling dromedary camel calves (*Camelus dromedarius*) in Kenya. *Vet. Parasitol.* 152, 194–201.

147. Bosco, A., Rinaldi, L., Cappelli, G., Saratsis, A., Nisoli, L., Cringoli, G., 2015. Metaphylactic treatment strategies with toltrazuril and diclazuril and growth performance of buffalo calves exposed to a natural *Eimeria* infection. *Vet. Parasitol.* 212, 408–410.

148. Boughton, D.C., 1943. Sulfaguanidine therapy in experimental bovine coccidiosis. *Am. J. Vet. Res.* 4, 66.

149. Bouts, T., Fox, M.T., Scheres, G., Chávez, A., 2003. Identification of gastro-intestinal nematodes and coccidia in wild vicunas (*Lama vicugna*) in Pampa Galeras, Peru. *Erkrankungen der Zootiere: Verhandlungsber. Int. Symp. Erkr. Zoo- und Wildtiere*, Rome, Italy, May 28–June 1, pp. 101–105. Symposiums.

150. Bouvier, G., 1967. Les coccidies rencontrées en Suisse chez le lièvre gris (*Lepus europaeus*). *Ann. Parasitol.* 42, 551–559.

151. Brandborg, L.L., Goldberg, S.B., Breidenbach, W.C., 1970. Human coccidiosis—A possible cause of malabsorption. The life cycle in small-bowel mucosal biopsies as a diagnostic feature. *N. Engl. J. Med.* 283, 1306–1313.

152. Braun, R., Eckert, J., Roditi, I., Smith, N., Wallach, M., 1992. Coccidiosis of poultry and farm animals. *Parasitol. Today* 8, 220–221.

153. Breed, D.G.J., Dorrestein, J., Schetters, T.P.M., Waart, L.V.D., Rijke, E., Vermeulen, A.N., 1997. Peripheral blood lymphocytes from *Eimeria tenella* infected chickens produce gamma-interferon after stimulation *in vitro*. *Parasite Immunol.* 19, 127–135.

154. Breed, D.G.J., Dorrestein, J., Vermeulen, A.N., 1996. Immunity to *Eimeria tenella* in chickens: Phenotypical and functional changes in peripheral blood T-cell subsets. *Avian Dis.* 40, 37–48.

155. Breed, D.G.J., Schetters, T.P.M., Verhoeven, N.A.P., Vermeulen, A.N., 1997. Characterization of phenotype related responsiveness of peripheral blood lymphocytes from *Eimeria tenella* infected chickens. *Parasite Immunol.* 19, 563–569.

156. Bromley, E., Leeds, N., Clark, J., McGregor, E., Ward, M., Dunn, M.J., Tomley, F., 2003. Defining the protein repertoire of microneme secretory organelles in the apicomplexan parasite *Eimeria tenella*. *Proteomics* 3, 1553–1561.

157. Brownlie, R., Allan, B., 2011. Avian toll-like receptors. *Cell Tissue Res.* 343, 121–130.

158. Broz, J., Frigg, M., 1987. Incompatibility between lasalocid and chloramphenicol in broiler chicks after a long-term simultaneous administration. *Vet. Res. Commun.* 11, 159–172.

159. Bryan, G.T., 1978. *Nitrofurans: Chemistry, Metabolism, Mutagenesis, and Carcinogenesis.* 214–215. Raven Press. New York.

160. Buehl, I.E., Prosl, H., Mundt, H.-C., Tichy, A.G., Joachim, A., 2006. Canine isosporosis—Epidemiology of field and experimental infections. *J. Vet. Med. B* 53, 482–487.

161. Bukovszki, V., Kočišová, A., 2015. Surveillance of rabbit parasitoses on selected farms in eastern Slovakia. *Folia Vet.* 59, 74–76.

162. Bun, S.D., Guo, Y.M., Guo, F.C., Ji, F.J., Cao, H., 2011. Influence of organic zinc supplementation on the antioxidant status and immune responses of broilers challenged with *Eimeria tenella*. *Poult. Sci.* 90, 1220–1226.

163. Bundina, L.A., Khrustalev, V.A., 2016. The first detection of *Eimeria leuckarti* in horses on the territory of the Russian Federation. *Russian J. Parasitol.* 35, 7–12 (in Russian).

164. Burke, J.M., Miller, J.E., Terrill, T.H., Orlik, S.T., Acharya, M., Garza, J.J., Mosjidis, J.A., 2013. Sericea lespdeza as an aid in the control of *Emeria* spp. in lambs. *Vet. Parasitol.* 193, 39–46.

165. Buss, S.N., Leber, A., Chapin, K., Fey, P.D., Bankowski, M.J., Jones, M.K., Rogatcheva, M., Kanack, K.J., Bourzac, K.M., 2015. Multicenter evaluation of the BioFire FilmArray Gastrointestinal Panel for etiologic diagnosis of infectious gastroenteritis. *J. Clin. Microbiol.* 53, 915–925.

166. Cafrune, M.M., Marín, R.E., Rigalt, F.A., Romero, S.R., Aguirre, D.H., 2009. Prevalence of *Eimeria macusaniensis* and *Eimeria ivitaensis* in South American camelids of Northwest Argentina. *Vet. Parasitol.* 162, 338–341.

167. Cafrune, M.M., Romero, S.R., Aguirre, D.H., 2014. Prevalence and abundance of *Eimeria* spp. infection in captive vicuñas (*Vicugna vicugna*) from the Argentinean Andean Altiplano. *Small Ruminant Res.* 120, 150–154.

168. Cai, X., Fuller, A.L., McDougald, L.R., Zhu, G., 2003. Apicoplast genome of the coccidian *Eimeria tenella*. *Gene* 321, 39–46.

169. Calandra, T., Bernhagen, J., Mitchell, R.A., Bucala, R., 1994. The macrophage is an important and previously unrecognized source of macrophage migration inhibitory factor. *J. Exp. Med.* 179, 1895–1902.

170. Cama, V.A., Ortega, Y.R., 2018. *Cyclospora cayetanensis*. In Ortega, Y.R. and Sterling, C.R. (Ed.), *Foodborne Parasites*. Springer International Publishing. New York, 2nd ed., 41–56.

171. Campos, R., Neto, V.A., Campos, L.L., 1969. Brote de isosporosis en niños de un orfelinato. *Bol. Chil. Parasitol.* 24, 127–129.

172. Cantacessi, C., Riddell, S., Morris, G.M., Doran, T., Woods, W.G., Otranto, D., Gasser, R.B., 2008. Genetic characterization of three unique operational taxonomic units of *Eimeria* from chickens in Australia based on nuclear spacer ribosomal DNA. *Vet. Parasitol.* 152, 226–234.

173. Caradonna, T., Marangi, M., Del Chierico, F., Ferrari, N., Reddel, S., Bracaglia, G., Normanno, G., Putignani, L., Giangaspero, A., 2017. Detection and prevalence of protozoan parasites in ready-to-eat packaged salads on sale in Italy. *Food Microbiol.* 67, 67–75.

174. Cardim, S.T., Seixas, M., Tabacow, V.B.D., Taroda, A., Carneiro, P.G., Martins, T.A., de Barros, L.D. et al., 2018. Prevalence of *Eimeria* spp. in calves from dairy farms in northern Paraná state, Brazil. *Rev. Bras. Parasitol. Vet.* 27, 119–123.

175. Carrau, T., Pérez, D., Silva, L.M., Macias, J., Martinez-Carrasco, C., Taubert, A., Hermosilla, C., Ruiz de Ybáñez, R., 2016. Postparturient rise in the excretion of *Eimeria* spp. in Manchega dairy sheep. *J. Vet. Med. Res.* 2, 1047.

176. Carrau, T., Silva, L.M.R., Pérez, D., Ruiz de Ybáñez, R., Taubert, A., Hermosilla, C., 2016. First description of an *in vitro* culture system for *Eimeria ovinoidalis* macromeront formation in primary host endothelial cells. *Parasitol. Int.* 65, 516–519.

177. Carreno, R.A., Schnitzler, B.E., Jeffries, A.C., Tenter, A.M., Johnson, A.M., Barta, J.R., 1998. Phylogenetic analysis of coccidia based on 18S rDNA sequence comparison indicates that *Isospora* is most closely related to *Toxoplasma* and *Neospora*. *J. Eukaryot. Microbiol.* 45, 184–188.

178. Casadevall, A., 2003. Antibody-mediated immunity against intracellular pathogens: Two-dimensional thinking comes full circle. *Infect. Immun.* 71, 4225–4228.

179. Casadevall, A., Pirofski, L.A., 2003. Antibody-mediated regulation of cellular immunity and the inflammatory response. *Trends Immunol.* 24, 474–478.

180. Casillas, S.M., Bennett, C., Straily, A., 2018. Multiple cyclosporiasis outbreaks—United States, 2018. *MMWR Morb. Mortal. Wkly. Rep.* 67, 1101–1111.

181. Castañón, C.A.B., Fraga, J.S., Fernandez, S., Gruber, A., Costa, L.F., 2007. Biological shape characterization for automatic image recognition and diagnosis of protozoan parasites of the genus *Eimeria*. *Pattern Recognition* 40, 1899–1910.

182. Castanon, J.I.R., 2007. History of the use of antibiotic as growth promoters in European poultry feeds. *Poult. Sci.* 86, 2466–2471.

183. Castillo, D.H., Chávez, V.A., Hoces, R.D., Casas, A.E., Rosadio, A.R., Wheeler, J.C., 2008. Contribución al estudio del parasitismo gastrointestinal en guanacos (*Lama guanicoe cacsilensis*). *Rev. Inv. Vet. Perú* 19, 168–175.

184. Catchpole, J., Harris, T.J., 1989. Interaction between coccidia and *Nematodirus battus* in lambs on pasture. *Vet. Rec.* 124, 603–605.

185. Catchpole, J., Maes, L., 1996. Is coccidiosis a problem in turkeys? In Anonymous (Ed.), *World Poultry. Misset International*. Doetinchem, the Netherlands, 30–33.

186. Catchpole, J., Norton, C.C., Gregory, M.W., 1993. Immunisation of lambs against coccidiosis. *Vet. Rec.* 132, 56–59.

187. Catchpole, J., Norton, C.C., Joyner, L.P., 1976. Experiments with defined multispecific coccidial infections in lambs. *Parasitology* 72, 137–147.

188. Cavalcante, A.C.R., Teixeira, M., Monteiro, J.P., Lopes, C.W.G., 2012. *Eimeria* species in dairy goats in Brazil. *Vet. Parasitol.* 183, 356–358.

189. CDC, 2004. Centers for Disease Control and Prevention. Outbreak of cyclosporiasis associated with snow peas—Pennsylvania, 2004. *MMWR (Morb. Mortal. Wkly. Rep.)* September 24, 2004, 53 (37), 876–878. https://cdc.gov/mmwr/preview/mmwrhtml/mm5337a6.htm (accessed June 20, 2019).

190. Cebra, C.K., 2015. North American experiences with coccidiosis in new world camelids. *VII Congreso Mundial en Camélidos sudamericanos*, Puno-Peru, 2015.

191. Cebra, C.K., Anderson, D., Tibary, A., Van Saun, R., Johnson, L.W., 2014. Parasitic gastroenteritis. In Anonymous (Ed.), *Llama and Alpaca Care, Medicine, Surgery, Reproduction, Nutrition, and Health Care*. Saunders Elsevier. Saint Louis, MO. 501–512.

192. Cebra, C.K., Mattson, D.E., Baker, R.J., Sonn, R.J., Dearing, P.L., 2003. Potential pathogens in feces from unweaned llamas and alpacas with diarrhea. *J. Am. Vet. Med. Assoc.* 223, 1806–1808.

193. Cebra, C.K., Stang, B.V., 2008. Comparison of methods to detect gastrointestinal parasites in llamas and alpacas. *J. Am. Vet. Med. Assoc.* 232, 733–741.

194. Cebra, C.K., Stang, B.V., Smith, C.C., 2012. Development of a nested polymerase chain reaction assay for the detection of *Eimeria macusaniensis* in camelid feces. *Am. J. Vet. Res.* 73, 13–18.

195. Cebra, C.K., Valentine, B.A., Schlipf, J.W., Bildfell, R.J., McKenzie, E., Waitt, L.H., Heidel, J.R. et al., 2007. *Eimeria macusaniensis* infection in 15 llamas and 34 alpacas. *J. Am. Vet. Med. Assoc.* 230, 94–100.

196. Cere, N., Humbert, J.F., Licois, D., Corvione, M., Afanassieff, M., Chanteloup, N., 1996. A new approach for the identification and the diagnosis of *Eimeria* media parasite of the rabbit. *Exp. Parasitol.* 82, 132–138.

197. Cere, N. Licois, D., Humbert, J.F., 1995. Study of the inter- and intraspecific variation of *Eimeria* spp. from the rabbit using random amplified polymorphic DNA. *Parasitol. Res.* 81, 324–328.

198. Certad, G., Arenas-Pinto, A., Pocaterra, L., Ferrara, G., Castro, J., Bello, A., Núñez, L., 2003. Isosporiasis in Venezuelan adults infected with human immunodeficiency virus: Clinical characterization. *Am. J. Trop. Med. Hyg.* 69, 217–222.

199. Cervantes-Valencia, M.E., Alcalá-Canto, Y., Sumano-Lopez, H., Ducoing-Watty, A.M., Gutierrez-Olvera, L., 2016. Effects of *Curcuma longa* dietary inclusion against *Eimeria* spp. in naturally-infected lambs. *Small Ruminant Res.* 136, 27–35.

200. Cha, J.O., Talha, A.F.S.M., Lim, C.W., Kim, B., 2014. Effects of glass bead size, vortexing speed and duration on *Eimeria acervulina* oocyst excystation. *Exp. Parasitol.* 138, 18–24.

201. Chacín-Bonilla, L., 2008. Transmission of *Cyclospora cayetanensis* infection: A review focusing on soil-borne cyclosporiasis. *Trans. Roy. Soc. Trop. Med. Hyg.* 102, 215–216.

202. Chacín-Bonilla, L., 2010. Epidemiology of *Cyclospora cayetanensis*: A review focusing in endemic areas. *Acta Trop.* 115, 181–193.

203. Chacin-Bonilla, L., 2017. *Cyclospora cayetanensis*. In Rose, J.B. and Jiménez-Cisneros, B. (Ed.), *Global Water Pathogens Project*. http://www.waterpathogens.org (R. Fayer and W. Jakubowski, [Eds] Part 3: Protists). http://www.waterpathogens.org/book/cyclospora-cayetanensis. Michigan State University, East Lansing, MI, UNESCO.

204. Chacín-Bonilla, L., Barrios, F., Sanchez, Y., 2007. Epidemiology of *Cyclospora cayetanensis* infection in San Carlos Island, Venezuela: Strong association between socio-economic status and infection. *Trans. Roy. Soc. Trop. Med. Hyg.* 101, 1018–1024.

205. Chacín-Bonilla, L., Estévez, J., Monsalve, F., Quijada, L., 2001. *Cyclospora cayetanensis* infections among diarrheal patients from Venezuela. *Am. J. Trop. Med. Hyg.* 65, 351–354.

206. Chacin-Bonilla, L., Mejia de Young, M., Estevez, J., 2003. Prevalence and pathogenic role of *Cyclospora cayetanensis* in a Venezuelan community. *Am. J. Trop. Med. Hyg.* 68, 304–306.

207. Chae, C., Kwon, D., Kim, O., Min, K., Cheon, D.S., Choi, C., Kim, B., Suh, J., 1998. Diarrhoea in nursing piglets associated with coccidiosis: Prevalence, microscopic lesions and coexisting microorganisms. *Vet. Rec.* 143, 417–420.

208. Chakravarty, M., Basu, S.P., 1947. On a new coccidium *Tyzzeria alleni* n. sp. from the intestine of the bird cottonteal. *Sci. Cult.* 12, 106.

209. Challey, J.R., Jeffers, T.K., 1973. Synergism between 4-hydroxyquinoline and pyridone coccidiostats. *J. Parasitol.* 59, 502–504.

210. Chan, G., Farzan, A., DeLay, J., McEwen, B., Prescott, J.F., Friendship, R.M., 2013. A retrospective study on the etiological diagnoses of diarrhea in neonatal piglets in Ontario, Canada, between 2001 and 2010. *Can. J. Vet. Res.* 77, 254–260.

211. Chandra, D., Ghosh, S.S., 1990. Sporulation pattern of coccidial oocysts of swine origin. *Indian J. Anim. Sci.* 60, 426–428.

212. Chapman, H.D., 1975. *Eimeria tenella* in chickens: Development of resistance to quinolone anticoccidial drugs. *Parasitology* 71, 41–49.

213. Chapman, H.D., 1978. Studies on the excystation of different species of *Eimeria in vitro*. *Z. Parasitenkd.* 56, 115–121.

214. Chapman, H.D., 1978. The effect of monensin on the immunity arising from repeated low-level infections with *Eimeria maxima, E. brunetti* and *E. tenella. Avian Pathol.* 7, 269–277.

215. Chapman, H.D., 1983. Field isolates of *Eimeria* resistant to arprinocid. *Vet. Parasitol.* 12, 45–50.

216. Chapman, H.D., 1984. Development by genetic recombination of a line of *Eimeria tenella* resistant to robenidine, decoquinate and amprolium. *Z. Parasitenkd.* 70, 437–441.

217. Chapman, H.D., 1986. Isolates of *Eimeria tenella*: Studies on resistance to ionophorous anticoccidial drugs. *Res. Vet. Sci.* 41, 281–282.

218. Chapman, H.D., 1992. Research note: Immunity to *Eimeria* in broilers reared on nicarbazin and salinomycin. *Poult. Sci.* 71, 577–580.

219. Chapman, H.D., 1993. Resistance to anticoccidial drugs in fowl. *Parasitol. Today* 9, 159–162.

220. Chapman, H.D., 1994. A review of the biological activity of the anticoccidial drug nicarbazin and its application for the control of coccidiosis in poultry. *Poult. Sci. Rev.* 5, 231–243.

221. Chapman, H.D., 1994. Sensitivity of field isolates of *Eimeria* to monensin following the use of a coccidiosis vaccine in broiler chickens. *Poult. Sci.* 73, 476–478.

222. Chapman, H.D., 1996. Administration of a coccidiosis vaccine to day-old turkeys via the eye and development of immunity to *Eimeria* species. *Poult. Sci.* 75, 1496–1497.

223. Chapman, H.D., 1997. Biochemical, genetic and applied aspects of drug resistance in *Eimeria* parasites of the fowl. *Avian Pathol.* 26, 221–244.

224. Chapman, H.D., 1998. Evaluation of the efficacy of anticoccidial drugs against *Eimeria* species in the fowl. *Int. J. Parasitol.* 28, 1141–1144.

225. Chapman, H.D., 1999. Anticoccidial drugs and their effects upon the development of immunity to *Eimeria* infections in poultry. *Avian Pathol.* 28, 521–535.

226. Chapman, H.D., 1999. The development of immunity to *Eimeria* species in broilers given anticoccidial drugs. *Avian Pathol.* 28, 155–162.

227. Chapman, H.D., 2001. Use of anticoccidial drugs in broiler chickens in the USA: Analysis for the years 1995 to 1999. *Poult. Sci.* 80, 572–580.

228. Chapman, H.D., 2003. Origins of coccidiosis research in the fowl—The first fifty years. *Avian Dis.* 47, 1–20.

229. Chapman, H.D., 2008. Coccidiosis in the turkey. *Avian Pathol.* 37, 205–223.

230. Chapman, H.D., 2009. A landmark contribution to poultry science—Prophylactic control of coccidiosis in poultry. *Poult. Sci.* 88, 813–815.

230a. Chapman, H.D., 2014. Milestones in avian coccidiosis research: A review. *Poul. Sci.* 93, 501–511.

231. Chapman, H.D., 2018. Applied strategies for the control of coccidiosis in poultry. *CAB Reviews* 13, no. 026.

232. Chapman, H.D., Barta, J.R., Blake, D., Gruber, A., Jenkins, M., Smith, N.C., Suo, X., Tomley, F.M., 2013. A selective review of advances in coccidiosis research. *Adv. Parasitol.* 83, 93–171.

233. Chapman, H.D., Barta, J.R., Hafeez, M.A., Matsler, P., Rathinam, T., Raccoursier, M., 2016. The epizootiology of *Eimeria* infections in commercial broiler chickens where anticoccidial drug programs were employed in six successive flocks to control coccidiosis. *Poult. Sci.* 95, 1774–1778.

234. Chapman, H.D., Cherry, T.E., 1997. Comparison of two methods of administering live coccidiosis vaccines to newly hatched chicks: Infectivity and development of immunity to *Eimeria* species. *Proceedings of the VIIth International Coccidiosis Concerence*, Oxford, UK, p. 133.

235. Chapman, H.D., Cherry, T.E., 1997. Eyespray vaccination: Infectivity and development of immunity to *Eimeria acervulina* and *Eimeria tenella*. *J. Appl. Poultry Res.* 6, 274–278.

236. Chapman, H.D., Cherry, T.E., Danforth, H.D., Richards, G., Shirley, M.W., Williams, R.B., 2002. Sustainable coccidiosis control in poultry production: The role of live vaccines. *Int. J. Parasitol.* 32, 617–629.

237. Chapman, H.D., Fitzcoy, S.H., 1996. Effect of roxarsone and bacitracin methylene disalicylate on the development of immunity to *Eimeria* in broilers given a live coccidiosis vaccine. *Poult. Sci.* 75, 1488–1492.

238. Chapman, H.D., Hacker, A.B., 1993. The effects of shuttle programs upon the growth of broilers and the development of immunity to *Eimeria* species. *Poult. Sci.* 72, 658–663.

239. Chapman, H.D., Jeffers, T.K., 2014. Vaccination of chickens against coccidiosis ameliorates drug resistance in commercial poultry production. *Int. J. Parasitol. Drugs Drug Resist.* 4, 214–217.

240. Chapman, H.D., Jeffers, T.K., 2015. Restoration of sensitivity to salinomycin in *Eimeria* following 5 flocks of broiler chickens reared in floor-pens using drug programs and vaccination to control coccidiosis. *Poult. Sci.* 94, 943–946.

241. Chapman, H.D., Jeffers, T.K., Williams, R.B., 2010. Forty years of monensin for the control of coccidiosis in poultry. *Poult. Sci.* 89, 1788–1801.

242. Chapman, H.D., Johnson, Z.B., 1992. Oocysts of *Eimeria* in the litter of broilers reared to eight weeks of age before and after withdrawal of lasalocid or salinomycin. *Poult. Sci.* 71, 1342–1347.

243. Chapman, H.D., Marsler, P., LaVorgna, M.W., 2004. The effects of salinomycin and roxarsone on the performance of broilers when included in the feed for four, five, or six weeks and infected with *Eimeria* species during the starter or grower phase of production. *Poult. Sci.* 83, 761–764.

244. Chapman, H.D., Roberts, B., Shirley, M.W., Williams, R.B., 2005. Guidelines for evaluating the efficacy and safety of live anticoccidial vaccines, and obtaining approval for their use in chickens and turkeys. *Avian Pathol.* 34, 279–290.

245. Chapman, M.P., 1948. The use of sulfaquinoxaline in the control of liver coccidiosis in domestic rabbits. *Vet. Med.* 43, 375–379.

246. Charles, S.D., Chopade, H.M., Ciszewski, D.K., Arther, R.G., Settje, T.L., Reinemeyer, C.R., 2007. Safety of 5% ponazuril (toltrazuril sulfone) oral suspension and efficacy against naturally acquired *Cystoisospora ohioensis*-like infection in beagle puppies. *Parasitol. Res.* 101, S137–S144.

247. Chartier, C., Paraud, C., 2012. Coccidiosis due to *Eimeria* in sheep and goats, a review. *Small Ruminant Res.* 103, 84–92.

248. Chartier, C., Pellet, M.P., Pors, I., 1992. Effects of toltrazuril on oocyst discharge and growth in kids with naturally-acquired coccidial infections. *Small Ruminant Res.* 8, 171–177.

249. Chauve, C.M., Gounel, J.M., Reynaud, M.C., 1991. Les coccidies du canard mulard. Bilan d'une premiere enquete realisee dans trois elevages du sud-ouest de la France. *Avian Pathol.* 20, 713–719.

250. Chauve, C.M., Reynaud, M.C., Gounel, J.M., 1992. Isolement de 2 coccidies du genre *Isospora* chez des canards en France. *Ann. Rech. Vet.* 23, 395–398.

251. Chauve, C.M., Reynaud, M.C., Gounel, J.M., 1993. *Isospora* sp from ducks. Infectivity for the goose, four anatids and the domestic fowl. *Vet. Res., Biomed. Central.* 24, 430–433.

252. Chauve, C.M., Reynaud, M.C., Gounel, J.M., 1994. Description d'*Eimeria mulardi* n. sp. chez le canard mulard. Etude de la phase endogene de son cycle evolutif avec mise en evidence cu developpement intranucleaire. *Parasite* 1, 15–22.

253. Chen, B.L., Feng, J.X., Ye, B.H., Chen, J.H., 1988. A clinical report of duck coccidiosis. *Poult. Husb. Dis. Control* 3, 28 (in Chinese).

254. Chen, H., Wiedmer, S., Hanig, S., Entzeroth, R., Kurth, M., 2013. Development of *Eimeria nieschulzi* (Coccidia, Apicomplexa) gamonts and oocysts in primary fetal rat cells. *J. Parasitol. Res.* 2013, 591520.

255. Chen, P., Lv, J., Zhang, J., Sun, H., Chen, Z., Li, H., Wang, F., Zhao, X., 2015. Evaluation of immune protective efficacies of *Eimeria tenella* EtMic1 polypeptides with different domain recombination displayed on yeast surface. *Exp. Parasitol.* 155, 1–7.

256. Chen, X., Gu, Y., Singh, K., Shang, C., Barzegar, M., Jiang, S., Huang, S., 2014. Maduramicin inhibits proliferation and induces apoptosis in myoblast cells. *PLOS ONE* 9, e115652.

257. Chen, Z., Wang, X., Zhao, N., Han, L., Wang, F., Li, H., Cui, Y., Zhao, X., 2018. Improving the immunogenicity and protective efficacy of the EtMIC2 protein against *Eimeria tenella* infection through random mutagenesis. *Vaccine* 36, 2435–2441.

258. Cheng, P., Wang, C., Lin, X., Zhang, L., Fei, C., Zhang, K., Zhao, J. et al., 2018. Pharmacokinetics of a novel triazine ethanamizuril in rats and broiler chickens. *Res. Vet. Sci.* 117, 99–103.

259. Chessum, B.S., 1972. Reactivation of *Toxoplasma* oocyst production in the cat by infection with *Isospora felis. Br. Vet. J.* 128, 33–36.

260. Chhabra, R.C., Mafukidze, R.T., 1992. Prevalence of coccidia in pigs in Zimbabwe. *Vet. Parasitol.* 41, 1–5.

261. Chigerwe, M., Middleton, J.R., Williams, F., Tyler, J.W., Kreeger, J.M., 2007. Atypical coccidiosis in South American camelids. *J. Vet. Diagn. Invest.* 19, 122–125.

262. Chineme, C.N., 1980. A case report of coccidiosis caused by *Eimeria cameli* in a camel (*Camelus dromedarius*) in Nigeria. *J. Wildl. Dis.* 16, 377–380.

263. Chobotar, B., Danforth, H.D., Entzeroth, R., 1993. Ultrastructural observations of host-cell invasion by sporozoites of *Eimeria papillata in vivo. Parasitol. Res.* 79, 15–23.

264. Chobotar, B., Hammond, D.M., 1969. Development of gametocytes and second asexual generation stages of *Eimeria auburnensis* in calves. *J. Parasitol.* 55, 1218–1228.

265. Chobotar, B., Hammond, D.M., Miner, M.L., 1969. Development of the first-generation schizonts of *Eimeria auburnensis. J. Parasitol.* 55, 385–397.

266. Choi, K.D., Lillehoj, H.S., Zalenga, D.S., 1999. Changes in local IFN-γ and TGF-β4 mRNA expression and intraepithelial lymphocytes following *Eimeria acervulina* infection. *Vet. Immunol. Immunopathol.* 71, 263–275.

267. Chow, Y.P., Wan, K.L., Blake, D.P., Tomley, F., Nathan, S., 2011. Immunogenic *Eimeria tenella* glycosylphosphatidylinositol-anchored surface antigens (SAGs) induce inflammatory responses in avian macrophages. *PLOS ONE* 6, e25233.

268. Christensen, J.P.B., Henriksen, S.A., 1994. Shedding of oocysts in piglets experimentally infected with *Isospora suis. Acta Vet. Scand.* 35, 165–172.

269. Christiansen, M., Madsen, H., 1948. *Eimeria bucephalae* n. sp. (Coccidia) pathogenic in goldeneye (*Buchephala clangula* L.) in Denmark. *Dan. Rev. Game Biol.* 1, 62–73.

270. Cinar, H.N., Gopinath, G., Jarvis, K., Murphy, H.R., 2015. The complete mitochondrial genome of the foodborne parasitic pathogen *Cyclospora cayetanensis. PLOS ONE* 10, e0128645.

271. Cinar, H.N., Qvarnstrom, Y., Wei-Pridgeon, Y., Li, W., Nascimento, F.S., Arrowood, M.J., Murphy, H.R. et al., 2016. Comparative sequence analysis of *Cyclospora cayetanensis* apicoplast genomes originating from diverse geographical regions. *Parasit. Vectors* 9, 611.

272. Cintra Ferreira, D.R., Veras De Barros, A., da Silva Barros, M.B., Rodrigues da Mota, A.E., Bianque de Oliveira, J., 2013. Parasitos gastrointestinais de equinos em três municípios pernambucanos. *Proc. 13th Jornada de ensino, pesquisa e extensão*, Recife, Brazil, December 9–13, 2013.

273. Cirak, V.Y., Senlik, B., Gulegen, E., 2011. Gastrointestinal parasites of camels (*Camelus dromedarius*) from Turkey and efficacy of doramectin against trichostrongyles. *J. Camel Prac. Res.* 18, 283–285.

274. Claeskens, M., Verdonck, W., Heesen, H., Froyman, R., Torres, A., 2007. A field study assessing control of broiler coccidiosis by Paracox vaccination or by Toltrazuril (Baycox) stand-alone treatment. *Parasitol. Res.* 101 (Suppl 1), 105–112.

275. Clark, E.L., Macdonald, S.E., Thenmozhi, V., Kundu, K., Garg, R., Kumar, S., Ayoade, S. et al., 2016. Cryptic *Eimeria* genotypes are common across the southern but not northern hemisphere. *Int. J. Parasitol.* 46, 537–544.

276. Clark, E.L., Tomley, F.M., Blake, D.P., 2017. Are *Eimeria* genetically diverse, and does it matter? *Trends Parasitol.* 33, 231–241.

277. Clark, L.K., 1980. Managing an outbreak of coccidiosis. *Proc. Am. Assoc. Swine Pract. Ames*, IA, 84.

278. Clark, W.N., Hammond, D.M., 1969. Development of *Eimeria auburnensis* in cell cultures. *J. Protozool.* 16, 646–654.

279. Clarkson, M.J., 1958. Life history and pathogenicity of *Eimeria adenoeides* Moore and Brown, 1951, in the turkey poult. *Parasitology* 48, 70–88.

280. Clarkson, M.J., 1959. The life history and pathogenicity of *Eimeria meleagridis* Tyzzer, 1927, in the turkey poult. *Parasitology* 49, 519–528.

281. Clarkson, M.J., 1959. The life history and pathogenicity of *Eimeria meleagrimitis* Tyzzer 1929, in the turkey poult. *Parasitology* 49, 70–82.

282. Coelho, W.M.D., do Amarante, A.F.T., Bresciani, K.D.S., 2012. Occurrence of gastrointestinal parasites in goat kids. *Rev. Bras. Parasitol. Vet.* 21, 65–67.

283. Cole, L.J., Hadley, P.B., Kirkpatrick, W.F., 1910. Blackhead in turkeys: A study in avian coccidiosis. In Anonymous (Ed.), *23rd Annual report of the Rhode Island Agricultural Experimental Station.* Bulletin No. 141. Providence, RI, 137–271.

284. Collaboration Research Group for Qinghaosu, 1977. A new sesquiterpene lactone—Qinghaosu. *Chin. Sci. Bull.* 3, 142 (in Chinese).

285. Collier, C.T., Hofacre, C.L., Payne, A.M., Anderson, D.B., Kaiser, P., Mackie, R.I., Gaskins, H.R., 2008. Coccidia-induced mucogenesis promotes the onset of necrotic enteritis by supporting *Clostridium perfringens* growth. *Vet. Immunol. Immunopathol.* 122, 104–115.

286. Collins, J.E., Dubey, J.P., Rossow, K.D., 1988. Hepatic coccidiosis in a calf. *Vet. Pathol.* 25, 98–100.

287. Conlogue, G., Foreyt, W.J., Wescott, R.B., 1984. Bovine coccidiosis: Protective effects of low-level infection and coccidiostat treatments in calves. *Am. J. Vet. Res.* 45, 863–866.

288. Constable, P.D., Hinchcliff, K., Done, S.H., Grünberg, W., 2012. *Coccidiosis. Veterinary Medicine: A Textbook of the Diseases of Cattle, Horses, Sheep, Pigs, and Goats.* Elsevier, St. Louis, MO. 11th ed., 401–408.

289. Conway, D.P., McKenzie, M.E., 2007. Poultry coccidiosis. In Anonymous (Ed.), *Diagnostic and Testing Procedures.* Blackwell Publishing. Oxford, UK. 3rd ed. 168p.

290. Cook, S.M., Higuchi, D.S., McGowan, A.L., Schrader, J.S., Withanage, G.S.K., Francis, M.J., 2010. Polymerase chain reaction-based identity assay for pathogenic turkey *Eimeria. Avian Dis.* 54, 1152–1156.

291. Cordero Ramirez, A., Huanca López, W., Díaz Fernández, P., López Sández, C.M., Panadero Fontán, R., Fernández Rodriguez, G., Lago, N., Morrondo Pelayo, P., Díez Baños, P., 2011. Infection by gastrointestinal parasites in alpacas (*Lama pacos*) from Southern Perú. *Proceedings of the XII Congreso Ibérico de Parasitología SOCEPA*, Spain, July 5–8, 2011, 214.

292. Cornelissen, A.W.C.A., Overdulve, J.P., van der Ploeg, M., 1984. Determination of nuclear DNA of five eucoccidian parasites, *Isospora* (*Toxoplasma*) *gondii, Sarcocystis cruzi, Eimeria tenella, E. acervulina* and *Plasmodium berghei*, with special reference to gamontogenesis and meiosis in *I. (T.) gondii. Parasitology* 88, 531–553.

293. Cornelissen, A.W.C.A., Verstegen, R., van den Brand, H., Perie, N.M., Eysker, M., Lam, T.J.G.M., Pijpers, A., 1995. An obervational study of *Eimeria* species in housed cattle on Dutch dairy farms. *Vet. Parasitol.* 56, 7–16.

294. Cornelissen, J.B.W.J., Swinkels, W.J.C., Boersma, W.A., Rebel, J.M.J., 2009. Host response to simultaneous infections with *Eimeria acervulina, maxima* and *tenella*: A cumulation of single responses. *Vet. Parasitol.* 162, 58–66.

295. Correa, L., Zapata, B., Soto-Gamboa, M., 2012. Gastrointestinal and blood parasite determination in the guanaco (*Lama guanicoe*) under semi-captivity conditions. *Trop. Anim. Health Prod.* 44, 11–15.

296. Correa, W.M., Correa, C.N.M., Langoni, H., Volpato, O.A., Tsunoda, K., 1983. Canine isosporosis. *Canine Practice* 10, 44–46.

297. Costa, P.S., Lopes, C.W.G., 1994. Hipnozoitas de *Cystoisospora felis* (Apicomplexa: Cystoisosporinae) em vísceras de coelhos. *Rev. Bras. Ciênc. Vet.* 1, 35–36.

298. Costarella, C.E., Anderson, D.E., 1999. Ileocecocolic intussusception in a one-month-old llama. *J. Am. Vet. Med. Assoc.* 214, 1672–1673.

299. Cotteleer, C., Fameree, L., 1981. Parasitoses occasionnelles et anticorps toxoplasmiques chez les équidés en Belgique. Cas particulier des coccidies. *Schweiz. Arch. Tierheilkd.* 123, 263–271.

300. Coudert, P., 1976. Les coccidioses intestinales du lapin: Comparaison du pouvoir pathogène d'*Eimeria intestinalis* avec trois autres *Eimeria. C.R. Acad. Sci Paris.* 282, 2219–2222.

301. Coudert, P., Licois, D., Drouet-Viard, F., 1995. *Eimeria* species and strains of rabbits. In Eckert, J., Braun, R., Shirley, M.W., and Coudert, P. (Ed.), *Guidelines on Techniques in Coccidiosis Research.* European Commission, Directorate-General XII, Science, Research and Development Environment Research Programme. 52–73.

302. Coudert, P., Licois, D., Provôt, F., Drouet-Viard, F., 1993. *Eimeria* sp. from the rabbit (*Oryctolagus cuniculus*): Pathogenicity and immunogenicity of *Eimeria intestinalis. Parasitol. Res.* 79, 186–190.

303. Coudert, P., Licois, D., Streun, A., 1979. Characterization of *Eimeria* species. I. Isolation and study of pathogenicity of a pure strain of *Eimeria perforans* (Leuckart, 1879; Sluiter and Swellengrebel, 1912). *Z. Parasitenkd.* 59, 227–234.

304. Courtney, C.H., Ernst, J.V., Benz, G.W., 1976. Redescription of oocysts of the bovine coccidia *Eimeria bukidnonensis* Tubangui 1931 and *E. wyomingensis* Huizinga and Winger 1942. *J. Parasitol.* 62, 372–376.

305. Cowper, B., Matthews, S., Tomley, F., 2012. The molecular basis for the distinct host and tissue tropisms of coccidian parasites. *Mol. Biochem. Parasitol.* 186, 1–10.

306. Cringoli, G., Guarino, A., Fusco, G., Veneziano, V., Rinaldi, L., 1998. Diffusion dynamics of *Eimeria* spp. in infected buffalo herds. *Parassitologia* 40 (Suppl. 1), 38.

307. Cringoli, G., Rinaldi, L., Veneziano, V., Capelli, G., Scala, A., 2004. The influence of flotation solution, sample dilution and the choice of McMaster slide area (volume) on the reliability of the McMaster technique in estimating the faecal egg counts of gastrointestinal strongyles and *Dicrocoelium dendriticum* in sheep. *Vet. Parasitol.* 123, 121–131.

308. Cui, N., Wang, X., Wang, Q., Li, H., Wang, F., Zhao, X., 2017. Effect of dual infection with *Eimeria tenella* and subgroup J avian leukosis virus on the cecal microbiome in specific-pathogen-free chicks. *Front. Vet. Sci.* 4, Article 177.

309. Cui, P., Liu, H., Fang, S., Gu, X., Wang, P., Liu, C., Tao, G., Liu, X., Suo, X., 2017. A new species of *Eimeria* (Apicomplexa: Eimeriidae) from Californian rabbits in Hebei Province, China. *Parasitol. Int.* 66, 677–680.

310. Cui, X.Z., Zheng, M.X., Zhang, Y., Liu, R.L., Yang, S.S., Li, S., Xu, Z.Y., Bai, R., Lv, Q.H., Zhao, W.L., 2016. Calcium homeostasis in mitochondrion-mediated apoptosis of chick embryo cecal epithelial cells induced by *Eimeria tenella* infection. *Res. Vet. Sci.* 104, 166–173.

311. Cui, Y.H., Zhang, Y., Yan, Y.J., 2010. Diagnosis and treatment of coccidiosis in duckling. *Jilin Anim. Sci. Vet. Med.* 31, 27 (in Chinese).

312. Current, W.L., 1987. Neonatal swine coccidiosis. *Anim. Health Nutr.* 42, 8–12.

313. Da Costa, P.S., Lopes, C.W.G., 1998. Avaliação do parasitismo por *Cystoisospora felis* (Wenyon, 1923) Frenkel, 1977 (Apicomplexa: Cystoisosporinae) em coelhos tipo carne. *Rev. Bras. Parasitol. Vet.* 7, 15–19.

314. Da Costa, P.S., Lopes, C.W.G., de Carvalho, E.C.Q., 2001. Patologia comparativa na infecção experimental por *Cystoisospora felis* (Apicomplexa: Cystoisosporinae) em coelhos do tipo carne. *R. Bras. Med. Vet.* 23, 215–218.

315. Dai, Y. Lin, M., Zhang, S., Fu, A., 1991. Hepatic coccidiosis in the goat. *Int. J. Parasitol.* 21, 381–382.

316. Dai, Y.B., Liu, X.Y., Liu, M., Tao, J.P., 2006. Pathogenic effects of the coccidium *Eimeria ninakohlyakimovae* in goats. *Vet. Res. Commun.* 30, 149–160.

317. Dalloul, R.A., Lillehoj, H.S., 2005. Recent advances in immunomodulation and vaccination strategies against coccidiosis. *Avian Dis.* 49, 1–8.

318. Damriyasa, I.M., 2001. Querschnittsstudie zu Parasitosen bei Zuchtsauen in südhessischen Betrieben. Dr. med. vet. thesis. Justus-Liebig University, Giessen.

319. Danforth, H.D., 1998. Use of live oocyst vaccines in the control of avian coccidiosis: Experimental studies and field trials. *Int. J. Parasitol.* 28, 1099–1109.

320. Danforth, H.D., Hammond, D.M., 1972. Stages of merogony in multinucleate merozoites of *Eimeria magna* Pérard, 1925. *J. Protozool.* 19, 454–457.

321. Danforth, H.D., Lee, E.H., Martin, A., Dekich, M., 1997. Evaluation of a gel-immunization technique used with two different Immucox vaccine formulations in battery and floor-pen trials with broiler chickens. *Parasitol. Res.* 83, 445–451.

322. Das, G., Atasoglu, C., Akbag, H.I., Tölü, C., Yurtman, I.Y., Savas, T., 2012. Effects of kefir on coccidial oocysts excretion and performance of dairy goat kids following weaning. *Trop. Anim. Health Prod.* 44, 1049–1055.

323. Das, M., Deka, D.K., Sarmah, A.K., Sarmah, P.C., Islam, S., 2017. Gastrointestinal parasitic infections in cattle and swamp buffalo of Guwahati, Assam, India. *Indian J. Anim. Res.* B-3427.

324. Dasgupta, T., Lee, E.H., 2000. A gel delivery system for coccidiosis vaccine: Uniformity of distribution of oocysts. *Can. Vet. J.* 41, 613–616.

325. Daugschies, A., 2006. Protozoeninfektionen des Schweines. In Schnieder, T. (Ed.), *Veterinärmedizinische Parasitologie*. Paul Parey, Berlin 6th ed., 359–368.

326. Daugschies, A., Agneessens, J., Goossens, L., Mengel, H., Veys, P., 2007. The effect of a metaphylactic treatment with diclazuril (Vecoxan) on the oocyst excretion and growth performance of calves exposed to a natural *Eimeria* infection. *Vet. Parasitol.* 149, 199–206.

327. Daugschies, A., Akimaru, M., Bürger, H.J., 1986. Experimentelle *Eimeria bovis*-Infektionen beim Kalb: 1. Parasitologische und klinische Befunde. *Dtsch. tierarztl. Wochenschr.* 93, 393–397.

328. Daugschies, A., Bangoura, B., Lendner, M., 2013. Inactivation of exogenous endoparasite stages by chemical disinfectants: Current state and perspectives. *Parasitol. Res.* 112, 917–932.

329. Daugschies, A., Bialek, R., Joachim, A., Mundt, H.C., 2001. Autofluorescence microscopy for the detection of nematode eggs and protozoa, in particular *Isospora suis*, in swine faeces. *Parasitol. Res.* 87, 409–412.

330. Daugschies, A., Imarom, S., Bollwahn, W., 1999. Differentiation of porcine *Eimeria* spp. by morphologic algorithms. *Vet. Parasitol.* 81, 201–210.

331. Daugschies, A., Imarom, S., Ganter, M., Bollwahn, W., 2004. Prevalence of *Eimeria* spp. in sows at piglet-producing farms in Germany. *J. Vet. Med. B* 51, 135–139.

332. Daugschies, A., Mundt, H.C., Letkova, V., 2000. Toltrazuril treatment of cystoisosporosis in dogs under experimental and field conditions. *Parasitol. Res.* 86, 797–799.

333. Daugschies, A., Najdrowski, M., 2005. Eimeriosis in cattle: Current understanding. *J. Vet. Med. B* 52, 417–427.

334. Davies, S.F.M., 1957. An outbreak of duck coccidiosis in Britain. *Vet. Rec.* 69, 1051–1052.

335. Davies, S.F.M., Joyner, L.P., Kendall, S.B., 1963. *Coccidiosis*. 1st ed. Oliver and Boyd, Edinburgh and London, 264p.

336. Davis, L.R., 1973. Techniques. In Hammond, D.M. and Long, P.L. (Ed.), *The Coccidia: Eimeria, Isospora, Toxoplasma, and Related Genera*. University Park Press. Baltimore, MD, 409–458.

337. Davis, L.R., Boughton, D.C., Bowman, G.W., 1955. Biology and pathogenicity of *Eimeria alabamensis* Christensen, 1941, an intranuclear coccidium of cattle. *Am. J. Vet. Res.* 16, 274–281.

338. Davis, L.R., Bowman, G.W., 1957. The endogenous development of *Eimeria zurnii*, a pathogenic coccidium of cattle. *Am. J. Vet. Res.* 18, 569–574.

339. Davis, L.R., Bowman, G.W., 1962. Schizonts and microgametocytes of *Eimeria auburnensis* Christensen and Porter, 1939, in calves. *J. Protozool.* 9, 424–427.

340. Davis, L.R., Bowman, G.W., 1964. Observations on the life cycle of *Eimeria bukidnonensis* Tubangui, 1931, a coccidium of cattle. *J. Protozool.* 11 (Suppl.), 17.

341. Davis, L.R., Bowman, G.W., Boughton, D.C., 1957. The endogenous development of *Eimeria alabamensis* Christensen 1941, an intranuclear coccidium of cattle. *J. Protozool.* 4, 219–225.

342. Davoodi, Z., Kojouri, G.A., 2014. Mineral, metalloid, and heavy metal status in sheep with clinical coccidiosis. *Comp. Clin. Path.* 24, 259–262.

343. de Górgolas, M., Fortés, J., Fernández Guerrero, M.L., 2001. *Cyclospora cayetanensis* cholecystitis in a patient with AIDS. *Ann. Intern. Med.* 134, 166.

343a. de la Fuente, C., Alunda, J.M., 1992. A quantitative study of *Eimeria* infections of goats from central Spain. *Vet. Parasitol.* 41, 7–15.

344. de la Fuente, C., Cuquerella, M., Carrera, L., Alunda, J.M., 1993. Effect of subclinical coccidiosis in kids on subsequent trichostrongylid infection after weaning. *Vet. Parasitol.* 45, 177–183.

345. De Meireles, G.S., da Silva, N.M.P., Galvão, G.S., Almeida, C.R.R., Flausino, W., Lopes, C.W.G., 2012. Surto de coccidiose em bezerros búfalos (*Bubalus bubalis*) por *Eimeria bareillyi* Gil et al., 1963 (Apicomplexa: Eimeriidae)—relato de casos. *Rev. Bras. Med. Vet.* 34, 116–120.

346. de Noronha, A.C.F., Starke-Buzetti, W.A., Duszynski, D.W., 2009. *Eimeria* spp. in Brazilian water buffalo. *J. Parasitol.* 95, 231–234.

347. de Souza Rodrigues, F., Cezar, A.S., de Menezes, F.R., Sangioni, L.A., Vogel, F.S.F., de Avila Botton, S., 2017. Efficacy and economic analysis of two treatment regimens using toltrazuril in lambs naturally infected with *Eimeria* spp. on pasture. *Parasitol. Res.* 116, 2911–2919.

348. de Souza, L.E.B., da Cruz, J.F., Teixeira Neto, M.R., Albuquerque, G.R., Melo, A.D.B., Tapia, D.M.T., 2015. Epidemiology of *Eimeria* infections in sheep raised extensively in a semiarid region of Brazil. *Braz. J. Vet. Parasitol.* 24, 410–415.

349. de Venevelles, P., Chich, J.F., Faigle, W., Loew, D., Labbé, M., Girard-Misguich, F., Péry, P., 2004. Towards a reference map of *Eimeria tenella* sporozoite proteins by two-dimensional electrophoresis and mass spectrometry. *Int. J. Parasitol.* 34, 1321–1331.

350. de Venevelles, P., Chich, J.F., Faigle, W., Lombard, B., Loew, D., Péry, P., Labbé, M., 2006. Study of proteins associated with the *Eimeria tenella* refractile body by a proteomic approach. *Int. J. Parasitol.* 36, 1399–1407.

351. de Waal, T., 2012. Advances in diagnosis of protozoan diseases. *Vet. Parasitol.* 189, 65–74.

352. Degen, W.G.J., van Daal, N., van Zuilekom, H.I., Burnside, J., Schijns, V.E.J.C., 2004. Identification and molecular cloning of functional chicken IL-12. *J. Immunol.* 172, 4371–4380.

353. Deger, S., Gül, A., Ayaz, E., Biçek, K., 2003. The prevalence of *Eimeria* species in goats in Van. *Turk. J. Vet. Anim. Sci.* 27, 439–442.

354. DeHovitz, J.A., Pape, J.W., Boncy, M., Johnson, W.D., 1986. Clinical manifestations and therapy of *Isospora belli* infection in patients with the acquired immunodeficiency syndrome. *N. Engl. J. Med.* 315, 87–90.

355. del Cacho, E., Gallego, M., Lee, S.H., Lillehoj, H.S., Quilez, J., Lillehoj, E.P., Sánchez-Acedo, C., 2012. Induction of protective immunity against *Eimeria tenella, Eimeria maxima, Eimeria acervulina* infections using dendritic cell-derived exosomes. *Infect. Immun.* 80, 1909–1916.

356. del Cacho, E., Gallego, M., Lee, S.H., Lillehoj, H.S., Quilez, J., Lillehoj, E.P., Sánchez-Acedo, C., 2011. Induction of protective immunity against *Eimeria tenella* infection using antigen-loaded dendritic cells (DC) and DC-derived exosomes. *Vaccine* 29, 3818–3825.

357. del Cacho, E., Gallego, M., Lillehoj, H.S., Quilez, J., Lillehoj, E.P., Ramo, A., Sánchez-Acedo, C., 2014. IL-17A regulates *Eimeria tenella* schizont maturation and migration in avian coccidiosis. *Vet. Res.* 45, 25.

358. del Cacho, E., Gallego, M., Lillehoj, H.S., Quilez, J., Lillehoj, E.P., Sánchez-Acedo, C., 2013. Tetraspanin-3 regulates protective immunity against *Eimeria tenella* infection following immunization with dendritic cell-derived exosomes. *Vaccine* 31, 4668–4674.

359. del Cacho, E., Gallego, M., Lillehoj, H.S., Quilez, J., Lillehoj, E.P., Sánchez-Acedo, C., 2016. Induction of protective immunity against experimental *Eimeria tenella* infection using serum exosomes. *Vet. Parasitol.* 224, 1–6.

360. del Cacho, E., Pagés, M., Gallego, M., Barbero, J.L., Monteagudo, L., Sánchez-Acedo, C., 2010. Meiotic chromosome pairing and bouquet formation during *Eimeria tenella* sporulation. *Int. J. Parasitol.* 40, 453–462.

361. del Cacho, E., Pages, M., Gallego, M., Monteagudo, L., Sánchez-Acedo, C., 2005. Synaptonemal complex karyotype of *Eimeria tenella*. *Int. J. Parasitol.* 35, 1445–1451.

362. Denyer, M.P., Pinheiro, D.Y., Garden, O.A., Shepherd, A.J., 2016. Missed, not missing: Phylogenomic evidence for the existence of avian FoxP3. *PLOS ONE* 11, e0150988.

363. Desser, S.S., 1978. Extraintestinal development of eimeriid coccidia in pigs and chamois. *J. Parasitol.* 64, 933–935.

364. DeVos, A.J., Hammond, D.M., Speer, C.A., 1972. Development of *Eimeria crandallis* Honess from sheep in cultured cells. *J. Protozool.* 19, 335–343.

365. Dhanabal, J., Selvadoss, P.P., Muthuswamy, K., 2014. Comparative study of the prevalence of intestinal parasites in low socioeconomic areas from South Chennai, India. *J. Parasitol. Res.* 2014, Article ID 630968.

366. Di Cerbo, A.R., Manfredi, M.T., Zanzani, S., Stradiotto, K., 2010. Gastrointestinal infection in goat farms on Lombardy (Northern Italy): Analysis on community and spatial distribution of parasites. *Small Ruminant Res.* 88, 102–112.

367. Di Gliullo, A.B., Cribari, M.S., Bava, A.J., Cicconetti, J.S., Collazos, R., 2000. *Cyclospora cayetanensis* in sputum and stool samples. *Rev. Inst. Med. Trop. São Paulo* 42, 115–117.

368. Diaferia, M., Veronesi, F., Morganti, G., Nisoli, L., Fioretti, D.P., 2013. Efficacy of toltrazuril 5% suspension (Baycox, Bayer) and diclazuril (Vecoxan, Janssen-Cilag) in the control of *Eimeria* spp. in lambs. *Parasitol. Res.* 112 (Suppl 1), S163–S168.

369. Díaz, P., Panadero, R., López, R., Cordero, A., Pérez-Creo, A., López, C.M., Fernandez, G., Díez-Baños, P., Morrondo, P., 2016. Prevalence and risk factors associated to *Eimeria* spp. infection in unweaned alpacas (*Vicugna pacos*) from Southern Peru. *Acta Parasitol.* 61, 74–78.

370. Dibner, J., Ivey, F.J., Knight, C.D., 1999. Direct delivery of live coccidiosis vaccine into the hatchling yolk sac. *World Poultry, Special Supplement Coccidiosis* (3), 28–29.

371. Dickinson, E.M., 1941. The effects of variable dosages of sporulated *Eimeria acervulina* oocysts on chickens. *Poult. Sci.* 20, 413–424.

372. Dickinson, E.M., Babcock, W.E., Osebold, J.W., 1951. Coccidial immunity studies in chickens, I. *Poult. Sci.* 30, 76–80.

373. Ding, J., Bao, W., Liu, Q., Yu, Q., Abdille, M.H., Wei, Z., 2008. Immunoprotection of chickens against *Eimeria acervulina* by recombinant α-tubulin protein. *Parasitol. Res.* 103, 1133–1140.

374. Ding, J., Qian, W., Liu, Q., Liu, Q., 2012. Multi-epitope recombinant vaccine induces immunoprotection against mixed infection of *Eimeria* spp. *Parasitol. Res.* 110, 2297–2306.

375. Dobson, S., Kar, B., Kumar, R., Adams, B., Barik, S., 2001. A novel tetratricopeptide repeat (TPR) containing PP5 serine/threonine protein phosphatase in the malaria parasite, *Plasmodium falciparum. BMC Microbiol.* 1, 31.

376. Doelling, V.W., Martin, A., Hutchins, J.E., Tyczkowski, J.K., 2001. Infectivity of *E. acervulina* oocysts, sporocysts and sporozoites with *in ovo* delivery. *Proceedings of the VIIIth International Coccidiosis Conference*, Sydney, Australia, pp. 163–164.

377. Dolenc, M., 1966. Contribution to the knowledge on the biology, pathogenicity and distribution of *Eimeria* (*Globidium*) *leuckarti* Reichenow, 1950. Vet. med. thesis. Bioteh niske Fakultete, University Ljubljana (in Slovenian).

378. Döller, P.C., Dietrich, K., Filipp, N., Brockmann, S., Dreweck, C., Vonthein, R., Wagner-Wiening, C., Wiedenmann, A., 2002. Cyclosporiasis outbreak in Germany associated with the consumption of salad. *Emerg. Infect. Dis.* 8, 992–994.

379. Domínguez, F., Moreno, J., Cejudo, F.J., 2001. The nucellus degenerates by a process of programmed cell death during the early stages of wheat grain development. *Planta* 213, 352–360.

380. Dong, H., Suo, X., Wang, M., Teng, K., 2006. Characteristics of a line of *Eimeria necatrix* after 16 successive passages of oocysts collected after peak oocyst production. *J. Parasitol.* 92, 1229–1234.

381. Dong, H., Yang, S., Zhao, Q., Han, H., Zhu, S., Zhu, X., Li, C. et al., 2016. Molecular characterization and protective efficacy of silent information regulator 2A from *Eimeria tenella. Parasit. Vectors* 9, 602.

382. Dong, X., Abdelnabi, G.H., Lee, S.H., Li, G., Jin, H., Lillehoj, H.S., Suo, X., 2011. Enhanced egress of intracellular *Eimeria tenella* sporozoites by splenic lymphocytes from coccidian-infected chickens. *Infect. Immun.* 79, 3465–3470.

383. Doonan, G.R., Brown, C.M., Mullaney, T.P., Brooks, D.B., Ulman's, E.G., Slanker, M.R., 1989. Monensin poisoning in horses—An international incident. *Can. Vet. J.* 30, 165–169.

384. Doran, D.J., 1970. Effect of age and freezing on development of *Eimeria adenoeides* and *E. tenella* sporozoites in cell culture. *J. Parasitol.* 56, 27–29.

385. Doran, D.J., 1970. *Eimeria tenella*: From sporozoites to oocysts in cell culture. *Proc. Helminthol. Soc. Wash.* 37, 84–92.

386. Doran, D.J., 1971. Comparative development of *Eimeria tenella* in primary cultures of kidney cells from the chicken, pheasant, partridge, and turkey. *J. Parasitol.* 57, 1376–1377.

387. Doran, D.J., 1971. Increasing the yield of *Eimeria tenella* oocysts in cell culture. *J. Parasitol.* 57, 891–900.

388. Doran, D.J., 1971. Survival and development of five species of chicken coccidia in primary chicken kidney cell cultures. *J. Parasitol.* 57, 1135–1137.

389. Doran, D.J., 1973. Cultivation of coccidia in avian embryos and cell culture. In Hammond, D.M. and Long, P.L. (Ed.), *The Coccidia. Eimeria, Isospora, Toxoplasma, and Related Genera*. University Park Press. Baltimore, MD, 183–254.

390. Doran, D.J., 1974. *Eimeria tenella*: Merozoite production in cultured cells and attempts to obtain development of culture-produced merozoites. *Proc. Helminthol. Soc. Wash.* 41, 169–173.

391. Doran, D.J., 1978. The life cycle of *Eimeria dispersa* Tyzzer, 1929 in turkeys. *J. Parasitol.* 25, 293–297.

392. Doran, D.J., Augustine, P.C., 1973. Comparative development of *Eimeria tenella* from sporozoites to oocysts in primary kidney cell cultures from gallinaceous birds. *J. Protozool.* 20, 658–661.

393. Doran, D.J., Augustine, P.C., 1976. *Eimeria tenella*: Comparative oocyst production in primary cultures of chicken kidney cells maintained in various media systems. *Proc. Helminthol. Soc. Wash.* 43, 126–128.

394. Doran, D.J., Augustine, P.C., 1977. *Eimeria dispersa* and *Eimeria gallopavonis*: Infectivity, survival, and development in primary chicken and turkey kidney cell cultures. *J. Protozool.* 24, 172–176.

395. Doran, D.J., Augustine, P.C., 1978. *Eimeria tenella*: Vitamin requirements for development in primary cultures of chicken kidney cells. *J. Protozool.* 25, 544–546.

396. Doran, D.J., Farr, M.M., 1965. Susceptibility of 1- and 3-day-old chicks to infection with the coccidium, *Eimeria acervulina. J. Protozool.* 12, 160–166.

397. Doran, D.J., Vetterling, J.M., 1967. Comparative cultivation of poultry coccidia in mammalian kidney cell cultures. *J. Protozool.* 14, 657–662.

398. Doré, M., Morin, M., 1987. Porcine neonatal coccidiosis: Evaluation of monensin as preventive therapy. *Can. Vet. J.* 28, 663–666.

399. Dowling, L., 1992. Ionophore toxicity in chickens: A review of pathology and diagnosis. *Avian Pathol.* 21, 355–368.

400. Driesen, S.J., Carland, P.G., Fahy, V.A., 1993. Studies on preweaning piglet diarrhoea. *Aust. Vet. J.* 70, 259–262.

401. Driesen, S.J., Fahy, V.A., Carland, P.G., 1995. The use of toltrazuril for the prevention of coccidiosis in piglets before weaning. *Aust. Vet. J.* 72, 139–141.

402. Drouet-Viard, F., Coudert, P., Licois, D., Boivin, M., 1997. Acquired protection of the rabbit (*Oryctolagus cuniculus*) against coccidiosis using a precocious line of *Eimeria magna*: Effect of vaccine dose and age at vaccination. *Vet. Parasitol.* 69, 197–201.

403. Drouet-Viard, F., Coudert, P., Licois, D., Boivin, M., 1997. Vaccination against *Eimeria magna* coccidiosis using spray dispersion of precocious line oocysts in the nest box. *Vet. Parasitol.* 70, 61–66.

404. Drouet-Viard, F., Coudert, P., Roux, C., Licois, D., Boivin, M., 1994. Etude de l'immunité transmise aux lapereaux par des femelles immunisées contre *Eimeria magna*. In Anonymous (Ed.), *Recherche Cunicole*. 45–52. Presented at 6. Journées, La Rochelle, FRA (December 6–7, 1994). https://prodinra.inra.fr/record/127421.

405. Drouet-Viard, F., Licois, D., Provôt, F., Coudert, P., 1994. The invasion of the rabbit intestinal tract by *Eimeria intestinalis* sporozoites. *Parasitol. Res.* 80, 706–707.

406. Du, A., Wang, S., 2005. Efficacy of a DNA vaccine delivered in attenuated *Salmonella typhimurium* against *Eimeria tenella* infection in chickens. *Int. J. Parasitol.* 35, 777–785.

407. Du, A., Wang, S., Hu, S., 2006. Safety, stability and immunogenicity of a DNA vaccine delivered in attenuated *Salmonella typhimurium* against *Eimeria tenella* infection in chickens. *Chin. J. Vet. Sci.* 26, 147–150 (in Chinese).

408. Duan, C., Tang, X., Zhang, S., Hu, D., Suo, X., Liu, X., 2018. Research progress on transgenic technology of *Eimeria. Acta Parasitol. Med. Entomol. Sinica* 25, 272–278 (in Chinese).

409. Dubey, J.P., 1975. Experimental *Isospora canis* and *Isospora felis* infection in mice, cats, and dogs. *J. Protozool.* 22, 416–417.

410. Dubey, J.P., 1975. *Isospora ohioensis* sp. n. proposed for *I. rivolta* of the dog. *J. Parasitol.* 61, 462–465.

411. Dubey, J.P., 1976. Reshedding of *Toxoplasma* oocysts by chronically infected cats. *Nature* 262, 213–214.

412. Dubey, J.P., 1977. Attempted transmission of feline coccidia from chronically infected queens to their kittens. *J. Am. Vet. Med. Assoc.* 170, 541–543.

413. Dubey, J.P., 1978. Effect of immunization of cats with *Isospora felis* and BCG on immunity to reexcretion of *Toxoplasma gondii* oocysts. *J. Protozool.* 25, 380–382.

414. Dubey, J.P., 1978. Life cycle of *Isospora ohioensis* in dogs. *Parasitology* 77, 1–11.

415. Dubey, J.P., 1978. Pathogenicity of *Isospora ohioensis* infection in dogs. *J. Am. Vet. Med. Assoc.* 173, 192–197.

416. Dubey, J.P., 1979. Life cycle of *Isospora rivolta* (Grassi, 1879) in cats and mice. *J. Protozool.* 26, 433–443.

417. Dubey, J.P., 1982. Induced *Toxoplasma gondii, Toxocara canis*, and *Isospora canis* infection in coyotes. *J. Am. Vet. Med. Assoc.* 181, 1268–1269.

418. Dubey, J.P., 1983. Immunity to sarcocystosis: Modifications of intestinal coccidiosis, and disappearance of sarcocysts in dairy goats. *Vet. Parasitol.* 13, 23–34.

419. Dubey, J.P., 1986. Coccidiosis in the gallbladder of a goat. *Proc. Helminthol. Soc. Wash.* 53, 277–281.

420. Dubey, J.P., 2010. *Toxoplasmosis of Animals and Humans.* 2nd ed. CRC Press, Boca Raton, FL, 1–313.

421. Dubey, J.P., 2014. Life cycle of *Cystoisospora felis* (Coccidia: Apicomplexa) in cats and mice. *J. Eukaryot. Microbiol.* 61, 637–643.

422. Dubey, J.P., 2018. A review of coccidiosis in South American camelids. *Parasitol. Res.* 117, 1999–2013.

423. Dubey, J.P., 2018. A review of coccidiosis in water buffaloes (*Bubalus bubalis*). *Vet. Parasitol.* 256, 50–57.

424. Dubey, J.P., 2018. A review of *Cystoisospora felis* and *C. rivolta*-induced coccidiosis in cats. *Vet. Parasitol.* 263, 34–48.

425. Dubey, J.P., 2018. Gametogony of *Eimeria macusaniensis* Guerrero, Hernandez, Bazalar and Alva, 1971 in llama (*Lama glama*). *Parasitology* 145, 1540–1547.

426. Dubey, J.P., 2018. Re-evaluation of endogenous development of *Eimeria bareillyi* Gill, Chhabra and Lall, 1963 in water buffalo (*Bubalus bubalis*). *Parasitology* 145, 1845–1852.

427. Dubey, J.P., 2019. Coccidiosis in humans—The past 100 years: A revision of the coccidia parasitic in man. *Parasitology*, https://www.cambridge.org./core/blog/author/j-pdubey/ (accessed July 29, 2019).

428. Dubey, J.P., 2019. Re-evaluation of merogony of a *Cystoisospora ohioensis*-like coccidian and its distinction from gametogony in the intestine of a naturally infected dog. *Parasitology* 146, 740–745.

429. Dubey, J.P., Almeria, S., 2019. *Cystoisospora belli* infections in humans—The past 100 years. *Parasitology.* 146; 1490–1527.

430. Dubey, J.P., Bauer, C., 2018. A review of *Eimeria* infections in horses and other equids. *Vet. Parasitol.* 256, 58–70.

431. Dubey, J.P., Calero-Bernal, R., Rosenthal, B.M., Speer, C.A., Fayer, R., 2016. *Sarcocystosis of Animals and Humans*, CRC Press, Boca Raton, FL,. 2nd ed., 1–481.

432. Dubey, J.P., Evason, K.J., Walther, Z., 2019. Endogenous development of *Cystoisospora belli* in intestinal and biliary epithelium of humans. *Parasitology* 146, 865–872.

433. Dubey, J.P., Frenkel, J.K., 1972. Extra-intestinal stages of *Isospora felis* and *I. rivolta* (Protozoa: Eimeriidae) in cats. *J. Protozool.* 19, 89–92.

434. Dubey, J.P., Greene, C.E., 2012. Enteric coccidiosis. In Greene, C.E. (Ed.), *Infectious Diseases of the Dog and Cat.* 4th ed., 828–839. Elsevier, St. Louis, Missouri

435. Dubey, J.P., Hemphill, A., Calero-Bernal, R., Schares, G., 2017. *Neosporosis in Animals.* CRC Press. Boca Raton, FL, 1–530.

436. Dubey, J.P., Houk, A.E., Verma, S.K., Calero-Bernal, R., Humphreys, J.G., Lindsay, D.S., 2015. Experimental transmission of *Cystoisospora felis*-like coccidium from bobcat (*Lynx rufus*) to the domestic cat (*Felis catus*). *Vet. Parasitol.* 211, 35–39.

437. Dubey, J.P., Jenkins, M.C., 2018. Re-evaluation of the life cycle of *Eimeria maxima* Tyzzer, 1929 in chickens (*Gallus domesticus*). *Parasitology* 145, 1051–1058.

438. Dubey, J.P., Lindsay, D.S., 2019. Coccidiosis in dogs—100 years of progress. *Vet. Parasitol.* 266, 34–55.

438a. Dubey, J.P., Lindsay, D.S., 2019. Re-evaluation of asynchronous asexual development of *Cystoisospora canis* in intestines of dogs. *J. Parasitol.* 105, 25–28.

439. Dubey, J.P., Lindsay, D.S., 2019. New observations allowing the differentiation of late asexual stages of *Cystoisospora canis* from developing microgamonts in the intestines of experimentally infected dogs. *J. Parasitol.* 105, 345–350.

440. Dubey, J.P., Mahrt, J.L., 1978. *Isospora neorivolta* sp. n. from the domestic dog. *J. Parasitol.* 64, 1067–1073.

441. Dubey, J.P., Mehlhorn, H., 1978. Extraintestinal stages of *Isospora ohioensis* from dogs in mice. *J. Parasitol.* 64, 689–695.

442. Dubey, J.P., Pande, B.P., 1963. A note on *Eimeria rajasthani* n. sp. (Protozoa: Eimeriidae) from the Indian camel (*Camelus dromedarius*). *Curr. Sci.* 32, 273–274.

443. Dubey, J.P., Pande, B.P., 1963. A preliminary note on *Eimeria battakhi* n. sp. (Protozoa: Eimeriidae) from domestic duck (*Anas platyrhynchos platyrhynchos domesticus*). *Curr. Sci.* 32, 329–331.

444. Dubey, J.P., Pande, B.P., 1963. On a coccidian schizont in the Indian domestic duck (*Anas platyrhynchos domesticus*). *J. Parasitol.* 49, 770.

445. Dubey, J.P., Pande, B.P., 1964. On eimerian oocysts recovered from Indian camel (*Camelus dromedarius*). *Indian J. Vet. Sci.* 34, 28–34.

446. Dubey, J.P., Schuster, R.K., Kinne, J., 2018. Gametogony of *Eimeria cameli* in small intestine of one-humped camel (*Camelus dromedarius*). *Parasitol. Res.* 117, 3633–3638.

447. Dubey, J.P., Schuster, R.K., 2018. A review of coccidiosis in old world camels. *Vet. Parasitol.* 262, 75–83.

448. Dubey, J.P., Weisbrode, S.E., Rogers, W.A., 1978. Canine coccidiosis attributed to an *Isospora ohioensis*-like organism: A case report. *J. Am. Vet. Med. Assoc.* 173, 185–191.

449. Dubey, J.P., Wouda, W., Muskens, J., 2008. Fatal intestinal coccidiosis in a three-week-old buffalo calf (*Bubalus bubalis*). *J. Parasitol.* 94, 1289–1294.

450. Dubey, J.P., Yabsley, M.J., 2010. *Besnoitia neotomofelis* n. sp. (Protozoa: Apicomplexa) from the southern plains woodrat (*Neotoma micropus*). *Parasitology* 137, 1731–1747.

451. Dunlap, J.S., 1970. *Eimeria leuckarti* infection in the horse. *J. Am. Vet. Med. Assoc.* 156, 623–625.

452. Dürr, U., 1972. Life cycle of *Eimeria stiedai*. *Acta Vet. Acad. Sci. Hung.* 22, 101–103.

453. Dürr, U., Pellérdy, L., 1969. The susceptibility of suckling rabbits to infection with coccidia. *Acta Vet. Acad. Sci. Hung.* 19, 453–462.

454. Duszynski, D.W., Couch, L., 2013. *The Biology and Identification of the Coccidia (Apicomplexa) of Rabbits of the World.* 1st ed. Elsevier Inc., 1–352.

455. Duszynski, D.W., Upton, S.J., Couch, L., 1999. The coccidia cf Suidae (swine). From: *Coccidia of the World.* http://biology.unm.edu/coccidia/artiodact3.html (accessed August 30, 2018).

456. Duszynski, D., Wilber, P.G., 1997. A guideline for the preparation of species descriptions in the Eimeriidae. *J. Parasitol.* 83, 333–336.

457. Dwivedi, K.K., Prasad, G., Saini, S., Mahajan, S., Lal, S., Baveja U.K., 2007. Enteric opportunistic parasites among HIV infected individuals: Associated risk factors and immune status. *Jpn. J. Infect. Dis.* 60, 76–81.

458. Eberhard, M.L., Nace, E.K., Freeman, A.R., Streit, T.G., da Silva, A.J., Lammie, P.J., 1999. *Cyclospora cayetanensis* infections in Haiti: A common occurrence in the absence of watery diarrhea. *Am. J. Trop. Med. Hyg.* 60, 584–586.

459. Eckert, J., Braun, R., Shirley, M.W., Coudert, P., 1995. *COST 89/820 Biotechnology: Guidelines on Techniques in Coccidiosis Research.* 306. European Commission Directorate-General XII, Science, Research and Development Environmental Research Programme.

460. Eckert, J., Taylor, M., Catchpole, J., Licois, D., Coudert, P., Bucklar, H., 1995. Identification of *Eimeria* species and strains: Morphological characterization of oocysts. In Eckert, J., Braun, R., Shirley, M.W., and Coudert, P. (Ed.), *COST 89/820 Biotechnology—Guidelines on Techniques in Coccidiosis Research.* European Commission Directorate-General XII, Science, Research and Development: Agriculture Biotechnology, Luxembourg, 103–119.

461. Edgar, S.A., 1953. Coccidiosis vaccination. *Poult. Ind.* 59, 6, 14.

462. Edgar, S.A., 1954. Control of cecal coccidiosis by active immunization. *Auburn Vet.* 10, 79–81, 116.

463. Edgar, S.A., 1954. Effect of temperature on the sporulation of oocysts of the protozoan, *Eimeria tenella*. *Trans. Am. Micros. Soc.* 73, 237–242.

464. Edgar, S.A., 1955. Sporulation of oocysts at specific temperatures and notes on the prepatent period of several species of avian coccidia. *J. Parasitol.* 41, 214–216.

465. Edgar, S.A., 1958. Control of coccidiosis of chickens and turkeys by immunization. *Poult. Sci.* 37, 1200.

466. Edgar, S.A., 1964. Stable coccidiosis immunization. United States Patent 3,147,186.

467. Edgar, S.A., 1986. Coccidiosis in turkeys: Biology and incidence. In McDougald, L.R., Joyner, L.P., and Long, P.L. (Ed.), *Research in Avian Coccidiosis, Proceedings of the Georgia Coccidiosis Conference*, 1985. University of Georgia. Athens, GA, 116–123.

468. Edgar, S.A., Bond, D.S., 1965. Turkey coccidia widely distributed in United States. *Highlights of Agricultural Research*, 12, 13. Agricultural Experiment Station, Auburn University, AL.

469. Edgar, S.A., King, D.F., Flanagan, C., 1952. *Breeding and immunizing chickens for resistance to coccidiosis. 62nd and 63rd Annual Report of the Alabama Polytechnic Institute of the Agricultural Experiment Station,* 36–37.

470. Edgar, S.A., Seibold, C.T., 1964. A new coccidium of chickens, *Eimeria mivati* sp. n. (Protozoa: Eimeriidae) with details of its life history. *J. Parasitol.* 50, 193–204.

471. Ehret, T., Spork, S., Dieterich, C., Lucius, R., Heitlinger, E., 2017. Dual RNA-seq reveals no plastic transcriptional response of the coccidian parasite *Eimeria falciformis* to host immune defenses. *BMC Genomics* 18, 686.

472. El Salahy, M., Monib, M., Arafa, M.I., 2000. Parasitological studies of some gasterointestinal parasites of camels in Assiut Governorate with special reference to zoonotic nematodes. *Assiut Vet. Med. J.* 43, 280–294.

473. El-Zawawy, L.A., El-Said, D., Ali, S.M., Fathy, F.M., 2010. Disinfection efficacy of sodium dichloroisocyanurate (NADCC) against common food-borne intestinal protozoa. *J. Egypt. Soc. Parasitol.* 40, 165–185.

474. El-Alfy, E., Abbas, I.E., Al-Kappany, Y., Al-Araby, M., Abu-Elwafa, S.A., Dubey, J.P., 2019. Prevalence of *Eimeria* species in water buffaloes (*Bubalus bubalis*) from Egypt and first report of *Eimerica bareillyi* oocysts. *J. Parasitol.* 105, 748–754.

475. El-Ashram, S., Aboelhadid, S.M., Kamel, A.A., Mahrous, L.N., Abdelwahab, K.H., 2019. Diversity of parasitic diarrhea associated with *Buxtonella sulcata* in cattle and buffalo calves with control of buxtonellosis. *Animals* 9, 259.

476. El-Khabaz, K.A.S., Abdel-Hakeem, S.S., Arfa, M.I., 2019. Protozoan and helminthes parasites endorsed by imported camels (*Camel dromedaries*) to Egypt. *J. Parasit. Dis.* 1–9. Doi: 10.1007/s12639-019-01138-y.

477. El-Manyawe, S.M., Iskander, A.R., 1994. A study on the gastrointestinal parasites of camels in Egypt. *J. Egypt. Vet. Med. Assoc.* 54, 225–230.

478. El-Shahawi, G.A., El-Fayomi, H.M., Abdel-Haleem, H.M., 2012. Coccidiosis of domestic rabbit (*Oryctolagus cuniculus*) in Egypt: Light microscopic study. *Parasitol. Res.* 110, 251–258.

479. El-Sherif, A.M., Abdel-Gawad, M.A., Lotfy, H.S., Shokier, K.A.M., 2000. Impact of gastrointestinal nematodes and some enteric protozoal affections on the health of buffalo calves. *Assiut Vet. Med. J.* 43, 260–270.

480. El-Sherry, S., Ogedengbe, M.E., Hafeez, M.A., Sayf-Al-Din, M., Gad, N., Barta, J.R., 2014. Re-description of a genetically typed, single oocyst line of the turkey coccidium, *Eimeria adenoeides* Moore and Brown, 1951. *Parasitol. Res.* 113, 3993–4004.

481. El-Sherry, S., Ogedengbe, M.E., Hafeez, M.A., Sayf-Al-Din, M., Gad, N., Barta, J.R., 2015. Sequence-based genotyping clarifies conflicting historical morphometric and biological data for 5 *Eimeria* species infecting turkeys. *Poult. Sci.* 94, 262–272.

482. El-Sherry, S., Ogedengbe, M.E., Hafeez, M.A., Sayf-Al-Din, M., Gad, N., Barta, J.R., 2017. Re-description of a genetically typed, single oocyst line of the turkey coccidium, *Eimeria dispersa* Tyzzer, 1929. *Parasitol. Res.* 116, 2661–2670.

483. El-Sherry, S., Ogedengbe, M.E., Hafeez, M.A., Sayf-Al-Din, M., Gad, N., Barta, J.R., 2019. Cecal coccidiosis in turkeys: Comparative biology of *Eimeria* species in the lower intestinal tract of turkeys using genetically typed, single oocyst-derived lines. *Parasitol. Res.* 118, 583–598.

484. El-Sherry, S., Rathinam, T., Hafeez, M.A., Ogedengbe, M.E., Chapman, H.D., Barta, J.R., 2014. Biological re-description of a genetically typed, single oocyst line of the turkey coccidium, *Eimeria meleagrimitis* Tyzzer 1929. *Parasitol. Res.* 113, 1135–1146.

485. Elbadr, A.M., Essa, M., Tolba, M., Metwally, A., Taher, G.A., 2010. Studis on coccidiosis of camel in Assiut Goveronate. *Minufiya Vet. J.* 7, 161–164.

486. Ellis, J., Revets, H., 1990. *Eimeria* species which infect the chicken contain virus-like RNA molecules. *Parasitology* 101, 163–169.

487. Ellis, J.T., Holmdahl, O.J.M., Ryce, C., Njenga, J.M., Harper, P.A.W., Morrison, D.A., 2000. Molecular phylogeny of *Besnoitia* and the genetic relationships among *Besnoitia* of cattle, wildebeest and goats. *Protist* 151, 329–336.

488. Elshahawy, I., Elgoniemy, A., 2018. An epidemiological study on endoparasites of domestic rabbits (*Oryctolagus cuniculus*) in Egypt with special reference to their health impact. *Sains Malaysiana* 47, 9–18.

489. Elshazly, A.M., Elsheikha, H.M., Soltan, D.M., Mohammad, K.A., Morsy, T.A., 2007. Protozoal pollution of surface water sources in Dakahlia Governorate, Egypt. *J. Egypt. Soc. Parasitol.* 37, 51–64.

490. Elwasila, M., 1983. A fine-structural comparison of the sporozoites of *Grellia* (*Eucoccidium*) *dinophili* in *Dinophilus gyrociliatus* and of *Isospora felis* in the mouse. *Z. Parasitenkd.* 69, 583–589.

491. Enemark, H.L., Dahl, J., Enemark, J.M.D., 2013. Eimeriosis in Danish dairy calves—Correlation between species, oocyst excretion and diarrhoea. *Parasitol. Res.* 112 (Suppl), S169–S176.

492. Enemark, H.L., Dahl, J., Enemark, J.M.D., 2015. Significance of timing on effect of metaphylactic toltrazuril treatment against eimeriosis in calves. *Parasitol. Res.* 114 (Suppl 1), S201–S212.

493. Engels, K., Beyer, C., Suárez Fernández, M.L., Bender, F., Gaßel, M., Unden, G., Marhöfer, R.J., Mottram, J.C., Selzer, P.M., 2010. Inhibition of *Eimeria tenella* CDK-related kinase 2: From target identification to lead compounds. *Chem. Med. Chem.* 5, 1259–1271.

494. Engidaw, S., Anteneh, M., Demis, C., 2015. Coccidiosis in small ruminants. *Afr. J. Basic Appl. Sci.* 7, 311–319.

495. Enigk, K., 1934. Zur Kenntnis des *Globidium cameli* und der *Eimeria cameli*. *Arch. Protistenkd.* 83, 371–380.

496. Epe, C., von Samson-Himmelstjerna, G., Wirtherle, N., von der Heyden, V., Welz, C., Beening, J., Radeloff, I., Hellmann, K., Schnieder, T., Krieger, K., 2005. Efficacy of toltrazuril as a metaphylactic and therapeutic treatment of coccidiosis in first-year grazing calves. *Parasitol. Res.* 97 (Suppl 1), S127–S133.

497. Erber, M., Jakob, H.J., Lee, P., 1984. Influence of *Isospora suis* on the diarrhoea syndrome in piglets. *Zentralbl. Bakteriol. Mikrobiol. Hyg. A* 258, 367–377.

498. Ernst, J.V., Benz, G.W., 1980. Attempts to produce experimental *Eimeria wyomingensis* infections in calves. *J. Parasitol.* 66, 625–629.

499. Ernst, J.V., Benz, G.W., 1981. Coccidiosis. *Curr. Top. Vet. Med. Anim. Sci.* 6, 377–392.

500. Ernst, J.V., Courtney, C.H., 1977. Prepatent and patent periods of the bovine coccidium *Eimeria subspherica* Christensen, 1941, with a redescription of the sporulated oocyst. *Proc. Helminthol. Soc. Wash.* 44, 97–98.

501. Ernst, J.V., Lindsay, D.S., Current, W.L., 1985. Control of *Isospora suis*-induced coccidiosis on a swine farm. *Am. J. Vet. Res.* 46, 643–645.

502. Ernst, J.V., Lindsay, D.S., Jarvinen, J.A., Todd, K.S., Jr., Bane, D.P., 1986. The sporulation time of *Isospora suis* oocysts from different sources. *Vet. Parasitol.* 22, 1–8.

503. Ernst, J.V., Stevens, R.O., Cooper, C., Jr., 1971. Redescription of oocysts of the bovine coccidium *Eimeria brasiliensis* Torres and Ramos, 1939. *Am. J. Vet. Res.* 32, 223–228.

504. Ernst, J.V., Todd, K.S., 1977. New geographic record and redescription of the sporulated oocyst of *Eimeria pellita* Supperer 1952 from Alabama cattle. *Proc. Helminthol. Soc. Wash.* 44, 221–223.

505. Esmaeilzadeh, M., Shamsfard, M., Kazemi, A., Khalafi, S.A., Altome, S.A., 2009. Prevalence of protozoa and gastrointestinal helminthes in stray cats in Zanjan Province, north-west of Iran. *Iran. J. Parasitol.* 4, 71–75.

506. Espino, L., Suarez, M.L., Miño, N., Goicoa, A., Fidalgo, L.E., Santamarina, G., 2003. Suspected lasalocid poisoning in three dogs. *Vet. Hum. Toxicol.* 45, 241–242.

507. Esvan, R., Suleková, L.F., Gabrielli, S., Biliotti, E., Palazzo, D., Spaziante, M., Taliani, G., 2018. Severe diarrhoea due to *Cystoisospora belli* infection in a Good syndrome patient. *Parasitol. Int.* 67, 413–414.

508. Eugster, A.K., Jones, L.P., 1985. Coccidiosis in horses. *Southwest. Vet.* 36, 197.

509. Eustis, S.L., Nelson, D.T., 1981. Lesions associated with coccidiosis in nursing piglets. *Vet. Pathol.* 18, 21–28.

509a. Eydal, M., 1994. Parasites of horses in Iceland. E.A.A.P./ Agricult. Soc. Iceland/Agric. Res. Inst. Iceland Symp. Proc. 1993. *Livestock Prod. Sci.* 40, 85.

510. Faber, J.E., Kollmann, D., Heise, A., Bauer, C., Failing, K., Bürger H.J., Zahner, H., 2002. *Eimeria* infections in cows in the periparturient phase and their calves: Oocyst excretion and levels of specific serum and colostrum antibodies. *Vet. Parasitol.* 104, 1–17.

511. Fabián, B.S.L., Daniel, G.A., Rodolfo, N.G., Herminio, T.C., 2014. Estudio coproparasitario y ectoparasitario en alpacas (*Vicugna pacos* Linnaeus, 1758) de Apolobamba, con nuevos registros de Phthiraptera (Insecta) e Ixodidae (Acari), La Paz—Bolivia. *J. Selva Andina Anim. Sci.* 2, 2–17.

512. Fagiolini, M., Lia, R.P., Laricchiuta, P., Cavicchio, P., Mannella, R., Cafarchia, C., Otranto, D., Finotello, R., Perrucci, S., 2010. Gastrointestinal parasites in mammals of two Italian zoological gardens. *J. Zoo Wildl. Med.* 41, 662–670.

513. Faizal, A.C.M., Rajapakse, R.P.V.J., 2001. Prevalence of coccidia and gastrointestinal nematode infections in cross bred goats in the dry areas of Sri Lanka. *Small Ruminant Res.* 40, 233–238.

514. Farr, M.M., 1964. Life cycle of *Eimeria gallopavonis* Hawkins in the turkey. *J. Parasitol.* 50 (3, sec. 2), 52.

515. Farr, M.M., 1965. Coccidiosis of the lesser scaup duck, *Aythya affinis* (Eyton, 1838) with a description of a new species, *Eimeria aythyae*. *Proc. Helminthol. Soc. Wash.* 32, 236–238.

516. Farr, M.M., Wehr, E.E., Shalkop, W.T., 1961. Pathogenicity of *Eimeria gallopavonis*. *Virginia J. Sci.* 12, 150–151.

517. Faust, E.C., Giraldo, L.E., Caicedo, G., Bonfante, R., 1961. Human isosporosis in the western hemisphere. *Am. J. Trop. Med. Hyg.* 10, 343–349.

518. Fayer, R., Frenkel, J.K., 1979. Comparative infectivity for calves of oocysts of feline coccidia: *Besnoitia, Hammondia, Cystoisospora, Sarcocystis*, and *Toxoplasma*. *J. Parasitol.* 65, 756–762.

519. Fayer, R., Gamble, H.R., Ernst, J.V., 1984. *Isospora suis*: Development in cultured cells with some cytological observations. *Proc. Helminthol. Soc. Wash.* 51, 154–159.

520. Fayer, R. Hammond, D.M., 1967. Development of first-generation schizonts of *Eimeria bovis* in cultured bovine cells. *J. Protozool.* 14, 764–772.

521. Fayer, R., Reid, W.M., 1982. Control of coccidiosis. In Long, P.L. (Ed.), *The Biology of the Coccidia*. University Park Press. Baltimore, MD, 453–487.

522. Fei, C., Fan, C., Zhao, Q., Lin, Y., Wang, X., Zheng, W., Wang, M. et al., 2013. Anticoccidial effects of a novel triazine nitromezuril in broiler chickens. *Vet. Parasitol.* 198, 39–44.

523. Feng, L., Nie, S.J., Huang, Y.H., Huang, X.D., Cai, H.F., Ma, D.X. Li, G.X., 2016. Cloning and expression of *Eimeria acervulina* Hsp90 gene and the immune protection of its DNA vaccine. *Chin. J. Vet. Med.* 52, 10–13 (in Chinese).

524. Feng, X.X., 2013. Diagnosis and treatment of a duck coccidiosis. *Nong Min Zhi Fu Zhi You.* 14, 218 (in Chinese).

525. Ferguson, D.J.P., Belli, S.I., Smith, N.C., Wallach, M.G., 2003. The development of the macrogamete and oocyst wall in *Eimeria maxima*: Immuno-light and electron microscopy. *Int. J. Parasitol.* 33, 1329–1340.

526. Ferguson, D.J.P., Birch-Andersen, A., Hutchinson, W.M., Siim, J.C., 1980. Ultrastructural observations showing enteric multiplication of *Cystoisospora (Isospora) felis* by endodyogeny. *Z. Parasitenkd.* 63, 289–291.

527. Ferguson, D.J.P., Birch-Andersen, A., Hutchison, W.M., Siim, J.C., 1980. Ultrastructural observations on macrogametogenesis and the structure of the macrogamete of *Isospora felis*. *Acta Pathol. Microbiol. Scand. B* 88, 161–168.

528. Ferguson, D.J.P., Birch-Andersen, A., Hutchison, W.M., Siim, J.C., 1980. Ultrastructural observations on microgametogenesis and the structure of the microgamete of *Isospora felis*. *Acta Pathol. Microbiol. Scand. B* 88, 151–159.

529. Fernando, M.A., 1982. Pathology and pathogenicity. In Long, P.L. (Ed.), *The Biology of the Coccidia*. University Park Press. Baltimore, MD, 387–327.

530. Ferreira, L.F., Coutinho, S.G., Argento, C.A., da Silva, J.R., 1962. Experimental human coccidial enteritis by *Isospora belli* Wenyon, 1923. A study based on the infection of 5 volunteers. *Hospital. (Rio J.)* 62, 795–804.

531. Fetterer, R.H., Barfield, R.C., Jenkins, M.C., 2015. Protection of broiler chicks housed with immunized cohorts against infection with *Eimeria maxima* and *E. acervulina*. *Avian Dis.* 59, 98–105.

532. Fetterer, R.H., Jenkins, M.C., Miska, K.B., Cain, G.D., 2010. Metam sodium reduces viability and infectivity of *Eimeria* oocysts. *J. Parasitol.* 96, 632–637.

533. Fetterer, R.H., Miska, K.B., Jenkins, M.C., Barfield, R.C., 2004. A conserved 19-kDa *Eimeria tenella* antigen is a profilin-like protein. *J. Parasitol.* 90, 1321–1328.

534. Fiege, N., Klatte, D., Kollmann, D., Zahner, H., Burger, H.J., 1992. *Eimeria bovis* in cattle: Colostral transfer of antibodies and immune response to experimental infections. *Parasitol. Res.* 78, 32–38.

535. Fisher, J.W., Kelley, G.L., Youssef, N.N., 1979. Development of *Eimeria dispersa* Tyzzer, 1929, from Bobwhite quail (*Colinis virginianus*), in bovine kidney cell cultures. *Z. Parasitenkd.* 59, 203–210.

536. Fitz-Coy, S.H., Edgar, S.A., 1989. *Eimeria mitis*: Immunogenicity and cross immunity of two isolates. *Avian Dis.* 33, 236–237.

537. Fitzgerald, P.R., 1962. Coccidia in hereford calves on summer and winter ranges and in feedlots in Utah. *J. Parasitol.* 48, 347–351.

538. Fitzgerald, P.R., 1967. Results of continuous low-level inoculations with *Eimeria bovis* in calves. *Am. J. Vet. Res.* 28, 659–665.

539. Fitzgerald, P.R., 1974. Results of blood transfusions from donor rabbits infected with *Eimeria stiedai* to recipient coccidia-free rabbits. *J. Protozool.* 21, 336–338.

540. Fitzgerald, P.R., 1980. The economic impact of coccidiosis in domestic animals. *Adv. Vet. Sci. Comp. Med.* 24, 121–143.

541. Fitzgerald, P.R., Mansfield, M.E., 1978. Ovine coccidiosis: Effect of the antibiotic monensin against *Eimeria ninakohlyakimovae* and other naturally occurring coccidia of sheep. *Am. J. Vet. Res.* 39, 7–10.

542. Fitzgerald, P.R., Mansfield, M.E., 1989. Effects of intermittent and continuous administration of decoquinate on bovine coccidiosis in male calves. *Am. J. Vet. Res.* 50, 961–964.

543. Flesch, M., 1883. Über ein Sporozoon beim Pferde. *Zoologischer Anzeiger* 6, 396–397.

544. Florião, M.M., Lopes, B.B., Berto, B.P., Lopes, C.W.G., 2016. New approaches for morphological diagnosis of bovine *Eimeria* species: A study on a subtropical organic dairy farm in Brazil. *Trop. Anim. Health Prod.* 48, 577–584.

545. Foreyt, W.J., 1987. Coccidiosis in sheep and goats. *Vet. Hum. Toxicol.* 29 (Suppl 1), 60–64.

546. Foreyt, W.J., 1990. Coccidiosis and cryptosporidiosis in sheep and goats. *Vet. Clin. North Am. Food Anim. Pract.* 6, 655–670.

547. Foreyt, W.J., Lagerquist, J., 1992. Experimental infections of *Eimeria alpacae* and *Eimeria punoensis* in llamas (*Lama glama*). *J. Parasitol.* 78, 906–909.

548. Foreyt, W.J., Rice, D.H., Wescott, R.B., 1986. Evaluation of lasalocid as a coccidiostat in calves: Titration, efficacy, and comparison with monensin and decoquinate. *Am. J. Vet. Res.* 47, 2031–2035.

549. Foster, A.O., 1949. The economic losses due to coccidiosis. *Ann. N. Y. Acad. Sci.* 52, 434–442.

550. Foster, A.O., Christensen, J.F., 1941. Treatment of coccidial infections of lambs with sulfaguanidine. *Proc. Helminthol. Soc. Wash.* 8, 33.

551. Founta, A., Papadopoulos, E., Chliounakis, S., Bampidis, V.A., Papazahariadou, M., 2018. Presence of endoparasites in the Greek buffalo (*Bubalus bubalis*) from Northern Greece. *J. Hellenic Vet. Med. Soc.* 69, 999–1003.

552. Fox, J.E., 1985. Coccidiosis in cattle. A review of coccidiosis: Its etiology, diagnosis and control. *Mod. Vet. Pract.* 66, 113–116.

553. Franson, J.C., Derksen, D.V., 1981. Renal coccidiosis in oldsquaws (*Clangula hyemalis*) from Alaska. *J. Wildl. Dis.* 17, 237–239.

554. Franzen, C., Müller, A., Bialek, R., Diehl, V., Salzberger, B., Fätkenheuer, G., 2000. Taxonomic position of the human intestinal protozoan parasite *Isospora belli* as based on ribosomal RNA sequences. *Parasitol. Res.* 86, 669–676.

555. Franzen, C., Müller, A., Salzberger, B., Hartmann, P., Diehl, V., Fätkenheuer, G., 1996. Uvitex 2B stain for the diagnosis of *Isospora belli* infections in patients with the acquired immunodeficiency syndrome. *Arch. Pathol. Lab. Med.* 120, 1023–1025.

556. Freire, R.B., Lopes, C.W., 1995. Determination of macrophage activity in albino mice experimentally infected with *Cystoisospora felis* (Wenyon, 1923) Frenkel, 1977 (Apicomplexa: Sarcocystidae). *Rev. Bras. Parasitol. Vet.* 4, 25–28.

557. Freire, R.B., Lopes, C.W.G., 1995. Avaliação da digestão enzimática por pepsina e tripsina na obtenção de hipnozoítas de *Cystoisospora felis* (Wenyon, 1923) Frenkel, 1977 (Apicomplexa: Sarcocystidae). *Rev. Bras. Parasitol. Vet.* 4, 21–23.

558. Freire, R.B., Lopes, C.W.G., 1996. Distribuição de hipnozoítas de *Cystoisospora felis* (Wenyon, 1923) Frenkel, 1977 (Apicomplexa: Sarcocystidae) em camundongos albinos experimentalmente infectados. *Rev. Bras. Parasitol. Vet.* 5, 23–28.

559. Frenkel, J.K., 1977. *Besnoitia wallacei* of cats and rodents: With a reclassification of other cyst-forming isosporoid coccidia. *J. Parasitol.* 63, 611–628.

560. Frenkel, J.K., Dubey, J.P., 1972. Rodents as vectors for feline coccidia, *Isospora felis* and *Isospora rivolta*. *J. Infect. Dis.* 125, 69–72.

561. Freudenschuss, B., Ruttkowski, B., Shrestha, A., Abd-Elfattah, A., Pagès, M., Ladingi, A., Joachim, A., 2018. Antibody and cytokine response to *Cystoisospora suis* infections in immune-competent young pigs. *Parasit. Vectors* 11, 390.

562. Friend, S.C.E., Stockdale, P.H.G., 1980. Experimental *Eimeria bovis* infection in calves: A histopathological study. *Can. J. Comp. Med.* 44, 129–140.

563. Frölich, S., Entzeroth, R., Wallach, M., 2012. Comparison of protective immune responses to apicomplexan parasites. *J. Parasitol. Res.* 2012, 852591.

564. Fry, M., Williams, R.B., 1984. Effects of decoquinate and clopidol on electron transport in mitochondria of *Eimeria tenella* (Apicomplexa: Coccidia). *Biochem. Pharmacol.* 33, 229–240.

565. Fu, A.Q., Wu, Q.F., 1989. A preliminary survey of duck coccidiosis in Yangzhou. *China Poultry.* 11, 32–35 (in Chinese).

566. Fugassa, M.H., Sardella, N.H., Taglioretti, V., Reinhard, K.J., Araújo, A., 2008. Eimeriid oocysts from archaeological samples in Patagonia, Argentina. *J. Parasitol.* 94, 1418–1420.

567. Fusco, G., Guarino, A., Merola, A., Veneziano, V., Cringoli, G., 1997. Natural diffusion of *Eimeria* spp. in buffalo calves. *Proceedings of the 5th World Buffalo Congress*, Royal Palace, Caserta, Italy, October 13–16, 1997, pp. 569–573.

568. Gabner, S., Worliczek, H.L., Witter, K., Meyer, F.R.L., Gerner, W., Joachim, A., 2014. Immune response to *Cystoisospora suis* in piglets: Local and systemic changes in T-cell subsets and selected mRNA transcripts in the small intestine. *Parasite Immunol.* 36, 277–291.

569. Gadde, U., Chapman, H.D., Rathinam, T., Erf, G.F., 2011. Cellular immune responses, chemokine, and cytokine profiles in turkey poults following infection with the intestinal parasite *Eimeria adenoeides*. *Poult. Sci.* 90, 2243–2250.

570. Gadde, U., Chapman, H.D., Rathinam, T.R., Erf, G.F., 2009. Acquisition of immunity to the protozoan parasite *Eimeria adenoeides* in turkey poults and the peripheral blood leukocyte response to a primary infection. *Poult. Sci.* 88, 2346–2352.

571. Gadde, U., Rathinam, T., Erf, G.F., Chapman, H.D., 2013. Acquisition of immunity to the protozoan parasite *Eimeria adenoeides* in turkey poults and cellular responses to infection. *Poult. Sci.* 92, 3149–3157.

572. Gadde, U., Rathinam, T., Lillehoj, H.S., 2015. Passive immunization with hyperimmune egg-yolk IgY as prophylaxis and therapy for poultry diseases—A review. *Anim. Health Res. Rev.* 16, 163–176.

573. Gajadhar, A.A., Cawthorn, R.J., Wobeser, G.A., Stockdale, P.H.G., 1983. Prevalence of renal coccidia in wild waterfowl in Saskatchewan. *Can. J. Zool.* 61, 2631–2633.

574. Gajadhar, A.A., Wobeser, G., Stockdale, P.H.G., 1983. Coccidia of domestic and wild waterfowl (Anseriformes). *Can. J. Zool.* 61, 1–24.

575. Gal, A., Harrus, S., Arcoh, I., Lavy, E., Aizenberg, I., Mekuzas-Yisaschar, Y., Baneth, G., 2007. Coinfection with multiple tick-borne and intestinal parasites in a 6-week-old dog. *Can. Vet. J.* 48, 619–622.

576. Galariri, R., Fioroni, L., Angelucci, F., Tovo, G.R., Cristofani, E., 2009. Simultaneous determination of eleven quinolones in animal feed by liquid chromatography with fluorescence and ultraviolet absorbance detection. *J. Chromatogr. A* 1216, 8158–8164.

577. Galiero, G., Consalvo, F., 1993. Indagine sulla presenza e diffusione delle malattie infettive e parassitarie tra vitelli bufalini in aziende da late. *Estratto da Selezione Veterinaria* 34, 1057–1063.

578. Galvan-Díaz, A.L., Herrera-Jaramillo, V., Santos-Rodriguez, Z.M., Delgado-Naranjo, M., 2008. Coloracıones Ziehl–Neelsen y Safranina modificadas para el diagnóstico de *Cyclospora cayetanensis*. *Rev. Salud Pública (Bogota.)* 10, 488–493.

579. Gao, J., Zhang, H.J., Wu, S.G., Yu, S.H., Yoon, I., Moore, D., Gao, Y.P., Yan, H.J., Qi, G.H., 2009. Effect of *Saccharomyces cerevisiae* fermentation product on immune functions of broilers challenged with *Eimeria tenella*. *Poult. Sci.* 88, 2141–2151.

580. Garcia, L.S., Arrowood, M., Kokoskin, E., Paltridge, G.P., Pillai, D.R., Procop, G.W., Ryan, N., Shimizu, R.Y., Visvesvara, G., 2018. Laboratory diagnosis of parasites from the gastrointestinal tract. *Clin. Microbiol. Rev.* 31, e00025–17.

581. Garcia-Campos, A., Power, C., O'Shaughnessy, J., Browne, C., Lawlor, A., McCarthy, G., O'Neill, E.J., de Waal, T., 2019. One-year parasitological screening of stray dogs and cats in County Dublin, Ireland. *Parasitology* 146, 746–752.

582. Gardiner, C.H., Fayer, R., Dubey, J.P., 1988. *An Atlas of Protozoan Parasites in Animal Tissues*. Agriculture handbook number 651. U.S. Department of Agriculture, Agriculture Research Service, Washington, DC.

583. Gareis-Waldburg, A., 2008. *Feldstudien zum Vorkommen von Endoparasiten bei Neuweltkameliden in Ecuador*. Dr. med. vet. thesis. Universität Leipzig.

584. Gargus, E.B., Sundermann, C.A., Lindsay, D.S., Blagburn, B.L., 1987. New observations on first-generation merogony of *Eimeria tuskegeensis* in *Sigmodon hispidus*. *J. Protozool.* 34, 256–258.

585. Gauly, M., Reeg, J., Bauer, C., Erhardt, G., 2004. Influence of production systems in lambs on the *Eimeria* oocyst output and weight gain. *Small Ruminant Res.* 55, 159–167.

586. Gazzinelli, R.T., Denkers, E.Y., 2006. Protozoan encounters with Toll-like receptor signalling pathways: Implicatıons for host parasitism. *Nat. Rev. Immunol.* 6, 895–906.

587. Gerlach, F., 2008. Kokzidiose beim Dromedar (*Camelus dromedarius*). Dr. med. vet. thesis. Freie Universität, Berlin.

588. Ghanem, M.M., Radwaan, M.E., Moustafa, A.M.M., Ebeid, M.H., 2008. Comparative therapeutic effect of toltrazuril, sulphadimidine and amprolium on *Eimeria bovis* and *Eimeria zuernii* given at different times following infection in buffalo calves (*Bubalus bubalis*). *Prev. Vet. Med.* 84, 161–170.

589. Giangaspero, A., Gasser, R.B., 2019. Human cyclosporiasis. *Lancet Infect. Dis.* 19, e226–e236.

590. Giangaspero, A., Marangi, M., Arace, E., 2015. *Cyclospora cayetanensis* travels in tap water on Italian trains. *J. Water Health* 13, 210–216.

591. Giangaspero, A., Marangi, M., Koehler, A.V., Papini, R., Normanno, G., Lacasella, V., Lonigro, A., Gasser, R.B., 2015. Molecular detection of *Cyclospora* in water, soil, vegetables and humans in southern Italy signals a need for improved monitoring by health authorities. *Int. J. Food Microbiol.* 211, 95–100.

592. Giannelli, A., Capelli, G., Joachim, A., Hinney, B., Losson, B., Kirkova, Z., René-Martellet, M. et al., 2017. Lungworms and gastrointestinal parasites of domestic cats: A European perspective. *Int. J. Parasitol.* 47, 517–528.

593. Gibbons, P., Love, D., Craig, T., Budke, C., 2016. Efficacy of treatment of elevated coccidial oocyst counts in goats using amprolium versus ponaxzuril. *Vet. Parasitol.* 218, 1–4.

594. Gibbs, G.M., Roelants, K., O'Bryan, M.K., 2008. The CAP superfamily: Cysteine-rich secretory proteins, antigen 5, and pathogenesis-related 1 proteins—Roles in reproduction, cancer, and immune defense. *Endocrine Reviews* 29, 865–897.

595. Gill, B.S., Chhabra, M.B., Lall, N.B., 1963. A new species of coccidium—*Eimeria bareillyi* n. sp., from buffaloes. *Arh. Protistenk.* 106, 571–574.

596. Gill, H.S., 1976. Incidence of *Eimeria* and *Infundibulorium* in camel. *Indian Vet. J.* 53, 897–898.

597. Girard, C., Morin, M., 1987. Amprolium and furazolidone as preventive treatment for intestinal coccidiosis of piglets. *Can. Vet. J.* 28, 667–669.

598. Godfray, H.C.J., Beddington, J.R., Crute, I.R., Haddad, L., Lawrence, D., Muir, J.F., Pretty, J., Robinson, S., Thomas, S.M., Toulmin, C., 2010. Food security: The challenge of feeding 9 billion people. *Science* 327, 812–818.

599. Gómez Martínez, E., Figuera, L., Guilarte, D.V., Simoni, Z., Díaz, M.T., Berrizbeitia, M., Cerrada, S., 2016. Primer reporte de *Cyclospora cayetanensis* en una comunidad indígena Kariña del municipio Sucre, estado Sucre, Venezuela. *Boletín de Malariología y Salud Ambiental* 56, 24–38.

600. Gomez-Bautista, M., Garcia, M.V., Rojo-Vazquez, F.A., 1986. The levels of total protein and protein fractions in the serum of rabbits infected with *Eimeria stiedai*. *Ann. Parasitol. Hum. Comp.* 61, 393–400.

601. Gomez-Bautista, M., Rojo-Vazquez, F.A., Alunda, J.M., 1987. The effect of the host's age on the pathology of *Eimeria stiedai* infection in rabbits. *Vet. Parasitol.* 24, 47–57.

602. Gong, Z., Yin, H., Ma, X., Liu, B., Han, Z., Gou, L., Cai, J., 2017. Widespread 5-methylcytosine in the genomes of avian coccidia and other apicomplexan parasites detected by an ELISA-based method. *Parasitol. Res.* 116, 1573–1579.

603. Goodwin, M.A., Brown, J., Bounous, D.I., 1998. Use of microscopic lesion scores, gross lesion scores and oocyst count scores to detect *Eimeria maxima* in chickens. *Avian Pathol.* 27, 405–408.

604. Gopinath, G.R., Cinar, H.N., Murphy, H.R., Durigan, M., Almeria, M., Tall, B.D., DaSilva, A.J., 2018. A hybrid reference-guided *de novo* assembly approach for generating *Cyclospora* mitochondrion genomes. *Gut Pathogens* 10, 15.

605. Gothe, R., Reichler, I., 1990. Artenspektrum und Befallshäufigkeit von Endoparasiten bei Mutterhündinnen und ihren Welpen in Süddeutschland. *Tierärztl. Prax.* 18, 61–64.

606. Gothe, R., Reichler, I., 1990. Zur Befallshäufigkeit von Kokzidien bei Hundefamilien unterschiedlicher Haltung und Rassen in Süddeutschland. *Tierärztl. Prax.* 18, 407–413.

607. Gousseff, W.F., 1935. Zur Frage der Coccidien der Einhufer. *Arch. Wiss. Prakt. Tierheilk.* 68, 67–73.

608. Gowen, B.B., Smee, D.F., Wong, M.H., Judge, J.W., Jung, K.H., Bailey, K.W., Pace, A.M., Rosenberg, B., Sidwell, R.W., 2006. Recombinant *Eimeria* protozoan protein elicits resistance to acute phlebovirus infection in mice but not hamsters. *Antimicrob. Agents Chemother.* 50, 2023–2029.

609. Graat, E.A.M., Henken, A.M., Ploeger, H.W., Noordhuizen, J.P.T.M., Vertommen, M.H., 1994. Rate and course of sporulation of oocysts of *Eimeria acervulina* under different environmental conditions. *Parasitology* 108, 497–502.

610. Graczyk, T.K., Ortega, Y.R., Conn, D.B., 1998. Recovery of waterborne oocysts of *Cyclospora cayetanensis* by Asian freshwater clams (*Corbicula fluminea*). *Am. J. Trop. Med. Hyg.* 59, 928–932.

611. Gräfner, G., Graubmann, H.D., Kron, A., 1978. Zur Epizootiologie der Rinderkokzidiose in Aufzucht- und Mastbetrieben. *Mh. Vet. Med.* 33, 910–912.

612. Gräfner, G., Graubmann, H.D., Schwartz, K., Hiepe, T., Kron, A., 1985. Weitere Untersuchungen zu Vorkommen, Epizootiologie und Bekämpfung der *Eimeria*-Kokzidiose des Rindes unter den Bedingungen der intensiven Stallhaltung. *Mh. Vet. Med.* 40, 41–44.

613. Gräfner, G., Weichelt, K., 1966. Die Kokzidien des Rindes im Bezirk Schwerin. *Mh. Vet. Med.* 21, 107–109.

614. Gregory, M.W., 1982. Some factors in the pathogenesis of intestinal coccidiosis in mammals. *Brit. Soc. Parasitol. Proc.* 85, R3.

615. Gregory, M.W., 1990. Pathology of coccidial infections. In Long, P.L. (Ed.), *Coccdiosis of Man and Domestic Animals*. CRC Press. Boca Raton, FL, 236–258.

616. Gregory, M.W., Catchpole, J., 1986. Coccidiosis in rabbits: The pathology of *Eimeria flavescens* infection. *Int. J. Parasitol.* 16, 131–145.

617. Gregory, M.W., Catchpole, J., 1987. Ovine coccidiosis: Pathology of *Eimeria ovinoidalis* infection. *Int. J. Parasitol.* 17, 1099–1111.

618. Gregory, M.W., Catchpole, J., 1989. Ovine coccidiosis: Heavy infection in young lambs increases resistance without causing disease. *Vet. Rec.* 124, 458–461.

619. Gregory, M.W., Catchpole, J., 1990. Ovine coccidiosis: The pathology of *Eimeria crandallis* infection. *Int. J. Parasitol.* 20, 849–860.

620. Gregory, M.W., Catchpole, J., Joyner, L.P., Parker, B.N.J., 1983. Observations on the epidemiology of coccidial infections in sheep under varying conditions of intensive husbandry including chemoprophylaxis with monensin. *Parasitology* 87, 421–427.

621. Gregory, M.W., Catchpole, J., Nolan, A., Hebert, C.N., 1989. Ovine coccidiosis: Studies on the pathogenicity of *Eimeria ovinoidalis* and *E. crandallis* in conventionally-reared lambs, including possible effects of passive immunity. *Dtsch. tierärztl. Wochenschr.* 96, 287–292.

622. Gregory, M.W., Catchpole, J., Norton, C.C., 1989. Observations on the endogenous stages of *Eimeria crandallis* in domestic lambs (*Ovis aries*). *Int. J. Parasitol.* 19, 907–914.

623. Gregory, M.W., Norton, C.C., Catchpole, J., 1987. Les coccidioses ovines. *Le Point Vétérinaire* 19, 29–40.

624. Greif, G., Harder, A., Haberkorn, A., 2001. Chemotherapeutic approaches to protozoa: Coccidiae—Current level of knowledge and outlook. *Parasitol. Res.* 87, 973–975.

625. Grès, V., Marchandeau, S., Landau, I., 2000. The biology and epidemiology of *Eimeria exigua*, a parasite of wild rabbits invading the host cell nucleus. *Parassitologia* 42, 219–225.

626. Grès, V., Marchandeau, S., Landau, I., 2002. Description d'une nouvelle espèce d'*Eimeria* (Coccidia, Eimeridea) chez le lapin de garenne *Oryctolagus cuniculus* en France. *Zoosystema* 24, 203–207.

627. Greve, E., 1985. *Isospora suis* species in a Danish SPF herd. *Nordisk Veterinaermed* 37, 140–144.

628. Grilo, M.L., de Carvalho, L.M.M., 2014. Coccidiose em ruminantes—pequenos agentes e grandes problemas nas diarreias parasitárias. *Vet. Med.* 1, 34–48.

629. Grumbles, L.C., Delaplane, J.P., Higgins, T.C., 1948. Continuous feeding of low concentrations of sulfaquinoxaline for the control of coccidiosis in poultry. *Poult. Sci.* 27, 605–608.

630. Gruvel, J., Graber, M., 1965. Quelques résultats d'enquêtes récentes ur la globidiose du dromadaire au Tchad. Note préliminaire. *Rev. Élev. Méd. vét. Pays Trop.* 18, 423–428.

631. Gualdi, V., Vezzoli, F., Luini, M., Nisoli, L., 2004. Efficacy of Baycox 5% and impact of coccidiosis due to *Isospora suis* on the growth of suckling piglets. In: *Proceedings 18th IPVS Congress*, Hamburg, vol.1, 269.

632. Guarino, A., Fusco, G., Bani, A., Veneziano, V., Cringoli, G., 1997. *Eimeria* spp. in buffalo breeding farms in southern Italy. *Proceedings of the 5th World Buffalo Congress*, Royal Palace, Caserta, Italy, October 13–16, 1997, pp. 565–568.

633. Guedes, A.C., Catalano, Z., Pérez, P., Molina, J.M., Muñoz, M.C., Ferrer, O., Hermosilla, C., Taubert, A., Lara, P., Ruiz, A., 2017. Immunoprotection against experimental infections with *Eimeria* spp in goat kids by using x-irradiated oocysts. *XX Congreso de la Sociedad Española de Parasitologia*, San Cristóbal de La Laguna—Tenerife, Spain, July 19–21, 2017.

634. Guerrero Diaz, C.A., Hernandez, J., Alva, M.J., 1967. Coccidiosis en alpacas. *Rev. Med. Vet.* 21, 59–68.

635. Guerrero, C.A., 1967. Coccidia (Protozoa: Eimeriidae) of the alpaca (*Lama pacos*). Masters thesis. University of Illinois, Urbana, Illinois.

636. Guerrero, C.A., 1967. Coccidia (Protozoa: Eimeriidae) of the alpaca *Lama pacos*. *J. Protozool.* 14, 613–616.

637. Guerrero, C.A., Alva, J., Bazalar, H., Tabacchi, L., 1970. Infección experimental de alpacas con *Eimeria lamae*. *Boletin Exptraordinario Instituto Veterinario de Investigaciones Tropicales y Altura* 4, 79–83.

638. Guerrero, C.A., Hernandez, J., Bazalar, H., Alva, J., 1971. *Eimeria macusaniensis* n. sp. (Protozoa: Eimeriidae) of the alpaca *Lama pacos*. *J. Protozool.* 18, 162–163.

639. Guiguet, M., Furco, A., Tattevin, P., Costagliola, D., Molina J.M., and the French Hospital Database on HIV Clinica. Epidemiology Group, 2007. HIV-associated *Isospora belli* infection: Incidence and risk factors in the French Hospital Database on HIV. *HIV Med.* 8, 124–130.

640. Gül, A.. 2007. The prevalence of *Eimeria* species in goats in Igdir. *Turk. J. Vet. Anim. Sci.* 31, 411–414.

641. Guo, A.. Cai, J., Gong, W., Yan, H., Luo, X., Tian, G., Zhang, S., Zhang, H., Zhu, G., Cai, X., 2013. Transcriptome analysis in chicken cecal epithelia upon infection by *Eimeria tenella in vivo*. *PLOS ONE* 8, e64236.

642. Guo, F.C., Kwakkel, R.P., Williams, C.B., Suo, X., Li, W.K., Verstegen, M.W., 2005. Coccidiosis immunization: Effects of mushroom and herb polysaccharides on immune responses of chickens infected with *Eimeria tenella*. *Avian Dis.* 49, 70–73.

643. Guo, F.C., Suo, X., Zhang, G.Z., Shen, J.Z., 2007. Efficacy of decoquinate against drug sensitive laboratory strains of *Eimeria tenella* and field isolates of *Eimeria* spp. in broiler chickens in China. *Vet. Parasitol.* 147, 239–245.

644. Guo, Y., Li, N., Ortega, Y.R., Zhang, L., Roellig, D.M., Feng, Y., Xiao, L., 2018. Population genetic characterization of *Cyclospora cayetanensis* from discrete geographical regions. *Exp. Parasitol.* 184, 121–127.

645. Guo, Y., Roellig, D.M., Li, N., Tang, K., Frace, M., Ortega, Y., Arrowood, M.J., et al., 2016. Multilocus sequence typing tool for *Cyclospora cayetanensis*. *Emerg. Infect. Dis.* 22, 1464–1467.

646. Guo, Y., Wang, Y., Wang, X., Zhang, L., Ortega, Y., Feng, Y., 2019. Mitochondrial genome sequence variation as a useful marker for assessing genetic heterogeneity among *Cyclospora cayetanensis* isolates and source-tracking. *Parasit. Vectors* 12, 47.

647. Gupta, A., Singh, N.K., Singh, H., Rath, S.S., 2016. Assessment of risk factors associated with prevalence of coccidiosis in dairy animals of Punjab. *J. Parasit. Dis.* 40, 1359–1364.

648. Gupta, R., Jindal, N., Narang, G., Gupta, R.P., Kapoor, P.K., 2012. Outbreaks of coccidiosis in rabbits in Haryana. *Haryana Vet.* 51, 111–113.

649. Gutiérrez-Blanco, E., Rodríguez-Vivas, R.I., Torres-Acosta, J.F.J., Tórtora-Pérez, J., López-Arellano, R., Ramírez-Cruz, G.T., Aguilar-Caballero, A.J., 2006. Effect of a sustained-release intra-ruminal sulfamethazine bolus on *Eimeria* spp. oocyst output and weight gain of naturally infected lambs in the Mexican tropics. *Small Ruminant Res.* 63, 242–248.

650. Guzman, V.B., Silva, D.A.O., Kawazoe, U., Mineo, J.R., 2003. A comparison between IgG antibodies against *Eimeria acervulina*, *E. maxima*, and *E. tenella* and oocyst shedding in broiler-breeders vaccinated with live anticoccidial vaccines. *Vaccine* 21, 4225–4233.

651. Haberkorn, A., Mundt, H.C., 1988. Untersuchungen an einem vielseitig einsetzbaren Kokzidiosetherapeutikum. *Prakt. Tierarzt* 69, 46–51.

652. Haberkorn, A., Stoltefuss, J., 1987. Studies on the activity spectrum of toltrazuril, a new anti-coccidial agent. *Vet. Med. Rev.* 1, 22–32.

653. Hackstein, J.H.P., Mackenstedt, U., Mehlhorn, H., Meijerink, J.P.P., Schubert, H., Leunissen, J.A.M., 1995. Parasitic apicomplexans harbor a chlorophyll a-D1 complex, the potential target for therapeutic triazines. *Parasitol. Res.* 81, 207–216.

654. Hafeez, M.A., Vrba, V., Barta, J.R., 2016. The complete mitochondrial genome sequence of *Eimeria innocua* (Eimeriidae, Coccidia, Apicomplexa). *Mitochondrial DNA A DNA Mapp. Seq. Anal.* 27, 2805–2806.

655. Hall, R.L., Jones, J.L., Herwaldt, B.L., 2011. Surveillance for laboratory-confirmed sporadic cases of cyclosporiasis—United States, 1997–2008. *MMWR Surveill. Summ.* 60, 1–11.

656. Hall, R.L., Jones, J.L., Hurd, S., Smith, G., Mahon, B.E., Herwaldt, B.L., 2012. Population-based active surveillance for *Cyclospora* infection—United States, Foodborne Diseases Active Surveillance Network (FoodNet), 1997–2009. *Clin. Infect. Dis.* 54 (Suppl 5), S411–S417.

657. Hamadejova, K., Vítovec, J., 2005. Occurrence of the coccidium *Isospora suis* in piglets. *Vet. Med. Czech.* 50, 159–163.

658. Hamid, P.H., Hirzmann, J., Kerner, K., Gimpl, G., Lochnit, G., Hermosilla, C.R., Taubert, A., 2015. *Eimeria bovis* infection modulates endothelial host cell cholesterol metabolism for successful replication. *Vet. Res.* 46, 100.

659. Hammond, D.M., 1973. Life cycles, development of coccidia. In Hammond, D.M. and Long, P.L. (Ed.), *The Coccidia, Eimeria, Isospora, Toxoplasma, and Related Genera*. University Park Press, Baltimore, MD, 45–79.

660. Hammond, D.M., Andersen, F.L., Miner, M.L., 1963. The occurrence of a second asexual generation in the life cycle of *Eimeria bovis* in calves. *J. Parasitol.* 49, 428–434.

661. Hammond, D.M., Bowman, G.W., Davis, L.R., Simms, B.T., 1946. The endogenous phase of the life cycle of *Eimeria bovis*. *J. Parasitol.* 32, 409–427.

662. Hammond, D.M., Chobotar, B., Ernst, J.V., 1968. Cytological observations on sporozoites of *Eimeria bovis* and *E. auburnensis*, and an *Eimeria* species from the Ord kangaroo rat. *J. Parasitol.* 54, 550–558.

663. Hammond, D.M., Clark, G.W., Miner, M.L., Trost, W.A., Johnson, A.E., 1959. Treatment of experimental bovine coccidiosis with multiple small doses and single large doses of sulfamethazine and sulfabromomethazine. *Am. J. Vet. Res.* 20, 708–713.

664. Hammond, D.M., Clark, W.N., Miner, M.L., 1961. Endogenous phase of the life cycle of *Eimeria auburnensis* in calves. *J. Parasitol.* 47, 591–596.

665. Hammond, D.M., Ernst, J.V., Chobotar, B., 1970. Composition and function of the substiedal body in the sporocysts of *Eimeria utahensis*. *J. Parasitol.* 56, 618–619.

666. Hammond, D.M., Fayer, R., Miner, M.L., 1969. Further studies on *in vitro* development of *Eimeria bovis* and attempts to obtain second-generation schizonts. *J. Protozool.* 16, 298–302.

667. Hammond, D.M., Shupe, J.L., Johnson, A.E., Fitzgerald, P.R., Thorne, J.L., 1956. Sulfaquinoxaline and sulfamerazine in the treatment of experimental infections with *Eimeria bovis* in calves. *Am. J. Vet. Res.* 17, 463–470.

668. Han, H., Xue, P., Dong, H., Zhu, S., Zhao, Q., Huang, B., 2016. Screening and characterization of apical membrane antigen 1 interacting proteins in *Eimeria tenella. Exp. Parasitol.* 170, 116–124.

669. Han, H.Y., Lin, J.J., Zhao, Q.P., Dong, H., Jiang, L.L., Xu, M.Q., Zhu, S.H., Huang, B., 2010. Identification of differentially expressed genes in early stages of *Eimeria tenella* by suppression subtractive hybridization and cDNA microarray. *J. Parasitol.* 96, 95–102.

670. Han, Q., Li, J., Gong, P., Gai, J., Li, S., Zhang, X., 2011. Virus-like particles in *Eimeria tenella* are associated with multiple RNA segments. *Exp. Parasitol.* 127, 646–650.

671. Han, X., Sun, F.L., 2008. Diagnosis and treatment of duck coccidiosis. *Tech. Advis. Anim. Husb.* 7, 114–115 (in Chinese).

672. Hänichen, T., Wiesner, H., Göbel, E., 1994. Zur Pathologie, Diagnostik und Therapie der Kokzidiose bei Wiederkäuern im Zoo. *Verhandlungsber. Int. Symp. Erkr. Zoo- und Wildtiere* 36, 375–380.

673. Hao, L., Liu, X., Zhou, X., Li, J., Suo, X., 2007. Transient transfection of *Eimeria tenella* using yellow or red fluorescent protein as a marker. *Mol. Biochem. Parasitol.* 153, 213–215.

674. Harder, A., Haberkorn, A., 1989. Possible mode of action of toltrazuril: Studies on two *Eimeria* species and mammalian and *Ascaris suum* enzymes. *Parasitol. Res.* 76, 8–12.

675. Harleman, J.H., Meyer, R.C., 1983. *Isospora suis* infection in piglets. A review. *Vet. Quart.* 5, 178–185.

676. Harleman, J.H., Meyer, R.C., 1984. Life cycle of *Isospora suis* in gnotobiotic and conventionalized piglets. *Vet. Parasitol.* 17, 27–39.

677. Harleman, J.H., Meyer, R.C., 1985. Pathogenicity of *Isospora suis* in gnotobiotic and conventionalised piglets. *Vet. Rec.* 116, 561–565.

678. Harper, C.K., Penzhorn, B.L., 1999. Occurrence and diversity of coccidia in indigenous, Saanen and crossbred goats in South Africa. *Vet. Parasitol.* 82, 1–9.

679. Hashem, F.G., 2012. Epidemiological studies on internal parasitic diseases in cattle and buffaloes in Giza Governorate. Masters thesis. University of Beni Suef, Faculty of Vet. Medicine, Egypt.

680. Hashemnia, M., Khodakaram-Tafti, A., Razavi, S.M., Nazifi, S., 2011. Changing patterns of acute phase proteins and inflammatory mediators in experimental caprine coccidiosis. *Korean J. Parasitol.* 49, 213–219.

681. Hashemnia, M., Khodakaram-Tafti, A., Razavi, S.M., Nazifi, S., 2012. Experimental caprine coccidiosis caused by *Eimeria arloingi*: Morphopathologic and electron microscopic studies. *Vet. Res. Commun.* 36, 47–55.

682. Hashemnia, M., Khodakaram-Tafti, A., Razavi, S.M., Nazifi, S., 2014. Hematological and serum biochemical analyses in experimental caprine coccidiosis. *J. Parasit. Dis.* 38, 116–123.

683. Hassum, I.C., de Menezes, R.C.A.A., 2005. Infecção natural por espécies do gênero *Eimeria* em pequenos ruminantes criados em dois munípios do estado do Rio de Janeiro. *Rev. Bras. Parasitol. Vet.* 14, 95–100.

684. Hauck, R., 2017. Interactions between parasites and the bacterial microbiota of chickens. *Avian Dis.* 61, 428–436.

685. Haug, A., Gjevre, A.G., Skjerve, E., Kaldhusdal, M., 2008. A survey of the economic impact of subclinical *Eimeria* infections in broiler chickens in Norway. *Avian Pathol.* 37, 333–341.

686. Haug, A., Williams, R.B., Larsen, S., 2006. Counting coccidial oocysts in chicken faeces: A comparative study of a standard McMaster technique and a new rapid method. *Vet. Parasitol.* 136, 233–242.

687. Hawkins, P.A., 1950. Coccidiosis in turkeys. Doctoral thesis. Michigan State College of Agriculture and Applied Science, Department of Animal Pathology, East Lansing, Michigan.

688. Hawkins, P.A., 1952. Coccidiosis in turkeys. Technical Bulletin 226, East Lansing, MI. Michigan State College Agricultural Experiment Station.

689. Hayat, C.S., Rukn-ud-Din, Hayat, B., Akhtar, M., 1994. Prevalence of coccidiosis in cattle and buffaloes with emphasis on age, breed, sex, season and management. *Pak. Vet. J.* 14, 214–217.

690. He, P., Li, J., Gong, P., Huang, J., Zhang, X., 2012. *Cystoisospora* spp. from dogs in China and phylogenetic analysis of its 18S and ITS1 gene. *Vet. Parasitol.* 190, 254–258.

691. He, X.L., Grigg, M.E., Boothroyd, J.C., Garcia, K.C., 2002. Structure of the immunodominant surface antigen from the *Toxoplasma gondii* SRS superfamily. *Nat. Struct. Biol.* 9, 606–611.

692. Heath, H.L., Blagburn, B.L., Elsasser, T.H., Pugh, D.G., Sanders, L.G., Sartin, E.A., Steele, B., Sartin, J.L., 1997. Hormonal modulation of the physiologic responses of calves infected with *Eimeria bovis. Am. J. Vet. Res.* 58, 891–896.

693. Hein, B., Lämmler, G., 1978. Veränderungen der Enzymaktivitäten im Serum bei *Eimeria stiedai* infizierten Kaninchen. *Z. Parasitenkd.* 57, 199–211.

694. Hein, H., 1968. Resistance in young chicks to reinfection by immunization with two doses of oocysts of *Eimeria acervulina. Exp. Parasitol.* 22, 12–18.

695. Hein, H., 1971. *Eimeria brunetti*: Cross infections in chickens immunized to *E. maxima. Exp. Parasitol.* 29, 367–374.

696. Hein, H.E., 1975. *Eimeria acervulina, E. brunetti,* and *E. maxima*: Immunity in chickens with low multiple doses of mixed oocysts. *Exp. Parasitol.* 38, 271–278.

697. Hein, H.E., 1976. *Eimeria acervulina, E. brunetti,* and *E. maxima*: Pathogenic effects of single or mixed infections with low doses of oocysts in chickens. *Exp. Parasitol.* 39, 415–421.

698. Heine, J., 1981. Die tryptische Organverdauung als Methode zum Nachweis extraintestinaler Stadien bei *Cystoisospora* spp.-Infektionen. *Berl. Münch. tierärztl. Wochenschr.* 94, 103–104.

699. Heitlinger, E., Spork, S., Lucius, R., Dieterich, C., 2014. The genome of *Eimeria falciformis*—Reduction and specialization in a single host apicomplexan parasite. *BMC Genomics* 15, 696.

700. Helmy, M.M.F., Rashed, L.A., Abdel-Fattah, H.S., 2006. Co-infection with *Cryptosporidium parvum* and *Cyclospora cayetanensis* in immunocompromised patients. *J. Egypt. Soc. Parasitol.* 36, 613–627.

701. Hemmert-Halswick, A., 1943. Infektion mit *Globidium leuckarti* beim Pferd. *Z. Veterinärkd.* 55, 192–199.

702. Henriksen, S.A., Christensen, J.P.B., 1992. Demonstration of *Isospora suis* oocysts in faecal samples. *Vet. Rec.* 131, 443–444.

703. Henry, A., Masson, G., 1932. Considérations sur le genre *Globidium*, *Globidium cameli* n. sp. parasite du dromadaire. *Ann. Soc. Belg. Med. Trop.* 10, 385–401.

704. Henry, S.C., Tokach, L.M., 1995. *Eimeria*-associated pathology in breeding gilts. *J. Swine Health Prod.* 3, 200–201.

705. Hermosilla, C., Barbisch, B., Heise, A., Kowalik, S., Zahner, H., 2002. Development of *Eimeria bovis in vitro*: Suitability of several bovine, human and porcine endothelial cell lines, bovine fetal gastrointestinal, Madin-Darby bovine kidney (MDBK) and African green monkey kidney (VERO) cells. *Parasitol. Res.* 88, 301–307.

706. Hermosilla, C., Bürger, H.J., Zahner, H., 1999. T cell responses in calves to a primary *Eimeria bovis* infection: Phenotypical and functional changes. *Vet. Parasitol.* 84, 49–64.

707. Hermosilla, C., Diakou, A., Psychas, V., Silva, L.M.R., Taubert, A., 2016. Fatal *Eimeria gilruthi*-induced abomasal coccidiosis: A still neglected parasitosis? *J. Vet. Med. Res.* 3, 1055.

708. Hermosilla, C., Stamm, I., Menge, C., Taubert, A., 2015. Suitable *in vitro* culture of *Eimeria bovis* meront II stages in bovine colonic epithelial cells and parasite-induced upregulation of CXCL10 and GM-CSF gene transcription. *Parasitol. Res.* 114, 3125–3136.

709. Hertzberg, H., Kohler, L., 2006. Prevalence and significance of gastrointestinal helminths and protozoa in South American camelids in Switzerland. *Berl. Münch. tierärztl. Wochenschr.* 119, 291–294.

710. Herwaldt, B.L., 2000. *Cyclospora cayetanensis*: A review, focusing on the outbreaks of cyclosporiasis in the 1990s. *Clin. Infect. Dis.* 31, 1040–1057.

711. Herwaldt, B.L., Ackers, M.L., the Cyclospora Working Group, 1997. An outbreak in 1996 of cyclosporiasis associated with imported raspberries. *N. Engl. J. Med.* 336, 1548–1556.

712. Hidalgo Argüello, M.R., Cordero del Campillo, M., 1987. Quantity of *Eimeria* spp. oocyst elimination in sheep. *Angew. Parasitol.* 28, 7–14.

713. Hidalgo Argüello, M.R., Cordero del Campillo, M., 1999. Parasitosis del aparato digestivo. In Cordero del Campillo, M. and Rojo-Vázquez, F.A. (Ed.), *Parasitología Veterinaria*. McGraw-Hill, Madrid, 195–212.

714. Hiepe, T., Romeyke, D., Jungmann, R., 1978. Studies of coccidia infections in calves under intensive rearing conditions and recommendations for their control. *Mh. Vet. Med.* 33, 904–910.

715. Higgins, R.J., 1988. Coccidiosis—An emerging disease of young pigs. *Vet. Ann.* 24, 49–64.

716. Hikosaka, K., Nakai, Y., Watanabe, Y., Tachibana, S., Arisue, N., Palacpac, N.M.Q., Toyama, T., et al., 2011. Concatenated mitochondrial DNA of the coccidian parasite *Eimeria tenella*. *Mitochondrion* 11, 273–278.

717. Hilali, M., Fatani, A., Al-Atiya, S., 1995. Isolation of tissue cysts of *Toxoplasma*, *Isospora*, *Hammondia* and *Sarcocystis* from camel (*Camelus dromedarius*) meat in Saudi Arabia. *Vet. Parasitol.* 58, 353–356.

718. Hilali, M., Nassar, A.M., El-Ghaysh, A., 1992. Camel (*Camelus dromedarius*) and sheep (*Ovis aries*) meat as a source of dog infection with some coccidian parasites. *Vet. Parasitol.* 43, 37–43.

719. Hill, J.E., Lomax, L.G., Lindsay, D.S., Lynn, B.S., 1985. Coccidosis caused by *Eimeria scabra* in a finishing hog. *J. Am. Vet. Med. Assoc.* 186, 981–983.

720. Hirani, N.D., Solanki, J.B., 2010. Prevalence of coccidia in rabbit in middle Gujarat. *Indian J. Field Vet.* 5 (3), 37–38.

721. Hirayama, K., Okamoto, M., Sako, T., Kihara, K., Okai, K., Taharaguchi, S., Yoshino, T., Taniyama, H., 2002. *Eimeria* organisms develop in the epithelial cells of equine small intestine. *Vet. Pathol.* 39, 505–508.

722. Hitchcock, M.M., Hogan, C.A., Budvytiene, I., Banaei, N., 2019. Reproducibility of positive results for rare pathogens on the FilmArray GI Panel. *Diagn. Microbiol. Infect. Dis.*, 95, 10–14.

723. Hnida, J.A., Duszynski, D.W., 1999. Cross-transmission studies with *Eimeria arizonensis*, *E. arizonensis*-like oocysts and *Eimeria langebarteli*: Host specificity at the genus and species level within the Muridae. *J. Parasitol.* 85, 873–877.

724. Hoan, T.D., Thao, D.T., Gadahi, J.A., Song, X., Xu, L., Yan, R., Li, X., 2014. Analysis of humoral immune response and cytokines in chickens vaccinated with *Eimeria brunetti* apical membrane antigen-1 (EbAMA1) DNA vaccine. *Exp. Parasitol.* 144, 65–72.

725. Hoan, T.D., Zhang, Z., Huang, J., Yan, R., Song, X., Xu, L., Li, X., 2016. Identification and immunogenicity of microneme protein 2 (EbMIC2) of *Eimeria brunetti*. *Exp. Parasitol.* 162, 7–17.

726. Hodgin, C., Schillhorn van Veen, T.W., Fayer, R., Richter, N., 1984. Leptospirosis and coccidial infection in a guanaco. *J. Am. Vet. Med. Assoc.* 185, 1442–1444.

727. Hofstetter, J.N., Nascimento, F.S., Park, S., Casillas, S., Herwaldt, B.L., Arrowood, M.J., Qvarnstrom, Y., 2019. Evaluation of multilocus sequence typing of *Cyclospora cayetanensis* based on microsatellite markers. *Parasite* 26, 3.

728. Hoge, C.W., Echeverria, P., Rajah, R., Jacobs, J., Malthouse, S., Chapman, E., Jimenez, L.M., Shlim, D.R., 1995. Prevalence of *Cyclospora* species and other enteric pathogens among children less than 5 years of age in Nepal. *J. Clin. Microbiol.* 33, 3058–3060.

729. Hoge, C.W., Shlim, D.R., Ghimire, M., Rabold, J.G., Pandey, P., Walch, A., Rajah, R., Gaudio, P., Echovorria, P., 1995. Placebo-controlled trial of co-trimoxazole for *Cyclospora* infections among travellers and foreign residents in Nepal. *Lancet* 345, 691–693.

730. Hoge, C.W., Shlim, D.R., Rajah, R., Triplett, J., Shear, M., Rabold, J.G., Echeverria, P., 1993. Epidemiology of diarrhoeal illness associated with coccidian-like organism among travellers and foreign residents in Nepal. *Lancet* 341, 1175–1179.

731. Holst, H., Svensson, C., 1994. Changes in the blood composition of calves during experimental and natural infections with *Eimeria alabamensis*. *Res. Vet. Sci.* 57, 377–383.

732. Hong, Y.H., Lillehoj, H.S., Dalloul, R.A., Min, W., Miska, K.B., Tuo, W., Lee, S.H., Han, J.Y., Lillehoj, E.P., 2006. Molecular cloning and characterization of chicken NK-lysin. *Vet. Immunol. Immunopathol.* 110, 339–347.

733. Hong, Y.H., Lillehoj, H.S., Lee, S.H., Dalloul, R.A., Lillehoj, E.P., 2006. Analysis of chicken cytokine and chemokine gene expression following *Eimeria acervulina* and *Eimeria tenella* infections. *Vet. Immunol. Immunopathol.* 114, 209–223.

734. Hong, Y.H., Lillehoj, H.S., Lee, S.H., Park, D.W., Lillehoj, E.P., 2006. Molecular cloning and characterization of chicken lipopolysaccharide-induced TNF-α factor (LITAF). *Dev. Comp. Immunol.* 30, 919–929.

735. Hong, Y.H., Lillehoj, H.S., Lillehoj, E.P., Lee, S.H., 2006. Changes in immune-related gene expression and intestinal lymphocyte subpopulations following *Eimeria maxima* infection of chickens. *Vet. Immunol. Immunopathol.* 114, 259–272.

736. Hooshmand-Rad, P., Svensson, C., Uggla, A., 1994. Experimental *Eimeria alabamensis* infection in calves. *Vet. Parasitol.* 53, 23–32.

737. Horton, G.M., Stockdale, P.H., 1981. Lasalocid and monensin in finishing diets for early weaned lambs with naturally occurring coccidiosis. *Am. J. Vet. Res.* 42, 433–436.

738. Horton-Smith, C., 1947. The treatment of hepatic coccidiosis in rabbits. *Br. Vet. J.* 103, 207–213.

739. Horton-Smith, C., 1948. The effect of sulphamezathine on the second generation schizonts of *Eimeria tenella*. *Trans. Roy. Soc. Trop. Med. Hyg.* 42, 11.

740. Horton-Smith, C., 1949. The acquisition of resistance to coccidiosis by chickens during treatment with sulphonamides. *Vet. Rec.* 19, 237–238.

741. Horton-Smith, C., Long, P.L., 1952. Nitrofurazone in the treatment of caecal coccidiosis in chickens. *Br. Vet. J.* 108, 47–57.

742. Horton-Smith, C., Long, P.L., 1966. The fate of the sporozoites of *Eimeria acervulina*, *Eimeria maxima* and *Eimeria mivati* in the caeca of the fowl. *Parasitology* 56, 569–574.

743. Houk, A.E., Lindsay, D.S., 2013. *Cystoisospora canis* (Apicomplexa: Sarcocystidae): Development of monozoic tissue cysts in human cells, demonstration of egress of zoites from tissue cysts, and demonstration of repeat monozoic tissue cyst formation by zoites. *Vet. Parasitol.* 197, 455–461.

744. Houk, A.E., O'Connor, T., Pena, H.F.J., Gennari, S.M., Zajac, A.M., Lindsay, D.S., 2013. Experimentally induced clinical *Cystoisospora canis* coccidiosis in dogs with prior natural patent *Cystoisospora ohioensis*-like or *C. canis* infections. *J. Parasitol.* 99, 892–895.

745. Hu, D., Suo, X., Liu, X., 2018. Current research progress in molecular biology of chicken coccidia in China. *Acta Parasitol. Med. Entomol. Sinica* 25, 262–271 (in Chinese).

746. Hu, D., Wang, C., Wang, S., Tang, X., Duan, C., Zhang, S., Suo, J., et al., 2018. Comparative transcriptome analysis of *Eimeria maxima* (Apicomplexa: Eimeriidae) suggests DNA replication activities correlating with its fecundity. *BMC Genomics* 19, 699.

747. Hu, T.W., Su, J.H., 1995. A discussion on diagnosis and treatment of duck coccidiosis. *Jiangxi Anim. Sci. Vet. Med.* 49, 44–45 (in Chinese).

748. Huang, C., Wen, F., Yue, L., Chen, R., Zhou, W., Hu, L., Chen, M., Wang, S., 2016. Exploration of fluorescence-based real-time loop-mediated isothermal amplification (LAMP) assay for detection of *Isospora suis* oocysts. *Exp. Parasitol.* 165, 1–6.

749. Huang, G., Tang, X., Bi, F., Hao, Z., Han, Z., Suo, J., Zhang, S., et al., 2018. *Eimeria tenella* infection perturbs the chicken gut microbiota from the onset of oocyst shedding. *Vet. Parasitol.* 258, 30–37.

750. Huang, G., Zhang, S., Zhou, C., Tang, X., Li, C., Wang, C., Tang, X., et al., 2018. Influence of *Eimeria falciformis* infection on gut microbiota and metabolic pathways in mice. *Infect. Immun.* 86, e00073–18.

751. Huang, J., Liu, T., Li, K., Song, X., Yan, R., Xu, L., Li, X., 2018. Proteomic analysis of protein interactions between *Eimeria maxima* sporozoites and chicken jejunal epithelial cells by shotgun LC-MS/MS. *Parasit. Vectors* 11, 226.

752. Huang, P., Weber, J.T., Sosin, D.M., Griffin, P.M., Long, E.G., Murphy, J.J., Kocka, F., Peters, C., Kallick, C., 1995. The first reported outbreak of diarrheal illness associated with *Cyclospora* in the United States. *Ann. Intern. Med.* 123, 409–414.

753. Huang, X., Liu, J., Tian, D., Li, W., Zhou, Z., Huang, J., Song, X., Xu, L., Yan, R., Li, X., 2018. The molecular characterization and protective efficacy of microneme 3 of *Eimeria mitis* in chickens. *Vet. Parasitol.* 258, 114–123.

754. Huang, X., Zou, J., Xu, H., Ding, Y., Yin, G., Liu, X., Suo, X., 2011. Transgenic *Eimeria tenella* expressing enhanced yellow fluorescent protein targeted to different cellular compartments stimulated dichotomic immune responses in chickens. *J. Immunol.* 187, 3595–3602.

755. Hughes, H.P.A., Whitmire, W.M., Speer, C.A., 1989. Immunity patterns during acute infection by *Eimeria bovis*. *J. Parasitol.* 75, 86–91.

756. Hussain, R., Mahmood, F., Khan, A., Mehmood, K., 2017. Prevalence and pathology of bovine coccidiosis in Faisalabad district, Pakistan. *Thai J. Vet. Med.* 47, 401–406.

757. Hussein, E.M., Abdul-Manaem, A.H., El-Attary, E.S.L., 2005. *Cyclospora cayetanensis* oocysts in sputum of a patient with active pulmonary tuberculosis, case report in Ismailia, Egypt. *J. Egypt. Soc. Parasitol.* 35, 787–793.

758. Hussein, E.M., Ahmed, S.A., Mokhtar, A.B., Elzagawy, S.M., Yahi, S.H., Hussein, A.M., El-Tantawey, F., 2018. Antiprotozoal activity of magnesium oxide (MgO) nanoparticles against *Cyclospora cayetanensis* oocysts. *Parasitol. Int.* 67, 666–674.

759. Hussein, E.M., El-Moamly, A.A., Dawoud, H.A., Fahmy, H., El-Shal, H.E., Sabek, N.A., 2007. Real-time PCR and flow cytometry in detection of *Cyclospora* oocysts in fecal samples of symptomatic and asymptomatic pediatrics patients. *J. Egypt. Soc. Parasitol.* 37, 151–170.

760. Hussein, H.S., Kasim, A.A., Shawa, Y.R., 1987. The prevalence and pathology of *Eimeria* infections in camels in Saudi Arabia. *J. Comp. Pathol.* 97, 293–297.

761. Hyuga, A., Matsumoto, J., 2016. A survey of gastrointestinal parasites of alpacas (*Vicugna pacos*) raised in Japan. *J. Vet. Med. Sci.* 78, 719–721.

762. Ibarra-Velarde, F., Alcala-Canto, Y., 2007. Downregulation of the goat β-defensin-2 gene by IL-4 in caprine intestinal epithelial cells infected with *Eimeria* spp. *Parasitol. Res.* 101, 613–618.

763. Idris, A.B., Bounous, D.I., Goodwin, M.A., Brown, J., Krushinskie, E.A., 1997. Lack of correlation between microscopic lesion scores and gross lesion scores in commercially grown broilers examined for small intestinal *Eimeria* spp. coccidiosis. *Avian Dis.* 41, 388–391.

764. Ilieff, A., 1997. Untersuchungen zur Verbreitung und zur Epidemiologie von enteropathogenen Infektionserregern bei durchfallkranken Saug- und Absatzferkeln. Dr. med. vet. thesis. Justus-Liebig Universitat, Gießen.

765. Imai, R.K., Barta, J.R., 2019. Distribution and abundance of *Eimeria* species in commercial turkey flocks across Canada. *Can. Vet. J.* 60, 153–159.

766. Indermühle, N.A., 1978. Endoparasitenbefall beim Schwein. *Schweiz. Arch. Tierheilk.* 120, 513–525.

767. Inoue, I., 1967. *Eimeria saitamae* n. sp.: A new cause of coccidiosis in domestic ducks (*Anas platyrhyncha var. domestica*). *Jpn. J. Vet. Sci.* 29, 209–215.

768. Inoue, I., Nomoto, S., Watanabe, F., Suzuki, M., 1965. An outbreak of coccidiosis among ducks in the field. *J. Jpn. Vet. Med. Assoc.* 18, 393–395 (in Japanese).

769. Inoue, I., Nomoto, S., Watanabe, F., Tsunoda, K., 1966. Life cycle of coccidia isolated from experimentally infected ducks. *J. Jpn. Vet. Med. Assoc.* 19, 158–160 (in Japanese).

770. Inoue, R., Tsukahara, T., Nakanishi, N., Ushida, K., 2005. Development of the intestinal microbiota in the piglet. *J. Gen. Appl. Microbiol.* 51, 257–265.

771. Iqbal, A., Tariq, K.A., Wazir, V.S., Singh, R., 2013. Antiparasitic efficacy of *Artemisia absinthium*, toltrazuril and amprolium against intestinal coccidiosis in goats. *J. Parasit. Dis.* 37, 88–93.

772. Islam, F.M.S., Rahman, M.H., Chowdhury, S.M.Z.H., 1992. Prevalence of parasites of water buffaloes in Bangladesh. *Asian J. Anim. Sci.* 5, 601–604.

773. Islam, K.M.S., Klein, U., Burch, D.G.S., 2009. The activity and compatibility of the antibiotic tiamulin with other drugs in poultry medicine—A review. *Poult. Sci.* 88, 2353–2359.

774. Isler, C.M., Bellamy, J.E.C., Wobeser, G.A., 1987. Pathogenesis of neurological signs associated with bovine enteric coccidiosis: A prospective study and review. *Can. J. Vet. Res.* 51, 261–270.

775. Jahanzaib, M.S., Avais, M., Khan, M.S., Atif, F.A., Ahmad, N., Ashraf, K., Zafar, M.U., 2017. Prevalence and risk factors of coccidiosis in buffaloes and cattle from Ravi River region, Lahore, Pakistan. *Buffalo Bull.* 36, 427–438.

776. Jakowlew, S.B., Dillard, P.J., Winokur, T.S., Flanders, K.C., Sporn, M.B., Roberts, A.B., 1991. Expression of transforming growth factor-βs 1–4 in chicken embryo chondrocytes and myocytes. *Dev. Biol.* 143, 135–148.

777. Jalila, A., Dorny, P., Sani, R., Salim, N.B., Vercruysse, J., 1998. Coccidial infections of goats in Selangor, peninsular Malaysia. *Vet. Parasitol.* 74, 165–172.

778. James, S., 1980. Thiamine uptake in isolated schizonts of *Eimeria tenella* and the inhibitory effects of amprolium. *Parasitology* 80, 313–322.

779. Jang, S.I., Kim, D.K., Lillehoj, H.S., Lee, S.H., Lee, K.W., Bertrand, F., Dupuis, L., Deville, S., Ben Arous, J., Lillehoj, E.P., 2013. Evaluation of Montanide ISA 71 VG adjuvant during profilin vaccination against experimental coccidiosis. *PLOS ONE* 8, e59786.

780. Jang, S.I., Lillehoj, H.S., Lee, S.H., Kim, D.K., Pagés, M., Hong, Y.H., Min, W., Lillehoj, E.P., 2011. Distinct immunoregulatory properties of macrophage migration inhibitory factors encoded by *Eimeria* parasites and their chicken host. *Vaccine* 29, 8998–9004.

781. Jang, S.I., Lillehoj, H.S., Lee, S.H., Lee, K.W., Lillehoj, E.P., Bertrand, F., Dupuis, L., Deville, S., 2011. Montanide IMS 1313 N VG PR nanoparticle adjuvant enhances antigen-specific immune responses to profilin following mucosal vaccination against *Eimeria acervulina*. *Vet. Parasitol.* 182, 163–170.

782. Jang, S.I., Lillehoj, H.S., Lee, S.H., Lee, K.W., Lillehoj, E.P., Bertrand, F., Dupuis, L., Deville, S., 2011. Mucosal immunity against *Eimeria acervulina* infection in broiler chickens following oral immunization with profilin in Montanide adjuvants. *Exp. Parasitol.* 129, 36–41.

783. Jang, S.I., Lillehoj, H.S., Lee, S.H., Lee, K.W., Park, M.S., Bauchan, G.R., Lillehoj, E.P., Bertrand, F., Dupuis, L., Deville, S., 2010. Immunoenhancing effects of Montanide ISA oil-based adjuvants on recombinant coccidia antigen vaccination against *Eimeria acervulina* infection. *Vet. Parasitol.* 172, 221–228.

784. Jarpa Gana, A., 1966. Coccidiosis humana. *Biologica* 39, 3–26.

785. Jarvinen, J.A., 1999. Prevalence of *Eimeria macusaniensis* (Apicomplexa: Eimeriidae) in midwestern *Lama* spp. *J. Parasitol.* 85, 373–376.

786. Jarvinen, J.A., 2008. Infection of llamas with stored *Eimeria macusaniensis* oocysts obtained from guanaco and alpaca feces. *J. Parasitol.* 94, 969–972.

787. Järvis, T., Mägi, E., Lassen, B., 2013. Outbreak of eimeriosis in an Estonian rabbit farm. *Vet. Med. Zoot.* 64, 11–15.

788. Jatau, I.D., Lawal, I.A., Kwaga, J.K.P., Tomley, F.M., Blake, D.P., Nok, A.J., 2016. Three operational taxonomic units of *Eimeria* are common in Nigerian chickens and may undermine effective molecular diagnosis of coccidiosis. *BMC Vet. Res.* 12, 86.

789. Jeffers, T.K., 1974. Genetic transfer of anticoccidial drug resistance in *Eimeria tenella*. *J. Parasitol.* 60, 900–904.

790. Jeffers, T.K., 1975. Attenuation of *Eimeria tenella* through selection for precociousness. *J. Parasitol.* 61, 1083–1090.

791. Jeffers, T.K., 1976. Genetic recombination of precociousness and anticoccidial drug resistance in *Eimeria tenella*. *Z. Parasitenkd.* 50, 251–255.

792. Jeffers, T.K., 1976. Reduction of anticoccidial drug resistance by massive introduction of drug-sensitive coccidia. *Avian Dis.* 20, 649–653.

793. Jeffers, T.K., Challey, J.R., 1973. Collateral sensitivity to 4-hydroxyquinolines in *Eimeria acervulina* strains resistant to meticlorpindol. *J. Parasitol.* 59, 624–630.

794. Jeffers, T.K., Long, P.L., 1985. *Eimeria tenella*: Immunogenicity of arrested sporozoites in chickens. *Exp. Parasitol.* 60, 175–180.

795. Jeffers, T.K., Tonkinson, L.V., Callender, M.E., 1988. Anticoccidial efficacy of narasin in battery cage trials. *Poult. Sci.* 67, 1043–1049.

796. Jeffery, G.M., 1956. Human coccidiosis in South Carolina. *J. Parasitol.* 42, 491–495.

797. Jelínková, A., Licois, D., Pakandl, M., 2008. The endogenous development of the rabbit coccidium *Eimeria exigua* Yakimoff, 1934. *Vet. Parasitol.* 156, 168–172.

798. Jenkins, M., Klopp, S., Ritter, D., Miska, K., Fetterer, R., 2010. Comparison of *Eimeria* species distribution and salinomycin resistance in commercial broiler operations utilizing different coccidiosis control strategies. *Avian Dis.* 54, 1002–1006.

799. Jenkins, M.C., Augustine, P.C., Barta, J.R., Castle, M.D., Danforth, H.D., 1991. Development of resistance to coccidiosis in the absence of merogonic development using X-irradiated *Eimeria acervulina* oocysts. *Exp. Parasitol.* 72, 285–293.

800. Jenkins, M.C., Augustine, P.C., Danforth, H.D., Barta, J.R., 1991. X-Irradiation of *Eimeria tenella* oocysts provides direct evidence that sporozoite invasion and early schizont development induce a protective immune response(s). *Infect. Immun.* 59, 4042–4048.

801. Jenkins, M.C., Chute, M.B., Danforth, H.D., 1997. Protection against coccidiosis in outbred chickens elicited by γ-irradiated *Eimeria maxima*. *Avian Dis.* 41, 702–708.

802. Jenkins, M.C., Miska, K., Klopp, S., 2006. Improved polymerase chain reaction technique for determining the species composition of *Eimeria* in poultry litter. *Avian Dis.* 50, 632–635.

803. Jenkins, M.C., Parker, C., Klopp, S., O'Brien, C., Miska, K., Fetterer, R., 2012. Gel-bead delivery of *Eimeria* oocysts protects chickens against coccidiosis. *Avian Dis.* 56, 306–309.

804. Jenkins, M.C., Parker, C., O'Brien, C., Persyn, J., Barlow, D., Miska, K., Fetterer, R., 2013. Protecting chickens against coccidiosis in floor pens by administering *Eimeria* oocysts using gel beads or spray vaccination. *Avian Dis.* 57, 622–626.

805. Jenkins, M.C., Parker, C., Ritter, D., 2017. *Eimeria* oocyst concentrations and species composition in litter from commercial broiler farms during anticoccidial drug or live *Eimeria* oocyst vaccine control programs. *Avian Dis.* 61, 214–220.

806. Jenkins, M.C., Seferian, P.G., Augustine, P.C., Danforth, H.D., 1993. Protective immunity against coccidiosis elicited by radiation-attenuated *Eimeria maxima* sporozoites that are incapable of asexual development. *Avian Dis.* 37, 74–82.

807. Jeong, J., Kim, W.H., Yoo, J., Lee, C., Kim, S., Cho, J.H., Jang, H.K., Kim, D.W., Lillehoj, H.S., Min, W., 2012. Identification and comparative expression analysis of interleukin 2/15 receptor β chain in chickens infected with *E. tenella*. *PLOS ONE* 7, e37704.

808. Jeyakumar, S., Kumar, B.G., Roy, K., Sunder, J., Kundu, A., 2009. Incidence of parasitic infection in livestock and poultry in Andaman. *Indian Vet. J.* 86, 1178–1179.

809. Jha, A.K., Uppal, B., Chadha, S., Bhalla, P., Ghosh, R., Aggarwal, P., Dewan, R., 2012. Clinical and microbiological profile of HIV/AIDS cases with diarrhea in north India. *J. Pathog.* 2012, Article ID 971958.

810. Ji, Z.G., 2017. Effective treatment of duck coccidiosis. *Contemp. Anim. Husb.* 373, 91–92 (in Chinese).

811. Jia, H.W., Li, D.G., Dai, C.L., Ding, R.F., 2010. Diagnosis and treatment of coccidiosis in juvenile mallard duck. *Contemp. Anim. Husb.* 199, 15–16 (in Chinese).

812. Jian, Y.L., Tu, Y.Q., Han, Q.S., Bai, Y., Luo, H.Q., Gao, Y.A., 2014. Epidemiological investigation of rabbit coccidiosis in Wenzhou area. *Acta Agric. Zhejiangensis* 26, 868–871 (in Chinese).

813. Jiang, J.S., Yin, P.Y., Lin, K.H., Li, A.X., Suo, X., Han, Q., 1990. Comparative experiment on the efficacy of diclazuril, maduramycin, lasalocid and narasin on duck coccidiosis. *Chin. J. Vet. Med.* 7, 10–11 (in Chinese).

814. Jiang, L., Lin, J., Han, H., Dong, H., Zhao, Q., Zhu, S., Huang, B., 2012. Identification and characterization of *Eimeria tenella* apical membrane antigen-1 (AMA1). *PLOS ONE* 7, e41115.

815. Jiang, Y., Yan, W., Wang, T., Suo, X., Xue, B., Qian, W., Yuan, L., 2013. Epidemiological investigation and *Eimeria* species identificaiton of rabbit coccidiosis in Henan Province. *Chin. Agric. Sci. Bull.* 29, 47–51.

816. Jiao, J., Yang, Y., Liu, M., Li, J., Cui, Y., Yin, S., Tao, J., 2018. Artemisinin and *Artemisia annua* leaves alleviate *Eimeria tenella* infection by facilitating apoptosis of host cells and suppressing inflammatory response. *Vet. Parasitol.* 254, 172–177.

817. Jing, B., Zhao, A., Tao, D.Y., 2010. A preliminary survey of duck coccidiosis in Kuerle. *Anim. Husb. Vet. Med.* 42, 104–105 (in Chinese).

818. Jing, F., Yin, G., Liu, X., Suo, X., Qin, Y., 2012. Large-scale survey of the prevalence of *Eimeria* infections in domestic rabbits in China. *Parasitol. Res.* 110, 1495–1500.

819. Jing, J., Liu, C., Zhu, S.X., Jiang, Y.M., Wu, L.C., Song, H.Y., Shao, Y.X., 2016. Pathological and ultrastructural observations and liver function analysis of *Eimeria stiedai*-infected rabbits. *Vet. Parasitol.* 223, 165–172.

820. Jirku, M., Jirku, M., Oborník, M., Lukeš, J., Modrý, D., 2009. A model for taxonomic work on homoxenous coccidia: Redescription, host specificity, and molecular phylogeny of *Eimeria ranae* Dobell, 1909, with a review of anuran-host *Eimeria* (Apicomplexa: Eimeriorina). *J. Eukaryot. Microbiol.* 56, 39–51.

821. Jirku, M., Modrý, D., Šlapeta, J.R., Koudela, B., Lukeš, J., 2002. The phylogeny of *Goussia* and *Choleoeimeria* (Apicomplexa; Eimeriorina) and the evolution of excystation structures in coccidia. *Protist* 153, 379–390.

822. Joachim, A., Altreuther, G., Bangoura, B., Charles, S., Daugschies, A., Hinney, B., Lindsay, D.S., Mundt, H.C., Ocak, M., Sotiraki, S., 2018. WAAVP guideline for evaluating the efficacy of anticoccidials in mammals (pigs, dogs, cattle, sheep). *Vet. Parasitol.* 253, 102–119.

823. Joachim, A., Mundt, H.C., 2011. Efficacy of sulfonamides and Baycox against *Isospora suis* in experimental infections of suckling piglets. *Parasitol. Res.* 109, 1653–1659.

824. Joachim, A., Ruttkowski, B., Sperling, D., 2018. Detection of *Cystoisospora suis* in faeces of suckling piglets—When and how? A comparison of methods. *Porcine Health Manag.* 4, 20.

825. Joachim, A., Ruttkowski, B., Zimmermann, M., Daugschies, A., Mundt, H.C., 2004. Detection of *Isospora suis* (Biester and Murray 1934) in piglet faeces—Comparison of microscopy and PCR. *J. Vet. Med. B Infect. Dis. Vet. Public Health* 51, 140–142.

826. Joachim, A., Schwarz, L., Hinney, B., Ruttkowski, B., Vogl, C., Mundt, H.C., 2014. Which factors influence the outcome of experimental infection with *Cystoisospora suis*? *Parasitol. Res.* 113, 1863–1873.

827. Joachim A., Shrestha, A., Freudenschuss, B., Palmieri, N., Hinney, B., Karembe, H., Sperling, D., 2018. Comparison of an injectable toltrazuril-gleptoferron (Forceris) and an oral toltrazuril (Baycox) + injectable iron dextran for the control of experimentally induced piglet cystoisosporosis. *Parasit. Vectors* 11, 206.

828. Jöckel, J., Wendt, B., Löffler, M., 1998. Structural and functional comparison of agents interfering with dihydroorotate, succinate and NADH oxidation of rat liver mitochondria. *Biochem. Pharmacol.* 56, 1053–1060.

829. Johnson, A.L., Stewart, J.E., Perkins, G.A., 2009. Diagnosis and treatment of *Eimeria macusaniensis* in an adult alpaca with signs of colic. *Vet. J.* 179, 465–467.

830. Johnson, J., Reid, W.M., Jeffers, T.K., 1979. Practical immunization of chickens against coccidiosis using an attenuated strain of *Eimeria tenella*. *Poult. Sci.* 58, 37–41.

831. Johnson, J.K., Long, P.L., McKenzie, M.E., 1986. The pathogenicity, immunogenicity and endogenous development of a precocious line of *Eimeria brunetti*. *Avian Pathol.* 15, 697–704.

832. Johnson, M.W., Fitzgerald, G.R., Welter, M.W., Welter, C.J., 1992. The six most common pathogens responsible for diarrhoea in newborn pigs. *Vet. Med.* 87, 382–386.

833. Johnson, W.T., 1923. Avian coccidiosis. *Poult. Sci.* 2, 146–163.

834. Johnson, W.T., 1930. Director's biennial report 1928–1930. *Oregon Agric. Coll. Exp. Stn.* 1–143.

835. Johnson, W.T., 1932. Immunity to coccidiosis in chickens, produced by inoculation through the ration. *J. Parasitol.* 19, 160–161.

835a. Johnson, W.T., 1938. Coccidiosis of the chicken with special reference to species. Oregon State Agricultural Experiment Station, Bulletin 358.

836. Johnstone, A.C., Pearce, H.G., Charleston, W.A.G., 1982. First report of *Eimeria leuckarti* infection in a horse in New Zealand. *N. Z. Vet. J.* 30, 104–105.

837. Jolley, W.R., Bardsley, K.D., 2006. Ruminant coccidiosis. *Vet. Clin. Food Anim.* 22, 613–621.

838. Jones, J.E., Solis, J., Hughes, B.L., Castaldo, D.J., Toler, J.E., 1990. Production and egg-quality responses of White Leghorn layers to anticoccidial agents. *Poult. Sci.* 69, 378–387.

839. Jongwutiwes, S., Putaporntip, C., Charoenkorn, M., Iwasaki, T., Endo, T., 2007. Morphologic and molecular characterization of *Isospora belli* oocysts from patients in Thailand. *Am. J. Trop. Med. Hyg.* 77, 107–112.

840. Jongwutiwes, S., Sampatanukul, P., Putaporntip, C., 2002. Recurrent isosporiasis over a decade in an immunocompetent host successfully treated with pyrimethamine. *Scand. J. Infect. Dis.* 34, 859–862.

841. Jonsson, N.N., Piper, E.K., Gray, C.P., Deniz, A., Constantinoiu, C.C., 2011. Efficacy of toltrazuril 5% suspension against *Eimeria bovis* and *Eimeria zuernii* in calves and observations on the associated immunopathology. *Parasitol. Res.* 109 (Suppl 1), S113–S128.

842. Joyner, L.P., 1958. Experimental *Eimeria mitis* infections in chickens. *Parasitology* 48, 101–112.

843. Joyner, L.P., 1969. Immunological variation between two strains of *Eimeria acervulina*. *Parasitology* 59, 725–732.

844. Joyner, L.P., Gregory, M.W., Norton, C.C., Done, J.T., Wells, G.W., 1981. Coccidiosis and coprophagy in pigs. *Vet. Rec.* 108, 264–265.

845. Joyner, L.P., Norton, C.C., 1969. A comparison of two laboratory strains of *Eimeria tenella*. *Parasitology* 59, 907–913.

846. Joyner, L.P., Norton, C.C., 1973. The immunity arising from continuous low-level infection with *Eimeria tenella*. *Parasitology* 67, 333–340.

847. Joyner, L.P., Norton, C.C., 1976. The immunity arising from continuous low-level infection with *Eimeria maxima* and *Eimeria acervulina*. *Parasitology* 72, 115–125.

848. Juckett, D.A., Aylsworth, C.F., Quensen, J.Q., 2008. Intestinal protozoa are hypothesized to stimulate immunosurveillance against colon cancer. *Med. Hypotheses* 71, 104–110.

849. Julander, J.G., Judge, J.W., Olsen, A.L., Rosenberg, B., Schafer, K., Sidwell, R.W., 2007. Prophylactic treatment with recombinant *Eimeria* protein, alone or in combination with an agonist cocktail, protects mice from Banzi virus infection. *Antiviral Res.* 75, 14–19.

850. Julian, R.J., Harrison, K.B., Richardson, J.A., 1976. Nervous signs in bovine coccidiosis. *Mod. Vet. Pract.* 57, 711–712, 716, 718.

851. Jung, C., Lee, C.Y.F., Grigg, M.E., 2004. The SRS superfamily of *Toxoplasma* surface proteins. *Int. J. Parasitol.* 34, 285–296.

852. Junker, K., Houwers, D.J., 2000. Diarree, pupsterfte en *Cystoïsospora*-species (coccidiose). *Tijdschr. Diergeneeskd.* 125, 582–584.

853. Jyoti, Singh, N.K., Juyal, P.D., Haque, M., Rath, S.S., 2012. Epidemiology of gastrointestinal parasites in buffalo calves of Punjab state. *J. Vet. Parasitol.* 26, 19–22.

854. Kahn, C.M., Line, S., 2010. *The Merck Veterinary Manual*. 10th ed. Merck & Co., Inc., New Jersey, USA, 1–2954.

855. Kaiser, P., Poh, T.Y., Rothwell, L., Avery, S., Balu, S., Pathania, U.S., Hughes, S., et al., 2005. A genomic analysis of chicken cytokines and chemokines. *J. Interferon Cytokine Res.* 25, 467–484.

856. Kakino, J., Shimura, O., Kagabu, Y., Itho, R., Satho, M., Maki, T., 1988. Outbreaks of diarrhea in nursing piglets presumably associated with *Isospora suis*. *J. Jpn. Vet. Med. Assoc.* 41, 478–481.

857. Kanamori, K., Manchanayake, T., Matsubayashi, M., Imai, N., Kobayashi, Y., Sasai, K., Shibahara, T., 2018. Genetic and histopathological identification of *Cystoisospora suis* in a post-weaned piglet with watery diarrhea. *Jpn. Agri. Res. Quart.* 52, 55–61.

858. Kant, V., Singh, P., Verma, P.K., Bais, I., Parmar, M.S., Gopal, A., Gupta, V., 2013. Anticoccidial drugs used in the poultry: An overview. *Science Int.* 1, 261–265.

859. Kanyari, P.W.N., 1993. The relationship between coccidial and helminth infections in sheep and goats in Kenya. *Vet. Parasitol.* 51, 137–141.

860. Karamon, J., Ziomko, I., Cencek, T., 2007. Prevalence of *Isospora suis* and *Eimeria* spp. in suckling piglets and sows in Poland. *Vet. Parasitol.* 147, 171–175.

861. Karawan, A.C., Jadaan, M., Al-Fatlawi, M.A., 2017. Diagnostic study of gastro-intestinal parasites in buffaloes of Diwanyiah Province. *Bas J. Vet. Res.* 16, 298312.

862. Kart, A., Bilgili, A., 2008. Ionophore antibiotics: Toxicity, mode of action and neurotoxic aspect of carboxylic ionophores. *J. Anim. Vet. Adv.* 7, 748–751.

863. Kasim, A.A., Hussein, H.S., al Shawa, Y.R., 1985. Coccidia in camels (*Camelus dromedarius*) in Saudi Arabia. *J. Protozool.* 32, 202–203.

864. Kawahara, F., Zhang, G., Mingala, C.N., Tamura, Y., Koiwa, M., Onuma, M., Nunoya, T., 2010. Genetic analysis and development of species-specific PCR assays based on ITS-1 region of rRNA in bovine *Eimeria* parasites. *Vet. Parasitol.* 174, 49–57.

865. Kawas, J.R., Andrade-Montemayor, H., Lu, C.D., 2010. Strategic nutrient supplementation of free-ranging goats. *Small Ruminant Res.* 89, 234–243.

866. Kawasmeh, Z.A., Elbihari, S., 1983. *Eimeria cameli* (Henry and Masson, 1932) Reichenow, 1952: Redescription and prevalence in the Eastern Province of Saudi Arabia. *Cornell Vet.* 73, 58–66.

867. Kawazoe, U., Chapman, H.D., Shaw, M., 1991. Sensitivity of field isolates of *Eimeria acervulina* to salinomycin, maduramicin, and a mixture of clopidol and methyl benzoquate in the chicken. *Avian Pathol.* 20, 439–446.

868. Keeton, S.T.N., Navarre, C.B., 2018. Coccidiosis in large and small ruminants. *Vet. Clin. Food Anim.* 34, 201–208.

869. Kelley, G.L., Hammond, D.M., 1970. Development of *Eimeria ninakohlyakimovae* from sheep in cell cultures. *J. Protozool.* 17, 340–349.

870. Kelley, G.L., Hammond, D.M., 1972. Fine structural aspects of early development of *Eimeria ninakohlyakimovae* in cultured cells. *Z. Parasitenkd.* 38, 271–284.

871. Kelley, G.L., Hammond, D.M., 1973. Fine structural aspects of nuclear division and merogony of *Eimeria ninakohlyakimovae* in cultured cells. *J. Parasitol.* 59, 1071–1079.

872. Kendall, S.B., McCullough, F.S., 1952. Relationships between sulphamezathine therapy and the acquisition of immunity to *Eimeria tenella*. *J. Comp. Pathol.* 62, 116–124.

873. Kennett, R.L., Kantor, S., Gallo, A., 1974. Efficacy studies with robenidine, a new type of anticoccidial, in the diet. *Poult. Sci.* 53, 978–986.

874. Keshavarz, K., McDougald, L.R., 1981. Influence of anticoccidial drugs on losses of broiler chickens from heat stress and coccidiosis. *Poult. Sci.* 60, 2423–2428.

875. Khan, M.N., Tauseef-ur-Rehman, Sajid, M.S., Abbas, R.Z., Zaman, M.A., Sikandar, A., Riaz, M., 2013. Determinants influencing prevalence of coccidiosis in Pakistani buffaloes. *Pak. Vet. J.* 33, 287–290.

876. Khedr, E.A.H., 2016. Studies on some protozoans infecting camels in Behera Province. Masters thesis. Alexandria University, Alexandria, Egypt.

877. Kheirandish, R., Nourollahi-Fard, S.R., Faryabi, Z., 2012. Prevalence and pathologic study of *Eimeria cameli* in slaughtered camels. *Eurasian J. Vet. Sci.* 28, 138–141.

878. Kheirandish, R., Nourollahi-Fard, S.R., Yadegari, Z., 2014. Prevalence and pathology of coccidiosis in goats in southeastern Iran. *J. Parasit. Dis.* 38, 27–31.

879. Khodakaram Tafti, A., Mansourian, M., 2008. Pathologic lesions of naturally occurring coccidiosis in sheep and goats. *Comp. Clin. Pathol.* 17, 87–91.

880. Khodakaram-Tafti, A., Hashemnia, M., 2017. An overview of intestinal coccidiosis in sheep and goats. *Revue Méd. Vét.* 167, 9–20.

881. Khodakaram-Tafti, A., Hashemnia, M., Razavi, S.M., Sharifiyazdi, H., Nazifi, S., 2013. Genetic characterization and phylogenetic analysis of *Eimeria arloingi* in Iranian native kids. *Parasitol. Res.* 112, 3187–3192.

882. Kim, D.K., Lillehoj, H.S., Hong, Y.H., Park, D.W., Lamont, S.J., Han, J.Y., Lillehoj, E.P., 2008. Immune-related gene expression in two *B*-complex disparate genetically inbred Fayoumi chicken lines following *Eimeria maxima* infection. *Poult. Sci.* 87, 433–443.

883. Kim, D.K., Lillehoj, H.S., Lee, S.H., Dominowski, P., Yancey, R.J., Lillehoj, E.P., 2012. Effects of novel vaccine/adjuvant complexes on the protective immunity against *Eimeria acervulina* and transcriptome profiles. *Avian Dis.* 56, 97–109.

884. Kim, M.J., Kim, W.H., Jung, H.C., Chai, J.W., Chai, J.Y., 2013. *Isospora belli* infection with chronic diarrhea in an alcololic patient. *Korean J. Parasitol.* 51, 207–212.

885. Kim, W.H., Jeong, J., Park, A.R., Yim, D., Kim, S., Chang, H.H., Yang, S.H., Kim, D.H., Lillehoj, H.S., Min, W., 2014. Downregulation of chicken interleukin-17 receptor A during *Eimeria* infection. *Infect. Immun.* 82, 3845–3854.

886. Kim, W.H., Jeong, J., Park, A.R., Yim, D., Kim, Y.H., Kim, K.D., Chang, H.H., Lillehoj, H.S., Lee, B.H., Min, W., 2012. Chicken IL-17F: Identification and comparative expression analysis in *Eimeria*-infected chickens. *Dev. Comp. Immunol.* 38, 401–409.

887. Kim, W.H., Lillehoj, H.S., 2019. Immunity, immunomodulation, and antibiotic alternatives to maximize the genetic potential of poultry for growth and disease response. *Anim. Feed Sci. Technol.* 250;41–50.

888. Kim, W.H., Lillehoj, H.S., Gay, C.G., 2016. Using genomics to identify novel antimicrobials. *Rev. Sci. Tech. Off. Int. Epiz.* 35, 95–103.

889. Kim, W.H., Lillehoj, H.S., Min, W., 2017. Evaluation of the immunomodulatory activity of the chicken NK-lysin-derived peptide cNK-2. *Sci. Rep.* 7, 45099.

890. Kim, W.H., Lillehoj, H.S., Min, W., 2019. Indole treatment alleviates intestinal tissue damage induced by chicken coccidiosis through activation of the aryl hydrocarbon receptor. *Front. Immunol.* 10, Article 560.

891. Kimbita, E.N., Silayo, R.S., Mwega, E.D., Mtau, A.T., Mroso, J.B., 2009. Studies on the *Eimeria* of goats at Magadu Dairy Farm SUA, Morogoro, Tanzania. *Trop. Anim. Health Prod.* 41, 1263–1265.

892. Kinnaird, J.H., Bumstead, J.M., Mann, D.J., Ryan, R., Shirley, M.W., Shiels, B.R., Tomley, F.M., 2004. EtCRK2, a cyclin-dependent kinase gene expressed during the sexual and asexual phases of the *Eimeria tenella* life cycle. *Int. J. Parasitol.* 34, 683–692.

892a. Kinne, J., Ali, M., Wernery, U., 2001. Camel coccidiosis caused by *Isospora orlovi* in the United Arab Emirates. *Emir. J. Agric. Sci.* 13, 62–65.

893. Kinne, J., Ali, M., Wernery, U., Dubey, J.P., 2002. Clinical large intestinal coccidiosis in camels (*Camelus dromedarius*) in the United Arab Emirates: Description of lesions, endogenous stages, and redescription of *Isospora orlovi*, Tsygankov, 1950 oocysts. *J. Parasitol.* 88, 548–552.

894. Kinne, J., Wernery, U., 1997. Severe outbreak of camel coccidiosis in the United Arab Emirates. *J. Camel Prac. Res.* 4, 261–265.

895. Kirino, Y., Tanida, M., Hasunuma, H., Kato, T., Irie, T., Horii, Y., Nonaka, N., 2015. Increase of *Clostridium perfringens* in association with *Eimeria* in haemorrhagic enteritis in Japanese beef cattle. *Vet. Rec.* 177, 202.

896. Kirkman, L.A., Deitsch, K.W., 2014. Recombination and diversification of the variant antigen encoding genes in the malaria parasite *Plasmodium falciparum*. *Microbiol. Spectr.* 2. doi: 10.1128/microbiolspec.MDNA3-0022-2014.

897. Kitajima, M., Haramoto, E., Iker, B.C., Gerba, C.P., 2014. Occurrence of *Cryptosporidium*, *Giardia*, and *Cyclospora* in influent and effluent water at wastewater treatment plants in Arizona. *Sci. Total Environ.* 484, 129–136.

898. Kitchen, D., Gaafar, S.M., 1974. *Eimeria leuckarti* in a horse from Indiana (a case report). *Vet. Med. Small Anim. Clin.* 69, 408–412.

899. Klesius, P.H., Kristensen, F., Elston, A.L., Williamson, O.C., 1977. *Eimeria bovis*: Evidence for a cell-mediated immune response in bovine coccidiosis. *Exp. Parasitol.* 41, 480–490.

900. Klimes, B., Rootes, D.G., Tanielian, Z., 1972. Sexual differentiation of merozoites of *Eimeria tenella*. *Parasitology* 65, 131–136.

901. Klotz, C., Marhöfer, R.J., Selzer, P.M., Lucius, R., Pogonka, T., 2005. *Eimeria tenella*: Identification of secretory and surface proteins from expressed sequence tags. *Exp. Parasitol.* 111, 14–23.

902. Kniel, K.E., Shearer, A.E.H., Cascarino, J.L., Wilkins, G.C., Jenkins, M.C., 2007. High hydrostatic pressure and UV light treatment of produce contaminated with *Eimeria acervulina* as a *Cyclospora cayetanensis* surrogate. *J. Food Prot.* 70, 2837–2842.

903. Koçkaya, M., Özsensoy, Y., 2016. Determination of some blood parameters and macro elements in coccidiosis affected Akkaraman Kangal lambs. *J. Asian Sci. Res.* 6, 138–142.

904. Koinari, M., Karl, S., Ryan, U., Lymbery, A.J., 2013. Infection levels of gastrointestinal parasites in sheep and goats in Papua New Guinea. *J. Helminthol.* 87, 409–415.

905. Kommuru, D.S., Barker, T., Desai, S., Burke, J.M., Ramsay, A., Mueller-Harvey, I., Miller, J.E., Mosjidis, J.A., Kamisetti, N., Terrill, T.H., 2014. Use of pelleted sericea lespedeza (*Lespedeza cuneata*) for natural control of coccidia and gastrointestinal nematodes in weaned goats. *Vet. Parasitol.* 204, 191–198.

906. Kong, F.Y., Ning, C.S., Yin, P.Y., 1994. A survey of drug resistance to coccidiostats of 15 field isolates of *Eimeria tenella* in China. *Acta Agr. Univ. Pekin.* 20, 302–308 (in Chinese).

907. Kong, Q.D., 2010. Diagnosis and treatment of duck coccidiosis. *Waterfowl World* 6, 31.

908. Koreeda, T., Kawakami, T., Okada, A., Hirashima, Y., Imai, N., Sasai, K., Tanaka, S., Matsubayashi, M., Shibahara, T., 2017. Pathogenic characteristics of a novel intranuclear coccidia in Japanese black calves and its genetic identification as *Eimeria subspherica*. *Parasitol. Res.* 116, 3243–3247.

909. Koskela, K., Kohonen, P., Salminen, H., Uchida, T., Buerstedde, J.M., Lassila, O., 2004. Identification of a novel cytokine-like transcript differentially expressed in avian γδ T cells. *Immunogenetics* 55, 845–854.

910. Koudela, B., Boková, A., 1998. Coccidiosis in goats in the Czech Republic. *Vet. Parasitol.* 76, 261–267.

911. Koudela, B., Gomez, E., Abreu, R., Vítovec, J., 1989. Porcine neonatal coccidiosis in Cuba. *Folia Parasitol.* 36, 31–32.

912. Koudela, B., Kucerová, S., 1999. Role of acquired immunity and natural age resistance on course of *Isospora suis* coccidiosis in nursing piglets. *Vet. Parasitol.* 82, 93–99.

913. Koudela, B., Kucerová, S., 2000. Immunity against *Isospora suis* in nursing piglets. *Parasitol. Res.* 86, 861–863.

914. Koudela, B., Vítovec, J., 1992. Biology and pathogenicity of *Eimeria spinosa* Henry, 1931 in experimentally infected pigs. *Int. J. Parasitol.* 22, 651–656.

915. Koudela, B., Vítovec, J., Šonková, J., Vobrová, D., 1986. Kokcidióza sajících selat chovaných ve velkochovu. *Vet. Med. (Praha)* 31, 725–732.

916. Koudela, B., Vodstrcilová, M., Klimes, B., Vladik, P., Vítovec, J., 1991. Pouziti antikokcidika tortrazuril (Baycox, Bayer) pri kokcidioze sajicich selat. *Vet. Med. (Praha)* 36, 657–663.

917. Kreiner, T., Worliczek, H.L., Tichy, A., Joachim, A., 2011. Influence of toltrazuril treatment on parasitological parameters and health performance of piglets in the field—An Austrian experience. *Vet. Parasitol.* 183, 14–20.

918. Kuhnert, Y., Schmäschke, R., Daugschies, A., 2006. Vergleich verschiedener Verfahren zur Untersuchung von Saugferkelkot auf *Isospora suis*. *Berl. Münch. tierärztl. Wochenschr.* 119, 282–286.

919. Kulkarni, S., Patsute, S., Sane, S., Chandane, M., Vidhate, P., Risbud, A., 2013. Enteric pathogens in HIV infected and HIV uninfected individuals with diarrhea in Pune. *Trans. Roy. Soc. Trop. Med. Hyg.* 107, 648–652.

920. Kumar, H., Kawai, T., Akira, S., 2011. Pathogen recognition by the innate immune. *Int. Rev. Immunol.* 30, 16–34.

921. Kumar, N., Rao, T.K.S., Varghese, A., Rathor, V.S., 2013. Internal parasite management in grazing livestock. *J. Parasit. Dis.* 37, 151–157.

922. Kumar, S., Ghorui, S.K., Patil, N.V., 2016. *Eimeria leuckarti* from dromedaries camel calves. *J. Camel Prac. Res.* 23, 91–94.

923. Kumar, S., Rani, S., Dadhich, H., Mathur, M., 2015. Occurrence and pathological study of intestinal coccidiosis in camels (*Camelus dromedarius*) of western Rajasthan. *J. Camel Prac. Res.* 22, 79–84.

924. Kundu, K., Garg, R., Kumar, S., Mandal, M., Tomley, F.M., Blake, D.P., Banerjee, P.S., 2017. Humoral and cytokine response elicited during immunisation with recombinant immune mapped protein-1 (EtIMP-1) and oocysts of *Eimeria tenella*. *Vet. Parasitol.* 244, 44–53.

925. Kupke, A., 1923. Untersuchungen über *Globidium leuckarti* Flesch. *Z. Infektionskrankh. Parasitäre Krankh. Hyg. Haustiere* 24, 210–223.

926. Kurnosova, O.P., 2013. Species structure and features of distribution of intestinal protozoa of pet animals in the city of Moscow. *Russian J. Parasitol.* 1, 10–17.

927. Kurnosova, O.P., Arisov, M.V., Odoyevskaya, I.M., 2019. Intestinal parasites of pets and other house-kept animals in Moscow. *Helminthologia* 56, 108–117.

928. Kusiluka, L.J.M., Kambarage, D.M., Harrison, L.J.S., Daborn, C.J., Matthewman, R.W., 1998. Prevalence and seasonal patterns of coccidial infections in goats in two ecoclimatic areas in Morogoro, Tanzania. *Small Ruminant Res.* 30, 85–91.

929. Kutuzov, M.A., Andreeva, A.V., Voyno-Yasenetskaya, T.A., 2005. Regulation of apoptosis signal-regulating kinase 1 (ASK1) by polyamine levels via protein phosphatase 5. *J. Biol. Chem.* 280, 25388–25395.

930. Kutzer, E., 1969. *Eimeria leuckarti*, ein seltener Parasit von Pferd und Esel. *Dtsch. tierärztl. Wochenschr.* 76, 35–37.

931. Kvicerová, J., Pakandl, M., Hypša, V., 2008. Phylogenetic relationships among *Eimeria* spp. (Apicomplexa, Eimeriidae) infecting rabbits: Evolutionary significance of biological and morphological features. *Parasitology* 135, 443–452.

932. Laczay, P., Simon, F., Móra, Z.S., Lehel, J., 1989. Zur Kompatibilität der neueren Ionophor-Antikokzidika mit anderen Chemotherapeutika bei Broilern. *Dtsch. Tierärztl. Wochenschr.* 96, 449–451.

933. Laczay, P., Simon, F., Szurop, I., Voros, G., Lehel, J., 1988. Study of the compatibility of CH-402 antioxidant with ionophore antibiotics and other chemotherapeutics in broilers. *Magyar Állatorvosok Lapja* 43, 627–630.

934. Lagrange-Xélot, M., Porcher, R., Sarfati, C., de Castro, N., Carel, O., Magnier, J.D., Delcey, V., Molina, J.M., 2008. Isosporiasis in patients with HIV infection in the highly active antiretroviral therapy era in France. *HIV Med.* 9, 126–130.

935. Lai, A., Dong, G., Song, D., Yang, T., Zhang, X., 2018. Responses to dietary levels of methionine in broilers medicated or vaccinated against coccidia under *Eimeria tenella*-challenged condition. *BMC Vet. Res.* 14, 140.

936. Lai, M., Zhou, R.Q., Huang, H.C., Hu, S.J., 2011. Prevalence and risk factors associated with intestinal parasites in pigs in Chongqing, China. *Res. Vet. Sci.* 91, 121–124.

937. Lal, K., Bromley, E., Oakes, R., Prieto, J.H., Sanderson, S.J., Kurian, D., Hunt, L., et al., 2009. Proteomic comparison of four *Eimeria tenella* life-cycle stages: Unsporulated oocyst, sporulated oocyst, sporozoite and second-generation merozoite. *Proteomics* 9, 4566–4576.

938. Lalonde, L.F., Gajadhar, A.A., 2011. Detection and differentiation of coccidian oocysts by real-time PCR and melting curve analysis. *J. Parasitol.* 97, 725–730.

939. Lalonde, L.F., Gajadhar, A.A., 2016. Optimization and validation of methods for isolation and real-time PCR identification of protozoan oocysts on leafy green vegetables and berry fruits. *Food Waterborne Parasitol.* 2, 1–7.

940. Lan, L., Zuo, B., Ding, H., Huang, Y., Chen, X., Du, A., 2016. Anticoccidial evaluation of a traditional Chinese medicine—*Brucea javanica*—in broilers. *Poult. Sci.* 95, 811–818.

941. Langkjaer, M., Roepstorff, A., 2008. Survival of *Isospora suis* oocysts under controlled environmental conditions. *Vet. Parasitol.* 152, 186–193.

942. Langrová, I., 2000. Seasonal prevalence of the coccidium *Eimeria leuckarti* and intensity of faecal oocyst output in various categories of horses in the Czech Republic. *Scientia Agriculturae Bohemica* 31, 123–129.

943. Lappin, M.R., 2010. Update on the diagnosis and management of *Isospora* spp infections in dogs and cats. *Top. Comp. Anim. Med.* 25, 133–135.

944. Larki, S., Alborzi, A., Chegini, R., Amiri, R., 2018. A preliminary survey on gastrointestinal parasites of domestic ducks in Ahvaz, Southwest Iran. *Iran. J. Parasitol.* 13, 137–144.

945. Lassen, B., Bangoura, B., Lepik, T., Orro, T., 2015. Systemic acute phase proteins response in calves experimentally infected with *Eimeria zuernii*. *Vet. Parasitol.* 212, 140–146.

946. Lassen, B., Østergaard, S., 2012. Estimation of the economical effects of *Eimeria* infections in Estonian dairy herds using a stochastic model. *Prev. Vet. Med.* 106, 258–265.

947. Lassen, B., Viltrop, A., Järvis, T., 2009. Herd factors influencing oocyst production of *Eimeria* and *Cryptosporidium* in Estonian dairy cattle. *Parasitol. Res.* 105, 1211–1222.

948. Lassen, B., Viltrop, A., Raaperi, K., Jarvis, T., 2009. *Eimeria* and *Cryptosporidium* in Estonian dairy farms in regard to age, species, and diarrhoea. *Vet. Parasitol.* 166, 212–219.

949. Láu, H.D., 1982. Eimerideos parasitos de búfalos no estado do Pará, Belém, EMBRAPA-CPATU. *Boletim de Pesquisa* 42, 11p.

950. Le Sueur, C., Mage, C., Mundt, H.C., 2009. Efficacy of toltrazuril (Baycox 5% suspension) in natural infections with pathogenic *Eimeria* spp. in housed lambs. *Parasitol. Res.* 104, 1157–1162.

951. Leathem, W.D., Burns, W.C., 1967. Effects of the immune chicken on the endogenous stages of *Eimeria tenella*. *J. Parasitol.* 53, 180–185.

952. Lebkowska-Wieruszewska, B.I., Kowalski, C.J., 2010. Sulfachlorpyrazine residues depletion in turkey edible tissues. *J. Vet. Pharmacol. Ther.* 33, 389–395.

953. Lee, E.H., Remmler, O., Fernando, M.A., 1977. Sexual differentiation in *Eimeria tenella* (Sporozoa: Coccidia). *J. Parasitol.* 63, 155–156.

954. Lee, E.H., Winder, N.C., 1981. *Eimeria acervulina* infections from each of the four sporocysts of a single oocyst. *Can. J. Comp. Med.* 45, 203–204.

955. Lee, J.T., Eckert, N.H., Ameiss, K.A., Stevens, S.M., Anderson, P.N., Anderson, S.M., Barri, A., McElroy, A.P., Danforth, H.D., Caldwell, D.J., 2011. The effect of dietary protein level on performance characteristics of coccidiosis vaccinated and nonvaccinated broilers following mixed-species *Eimeria* challenge. *Poult. Sci.* 90, 1916–1925.

956. Lee, M.B., Lee, E.H., 2001. Coccidial contamination of raspberries: Mock contamination with *Eimeria acervulina* as a model for decontamination treatment studies. *J. Food Prot.* 64, 1854–1857.

957. Lee, R.P., 1954. The occurrence of the coccidian *Eimeria bukidnorensis* Tubangui 1931, in Nigerian cattle. *J. Parasitol.* 40, 464–466.

958. Lee, R.P., Armour, J., 1958. A note on *Eimeria braziliensis* Torres and Ramos 1939 and its relationship to *Eimeria bohmi* Supperer 1952. *J. Parasitol.* 44, 302–304.

959. Lee, R.P., Armour, J., 1959. The coccidia oocysts of Nigerian cattle. *Br. Vet. J.* 115, 6–17.

960. Lee, S., Fernando, M.A., 1998. Intracellular localization of viral RNA in *Eimeria necatrix* of the domestic fowl. *Parasitol. Res.* 84, 601–606.

961. Lee, S., Fernando, M.A., Nagy, E., 1996. dsRNA associated with virus-like particles in *Eimeria* spp. of the domestic fowl. *Parasitol. Res.* 82, 518–523.

962. Lee, S., Kim, J., Cheon, D.S., Moon, E.A., Seo, D.J., Jung, S., Shin, H., Choi, C., 2018. Identification of *Cystoisospora ohioensis* in a diarrheal dog in Korea. *Korean J. Parasitol.* 56, 371–374.

963. Lee, S.H., Dong, X., Lillehoj, H.S., Lamont, S.J., Suo, X., Kim, D.K., Lee, K.W., Hong, Y.H., 2016. Comparing the immune responses of two genetically *B*-complex disparate Fayoumi chicken lines to *Eimeria tenella*. *Br. Poult. Sci.* 57, 165–171.

964. Lee, S.H., Lillehoj, H.S., Jang, S.I., Lee, K.W., Kim, D.K., Lillehoj, E.P., Yancey, R.J., Dominowski, P.J., 2012. Evaluation of novel adjuvant *Eimeria* profilin complex on intestinal host immune responses against live *E. acervulina* challenge infection. *Avian Dis.* 56, 402–405.

965. Leek, R.G., Fayer, R., McLoughlin, D.K., 1976. Effect of monensin on experimental infections of *Eimeria ninakohlyakimovae* in lambs. *Am. J. Vet. Res.* 37, 339–341.

966. Leguia, G.P., Casas, E.A., 1998. *Eimeria ivitaensis* n. sp (Protozoa: Eimeriidae) en alpacas (*Lama pacos*). *Rev. Peru. Parasitol.* 13, 59–61.

967. Leibovitz, L., 1968. *Wenyonella philiplevinei*, n. sp., a coccidial organism of the White Pekin duck. *Avian Dis.* 12, 670–681.

968. Lemaitre, B., 2004. The road to toll. *Nat. Rev. Immunol.* 4, 521–527.

969. LeMay, M.A., Genteman, K.C., Weber, F.H., Lewis, D.O., Evans, N.A., 2001. Efficacy of *in ovo* vaccination with single and mixed species of live *Eimeria* oocysts. *Proceedings of the VIIIth International Coccidiosis Conference*, Sydney, Australia, p. 107.

970. Lenghaus, C., O'Callaghan, M.G., Rogers, C., 2004. Coccidiosis and sudden death in an adult alpaca (*Lama pacos*). *Aust. Vet. J.* 82, 711–712.

971. Lepp, D.L., Todd, K.S., 1974. Life cycle of *Isospora canis* Nemeséri, 1959 in the dog. *J. Protozool.* 21, 199–206.

972. Levine, A.S., Ivens, V., 1970. *The Coccidian Parasites (Protozoa, Sporozoa) of Ruminants*. University of Illinois Press. Urbana, IL, 1–278.

973. Levine, N.D., 1973. Introduction, history, and taxonomy. In Hammond, D.M. and Long, P.L. (Ed.), *The Coccidia, Eimeria, Isospora, Toxoplasma, and Related Genera*. University Park Press. Baltimore, MD, 1–22.

974. Levine, N.D., 1973. *Protozoan Parasites of Domestic Animals and of Man*. 2nd ed. Burgess Publishing Company, Minneapolis, Minnesota, USA, 1–406.

975. Levine, N.D., 1982. Taxonomy and life cycle of coccidia. In Long, P.L. (Ed.), *The Biology of Coccidia*. Edward Arnold. London. 1–34.

976. Levine, N.D., 1988. Progress in taxonomy of the apicomplexan protozoa. *J. Protozool.* 35, 518–520.

977. Levine, N.D., Corliss, J.O., Cox, F.E.G., Deroux, G., Grain, J., Honigberg, B.M., Leedale, G.F., et al., 1980. A newly revised classificaiton of the protozoa. *J. Protozool.* 27, 37–58.

978. Levine, N.D., Ivens, V., 1967. The sporulated oocysts of *Eimeria illinoisensis* n. sp. and of other species of *Eimeria* of the ox. *J. Protozool.* 14, 351–360.

979. Levine, N.D., Ivens, V., 1986. *The Coccidian Parasites (Protozoa, Apicomplexa) of Artiodactyla*. University of Illinois Press. Urbana, IL, 1–265.

980. Levine, P., 1939. The effect of sulfanilamide on the course of experimental avian coccidiosis. *Cornell Vet.* 29, 430–439.

981. Levine, P.P., 1938. *Eimeria hagani* n. sp. (Protozoa: Eimeriidae) a new coccidium of the chicken. *Cornell Vet.* 28, 263–266.

982. Levine, P.P., 1941. The coccidiostatic effect of sulfaguanidine (sulfanilyl guanidine). *Cornell Vet.* 31, 107.

983. Levine, P.P., 1942. A new coccidium pathogenic for chickens, *Eimeria brunetti* n. sp. (Protozoa: Eimeriidae). *Cornell Vet.* 32, 430–439.

984. Lew, A.E., Anderson, G.R., Minchin, C.M., Jeston, P.J., Jorgensen, W.K., 2003. Inter- and intra-strain variation and PCR detection of the internal transcribed spacer 1 (ITS-1) sequences of Australian isolates of *Eimeria* species from chickens. *Vet. Parasitol.* 112, 33–50.

985. Li, C., Gu, X., Lu, C., Liao, Q., Liu, X., Suo, X., 2018. Studies on the prevalence of chicken coccidiosis in China. *Acta Parasitol. Med. Entomol. Sinica* 25, 230–241 (in Chinese).

986. Li, C.B., Xie, H., Wu, W.W., Hou, X., 2015. Diagnosis and treatment of coccidiosis in juvenile Muscovy duck. *China Anim. Health* 17, 43–44 (in Chinese).

987. Li, G.Q., Kanu, S., Xiao, S.M., Xiang, F.Y., 2005. Responses of chickens vaccinated with a live attenuated multi-valent ionophore-tolerant *Eimeria* vaccine. *Vet. Parasitol.* 129, 179–186.

988. Li, J., Feng, J.M., Tan, W.L., 1990. A case report of duck coccidiosis. *Guangxi Anim. Sci. Vet. Med.* 6, 28 (in Chinese).

989. Li, J., Gu, W., Tao, J., Liu, Z., 2009. The effects of S-nitroso-glutathione on the activities of some isoenzymes in *Eimeria tenella* oocysts. *Vet. Parasitol.* 162, 236–240.

990. Li, J., Xing, T., Wang, L., Tao, J., Liu, Z., 2010. Inhibitory effect of S-nitroso-glutathione on *Eimeria tenella* oocysts was mainly limited to the early stages of sporogony. *Vet. Parasitol.* 173, 64–69.

991. Li, J.G., Liu, Z.P., Tao, J.P., 2008. The effects of nitric oxide donors on the sporulation of *Eimeria tenella* oocysts. *Vet. Parasitol.* 154, 336–340.

992. Li, K., Zhao, H.M., 2013. Comparative experiment on the efficacy of ionic antibiotics on duck coccidiosis. *Heilongjiang Anim. Sci. Vet. Med.* 18, 103–104 (in Chinese).

993. Li, S., Zheng, M.X., Xu, H.C., Cui, X.Z., Zhang, Y., Zhang, L., Yang, S.S., Xu, Z.Y., Bai, R., Sun, X.G., 2017. Mitochondrial pathways are involved in *Eimeria tenella*-induced apoptosis of chick embryo cecal epithelial cells. *Parasitol. Res.* 116, 225–235.

994. Li, W.C., Zhang, X.K., Du, L., Pan, L., Gong, P.T., Li, J.H., Yang, J., Li, H., Zhang, X.C., 2013. *Eimeria maxima*: Efficacy of recombinant *Mycobacterium bovis* BCG expressing apical membrane antigen1 against homologous infection. *Parasitol. Res.* 112, 3825–3833.

995. Li, Y., Wang, Y., Tao, G., Cui, Y., Suo, X., Liu, X., 2016. Prophylactic and therapeutic efficacy of ponazuril against rabbit coccidiosis. *Proceedings 11th World Rabbit Congress*, Qingdao, China, June 15–18, 2016, 567–570.

996. Li, Y., Zhang, X., Jia, Q., Geng, T., Zhang, Z., Ding, D., 2017. Immune enhancing effects of recombinant plasmid pcDNA3-IL-2 on chicken coccidiosis vaccine. *Chin. J. Vet. Sci.* 37, 456–460 (in Chinese).

997. Li, Z., Tang, X., Suo, J., Qin, M., Yin, G., Liu, X., Suo, X., 2015. Transgenic *Eimeria mitis* expressing chicken interleukin 2 stimulated higher cellular immune response in chickens compared with the wild-type parasites. *Front. Microbiol.* 6, 533.

998. Licois, D., Coudert, P., Bahagia, S., Rossi, G.L., 1992. Endogenous development of *Eimeria intestinalis* in rabbits (*Oryctolagus cuniculus*). *J. Parasitol.* 78, 1041–1048.

999. Licois, D., Coudert, P., Boivin, M., Drouet-Viard, F., Provôt, F., 1990. Selection and characterization of a precocious line of *Eimeria intestinalis*, an intestinal rabbit coccidium. *Parasitol. Res.* 76, 192–198.

1000. Licois, D., Coudert, P., Drouet-Viard, F., Boivin, M., 1994. *Eimeria* media: Selection and characterization of a precocious line. *Parasitol. Res.* 80, 48–52.

1001. Licois, D., Coudert, P., Drouet-Viard, F., Boivin, M., 1995. *Eimeria magna*: Pathogenicity, immunogenicity and selection of a precocious line. *Vet. Parasitol.* 60, 27–35.

1002. Licois, D., Coudert, P., Mongin, P., 1978. Changes in hydromineral metabolism in diarrhoeic rabbits. 1. A study of the changes in water metabolism. *Ann. Rech. Vét.* 9, 1–10.

1003. Licois, D., Coudert, P., Mongin, P., 1978. Changes in hydromineral metabolism in diarrhoeic rabbits. 2. Study of the modifications of electrolyte metabolism. *Ann. Rech. Vét.* 9, 453–464.

1004. Licois, D., Guillot, J.F., 1980. Évolution du nombre de colibacilles chez des lapereaux atteints de coccidiose intestinale. *Rec. Méd. Vét.* 156, 555–560.

1005. Licois, D., Mongin, P., 1980. Hypothèse sur la pathogénie de la diarrhée chez le lapin à partir de l'étude des contenus intestinaux. *Reprod. Nutr. Dévelop.* 20, 1209–1216.

1006. Lillehoj, H.S., 1986. Immune response during coccidiosis in SC and FP chickens. I. *In vitro* assessment of T cell proliferation response to stage-specific parasite antigens. *Vet. Immunol. Immunopathol.* 13, 321–330.

1007. Lillehoj, H.S., 1987. Effects of immunosuppression on avian coccidiosis: Cyclosporin A but not hormonal bursectomy abrogates host protective immunity. *Infect. Immun.* 55, 1616–1621.

1008. Lillehoj, H.S., 1989. Intestinal intraepithelial and splenic natural killer cell responses to eimerian infections in inbred chickens. *Infect. Immun.* 57, 1879–1884.

1009. Lillehoj, H.S., 1994. Analysis of *Eimeria acervulina*-induced changes in the intestinal T lymphocyte subpopulations in two chicken strains showing different levels of susceptibility to coccidiosis. *Res. Vet. Sci.* 56, 1–7.

1010. Lillehoj, H.S., 1998. Role of T lymphocytes and cytokines in coccidiosis. *Int. J. Parasitol.* 28, 1071–1081.

1011. Lillehoj, H.S., Bacon, L.D., 1991. Increase of intestinal intraepithelial lymphocytes expressing CD8 antigen following challenge infection with *Eimeria acervulina*. *Avian Dis.* 35, 294–301.

1012. Lillehoj, H.S., Choi, K.D., 1998. Recombinant chicken interferon-gamma-mediated inhibition of *Eimeria tenella* development in vitro and reduction of oocyst production and body weight loss following *Eimeria acervulina* challenge infection. *Avian Dis.* 42, 307–314.

1013. Lillehoj, H.S., Choi, K.D., Jenkins, M.C., Vakharia, V.N., Song, K.D., Han, J.Y., Lillehoj, E.P., 2000. A recombinant *Eimeria* protein inducing interferon-γ production: Comparison of different gene expression systems and immunization strategies for vaccination against coccidiosis. *Avian Dis.* 44, 379–389.

1014. Lillehoj, H.S., Jang, S.I., Lee, S.H., Lillehoj, E.P., 2015. Avian coccidiosis as a prototype intestinal disease—Host protective immunity and novel disease control strategies. In Niewold, T.A. (Ed.), *Intestinal Health: Key to Optimize Production.* Wageningen Academic Publishers. Gelderland, the Netherlands, 69–113.

1015. Lillehoj, H.S., Li, G., 2004. Nitric oxide production by macrophages stimulated with coccidia sporozoites, lipopolysaccharide, or interferon-γ, and its dynamic changes in SC and TK strains of chickens infected with *Eimeria tenella*. *Avian Dis.* 48, 244–253.

1016. Lillehoj, H.S., Lillehoj, E.P., 2000. Avian coccidiosis. A review of acquired intestinal immunity and vaccination strategies. *Avian Dis.* 44, 408–425.

1017. Lillehoj, H.S., Min, W., Dalloul, R.A., 2004. Recent progress on the cytokine regulation of intestinal immune responses to *Eimeria*. *Poult. Sci.* 83, 611–623.

1018. Lillehoj, H.S., Trout, J.M., 1996. Avian gut-associated lymphoid tissues and intestinal immune responses to *Eimeria* parasites. *Clin. Microbiol. Rev.* 9, 349–360.

1019. Lim, L., McFadden, G.I., 2010. The evolution, metabolism and functions of the apicoplast. *Phil. Trans. R. Soc. B* 365, 749–763.

1020. Lima, J D., 2004. Coccidiose dos ruminantes domésticos. *Rev. Bras. Parasitol. Vet.* 13 Supp. 1, 9–13.

1021. Lima, J.D., de Oliveira, A.R.S., Martins, N.E., Boretti, L.P., 1983. Coccidiosis in unweaned piglets in Minas Gerais. *Arq. Bras. Med. Vet. Zootec.* 35, 33–40.

1022. Lin, H.Y., Li, M.W., Xu, F.Z., 2006. A preliminary survey of duck coccidiosis in Zhangjiang, Quangdong. *Poultry Husb. Dis. Control* 7, 21–22 (in Chinese).

1023. Lin, K., Xiong, D., 1981. A preliminary investigation of the coccidian species of chicken in the Peking area. *Acta Agr. Univ. Pekin.* 1–11 (in Chinese).

1024. Lin, K.E., Yin, P.Y., Jiang, J.S., Liu, G.Y., Fan, G.X., Chen, J.J., Duan, J.F., 1982. An outbreak of duck coccidiosis in Beijing. *Chin. J. Vet. Med.* 3, 7–9 (in Chinese).

1025. Lin, K.E., Yin, P.Y., Suo, X., Liu, Q., Zhang, L.X., 2004. Comparative experiment on the efficacy on five ionic antibiotics against domestic coccidiosis. *Chin. J. Vet. Med.* 40, 63–64 (in Chinese).

1026. Lin, Q., Yu, S., Chen, X., Pan, G., Wang, T., Li, T., 2002. The establishment of *E. tenella* single-oocyst isolation technique and its pathogenicity in chicken. *J. Northwest Sci-Tech Univ. Agr. Forest.* 30, 35–37 (in Chinese).

1027. Lin, R.Q., Lillehoj, H.S., Lee, S.K., Oh, S., Panebra, A., Lillehoj, E.P., 2017. Vaccination with *Eimeria tenella* elongation factor-1α recombinant protein induces protective immunity against *E. tenella* and *E. maxima* infections. *Vet. Parasitol.* 243, 79–84.

1028. Lin, R.Q., Qiu, L.L., Liu, G.H., Wu, X.Y., Weng, Y.B., Xie, W.Q., Hou, J., et al., 2011. Characterization of the complete mitochondrial genomes of five *Eimeria* species from domestic chickens. *Gene* 480, 28–33.

1029. Lin, Z.W., 2009. A clinical report of *Tyzzeria perniciosa* in juvenile Muscovy duck. *Fujian J. Anim. Sci. Vet. Med.* 31, 59–60 (in Chinese).

1030. Lindenthal, C., Klinkert, M.Q., 2002. Identification and biochemical characterisation of a protein phosphatase 5 homologue from *Plasmodium falciparum*. *Mol. Biochem. Parasitol.* 120, 257–268.

1031. Lindsay, D.S., 1989. Diagnosing and controlling *Isospora suis* in nursing pigs. *Vet. Med.* 84, 443–448.

1032. Lindsay, D.S., Blagburn, B.L., 1987. Development of *Isospora suis* from pigs in primary porcine and bovine cell cultures. *Vet. Parasitol.* 24, 301–304.

1033. Lindsay, D.S., Blagburn, B.L., 1994. Biology of mammalian *Isospora*. *Parasitol. Today* 10, 214–220.

1034. Lindsay, D.S., Blagburn, B.L., Boosinger, T.R., 1987. Experimental *Eimeria debliecki* infections in nursing and weaned pigs. *Vet. Parasitol.* 25, 39–45.

1035. Lindsay, D.S., Blagburn, B.L., Current, W.L., Ernst, J.V., 1985. Development of the swine coccidium *Eimeria debliecki* Douwes, 1921 in mammalian cell cultures. *J. Protozool.* 32, 669–671.

1036. Lindsay, D.S., Blagburn, B.L., Powe, T.A., 1992. Enteric coccidial infections and coccidiosis in swine. *Comp. Cont. Edu. Pract. Vet.* 14, 698–702.

1037. Lindsay, D.S., Blagburn, B.L., Toivio-Kinnucan, M., 1991. Ultrastructure of developing *Isospora suis* in cultured cells. *Am. J. Vet. Res.* 52, 471–473.

1038. Lindsay, D.S., Butler, J.M., Rippey, N.S., Blagburn, B.L., 1996. Demonstration of synergistic effects of sulfonamides and dihydrofolate reductase/thymidylate synthase inhibitors against *Neospora caninum* tachyzoites in cultured cells, and characterization of mutants resistant to pyrimethamine. *Am. J. Vet. Res.* 57, 68–72.

1039. Lindsay, D.S., Current, W.L., Ernst, J.V., 1982. Sporogony of *Isospora suis* Biester, 1934 of swine. *J. Parasitol.* 68, 861–865.

1040. Lindsay, D.S., Current, W.L., Ernst, J.V., Stuart, B.P., 1983. Diagnosis of neonatal porcine coccidiosis caused by *Isospora suis*. *Vet. Med. Small Anim. Clin.* 87, 89–94.

1041. Lindsay, D.S., Current, W.L., Haynes, T.B., 1983. Comparative development of *Isospora suis* in piglets, chicken embryos, and cell culture. *Proceedings, Fourth International Symposium on Neonatal Diarrhea October 3–5, 1983. University of Saskatchewan*, Saskatoon, Saskatchewan, Canada, 333–341.

1042. Lindsay, D.S., Current, W.L., Taylor, J.R., 1985. Effects of experimentally induced *Isospora suis* infection on morbidity, mortality, and weight gains in nursing pigs. *Am. J. Vet. Res.* 46, 1511–1512.

1043. Lindsay, D.S., Dubey, J.P., Blagburn, B.L., 1997. Biology of *Isospora* spp. from humans, nonhuman primates, and domestic animals. *Clin. Microbiol. Rev.* 10, 19–34.

1044. Lindsay, D.S., Dubey, J.P., Fayer, R., 1990. Extraintestinal stages of *Eimeria bovis* in calves and attempts to induce relapse of clinical disease. *Vet. Parasitol.* 36, 1–9.

1045. Lindsay, D.S., Dubey, J.P., Toivio-Kinnucan, M.A., Michiels, J.F., Blagburn, B.L., 1997. Examination of extraintestinal tissue cysts of *Isospora belli*. *J. Parasitol.* 83, 620–625.

1046. Lindsay, D.S., Ernst, J.V., Benz, G.W., Current, W.L., 1988. The sexual stages of *Eimeria wyomingensis* Huizinga and Winger, 1942, in experimentally infected calves. *J. Parasitol.* 74, 833–837.

1047. Lindsay, D.S., Ernst, J.V., Current, W.L., Stuart, B.P., Stewart, T.B., 1984. Prevalence of oocysts of *Isospora suis* and *Eimeria* spp. from sows on farms with and without a history of neonatal coccidiosis. *J. Am. Vet. Med. Assoc.* 185, 419–421.

1048. Lindsay, D.S., Houk, A.E., Mitchell, S.M., Dubey, J.P., 2014. Developmental biology of *Cystoisospora* (Apicomplexa: Sarcocystidae) monozoic tissue cysts. *J. Parasitol.* 100, 392–398.

1049. Lindsay, D.S., Neiger, R., Hildreth, M., 2002. Porcine enteritis associated with *Eimeria spinosa* Henry, 1931 infection. *J. Parasitol.* 88, 1262–1263.

1050. Lindsay, D.S., Quick, D.P., Steger, A.M., Toivio-Kinnucan, M.A., Blagburn, B.L., 1998. Complete development of the porcine coccidium *Isospora suis* Biester, 1934 in cell cultures. *J. Parasitol.* 84, 635–637.

1051. Lindsay, D.S., Stuart, B.P., Wheat, B.E., Ernst, J.V., 1980. Endogenous development of the swine coccidium, *Isospora suis* Biester 1934. *J. Parasitol.* 66, 771–779.

1052. Ling, K.H., Rajandream, M.A., Rivailler, P., Ivens, A., Yap, S.J., Madeira, A.M.B.N., Mungall, K., et al., 2007. Sequencing and analysis of chromosome 1 of *Eimeria tenella* reveals a unique segmental organization. *Genome Res.* 17, 311–319.

1053. Lipscomb, T.P., Dubey, J.P., Pletcher, J.M., Altman, N.H., 1989. Intraheptic biliary coccidiosis in a dog. *Vet. Pathol.* 26, 343–345.

1054. Liu, C.M., Hermann, T.E., Downey, A., Prosser, B.L.T., Schildknecht, E., Palleroni, N.J., Westley, J.W., Miller, P.A., 1983. Novel polyether antibiotics X-14868A, B, C, and D produced by a *Nocardia*. Discovery, fermentation, biological as well as ionophore properties and taxonomy of the producing culture. *J. Antibiot. (Tokyo)* 36, 343–350.

1055. Liu, D., Cao, L., Zhu, Y., Deng, C., Su, S., Xu, J., Jin, W., Li, J., Wu, L., Tao, J., 2014. Cloning and characterization of an *Eimeria necatrix* gene encoding a gametocyte protein and associated with oocyst wall formation. *Parasit. Vectors* 7, 27.

1056. Liu, D., Li, J., Cao, L., Wang, S., Han, H., Wu, Y., Tao, J., 2014. Analysis of differentially expressed genes in two immunologically distinct strains of *Eimeria maxima* using suppression subtractive hybridization and dot-blot hybridization. *Parasit. Vectors* 7, 259.

1057. Liu, G.H., Hou, J., Weng, Y.B., Song, H.Q., Li, S., Yuan, Z.G., Lin, R.Q., Zhu, X.Q., 2012. The complete mitochondrial genome sequence of *Eimeria mitis* (Apicomplexa: Coccidia). *Mitochondrial DNA* 23, 341–343.

1058. Liu, G.H., Tian, S.Q., Cui, P., Fang, S.F., Wang, C.R., Zhu, X.Q., 2015. The complete mitochondrial genomes of five *Eimeria* species infecting domestic rabbits. *Exp. Parasitol.* 159, 67–71.

1059. Liu, J., Liu, X., Cai, J., Suo, X., 2018. Early research in coccidiosis in China. *Acta Parasitol. Med. Entomol. Sinica* 4, 1–12 (in Chinese).

1060. Liu, L., 2014. A case report of duck coccidiosis. *Modern Anim. Husb. Technol.* 5, 217 (in Chinese).

1061. Liu, L., Chen, H., Fei, C., Wang, X., Zheng, W., Wang, M., Zhang, K., Zhang, L., Li, T., Xue, F., 2016. Ultrastructural effects of acetamizuril on endogenous phases of *Eimeria tenella*. *Parasitol. Res.* 115, 1245–1252.

1062. Liu, L., Huang, X., Liu, J., Li, W., Ji, Y., Tian, D., Tian, L., et al., 2017. Identification of common immunodominant antigens of *Eimeria tenella*, *Eimeria acervulina* and *Eimeria maxima* by immunoproteomic analysis. *Oncotarget* 8, 34935–34945.

1063. Liu, L., Xu, L., Yan, F., Yan, R., Song, X., Li, X., 2009. Immunoproteomic analysis of the second-generation merozoite proteins of *Eimeria tenella*. *Vet. Parasitol.* 164, 173–182.

1064. Liu, L.H., 1999. Diagnosis and treatment of coccidiosis in duckling. *Chin. J. Anim. Infect. Dis.* 3, 64 (in Chinese).

1065. Liu, L.L., Chen, Z.G., Mi, R.S., Zhang, K.Y., Liu, Y.C., Jiang, W., Fei, C.Z., Xue, F.Q., Li, T., 2016. Effect of acetamizuril on enolase in second-generation merozoites of *Eimeria tenella*. *Vet. Parasitol.* 215, 88–91.

1066. Liu, Q., Chen, Z., Shi, W., Sun, H., Zhang, J., Li, H., Xiao, Y., Wang, F., Zhao, X., 2014. Preparation and initial application of monoclonal antibodies that recognize *Eimeria tenella* microneme proteins 1 and 2. *Parasitol. Res.* 113, 4151–4161.

1067. Liu, R., Ma, X., Liu, A., Zhang, L., Cai, J., Wang, M., 2014. Identification and characterization of a cathepsin-L-like peptidase in *Eimeria tenella*. *Parasitol. Res.* 113, 4335–4348.

1068. Liu, S., Wang, L., Zheng, H., Xu, Z., Roellig, D.M., Li, N., Frace, M.A., et al., 2016. Comparative genomics reveals *Cyclospora cayetanensis* possesses coccidia-like metabolism and invasion components but unique surface antigens. *BMC Genomics* 17, 316.

1069. Liu, T., Huang, J., Ehsan, M., Wang, S., Fei, H., Zhou, Z., Song, X., Yan, R., Xu, L., Li, X., 2018. Protective immunity against *Eimeria maxima* induced by vaccines of Em14–3–3 antigen. *Vet. Parasitol.* 253, 79–86.

1070. Liu, X., Gong, Z., Ma, X., Qu, Z., Han, Z., Liu, B., Yuan, R., Yang, X., Cai, J., 2017. Expression profiling of polypeptide: N-acetylgalactosaminyl-transferase T2 during *Eimeria tenella* development cycle. *Acta Vet. Zootech. Sinica* 48, 2173–2180 (in Chinese).

1071. Liu, X., Shi, T., Ren, H., Su, H., Yan, W., Suo, X., 2008. Restriction enzyme-mediated transfection improved transfection efficiency *in vitro* in Apicomplexan parasite *Eimeria tenella*. *Mol. Biochem. Parasitol.* 161, 72–75.

1072. Logan, N.B., McKenzie, M.E., Conway, D.P., Chappel, L.R., Hammet, N.C., 1993. Anticoccidial efficacy of semduramicin. 2. Evaluation against field isolates including comparisons with salinomycin, maduramicin, and monensin in battery tests. *Poult. Sci.* 72, 2058–2063.

1073. Long, E.G., White, E.H., Carmichael, W.W., Quinlisk, P.M., Raja, R., Swisher, B.L., Daugharty, H., Cohen, M.T., 1991. Morphologic and staining characteristics of a *Cyanobacterium*-like organism associated with diarrhea. *J. Infect. Dis.* 164, 199–202.

1074. Long, P.L., 1968. The pathogenic effects of *Eimeria praecox* and *E. acervulina* in the chicken. *Parasitology* 58, 691–700.

1075. Long, P.L., 1972. *Eimeria tenella*: Reproduction, pathogenicity and immunogenicity of a strain maintained in chick embryos by serial passage. *J. Comp. Pathol.* 82, 429–437.

1076. Long, P.L., 1973. Endogenous stages of a "chick embryo-adapted" strain of *Eimeria tenella*. *Parasitology* 66, 55–62.

1077. Long, P.L., 1973. Pathology and pathogenicity of coccidial infections. In Hammond, D.M. and Long, P.L. (Ed.), *The Coccidia: Eimeria, Isospora, Toxoplasma, and Related Genera*. University Park Press. Baltimore, MD, 253–294.

1078. Long, P.L., 1974. Experimental infection of chickens with two species of *Eimeria* isolated from the Malaysian jungle fowl. *Parasitology* 69, 337–347.

1079. Long, P.L., 1974. Further studies on the pathogenicity and immunogenicity of an embryo-adapted strain of *Eimeria tenella*. *Avian Pathol.* 3, 255–268.

1080. Long, P.L., Joyner, L.P., 1984. Problems in the identification of species of *Eimeria*. *J. Protozool.* 31, 535–541.

1081. Long, P.L., Millard, B.J., 1979. *Eimeria*: Further studies on the immunisation of young chickens kept in litter pens. *Avian Pathol.* 8, 213–228.

1082. Long, P.L., Millard, B.J., 1979. Immunological differences in *Eimeria maxima*: Effect of a mixed immunizing inoculum on heterologous challenge. *Parasitology* 79, 451–457.

1083. Long, P.L., Millard, B.J., 1979. Studies on *Eimeria dispersa* Tyzzer 1929 in turkeys. *Parasitology* 78, 41–51.

1084. Long, P.L., Millard, B.J., Joyner, L.P., Norton, C.C., 1976. A guide to laboratory techniques used in the study and diagnosis of avian coccidiosis. *Folia Vet. Lat.* 6, 201–217.

1085. Long, P.L., Millard, B.J., Shirley, M.W., 1977. Strain variation within *Eimeria meleagrimitis* from the turkey. *Parasitology* 75, 177–182.

1086. Long, P.L., Millard, B.J., Smith, K.M., 1979. The effect of some anticoccidial drugs on the development of immunity to coccidiosis in field and laboratory conditions. *Avian Pathol.* 8, 453–467.

1087. Long, P.L., Tompkins, R.V., Millard, B.J., 1975. Coccidiosis in broilers: Evaluation of infection by the examination of broiler house litter for oocysts. *Avian Pathol.* 4, 287–294.

1088. Lopes, W.D.Z., Carvalho, R.S., Pereira, V., Martinez, A.C., Cruz, B.C., Teixeira, W.F., Maciel, W.G., et al., 2014. Efficacy of sulfadoxine + trimethoprim compared to managment measures for the control of *Eimeria* parasitism in naturally infected and clinically asymptomatic sheep that were maintained in a feedlot. *Small Ruminant Res.* 116, 37–43.

1089. Lopez, A.S., Bendik, J.M., Alliance, J.Y., Roberts, J.M., da Silva, A.J., Moura, I.N.S., Arrowood, M.J., Eberhard, M.L., Herwaldt, B.L., 2003. Epidemiology of *Cyclospora cayetanensis* and other intestinal parasites in a community in Haiti. *J. Clin. Microbiol.* 41, 2047–2054.

1090. López-Osorio, S., Silva, L.M.R., Taubert, A., Chaparro-Gutiérrez, J.J., Hermosilla, C.R., 2018. Concomitant *in vitro* development of *Eimeria zuernii*- and *Eimeria bovis*-macromeronts in primary host endothelial cells. *Parasitol. Int.* 67, 742–750.

1091. Lotze, J.C., 1952. The pathogenicity of the coccidian parasite, *Eimeria arloingi*, in domestic sheep. *Cornell Vet.* 42, 510–517.

1092. Lotze, J.C., 1954. The pathogenicity of the coccidian parasite, *Eimeria ninae-kohl-yakimovi*, Yakiniov and Rastegaeva, 1930, in domestic sheep. *Proceedings 90th Annu. Meet. Amer. Vet. Med. Ass.* 141–146.

1093. Lotze, J.C., Leek, R.G., Shalkop, W.T., Behin, R., 1961. Coccidial parasites in the "wrong host" animal. *J. Parasitol.* 47, 34.

1094. Lotze, J.C., Shalkop, W.T., Leek, R.G., Behin, R., 1964. Coccidial schizonts in mesenteric lymph nodes of sheep and goats. *J. Parasitol.* 50, 205–208.

1095. Love, D., Gibbons, P., Fajt, V., Jones, M., 2015. Pharmacokinetics of single-dose oral ponazuril in weanling goats. *J. Vet. Pharmacol. Therap.* 39, 305–308.

1096. Lu, G., 1994. A preliminary survey of duck coccidiosis in Chaohu. *Chin. J. Anim. Infect. Dis.* 2, 28–32 (in Chinese).

1097. Lu, H.H., Zhang, Y.H., Zhu, X.H., 2009. Diagnosis and treatment of Muscovy duck coccidiosis. *Shanghai J. Anim. Husb. Vet. Med.* 3, 106 (in Chinese).

1098. Lu, S.M., Yin, P.Y., Jiang, J.S., 1985. The efficacy of sulfonamides on treating *Tyzzeria perniciosa* in Pekin duck. *Chin. J. Vet. Med.* 21, 9–10 (in Chinese).

1099. Luis Enrique, J.P., Moreno, L.R., Núñez Fernández, F.A., Millán, I.A., Rivero, L.R., González, F.R., Pérez Rodríguez, J.C., 2018. Prevalence of intestinal parasitic infections in dogs from Havana, Cuba: Risk of zoonotic infections to humans. *Anim. Husb. Dairy Vet. Sci.* 2, 1–5.

1100. Lund, E.E., 1954. The effect of sulfaquinoxaline on the course of *Eimeria stiedae* infections in the domestic rabbit. *Exp. Parasitol.* 3, 497–503.

1101. Lv, L., Huang, B., Zhao, Q., Zhao, Z., Dong, H., Zhu, S., Chen, T., Yan, M., Han, H., 2018. Identification of an interaction between calcium-dependent protein kinase 4 (EtCDPK4) and serine protease inhibitor (EtSerpin) in *Eimeria tenella*. *Parasit. Vectors* 11, 259.

1102. Lyons, E.T., Drudge, J.H., Tolliver, S.C., 1988. Natural infection with *Eimeria leuckarti*: Prevalence of oocysts in feces of horse foals on several farms in Kentucky during 1986. *Am. J. Vet. Res.* 49, 96–98.

1103. Lyons, E.T., Tolliver, S.C., 2004. Prevalence of parasite eggs (*Strongyloides westeri*, *Parascaris equorum*, and strongyles) and oocysts (*Eimeria leuckarti*) in the feces of Thoroughbred foals on 14 farms in central Kentucky in 2003. *Parasitol. Res.* 92, 400–404.

1104. Lyons, E.T., Tolliver, S.C., Collins, S.S., 2006. Field studies on endoparasites of Thoroughbred foals on seven farms in central Kentucky in 2004. *Parasitol. Res.* 98, 496–500.

1105. Lyons, E.T., Tolliver, S.C., Rathgeber, R.A., Collins, S.S., 2007. Parasite field study in central Kentucky on thoroughbred foals (born in 2004) treated with pyrantel tartrate daily and other parasiticides periodically. *Parasitol. Res.* 100, 473–478.

1106. Ma, C., Zhang, L., Gao, M., Ma, D., 2017. Construction of *Lactococcus lactis* expressing secreted and anchored *Eimeria tenella* 3-1E protein and comparison of protective immunity against homologous challenge. *Exp. Parasitol.* 178, 14–20.

1107. Ma, D., Gao, M., Dalloul, R.A., Ge, J., Ma, C., Li, J., 2013. Protective effects of oral immunization with live *Lactococcus lactis* expressing *Eimeria tenella* 3-1E protein. *Parasitol. Res.* 112, 4161–4167.

1108. Macdonald, S.E., Nolan, M.J., Harman, K., Boulton, K., Hume, D.A., Tomley, F.M., Stabler, R.A., Blake, D.P., 2017. Effects of *Eimeria tenella* infection on chicken caecal microbiome diversity, exploring variation associated with severity of pathology. *PLOS ONE* 12, e0184890.

1109. Macrelli, M., Dunnett, L., Mitchell, S., Carson, A., 2019. Coccidiosis in sheep. *Vet. Rec.* 184, 549–550.

1110. Madibela, O.R., Kelemogile, K.M., 2008. Exposure of *Melia azedarach* fruits to *Eimeria* lowers oocyst output in yearling Tswana goats. *Small Ruminant Res.* 76, 207–210.

1111. Madsen, P., Henriksen, S.A., Larsen, K., 1994. Prophylactic treatment of *Isospora suis* coccidiosis in piglets with toltrazuril in a special oral suspension. *Proc. 13th IPVS Congress*, Bangkok, Thailand, 256–257.

1112. Maes, D., Vyt, P., Rabaeys, P., Gevaert, D., 2007. Effects of toltrazuril on the growth of piglets in herds without clinical isosporosis. *Vet. J.* 173, 197–199.

1113. Maes, L., Coussement, W., Vanparijs, O., Marsboom, R., 1988. *In vivo* action of the anticoccidial diclazuril (Clinacox) on the developmental stages of *Eimeria tenella*: A histological study. *J. Parasitol.* 74, 931–938.

1114. Mahmoud, O.M., Haroun, E.M., Magzoub, M., Omer, O.H., Sulman, A., 1998. Coccidial infection in camels of Gassim region, Central Saudi Arabia. *J. Camel Prac. Res.* 5, 257–260.

1115. Mahran, O.M., 2006. Some epidemiological and parasitological studies on prevalence of gastrointestinal parasites of dromedary camels at Shalatin Region, Red Sea Governorate, Egypt and trails of treatment. *Assiut Vet. Med. J.* 52, 149–162.

1116. Mahrt, J.L., 1967. Endogenous stages of the life cycle of *Isospora rivolta* in the dog. *J. Protozool.* 14, 754–759.

1117. Mai, K., Sharman, P.A., Walker, R.A., Katrib, M., de Souza, D., McConville, M.J., Wallach, M.G., Belli, S.I., Ferguson, D.J.P., Smith, N.C., 2009. Oocyst wall formation and composition in coccidian parasites. *Mem. Inst. Oswaldo Cruz* 104, 281–289.

1118. Mai, T., Yin, N., Wang, Y.P., Yan, J.W., 2015. China's waterfowl industry: Status quo and production policies—From the perspective of utilization of domestic and international resources. *Guangdong Agric. Sci.* 42, 178–186 (in Chinese).

1119. Main, D.C., Creeper, J.H., 1999. Coccidiosis of Brunner's glands in feral goats. *Aust. Vet. J.* 77, 49.

1120. Mamun, M.A.A., Begum, N., Mondal, M.M.H., 2011. A coprological survey of gastro-intestinal parasites of water buffaloes (*Bubalus bubalis*) in Kurigram district of Bangladesh. *J. Bangladesh Agril. Univ.* 9, 103–109.

1121. Männer, K., Matuschka, F.R., Seehawer, J., 1981. Einfluß einer Monoinfektion mit *Isospora suis* und ihre Behandlung mit Halofuginon und Lasalocid auf die Aufzuchtleistungen, Verdauungskoeffizienten und die stoffliche Zusammensetzung der Ganztierkörper frühabgesetzter Ferkel. *Berl. Münch. tierärztl. Wochenschr.* 94, 25–33.

1122. Mao, L.S., Wang, H.D., 2012. Diagnosis and treatment of Muscovy duck coccidiosis. *Zheijiang Anim. Sci. Vet. Med.* 37, 32 (in Chinese).

1123. Maphosa, V., Masika, P.J., 2012. *In vivo* validation of *Aloe ferox* (Mill). *Elephantorrhiza elephantina* Bruch. Skeels. and *Leonotis leonurus* (L) R. BR as potential anthelminthics and antiprotozoals against mixed infections of gastrointestinal nematodes in goats. *Parasitol. Res.* 110, 103–108.

1124. Maratea, K.A., Miller, M.A., 2007. Abomasal coccidiosis associated with proliferative abomasitis in a sheep. *J. Vet. Diagn. Invest.* 19, 118–121.

1125. Marhöfer, R.J., Mottram, J.C., Selzer, P.M., 2013. Protein kinases as suitable targets for combating *Eimeria* spp. In Doerig, C., Späth, G., and Wiese, M. (Ed.), *Parotein Phosphorylation in Parasites*. Wiley-VCH Verlag GmbH & Co. KGaA. Weinheim, Germany, 317–336.

1126. Markus, M.B., 1983. The hypnozoite of *Isospora canis*. *S. Afr. J. Sci.* 79, 117.

1127. Maron, M.I., Magle, C.T., Czesny, B., Turturice, B.A., Huang, R., Zheng, W., Vaidya, A.B., Williamson, K.C., 2016. Maduramicin rapidly eliminates malaria parasites and potentiates the gametocytocidal activity of the pyrazoleamide PA21A050. *Antimicrob. Agents Chemother.* 60, 1492–1499.

1128. Marquardt, W.C., 1959. The morphology and sporulation of the oocyst of *Eimeria brazilensis*, Torres and Ildefonso Ramos 1939, of cattle. *Am. J. Vet. Res.* 20, 742–746.

1129. Marquardt, W.C., 1960. Effect of high temperature on sporulation of *Eimeria zurnii*. *Exp. Parasitol.* 10, 58–65.

1130. Marquardt, W.C., 1973. Host and site specificity in the coccidia. In Hammond, D.M. and Long, P.L. (Ed.), *The Coccidia: Eimeria, Isospora, Toxoplasma, and Related Genera*. University Park Press. Baltimore, MD, 23–43.

1131. Marreros, N., Frey, C.F., Willisch, C.S., Signer, C., Ryser-Degiorgis, M.P., 2012. Coprological analyses on apparently healthy Alpine ibex (*Capra ibex ibex*) from two Swiss colonies. *Vet. Parasitol.* 186, 382–289.

1132. Martin, A.G., Danforth, H.D., Barta, J.R., Fernando, M.A., 1997. Analysis of immunological cross-protection and sensitivities to anticoccidial drugs among five geographical and temporal strains of *Eimeria maxima*. *Int. J. Parasitol.* 27, 527–533.

1133. Martineau, G.P., del Castillo, J., 2000. Epidemiological, clinical and control investigations on field porcine coccidiosis: Clinical, epidemiological and parasitological paradigms? *Parasitol. Res.* 86, 834–837.

1134. Martino, P.E., Parrado, E., Sanguinetti, R., Espinoza, C., Debenedetti, R., Di Benedetto, N.M., Cisterna, C., Gómez, P., 2009. Short communication: Massive mortality in rabbits by maduramicin poisoning. *World Rabbit Sci.* 17, 45–48.

1135. Mathea, J., 1993. Vorkommen von *Isospora suis* und *Cryptosporidium parvum* beim Ferkel in Schweinebeständen mit unterschiedlichen Haltungsbedingungen. Dr. med. vet. thesis. Free Univ., Berlin.

1136. Mathis, G.F., 1989. Epidemiology of coccidia isolated from turkey farms on an amprolium anticoccidial program. *Poult. Sci.* 68 (Suppl 1), 90.

1137. Mathis, G.F., 1999. The influence of the coccidiosis vaccine, Coccivac-Bw, on compensatory weight gain of broiler chickens in comparison with the anticoccidial, salinomycin. *Poult. Sci.* 12 (Suppl 1), 117.

1138. Mathis, G.F., Broussard, C., 2006. Increased level of *Eimeria* sensitivity to diclazuril after using a live coccidial vaccine. *Avian Dis.* 50, 321–324.

1139. Mathis, G.F., Newman, L.J., Fitz-Coy, S., Lumpkins, B., Charette, R., 2018. Comparison of breeder/layer coccidiosis vaccines: Part 2: Onset of immunity—Attenuated vaccines. *J. Appl. Poult. Res.* 27, 38–44.

1140. Matjila, P.T., Penzhorn, B.L., 2002. Occurrence and diversity of bovine coccidia at three localities in South Africa. *Vet. Parasitol.* 104, 93–102.

1141. Matos, L., Muñoz, M.C., Molina, J.M., Ferrer, O., Rodríguez, F., Pérez, D., López, A.M., et al., 2017. Humoral immune responses of experimentally *Eimeria ninakholyakimovae*-infected goat kids. *Comp. Immunol. Microbiol. Infect. Dis.* 51, 60–65.

1142. Matos, L., Muñoz, M.C., Molina, J.M., Rodríguez, F., Perez, D., Lopez, A., Ferrer, O., Hermosilla, C., Taubert, A., Ruiz, A., 2017. Protective immune responses during prepatency in goat kids experimentally infected with *Eimeria ninakohlyakimovae*. *Vet. Parasitol.* 242, 1–9.

1143. Matos, L., Muñoz, M.C., Molina, J.M., Rodríguez, F., Pérez, D., López, A.M., Hermosilla, C., Taubert, A., Ruiz, A., 2018. Age-related immune response to experimental infection with *Eimeria ninakohlyakimovae* in goat kids. *Res. Vet. Sci.* 118, 155–163.

1144. Matos, M.N., Cazorlia, S.I., Schulze, K., Ebensen, T., Guzmán, C.A., Malchiodi, E.L., 2017. Immunization with Tc52 or its amino terminal domain adjuvanted with c-di-AMP induces Th17+Th1 specific immune responses and confers protection against *Trypanosoma cruzi*. *PLOS Negl. Trop. Dis.* 11, e0005300.

1145. Matsche, M.A., Adams, C.R., Blazer, V.S., 2019. Newly described coccidia *Goussia bayae* from white perch *Morone americana*: Morphology and phylogentics support emerging taxonomy of *Goussia* within piscine hosts. *J. Parasitol.* 105, 1–10.

1146. Matsler, P.L., Chapman, H.D., 2006. Characterization of a strain of *Eimeria meleagridis* from the turkey. *Avian Dis.* 50, 599–604.

1147. Matsubayashi, H., Nozawa, T., 1948. Experimental infection of *Isospora hominis* in man. *Am. J. Trop. Med. Hyg.* 28, 633–637.

1148. Matsubayashi, M., Carreno, R.A., Tani, H., Yoshiuchi, R., Kanai, T., Kimata, I., Uni, S., Furuya, M., Sasai, K., 2011. Phylogenetic identification of *Cystoisospora* spp. from dogs, cats, and raccoon dogs in Japan. *Vet. Parasitol.* 176, 270–274.

1149. Matsubayashi, M., Kawahara, F., Hatta, T., Yamagishi, J., Miyoshi, T., Anisuzzaman, Sasai, K., Isobe, T., Kita, K., Tsuji, N., 2016. Transcriptional profiles of virulent and precocious strains of *Eimeria tenella* at sporozoite stage; novel biological insight into attenuated asexual development. *Infect. Genet. Evol.* 40, 54–62.

1150. Matsubayashi, M., Takayama, H., Kusumoto, M., Murata, M., Uchiyama, Y., Kaji, M., Sasai, K., Yamaguchi, R., Shibahara, T., 2016. First report of molecular identification of *Cystoisospora suis* in piglets with lethal diarrhea in Japan. *Acta Parasitol.* 61, 406–411.

1151. Matsui, T., Ito, S., Fujino, T., Morii, T., 1993. Infectivity and sporogony of *Caryospora*-type oocysts of *Isospora rivolta* obtained by heating. *Parasitol. Res.* 79, 599–602.

1152. Matsui, T., Morii, T., Iijima, T., Kobayashi, F., Fujino, T., 1989. Transformation of oocysts from several coccidian species by heat treatment. *Parasitol. Res.* 75, 264–267.

1153. Matsuoka, T., Callender, M.E., Shumard, R.F., 1969. Embryonic bovine tracheal cell line for *in vitro* cultivation of *Eimeria tenella*. *Am. J. Vet. Res.* 30, 1119–1122.

1154. Matsuoka, T., Novilla, M.N., Thomson, T.D., Donoho, A.L., 1996. Review of monensin toxicosis in horses. *J. Equine Vet. Sci.* 16, 8–15.

1155. Matuschka, F.R., Heydorn, A.O., 1980. Die Entwicklung von *Isospora suis* Biester und Murray 1934 (Sporozoa: Coccidia: Eimeriidae) im Schwein. *Zool. Beitr.* 26, 405–476.

1156. Matuschka, F.R., Männer, K., 1981. Die Entwicklung experimentell mit *Isospora suis* infizierter Absatzferkel als Modellfall für die Wirksamkeit von Lasalocid und Halofuginon auf Kokzidien. *Zbl. Bakt. Hyg., I. Abt. Orig. A* 248, 565–574.

1157. McCalla, D.R., 1983. Mutagenicity of nitrofuran derivatives: A review. *Environ. Mutagen.* 5, 745–765.

1158. McCullough, J.L., Maren, T.H., 1974. Dihydropteroate synthetase from *Plasmodium berghei*: Isolation, properties, and inhibition by dapsone and sulfadiazine. *Mol. Pharmacol.* 10, 140–145.

1159. McDonald, V., Rose, M.E., 1987. *Eimeria tenella* and *E. necatrix*: A third generation of schizogony is an obligatory part of the developmental cycle. *J. Parasitol.* 73, 617–622.

1160. McDonald, V., Shirley, M.W., 2009. Past and future: Vaccination against *Eimeria*. *Parasitology* 136, 1477–1489.

1161. McDonald, V., Wisher, M.H., Rose, M.E., Jeffers, T.K., 1988. *Eimeria tenella*: Immunological diversity between asexual generations. *Parasite Immunol.* 10, 649–660.

1162. McDougald, L.R., 1978. Monensin for the prevention of coccidiosis in calves. *Am. J. Vet. Res.* 39, 1748–1749.

1163. McDougald, L.R., 1979. Attempted cross-transmission of coccidia between sheep and goats and description of *Eimeria ovinoidalis* sp. n. *J. Protozool.* 26, 109–113.

1164. McDougald, L.R., da Silva, J.M.L., Solis, J., Braga, M., 1987. A survey of sensitivity to anticoccidial drugs in 60 isolates of coccidia from broiler chickens in Brazil and Argentina. *Avian Dis.* 31, 287–292.

1165. McDougald, L.R., Fitz-Coy, S.H., 2013. Coccidiosis. In Swayne, D.E., Glisson, J.R., McDougald, L.R., Nolan, L.K., Suarez, D.L., and Nair, V.L. (Ed.), *Diseases of Poultry*. Wiley-Blackwell. New York, 13th ed., 1148–1166.

1166. McDougald, L.R., Fuller, L., Solis, J., 1986. Drug-sensitivity of 99 isolates of coccidia from broiler farms. *Avian Dis.* 30, 690–694.

1167. McDougald, L.R., Jeffers, T.K., 1976. *Eimeria tenella* (Sporozoa, Coccidia): Gametogony following a single asexual generation. *Science* 192, 258–259.

1168. McLoughlin, D.K., Chute, M.B., 1978. Robenidine resistance in *Eimeria tenella*. *J. Parasitol.* 64, 874–877.

1169. McQueary, C.A., Worley, D.E., Catlin, J.E., 1977. Observations on the life cycle and prevalence of *Eimeria leuckarti* in horses in Montana. *Am. J. Vet. Res.* 38, 1673–1674.

1170. Medzhitov, R., 2001. Toll-like receptors and innate immunity. *Nat. Rev. Immunol.* 1, 135–145.

1171. Mehlhorn, H., Greif, G., 2016. Baycox. In Mehlhorn, H. (Ed.), *Encyclopedia of Parasitology*. Springer. Berlin, Germany, 299–300.

1172. Mehlhorn, H., Markus, M.B., 1976. Electron microscopy of stages of *Isospora felis* of the cat in the mesenteric lymph node of the mouse. *Z. Parasitenkd.* 51, 15–24.

1173. Mehlhorn, H., Ortmann-Falkenstein, G., Haberkorn, A., 1984. The effects of sym. triazinones on developmental stages of *Eimeria tenella*, *E. maxima* and *E. acervulina*: A light and electron microscopical study. *Z. Parasitenkd.* 70, 173–182.

1174. Mehlhorn, H., Pooch, H., Raether, W., 1983. The action of polyether ionophorous antibiotics (monensin, salinomycin, lasalocid) on developmental stages of *Eimeria tenella* (Coccidia, Sporozoa) *in vivo* and *in vitro*: Study by light and electron microscopy. *Z. Parasitenkd.* 69, 457–471.

1175. Melo, P.S., de Carvalho Filho, P.R., de Oliveira, F.C.R., Flausino, W., Lopes, C.W.G., 2003. Hypnozoites of *Cystoisospora felis* (Wenyon, 1923) Frenkel, 1977

(Apicomplexa: Cystoisosporinae) in swine (*Sus scrofa domesticus*) visceras: A new intermediate host. *Rev. Bras. Parasitol. Vet.* 12, 103–107.

1176. Melo, P.S., de Carvalho Filho, P.R., Lopes, C.W.G., Flausino, W., de Oliveira, F.C.R., 2003. Hypnozoites of *Cystoiospora felis* (Wenyon, 1923) Frenkel, 1977 (Apicomplexa: Cystoisosporinae) isolated from piglets experimentally infected. *Rev. Bras. Parasitol. Vet.* 12, 82–84.

1177. Mengel, H., Krüger, M., Krüger, M.U., Westphal, B., Swidsinski, A., Schwarz, S., Mundt, H.C., Dittmar, K., Daugschies, A., 2012. Necrotic enteritis due to simultaneous infection with *Isospora suis* and clostridia in newborn piglets and its prevention by early treatment with toltrazuril. *Parasitol. Res.* 110, 1347–1355.

1178. Menyaylova, I.S., Gaponov, S.P., 2012. Intestinal parasite invasions of carnivores in the city of Voronezh. *Russian J. Parasitol.* 2, 30–33.

1179. Meyer, C., Joachim, A., Daugschies, A., 1999. Occurrence of *Isospora suis* in larger piglet production units and on specialized piglet rearing farms. *Vet. Parasitol.* 82, 277–284.

1180. Meyer, C.M., 1998. Vorkommen und Bedeutung von *Isospora suis* Biester und Murray 1934 in intensiv geführten Ferkelerzeugerbetrieben und in der spezialisierten Ferkelaufzucht. Dr. med. vet. thesis, Tierärztliche Hochschule, Hannover.

1181. Michiels, J.F., Hofman, P., Bernard, E., Saint Paul, M.C., Boissy, C., Mondain, V., Lefichoux, Y., Loubiere, R., 1994. Intestinal and extraintestinal *Isospora belli* infection in an AIDS patient. A second case report. *Pathol. Res. Pract.* 190, 1089–1093.

1182. Min, W., Kim, W.H., Lillehoj, E.P., Lillehoj, H.S., 2013. Recent progress in host immunity to avian coccidiosis: IL-17 family cytokines as sentinels of the intestinal mucosa. *Dev. Comp. Immunol.* 41, 418–428.

1183. Min, W., Lillehoj, H.S., 2002. Isolation and characterization of chicken interleukin-17 cDNA. *J. Interferon Cytokine Res.* 22, 1123–1128.

1184. Min, W., Lillehoj, H.S., 2004. Identification and characterization of chicken interleukin-16 cDNA. *Dev. Comp. Immunol.* 28, 153–162.

1185. Min, W., Lillehoj, H.S., Fetterer, R.H., 2002. Identification of an alternatively spliced isoform of the common cytokine receptor γ chain in chickens. *Biochem. Biophys. Res. Commun.* 299, 321–327.

1186. Miner, M.L., Jensen, J.B., 1976. Decoquinate in the control of experimentally induced coccidiosis of calves. *Am. J. Vet. Res.* 37, 1043–1045.

1187. Mirani, A.H., Shah, M.G.U., Mirbahar, K.B., Khan, M.S., Lochi, G.M., Khan, I.U., Alam, F., Hasan, S.M., Tariq, M., 2012. Prevalence of coccidiosis and other gastointestinal nematode species in buffalo calves at Hyderabad, Sindh, Pakistan. *Afr. J. Microbiol. Res.* 6, 6291–6294.

1188. Mirza, M.Y., Al-Rawas, A.Y., 1976. Coccidia (Protozoa Eimeridiae) from camels (*Camelus dromedarius*) in Iraq. *Bull. Biol. Res. Center* 7, 24–31.

1188a. Miska, K.B., Fetterer, R.H., Rosenberg, G.H., 2008. Analysis of transcripts from intracellular stages of *Eimeria acervulina* using expressed sequence tags. *J. Parasitol.* 94, 462–466.

1189. Miska, K.B., Schwarz, R.S., Jenkins, M.C., Rathinam, T., Chapman, H.D., 2010. Molecular characterization and phylogenetic analysis of *Eimeria* from turkeys and gamebirds: Implications for evolutionary relationships in Galliform birds. *J. Parasitol.* 96, 982–986.

1190. Mitchell, E.S.E., Smith, R.P., Ellis-Iversen, J., 2012. Husbandry risk factors associated with subclinical coccidiosis in young cattle. *Vet. J.* 193, 119–123.

1191. Mitchell, S.M., Zajac, A.M., Charles, S., Duncan, R.B., Lindsay, D.S., 2007. *Cystoisospora canis* Neméséri, 1959 (syn. *Isospora canis*), infections in dogs: Clinical signs, pathogenesis, and reproducible clinical disease in beagle dogs fed oocysts. *J. Parasitol.* 93, 345–352.

1192. Mitrovic, M., Schildknecht, E.G., 1974. Anticoccidial activity of Lasalocid (X-537A) in chicks. *Poult. Sci.* 53, 1448–1455.

1193. Miyazaki, Y., Shibuya, M., Sugawara, H., Kawaguchi, O., Hirose, C., Nagatsu, J., Esumi, S., 1974. Salinomycin, a new polyether antibiotic. *J. Antibiot. (Tokyo)* 27, 814–821.

1194. Mo, P., Ma, Q., Zhao, X., Cheng, N., Tao, J., Li, J., 2014. Apoptotic effects of antimalarial artemisinin on the second generation merozoites of *Eimeria tenella* and parasitized host cells. *Vet. Parasitol.* 206, 297–303.

1195. Mohamaden, W.I., Sallam, N.H., Abouelhassan, E.M., 2018. Prevalence of *Eimeria* species among sheep and goats in Suez Governorate, Egypt. *Int. J. Vet. Sci. Med.* 6, 65–72.

1196. Mohammed, O.A.S., 2013. Studies on coccidial parasites. Doctoral thesis. Zagazig University, Egypt.

1197. Mohanty, I., Panda, P., Sahu, S., Dash, M., Narasimham, M.V., Padhi, S., Parida, B., 2013. Prevalence of isosporiasis in relation to CD4 cell counts among HIV-infected patients with diarrhea in Odisha, India. *Adv. Biomed Res.* 2, 61.

1198. Mohebali, M., Zarei, Z., Khanaliha, K., Kia, E.B., Motavalli-Haghi, A., Davoodi, J., Tarighi, F., Khodabakhsh, M., Rezaeian, M., 2019. Intestinal protozoa in domestic cats (Carnivora: Felidae, *Felis catus*) in Northwestern Iran: A cross-sectional study with prevalent of microsporidian and coccidian parasites. *Iran. J. Parasitol.* 14, 136–142.

1199. Mollenhauer, H.H., Morré, D.J., Rowe, L.D., 1990. Alteration of intracellular traffic by monensin, mechanism, specificity and relationship to toxicity. *Biochem. Biophys. Acta (BBA)—Rev. Biomembranes* 1031, 225–246.

1200. Molnár, K., Ostoros, G., Dunams-Morel, D., Rosenthal, B.M., 2012. *Eimeria* that infect fish are diverse and are related to, but distinct from, those that infect terrestrial vertebrates. *Infect. Genet. Evol.* 12, 1810–1815.

1201. Moore, E.N., Brown, J.A., 1951. A new coccidium pathogenic for turkeys, *Eimeria adenoeides* n. sp. (Protozoa: Eimeriidae). *Cornell Vet.* 41, 124–135.

1202. Moore, E.N., Brown, J.A., 1952. A new coccidium of turkeys, *Eimeria innocua* n. sp. (Protozoa: Eimeriidae). *Cornell Vet.* 42, 395–402.

1203. Moore, E.N., Brown, J.A., Carter, R.D., 1954. A new coccidium of turkeys, *Eimeria subrotunda* n. sp. (Protozoa: Eimeriidae). *Poult. Sci.* 33, 925–929.

1204. Morein, B., Abusugra, I., Blomqvist, G., 2002. Immunity in neonates. *Vet. Immunol. Immunopathol.* 87, 207–213.

1205. Morgan, J.A.T., Godwin, R.M., 2017. Mitochondrial genomes of Australian chicken *Eimeria* support the presence of ten species with low genetic diversity among strains. *Vet. Parasitol.* 243, 58–66.

1206. Morin, M., Robinson, Y., Turgeon, D., 1980. Intestinal coccidiosis in baby pig diarrhea. *Can. Vet. J.* 21, 65.

1207. Morin, M., Turgeon, D., Jolette, J., Robinson, Y., Phaneuf, J.B., Sauvageau, R., Beauregard, M., Teuscher, E., Higgins, R., Larivière, S., 1983. Neonatal diarrhea of pigs in Quebec: Infectious causes of significant outbreaks. *Can. J. Comp. Med.* 47, 11–17.

1208. Morris, A., Shanmugasundaram, R., McDonald, J., Selvaraj, R.K., 2015. Effect of *in vitro* and *in vivo* 25-hydroxyvitamin D treatment on macrophages, T cells, and layer chickens during a coccidia challenge. *J. Anim. Sci.* 93, 2894–2903.

1209. Morrsy, N.G., 1997. A study on *Eimeria* species infecting camels (*Camelus dromedarius*) in Egypt. *Vet. Med. J., Giza* 45, 499–507.

1210. Moskvira, T.V., Zheleznova, L.V., 2017. Parasitic diseases of dogs and cats in the city of Vladivostok. *Russian J. Parasitol.* 39, 55–58.

1211. Müller, A., Bialek, R., Fätkenheuer, G., Salzberger, B., Diehl, V., Franzen, C., 2000. Detection of *Isospora belli* by polymerase chain reaction using primers based on small-subunit ribosomal RNA sequences. *Eur. J. Clin. Microbiol. Infect. Dis.* 19, 631–634.

1212. Müller, B.E.G., De Vos, A.J., Hammond, D.M., 1973. *In vitro* development of first-generation schizonts of *Eimeria canadensis* (Bruce, 1921). *J. Protozool.* 20, 293–297.

1213. Müller, J., Hemphill, A., 2016. Drug target identification in protozoan parasites. *Expert Opin. Drug Discov.* 11, 815–824.

1214. Mundt, H.C., Cohnen, A., Daugschies, A., Joachim, A., Prosl, H., Schmäschke, R., Westphal, B., 2005. Occurrence of *Isospora suis* in Germany, Switzerland and Austria. *J. Vet. Med. B* 52, 93–97.

1215. Mundt, H.C., Daugschies, A., Uebe, F., Rinke, M., 2003. Efficacy of toltrazuril against artificial infections with *Eimeria bovis* in calves. *Parasitol. Res.* 90 (Suppl 3), S166–S167.

1216. Mundt, H.C., Daugschies, A., Wüstenberg, S., Zimmermann, M., 2003. Studies on the efficacy of toltrazuril, diclazuril and sulphadimidine against artificial infection with *Isospora suis* in piglets. *Parasitol. Res.* 90 (Suppl 3), S160–S162.

1217. Mundt, H.C., Dittmar, K., Daugschies, A., Grzonka, E., Bangoura, B., 2009. Study of the comparative efficacy of toltrazuril and diclazuril against ovine coccidiosis in housed lambs. *Parasitol. Res.* 105 (Suppl 1), S141–S150.

1218. Mundt, H.C., Joachim, A., Becka, M., Daugschies, A., 2006. *Isospora suis*: An experimental model for mammalian intestinal coccidiosis. *Parasitol. Res.* 98, 167–175.

1219. Mundt, H.C., Mundt-Wüstenberg, S., Daugschies, A., Joachim, A., 2007. Efficacy of various anticoccidials against experimental porcine neonatal isosporosis. *Parasitol. Res.* 100, 401–411.

1220. Mundt, H.-C., Bangoura, B., Mengel, H., Keidel, J., Daugschies, A., 2005. Control of clinical coccidiosis of calves due to *Eimeria bovis* and *Eimeria zuernii* with toltrazuril under field conditions. *Parasitol. Res.* 97 (Suppl 1), S134–S142.

1221. Mundt, H.-C., Bangoura, B., Rinke, M., Rosenbruch, M., Daugschies, A., 2005. Pathology and treatment of *Eimeria zuernii* coccidiosis in calves: Investigations in an infection model. *Parasitol. Int.* 54, 223–230.

1222. Muñoz-Caro, T., Mena Huertas, S.J., Conejeros, I., Alarcón, P., Hidalgo, M.A., Burgos, R.A., Hermosilla, C., Taubert, A., 2015. *Eimeria bovis*-triggered neutrophil extracellular trap formation is CD11b-, ERK 1/2-, p38 MAP kinase- and SOCE-dependent. *Vet. Res.* 46, 23.

1223. Murphy, H.R., Almeria, S., da Silva, A.J., 2017. BAM 19b: Molecular detection of *Cyclospora cayetanensis* in fresh produce using real-time PCR. https://www.fda.gov/food/laboratory-methods-food-safety/bam-19b-molecular-detection-Cyclospora-cayetanensis-fresh-produce-using-real-time-pcr.

1224. Murphy, H.R., Cinar, H.N., Gopinath, G., Noe, K.E., Chatman, L.D., Miranda, N.E., Wetherington, J.H., et al., 2018. Interlaboratory validation of an improved method for detection of *Cyclospora cayetanensis* in produce using a real-time PCR assay. *Food Microbiol.* 69, 170–178.

1225. Murphy, H.R., Lee, S., da Silva, A.J., 2017. Evaluation of an improved U.S. Food and Drug Administration method for the detection of *Cyclospora cayetanensis* in produce using real-time PCR. *J. Food Prot.* 80, 1133–1144.

1226. Murphy, S.C., Hoogestraat, D.R., Sengupta, D.J., Prentice, J., Chakrapani, A., Cookson, B.T., 2011. Molecular diagnosis of cystoisosporiasis using extended-range PCR screening. *J. Mol. Diagn.* 13, 359–362.

1227. Nachman, K.E., Baron, P.A., Raber, G., Francesconi, K.A., Navas-Acien, A., Love, D.C., 2013. Roxarsone, inorganic arsenic, and other arsenic species in chicken: A U.S.-based market basket sample. *Environ. Health Perspect.* 121, 818–824.

1228. Naciri-Bontemps, M., 1976. Reproduction of the cycle of coccidia *Eimeria acervulina* (Tyzzer, 1929) in cell cultures of chicken kidneys. *Ann. Rech. Vet.* 7, 223–230.

1229. Nahavandi, K.H., Mahvi, A.H., Mohebali, M., Keshavarz, H., Rezaei, S., Mirjalali, H., Elikaei, S., Rezaeian, M., 2016. Molecular typing of *Eimeria ahsata* and *E. crandallis* isolated from slaughterhouse wastewater. *Jundishapur J. Microbiol.* 9, e34140.

1230. Nain, N., Gupta, S.K., Sangwan, A.K., Gupta, S., 2017. Prevalence of *Eimeria* species in buffalo calves of Haryana. *Haryana Vet.* 56, 5–8.

1231. Nakayima, J., Kabasa, W., Aleper, D., Okidi, D., 2017. Prevalence of endo-parasites in donkeys and camels in Karamoja sub-region, North-eastern Uganda. *J. Vet. Med. Anim. Health* 9, 11–15.

1232. Nalbantoglu, S., Sari, B., Cicek, H., Karaer, Z., 2008. Prevalence of coccidian species in the water buffalo (*Bubalus bubalis*) in the province of Afyon, Turkey. *Acta Vet. Brno* 77, 111–116.

1233. Narnaware, S.D., Kumar, S., Dahiya, S.S., Patil, N.V., 2017. Concurrent infection of coccidiosis and haemonchosis in a dromedary camel calf from Rajasthan, India. *J. Camel Prac. Res.* 24, 225–228.

1234. Nation, P.N., Wobeser, G., 1977. Renal coccidiosis in wild ducks in Saskatchewan. *J. Wildl. Dis.* 13, 370–375.

1235. Naujokat, C., Fuchs, D., Opelz, G., 2010. Salinomycin in cancer: A new mission for an old agent. *Mol. Med. Rep.* 3, 555–559.

1236. Negm, A.Y., 2003. Human pathogenic protozoa in bivalves collected from local markets in Alexandria. *J. Egypt. Soc. Parasitol.* 33, 991–998.

1237. Neméséri, L., 1960. Beiträge zur Ätiologie der Coccidiose der Hunde. I. *Isospora canis* sp. n. *Acta Veterinaria* 10, 95–99.

1238. Ng, E., Markell, E.K., Fleming, R.L., Fried, M., 1984. Demonstration of *Isospora belli* by acid-fast stain in a patient with acquired immune deficiency syndrome. *J. Clin. Microbiol.* 20, 384–386.

1239. Ng, S.T., Jangi, M.S., Shirley, M.W., Tomley, F.M., Wan, K.L., 2002. Comparative EST analyses provide insights into gene expression in two asexual developmental stages of *Eimeria tenella*. *Exp. Parasitol.* 101, 168–173.

1240. Niestrath, M., Takla, M., Joachim, A., Daugschies, A., 2002. The role of *Isospora suis* as a pathogen in conventional piglet production in Germany. *J. Vet. Med. B* 49, 176–180.

1241. Niilo, L., 1970. Experimental winter coccidiosis in sheltered and unsheltered calves. *Can. J. Comp. Med.* 34, 20–25.

1242. Nilsson, O., 1988. *Isospora suis* in pigs with post weaning diarrhoea. *Vet. Rec.* 122, 310–311.

1243. Noack, S., Chapman, H.D., Selzer, P.M., 2019. Anticoccidial drugs of the livestock industry. *Parasitol. Res.* 118, 2009–2026.

1244. Nolan, A., Goldring, O.L., Catchpole, J., Gregory, M.W., Joyner, L.P., 1987. Demonstration of antibodies to *Eimeria* species in lambs by an enzyme-linked immunosorbent assay. *Res. Vet. Sci.* 42, 119–123.

1245. Nolan, M.J., Tomley, F.M., Kaiser, P., Blake, D.P., 2015. Quantitative real-time PCR (qPCR) for *Eimeria tenella* replication—Implications for experimental refinement and animal welfare. *Parasitol. Int.* 64, 464–470.

1246. Norcross, M.A., Siegmund, O.H., Fraser, C.M., 1974. Amprolium for coccidiosis in cattle: A review of efficacy and safety. *Vet. Med. Small Anim. Clin.* 69, 459.

1247. Norton, C.C., Catchpole, J., Joyner, L.P., 1979. Redescriptions of *Eimeria irresidua* Kessel and Jankiewicz, 1931 and *E. flavescens* Marotel and Guilhon, 1941 from the domestic rabbit. *Parasitology* 79, 231–248.

1248. Norton, C.C., Catchpole, J., Rose, M.E., 1977. *Eimeria stiedai* in rabbits: The presence of an oocyst residuum. *Parasitology* 75, 1–7.

1249. Norton, C.C., Chard, M.J., 1983. The oocyst sporulation time of *Eimeria* species from the fowl. *Parasitology* 86, 193–198.

1250. Norton, C.C., Hein, H.E., 1976. *Eimeria maxima*: A comparison of two laboratory strains with a fresh isolate. *Parasitology* 72, 345–354.

1251. Norton, C.C., Joyner, L.P., 1986. Avian coccidiosis: The administration of encapsulated oocysts. *Parasitology* 92 (Pt 3), 499–510.

1252. Nourollahi-Fard, S.R., Khedri, J., Ghashghaei, O., Mohammadyari, N., Sharifi, H., 2016. The prevalence of ovine *Eimeria* infection in Rudsar, North of Iran (2011–2012). *J. Parasit. Dis.* 40, 954–957.

1253. Novaes, J., Rangel, L.T.L.D., Ferro, M., Abe, R.Y., Manha, A.P.S., de Mello, J.C.M., Varuzza, L., Durham, A.M., Madeira, A.M.B.N., Gruber, A., 2012. A comparative transcriptome analysis reveals expression profiles conserved across three *Eimeria* spp. of domestic fowl and associated with multiple developmental stages. *Int. J. Parasitol.* 42, 39–48.

1254. Novicky, R., 1945. Swine coccidiosis in Venezuela. *J. Am. Vet. Med. Assoc.* 107, 400–403.

1255. Nurhidayah, N., Satrija, F., Retnani, E.B., 2019. Gastrointestinal parasitic infection of swamp buffalo in Banten Province, Indonesia: Prevalence, risk factor, and its impact on production performance. *Trop. Anim. Sci. J.* 41, 6–12.

1256. O'Brien, C.R., Pope, S.E., Malik, R., 2002. Vomiting, diarrhoea and inappetence in a young cat with hypoproteinaemia. *Aust. Vet. J.* 80, 544–551.

1257. O'Neill, P.A., 1976. Observations on *Isospora suis* infection in a minimal disease pig herd. *Vet. Rec.* 98, 321–323.

1258. Oakes, R.D., Kurian, D., Bromley, E., Ward, C., Lal, K., Blake, D.P., Reid, A.J., et al., 2013. The rhoptry proteome of *Eimeria tenella* sporozites. *Int. J. Parasitol.* 43, 181–188.

1259. Obayes, H.H., Al-Rubaie, H.M.A., Zayer, A.A.J., Radhy, A.M., 2016. Detection the prevalence of some gastrointestinal protozoa in buffaloes of Babylon Governorate. *Basrah J. Vet. Res.* 15, 294–303.

1260. Oborník, M., Jirku, M., Šlapeta, J.R., Modrý, D., Koudela, B., Lukeš, J., 2002. Notes on coccidian phylogeny, based on the apicoplast small subunit ribosomal DNA. *Parasitol. Res.* 88, 360–363.

1261. Oda, K., Nishida, Y., 1991. Prepatent and patent periods, and production and sporulation of oocysts of *Eimeria* subspherica isolated in Japan. *J. Vet. Med. Sci.* 53, 615–619.

1262. Odden, A., Denwood, M.J., Stuen, S., Robertson, L.J., Ruiz, A., Hamnes, I.S., Hektoen, L., Enemark, H.L., 2018. Field evaluation of anticoccidial efficacy: A novel approach demonstrates reduced efficacy of toltrazuril against ovine *Eimeria* spp. in Norway. *Int. J. Parasitol. Drugs Drug Resist.* 8, 304–311.

1263. Odden, A., Enemark, H.L., Robertson, L.J., Ruiz, A., Hektoen, L., Stuen, S., 2017. Treatment against coccidiosis in Norwegian lambs and potential risk factors for development of anticoccidial resistance—A questionnaire-based study. *Parasitol. Res.* 116, 1237–1245.

1264. Odden, A., Enemark, H.L., Ruiz, A., Robertson, L.J., Ersdal, C., Nes, S.K., Tømmerberg, V., Stuen, S., 2018. Controlled efficacy trial confirming toltrazuril resistance in a field isolate of ovine *Eimeria* spp. *Parasit. Vectors* 11, 394.

1265. Oehme, F.W., Pickrell, J.A., 1999. An analysis of the chronic oral toxicity of polyether ionophore antibiotics in animals. *Vet. Hum. Toxicol.* 41, 251–257.

1266. Ogedengbe, J.D., Ogedengbe, M.E., Hafeez, M.A., Barta, J.R., 2015. Molecular phylogenetics of eimeriid coccidia (Eimeriidae, Eimeriorina, Apicomplexa, Alveolata): A preliminary multi-gene and multi-genome approach. *Parasitol. Res.* 114, 4149–4160.

1267. Ogedengbe, M.E., El-Sherry, S., Whale, J., Barta, J.R., 2014. Complete mitochondrial genome sequences from five *Eimeria* species (Apicomplexa; Coccidia; Eimeriidae) infecting domestic turkeys. *Parasit. Vectors* 7, 335.

1268. Ogedengbe, M.E., Hafeez, M.A., Barta, J.R., 2013. Sequencing the complete mitochondrial genome of *Eimeria mitis* strain USDA 50 (Apicomplexa: Eimeriidae) suggests conserved start positions for mtCOI- and mtCOIII-coding regions. *Parasitol. Res.* 112, 4129–4136.

1269. Ogedengbe, M.E., Ogedengbe, J.D., Whale, J.C., Elliot, K., Juárez-Estrada, M.A., Barta, J.R., 2016. Molecular phylogenetic analyses of tissue coccidia (sarcocystidae; apicomplexa) based on nuclear 18 s RDNA and mitochondrial COI sequences confirms the paraphyly of the genus *Hammondia*. *Parasitol. Open* 2, e2.

1270. Ogedengbe, M.E., Qvarnstrom, Y., da Silva, A.J., Arrowood, M.J., Barta, J.R., 2015. A linear mitochondrial genome of *Cyclospora cayetanensis* (Eimeriidae, Eucoccidiorida, Coccidiasina, Apicomplexa) suggests the ancestral start position within mitochondrial genomes of eimeriid coccidia. *Int. J. Parasitol.* 45, 361–365.

1271. Okumu, P.O., Gathumbi, P.K., Karanja, D.N., Mande, J.D., Wanyoike, M.M., Gachuiri, C.K., Kiarie, N., Mwanza, R.N., Borter, D.K., 2014. Prevalence, pathology and risk factors for coccidiosis in domestic rabbits (*Oryctolagus cuniculus*) in selected regions in Kenya. *Vet. Quart.* 34, 205–210

1272. Oliveira, F.C.R., Albuquerque, G.R., Munhoz, A.D., Lopes, C.W.G., Massad, F.V., 2001. Hipnozoítas de *Cystoisospora ohioensis* (Dubey, 1975) Frenkel, 1977 (Apicomplexa: Cystoisosporinae) recuperados de órgãos de camundongos através da digestão péptica. *Rev. Bras. Parasitol. Vet.* 10, 29–35.

1273. Oliveira, U.C., Fraga, J.S., Licois, D., Pakandl, M., Gruber, A., 2011. Development of molecular assays for the identification of the 11 *Eimeria* species of the domestic rabbit (*Oryctolagus cuniculus*). *Vet. Parasitol.* 176, 275–280.

1274. Oliveira-Silva, M.B., Lages-Silva, E., Resende, D.V., Prata, A., Ramirez, L.E., Frenkel, J.K., 2006. *Cystoisospora belli*: *In vitro* multiplication in mammalian cells. *Exp. Parasitol.* 114, 189–192.

1275. Olson, M.E., 1985. Coccidiosis caused by *Isospora ohioensis*-like organisms in three dogs. *Can. Vet. J.* 26, 112–114.

1276. Olusegun, A.F., Okaka, C.E., Machado, R.L.D., 2009. Isosporiasis in HIV/AIDS patients in Edo State, Nigeria. *Malays. J. Med. Sci.* 16, 41–44.

1277. Omata, Y., Oikawa, H., Kanda, M., Mikazuki, K., Claveria, F.G., Dilorenzo, C., Takehara, T., Saito, A., Suzuki, N, 1991. Humoral immune response to *Isospora felis* and *Toxoplasma gondii* in cats experimentally inoculated with *Isospora felis*. *J. Vet. Med. Sci.* 53, 1071–1073.

1278. Omata, Y., Oikawa, H., Kanda, M., Mikazuki, K., Nakabayashi, T., Suzuki, N., 1990. *Isospora felis*: Possible evidence for transmission of parasites from chronically infected mother cats to kittens. *Jpn. J. Vet. Sci.* 52, 665–666.

1279. Omata, Y., Oikawa, H., Kanda, M., Mikazuki, K., Takehara, T., Venturini, C., Saito, A., Suzuki, N., 1991. Enhancement of humoral immune response of *Isospora felis*-infected cats after inoculation with *Toxoplasma gondii*. *J. Vet. Med. Sci.* 53, 163–165.

1280. Onawunmi, O.A., Todd, A.C., 1976. Suppression and control of experimentally induced porcine coccidiosis with chlortetracycline combination, buquinolate, and lincomycin hydrochloride. *Am. J. Vet. Res.* 37, 657–660.

1281. Orozco-Mosqueda, G.E., Martínez-Loya, O.A., Ortega, Y.R., 2014. *Cyclospora cayetanensis* in a pediatric hospital in Morelia, México. *Am. J. Trop. Med. Hyg.* 91, 537–540.

1282. Ortega, Y.R., Gilman, R.H., Sterling, C.R., 1994. A new coccidian parasite (Apicomplexa: Eimeriidae) from humans. *J. Parasitol.* 80, 625–629.

1283. Ortega, Y.R., Nagle, R., Gilman, R.H., Watanabe, J., Miyagui, J., Quispe, H., Kanagusuku, P., Roxas, C., Sterling, C.R., 1997. Pathologic and clinical findings in patients with cyclosporiasis and a description of intracellular parasite life-cycle stages. *J. Infect. Dis.* 176, 1584–1589.

1284. Ortega, Y.R., Robertson, L.J., 2017. *Cyclospora cayetanensis as a Foodborne Pathogen (Springer Briefs in Food, Health, and Nutrition)*. Springer. Berlin, Germany, 1–65.

1285. Ortega, Y.R., Sanchez, R., 2010. Update on *Cyclospora cayetanensis*, a food-borne and waterborne parasite. *Clin. Microbiol. Rev.* 23, 218–234.

1286. Ortega, Y.R., Sterling, C.R., 1996. *Cyclospora cayetanensis*: Epidemiology and diagnosis. *Clin. Microbiol. Newsletter* 18, 169–172.

1287. Ortega, Y.R., Sterling, C.R., Gilman, R.H., 1998. *Cyclospora cayetanensis. Adv. Parasitol.* 40, 399–418.

1288. Ortega, Y.R., Sterling, C.R., Gilman, R.H., Cama, V.A., Díaz, F., 1993. *Cyclospora* species: A new protozoan pathogen of humans. *N. Engl. J. Med.* 328, 1308–1312.

1289. Ortuño, A., Castellà, J., 2011. Intestinal parasites in shelter dogs and risk factors associated with the facility and its management. *Israel J. Vet. Med.* 66, 103–107.

1290. Oruc, E., 2007. Histopathological findings in naturally occurring biliary coccidiosis in a goat kid. *Vet. Rec.* 160, 93.

1291. Otten, A., 1995. Untersuchungen zur Epizootiologie und pathogenen Bedeutung von Infektionen mit *Isospora suis* in zehn Ferkelerzeugerbetrieben in Nordrhein-Westfalen. Doctoral Thesis. Hannover, TiHo.

1292. Otten, A., Takla, M., Daugschies, A., Rommel, M., 1996. Untersuchungen zur Epizootiologie und pathogenen Bedeutung von Infektionen mit *Isospora suis* in zehn Ferkelerzeugerbetrieben in Nordrhein-Westfalen. *Berl. Münch. tierärztl. Wochenschr.* 109, 220–223.

1293. Ovington, K.S., Alleva, L.M., Kerr, E.A., 1995. Cytokines and immunological control of *Eimeria* spp. *Int. J. Parasitol.* 25, 1331–1351.

1294. Owen, D., 1970. Life cycle of *Eimeria stiedae*. *Nature* 227, 304.

1295. Ozmen, O., Adanir, R., Haligur, M., 2012. Immunohistochemical detection of the cytokine and chemokine expression in the gut of lambs and kids with coccidiosis. *Small Ruminant Res.* 105, 345–350.

1296. Pacheco, F.T.F., Silva, R.K.N.R., Martins, A.S., Oliveira, R.R., Alcântara-Neves, N.M., Silva, M.P., Soares, N.M., Teixeira, M.C.A., 2013. Differences in the detection of *Cryptosporidium* and *Isospora (Cystoisospora)* oocysts according to the fecal concentration or staining method used in a clinical laboratory. *J. Parasitol.* 99, 1002–1008.

1297. Padilla, M.A., Romero, J.R.M., 2007. Survey of *Eimera* in water buffaloes (*Bubalus bubalis* L.) in Laguna and Cavite Provinces. *Philippine J. Vet. Anim. Sci.* 33, 83–91.

1298. Pakandl, M., 1986. Efficacy of salinomycin, monensin and lasalocid against spontaneous *Eimeria* infection in rabbits. *Folia Parasitol. (Praha)* 33, 195–198.

1299. Pakandl, M., 2005. Selection of a precocious line of the rabbit coccidium *Eimeria flavescens* Marotel and Guilhon (1941) and characterisation of its endogenous cycle. *Parasitol. Res.* 97, 150–155.

1300. Pakandl, M., 2009. Coccidia of rabbit: A review. *Folia Parasitol. (Praha)* 56, 153–166.

1301. Pakandl, M., Cerník, F., Coudert, P., 2003. The rabbit coccidium *Eimeria flavescens* Marotel and Guilhon, 1941: An electron microscopic study of its life cycle. *Parasitol. Res.* 91, 304–311.

1302. Pakandl, M., Coudert, P., 1999. Life cycle of *Eimeria vejdovskyi* Pakandl, 1988: Electron microscopy study. *Parasitol. Res.* 85, 850–854.

1303. Pakandl, M., Coudert, P., Licois, D., 1993. Migration of sporozoites and merogony of *Eimeria coecicola* in gut-associated lymphoid tissue. *Parasitol. Res.* 79, 593–598.

1304. Pakandl, M., Drouet-Viard, F., Coudert, P., 1995. How do sporozoites of rabbit *Eimeria* species reach their target cells? *C. R. Acad. Sci. III* 318, 1213–1217.

1305. Pakandl, M., Eid, A.N., Licois, D., Coudert, P., 1996. *Eimeria magna* Pérard, 1925: Study of the endogenous development of parental and precocious strains. *Vet. Parasitol.* 65, 213–222.

1306. Pakandl, M., Gaca, K., Drouet-Viard, F., Coudert, P., 1996. *Eimeria coecicola* Cheissin 1947: Endogenous development in gut-associated lymphoid tissue. *Parasitol. Res.* 82, 347–351.

1307. Pakandl, M., Gaca, K., Licois, D., Coudert, P., 1996. *Eimeria media* Kessel 1929: Comparative study of endogenous development between precocious and parental strains. *Vet. Res.* 27, 465–472.

1308. Pakandl, M., Hlásková, L., 2007. The reproduction of *Eimeria flavescens* and *Eimeria intestinalis* in suckling rabbits. *Parasitol. Res.* 101, 1435–1437.

1309. Pakandl, M., Hlásková, L., Poplštein, M., Chromá, V., Vodička, T., Salát, J., Mucksová, J., 2008. Dependence of the immune response to coccidiosis on the age of rabbit suckling. *Parasitol. Res.* 103, 1265–1271.

1310. Pakandl, M., Hlásková, L., Poplštein, M., Nevečeřalova, M., Vodička, T., Salát, J., Mucksová, J., 2008. Immune response to rabbit coccidiosis: A comparison between infections with *Eimeria flavescens* and *E. intestinalis*. *Folia Parasitol. (Praha)* 55, 1–6.

1311. Pakandl, M., Jelínková, A., 2006. The rabbit coccidium *Eimeria piriformis*: Selection of a precocious line and life-cycle study. *Vet. Parasitol.* 137, 351–354.

1312. Pakandl, M., Licois, D., Coudert, P., 2001. Electron microscopic study on sporocysts and sporozoites of parental strains and precocious lines of rabbit coccidia *Eimeria intestinalis, E. media* and *E. magna*. *Parasitol. Res.* 87, 63–66.

1313. Pakandl, M., Sewald, B., Drouet-Viard, F., 2006. Invasion of the intestinal tract by sporozoites of *Eimeria coecicola* and *Eimeria intestinalis* in naive and immune rabbits. *Parasitol. Res.* 98, 310–316.

1314. Palacios, C.E., Rosa Perales, C., Alfonso Chavera, C., y Teresa López, U., 2005. Caracterización anátomo-histopatológica de enteropatías causantes de mortalidad en crías de alpaca. *Rev. Inv. Vet. Perú* 16, 34–40.

1315. Palacios, C.E., Luis Tabacchi, N., Alfonso Chavera, C., Teresa López, U., Gilberto Santillán, A., Nieves Sandoval Ch., Danilo Pezo, C., y Rosa Perales, C., 2004. Eimeriosis en crías de alpacas: estudio anátomo histopatológico. *Rev. Inv. Vet. Perú* 15, 174–178.

1316. Palacios, C.A., Perales, R.A., Chavera, A.E., Lopez, M.T., Braga, W.U., Moro, M., 2006. *Eimeria macusaniensis* and *Eimeria ivitaensis* co-infection in fatal cases of diarrhoea in young alpacas (*Lama pacos*) in Peru. *Vet. Rec.* 158, 344–345.

1317. Palmer, D., 2013. Detection of trematode eggs and *Eimeria leuckarti*—Sedimentation method (test)—faecal samples. *Dept. Agricult. Food Western Australia.* PAM 26. Issue no. 16, 1–10.

1318. Palmieri, N., Shrestha, A., Ruttkowski, B., Beck, T., Vogl, C., Tomley, F., Blake, D.P., Joachim, A., 2017. The genome of the protozoan parasite *Cystoisospora suis* and a reverse vaccinology approach to identify vaccine candidates. *Int. J. Parasitol.* 47, 189–202.

1319. Pan, H., Halper, J., 2003. Cloning, expression, and characterization of chicken transforming growth factor β4. *Biochem. Biophys. Res. Commun.* 303, 24–30.

1320. Pande, B.P., Bhatia, B.B., Chauhan, P.P.S., 1971. Sexual stages and associated lesion in *Eimeria bareillyi* of buffalo calves. *Indian J. Anim. Sci.* 41, 151–154.

1321. Pape, J.W., Verdier, R.I., Boncy, M., Boncy, J., Johnson, W.D., Jr., 1994. *Cyclospora* infection in adults infected with HIV. Clinical manifestations, treatment, and prophylaxis. *Ann. Intern. Med.* 121, 654–657.

1322. Pape, J.W., Verdier, R.I., Johnson, W.D., Jr., 1989. Treatment and prophylaxis of *Isospora belli* infection in patients with the acquired immunodeficiency syndrome. *N. Engl. J. Med.* 320, 1044–1047.

1323. Parent, E., Fernandez, D., Boulianne, M., 2018. The use of a live non-attenuated coccidiosis vaccine modifies *Eimeria* spp. excretion in commercial antibiotic-free broiler chicken flocks compared to conventional shuttle anticoccidial programs. *Poult. Sci.* 97, 2740–2744.

1324. Parker, R.J., Jones, G.W., 1990. Destruction of bovine coccidial oocysts in simulated cattle yards by dry tropical winter weather. *Vet. Parasitol.* 35, 269–272.

1325. Partani, A.K., Kumar, D., Manohar, G.S., 1999. Prevalence of *Eimeria* infection in camels (*Camelus dromedarius*) at Bikaner (Rajasthan). *J. Camel Prac. Res.* 6, 69–71.

1326. Passafaro, T.L., Carrera, J.P.B., dos Santos, L.L., Raidan, F.S.S., dos Santos, D.C.C., Cardoso, E.P., Leite, R.C., Toral, F.L.B., 2015. Genetic analysis of resistance to ticks, gastrointestinal nematodes and *Eimeria* spp. in Nellore cattle. *Vet. Parasitol.* 210, 224–234.

1327. Pastor-Fernández, I., Kim, S., Billington, K., Bumstead, J., Marugán-Hernández, V., Küster, T., Ferguson, D.J.P., Vervelde, L., Blake, D.P., Tomley, F.M., 2018. Development of cross-protective *Eimeria*-vectored vaccines based on apical membrane antigens. *Int. J. Parasitol.* 48, 505–518.

1328. Patnaik, M.M., Pande, B.P., 1965. Some observations on the endogenous stages of species of *Eimeria* and related lesions in naturally infected buffalo-calves (*Bubalus bubalis*). *Indian J. Vet. Sci.* 35, 33–46.

1329. Patterson, F.D., 1933. Cross-infection experiments with coccidia of birds. *Cornell Vet.* 23, 249.

1330. Patton, W.H., 1965. *Eimeria tenella*: Cultivation of the asexual stages in cultured animal cells. *Science* 150, 767–769.

1331. Paula, J.P.L., Leal, P.V., Pupin, R.C., Lima, S.C., Souza, M.A.S., Santos, A.A., Lemos, R.A.A., Gomes, D.C., 2018. Healing of brain lesions in sheep recovered from amprolium-induced polioencephalomacia. *Pesq. Vet. Bras.* 38, 806–810.

1332. Pecka, Z., 1992. Life cycle and ultrastructure of *Eimeria stigmosa*, the intranuclear coccidian of the goose (*Anser anser domesticus*). *Folia Parasitol. (Praha)* 39, 105–114.

1333. Pecka, Z., 1992. The life cycle of *Eimeria danailovi* from ducks. *Folia Parasitol. (Praha)* 39, 13–18.

1334. Peek, H.W., Landman, W.J.M., 2003. Resistance to anticoccidial drugs of Dutch avian *Eimeria* spp. field isolates originating from 1996, 1999 and 2001. *Avian Pathol.* 32, 391–401.

1335. Peek, H.W., Landman, W.J.M., 2006. Higher incidence of *Eimeria* spp. field isolates sensitive for diclazuril and monensin associated with the use of live coccidiosis vaccination with Paracox-5 in broiler farms. *Avian Dis.* 50, 434–439

1336. Peek, H.W., Landman, W.J.M., 2011. Coccidiosis in poultry: Anticoccidial products, vaccines and other prevention strategies. *Vet. Quart.* 31, 143–161.

1337. Peek, H.W., ter Veen, C., Dijkman, R., Landman, W.J.M., 2017. Validation of a quantitative *Eimeria* spp. PCR for fresh droppings of broiler chickens. *Avian Pathol.* 46, 615–622.

1338. Peeters, J.E., Charlier, G., Antoine, O., Mammerickx, M., 1984. Clinical and pathological changes after *Eimeria intestinalis* infection in rabbits. *Zentralbl. Veterinärmed. B* 31, 9–24.

1339. Peeters, J.E., Geeroms, R., 1986. Efficacy of toltrazuril against intestinal and hepatic coccidiosis in rabbits. *Vet. Parasitol.* 22, 21–35.

1340. Peeters, J.E., Geeroms, R., 1989. Efficacy of diclazuril against robenidine resistant *Eimeria magna* in rabbits. *Vet. Rec.* 124, 589–590.

1341. Peeters, J.E., Geeroms, R., Antoine, O., Mammerickx, M., Halen, P., 1981. Efficacy of narasin against hepatic and intestinal coccidiosis in rabbits. *Parasitology* 83, 293–301.

1342. Pegg, E., Doyle, K., Clark, E.L., Jatau, I.D., Tomley, F.M., Blake, D.F., 2016. Application of a new PCR-RFLP panel suggests a restricted population structure for *Eimeria tenella* in UK and Irish chickens. *Vet. Parasitol.* 229, 60–67.

1343. Pellerdy, L., 1974. Coccidia and coccidiosis. Verlag Paul Parey. Berlin, Germany, 2nd ed., 1–959.

1344. Pellérdy, L., Dürr, U., 1970. Zum endogenen Entwicklungszyklus von *Eimeria stiedai* (Lindemann, 1865) Kisskalt & Hartmann, 1907. *Acta Vet. Acad. Sci. Hung.* 20, 227–244.

1345. Temesgen, T.T., Tysnes, K.R., Robertson, L.J., 2019. A New protocol for molecular detection of *Cyclospora cayetanensis* as contaminants of berry fruits. *Front. Microbiol.* 10, 1939.

1346. Penner, L.R., 1956. Studies on renal coccidiosis of wild ducks from Long Island Sound. *J. Protozool.* 3, 10–11.

1347. Penzhorn, B.L., De Cramer, K.G.M., Booth, L.M., 1992. Coccidial infection in German shepherd dog pups in a breeding unit. *J. S. Afr. Vet. Assoc.* 63, 27–29.

1348. Penzhorn, B.L., Knapp, S.E., Speer, C.A., 1994. Enteric coccidia in free-ranging American bison (*Bison bison*) in Montana. *J. Wildl. Dis.* 30, 267–269.

1349. Penzhorn, B.L., Rognlie, M.C., Hall, L.L., Knapp, S.E., 1994. Enteric coccidia of Cashmere goats in southwestern Montana, USA. *Vet. Parasitol.* 55, 137–142.

1350. Perelman, B., Abarbanel, J.M., Gur-Lavie, A., Meller, Y., Elad, T., 1986. Clinical and pathological changes caused by the interaction of lasalocid and chloramphenicol in broiler chickens. *Avian Pathol.* 15, 279–288.

1351. Pérez, D., Muñoz, M.C., Molina, J.M., Muñoz-Caro, T., Silva, L.M.R., Taubert, A., Hermosilla, C., Ruiz, A., 2016. *Eimeria ninakohlyakimovae* induces NADPH oxidase-dependent monocyte extracellular trap formation and upregulates IL-12 and TNF-α, IL-6 and CCL2 gene transcription. *Vet. Parasitol.* 227, 143–150.

1352. Pérez-Fonseca, A., Alcala-Canto, Y., Salem, A.Z.M., Alberti-Navarro, A.B., 2016. Anticoccidial efficacy of naringenin and a grapefruit peel extract in growing lambs naturally-infected with *Eimeria* spp. *Vet. Parasitol.* 232, 58–65.

1353. Periz, J., Ryan, R., Blake, D.P., Tomley, F.M., 2009. *Eimeria tenella* microneme protein EtMIC4: Capture of the full-length transcribed sequence and comparison with other microneme proteins. *Parasitol. Res.* 104, 717–721.

1354. Petry, G., Kruedewagen, E., Kampkoetter, A., Krieger, K., 2011. Efficacy of emodepside/toltrazuril suspension (Procox oral suspension for dogs) against mixed experimental *Isospora felis/Isospora rivolta* infection in cats. *Parasitol. Res.* 109(Suppl 1), S29–S36.

1355. Pham, D., 2009. Chronic intermittent diarrhea in a 14-month-old Abyssinian cat. *Can. Vet. J.* 50, 85–87.

1356. Pichler, V., 2010. Endoparasitenstatus von Neuweltkameliden in Niederösterreich und der Steiermark. Dr. Vet. Med. thesis. Veterinärmedizinische Universität Vienna.

1357. Pinckney, R.D., Lindsay, D.S., Toivio-Kinnucan, M.A., Blagburn, B.L., 1993. Ultrastructure of *Isospora suis* during excystation and attempts to demonstrate extraintestinal stages in mice. *Vet. Parasitol.* 47, 225–233.

1358. Pines, M., Vlodavsky, I., Nagler, A., 2000. Halofuginone: From veterinary use to human therapy. *Drug Develop. Res.* 50, 371–378.

1359. Platzer, B., Prosl, H., Cieslicki, M., Joachim, A., 2005. Epidemiology of *Eimeria* infections in an Austrian milking sheep flock and control with diclazuril. *Vet. Parasitol.* 129, 1–9.

1360. Plitt, A., Imarom, S., Joachim, A., Daugschies, A., 1999. Interactive classification of porcine *Eimeria* spp. by computer-assisted image analysis. *Vet. Parasitol.* 86, 105–112.

1361. Pommier, P., Keïta, A., Wessel-Robert, S., Dellac, B., Mundt, H.C., 2003. Efficacy of toltrazuril in the prevention and the treatment of suckling piglets coccidiosis: Results of two field trials. *Rev. Med. Vet.* 1, 41–46.

1362. Poplstein, M., Vrba, V., 2011. Description of the two strains of turkey coccidia *Eimeria adenoeides* with remarkable morphological variability. *Parasitology* 138, 1211–1216.

1363. Postoli, R., Robaj, A., Ceroni, V., Zalla, P., Andoni, E., Caushi, A., 2010. Epidemiological study on the prevalence of endoparasites of equines in Albania. *Veterinaria (Sarajevo)* 59, 37–45.

1364. Poston, R.M., Carter, A.L., Marin, A., Hutchins, J.E., Avakian, A.P., LeMay, M.A., Genteman, K.C., Weber, F.H., Doelling, V.W., 2001. Efficacy of a coccidiosis vaccine delivered *in ovo* to commercial broilers. *Proceedings of the VIIIth International Coccidiosis Conference*, Sydney, Australia, pp. 128–129.

1365. Pravinbhai, P.K., 2017. Epidemiological studies on gastrointestinal parasitic infections of camel population in hyper arid partially irrigated zone of Rajasthan. Masters thesis, Bikaner Rajasthan University of Veterinary and Animal Sciences. 69 pages.

1366. Price, K.R., Hafeez, M.A., Bulfon, J., Barta, J.R., 2016. Live *Eimeria* vaccination success in the face of artificial non-uniform vaccine administration in conventionally reared pullets. *Avian Pathol.* 45, 82–93.

1367. Pyziel, A.M., Józwikowski, M., Demiaszkiewicz, A.W., 2014. Coccidia (Apicomplexa: Eimeriidae) of the lowland European bison *Bison bonasus bonasus* (L.). *Vet. Parasitol.* 202, 138–144.

1368. Pyziel, A.M., Kowalczyk, R., Demiaszkiewicz, A.W., 2011. The annual cycle of shedding *Eimeria* oocysts by European bison (*Bison bonasus*) in the Bialowieza Primeval Forest, Poland. *J. Parasitol.* 97, 737–739.

1369. Qiao, J., Meng, Q.L., Cai, X.P., Tian, G.F., Chen, C.F., Wang, J.W., Wang, W.S., Zhang, Z.C., Cai, K.J., Yang, L.H., 2012. Prevalence of coccidiosis in domestic rabbits (*Oryctolagus cuniculus*) in northwest China. *J. Anim. Vet. Adv.* 11, 517–520.

1370. Qin, M., Liu, X.Y., Tang, X.M., Suo, J.X., Tao, G.R., Suo, X., 2014. Transfection of *Eimeria mitis* with yellow fluorescent protein as reporter and the endogenous development of the transgenic parasite. *PLOS ONE* 9, e114188.

1371. Qin, M., Tang, X., Yin, G., Liu, X., Suo, J., Tao, G., El-Ashram, S., Li, Y., Suo, X., 2016. Chicken IgY Fc expressed by *Eimeria mitis* enhances the immunogenicity of *E. mitis. Parasit. Vectors* 9, 164.

1372. Qin, Z., Arakawa, A., Baba, E., Fukata, T., Sasai, K., 1996. Effect of *Eimeria tenella* infection on the production of *Salmonella enteritidis*-contaminated eggs and susceptibility of laying hens to *S. enteritidis* infection. *Avian Dis.* 40, 361–367.

1373. Qin, Z., Kong, F., Arakawa, A., 1999. *Eimeria tenella* infection induces recrudescence of previous *Salmonella enteritidis* infection in chickens. *J. Chin. Agr. Univ.* 4 (Suppl), 93–97 (in Chinese).

1374. Qin, Z., Kong, F., Arakawa, A., 2000. Effect of *Eimeria tenella* infection on the population of some cecal intestinal flora. *Acta Vet. Zootech. Sinica* 31, 78–82 (in Chinese).

1375. Qin, Z., Kong, F., Arakawa, A., 2000. Effects of *Eimeria tenella* infection on the population of some cecal facultative anaerobic flora. *Acta Parasitol. Med. Entomol. Sinica* 7, 76–79 (in Chinese).

1376. Qin, Z., Kong, F., Arakawa, A., Baba, E., 1998. Enhancing effect of *Eimeria tenella* infection on *Salmonella enteritidis* in chickens. *J. China Agric. Univ.* 3 (suppl), 25–31 (in Chinese).

1377. Qin, Z.R., Kong, F., Arakawa, A., Fukata, T., 1999. Effect of *Eimeria tenella* infection on the cecal population of beneficial normal bacteria. *J. Microbiol. China* 26, 106–109 (in Chinese).

1378. Quick, D.P., Steger, A.M., Welter, C.J., Welter, L.M., Welter, M.W., 1998. *Isospora suis Vaccine*. Ambico Inc https://patents.google.com/patent/EP0832237A1/en (accessed September 8, 2018).

1379. Quiroz-Castañeda, R.E., Dantán-González, E., 2015. Control of avian coccidiosis: Future and present natural alternatives. *Biomed Res. Int.* 2015, 430610.

1380. Qvarnstrom, Y., Wei-Pridgeon, Y., Li, W., Nascimento, F.S., Bishop, H.S., Herwaldt, B.L., Moss, D.M., et al. 2015. Draft genome sequences from *Cyclospora cayetanensis* oocysts purified from a human stool sample. *Genome Announc.* 3, e01324–15.

1381. Radavelli, W.M., Pazinato, R., Klauck, V., Volpato, A., Balzan, A., Rossett, J., Cazarotto, C.J., et al. 2014. Occurrence of gastrointestinal parasites in goats from the Western Santa Catarina, Brazil. *Braz. J. Vet. Parasitol.* 23, 101–104.

1382. Radostits, O.M., Stockdale, P.H.G., 1980. A brief review of bovine coccidiosis in Western Canada. *Can. Vet. J.* 21, 227–230.

1383. Rahman, W.A., 1994. Effect of subclinical *Eimeria* species infections in tropical goats subsequently challenged with caprine *Haemonchus contortus. Vet. Rec.* 134, 235–237.

1384. Raisinghani, P.M., Manohar, G.S., Yadav, J.S., 1987. *Isospora* infection in the Indian camel *Camelus dromedarius. Indian J. Parasitol.* 11, 93–94.

1385. Rajput, N., Ali, S., Naeem, M., Khan, M.A., Wang, T., 2014. The effect of dietary supplementation with the natural carotenoids curcumin and lutein on pigmentation, oxidative stability and quality of meat from broiler chickens affected by a coccidiosis challenge. *Br. Poult. Sci.* 55, 501–509.

1386. Rakhshandehroo, E., Razavi, S.M., Nazifi, S., Farzaneh, M., Mobarraei, N., 2013. Dynamics of the enzymatic antioxidants during experimental caprine coccidiosis. *Parasitol. Res.* 112, 1437–1441.

1387. Ramachandran Iyer, P.K., Ramachandran, S., Joshi, T.P., 1968. An outbreak of haemorrhagic gastro-enteritis in camels (*Camelus dromedarius*). *Ann. Soc. Belg. Med. Trop.* 43, 5–14.

1388. Ramadan, M.Y., Khater, H.F., Abd El Hay, A.R., Abo Zekry, A.M., 2015. Studies on parasites that cause diarrhea in calves. *Benha Vet. Med. J.* 29, 214–219.

1389. Ramírez, A., Valbuena, R., Ochoa, K., Uzcátegui, D., Gil, M., Chacín, E., Simoes, D., Ramírez, R., Cubillán, F.A., 2013. Coccidiosis (*Eimeria* spp.) en búfalos (*Bubalus bubalis*) del municipio Colón, edo. *Zulia, Venezuela. Revista Cientifica, FCV-LUZ* 23, 191–197.

1390. Ramirez, L., Berto, B.P., Teixeira Filho, W.L., Flausino, W., De Meireles, G.S., Rodrigues, J.S., Almeida, C.R.R., Lopes, C.W.G., 2009. *Eimeria bareillyi* from the domestic water buffalo, *Bubalus bubalis*, in the state of Rio de Janeiro, Brazil. *Rev. Bras. Med. Vet.* 31, 261–264.

1391. Randelzhofer, A., 1990. Inzidenz und Artenspektrum von Endoparasiten bei Mutterschweinen und ihren Ferkeln in unterschiedlichen Haltungs- und Betriebsformen. Dr. med. vet. thesis, Ludwig Maximilian University, Munich.

1392. Rangarao, G.S.C., Sharma, R.L., 1997. Intestinal coccidiosis due to *Eimeria rajasthani* in Camel (*Camelius dromedarius*). *Indian Vet. J.* 74, 427–428.

1393. Rathinam, T., Gadde, U., Chapman, H.D., 2015. Molecular detection of field isolates of turkey *Eimeria* by polymerase chain reaction amplification of the cytochrome c oxidase I gene. *Parasitol. Res.* 114, 2795–2799.

1394. Raue, K., Heuer, L., Böhm, C., Wolken, S., Epe, C., Strube, C., 2017. 10-year parasitological examination results (2003 to 2012) of faecal samples from horses, ruminants, pigs, dogs, cats, rabbits and hedgehogs. *Parasitol. Res.* 116, 3315–3330.

1395. Rauscher, B.A., Schäfer-Somi, S., Ehling-Schulz, M., Möstl, K., Handl, S., Hinney, B., Spergser, J., Schaper, R., Joachim, A., 2013. Control of canine endoparasites, especially *Isospora* spp., with Procox in naturally infected puppies: Parasitological, bacteriological and health parameters. *Open J. Vet. Med.* 3, 121–130.

1396. Ravenel, J.M., Suggs, J.L., Legerton, C.W., 1976. Human coccidiosis. Recurrent diarrhea of 26 years duration due *Isospora belli*: A case report. *J. South Carolina Med. Assoc.* 72, 217–219.

1397. Rawdon, T., McFadden, A., King, C., Mitchell, V., Howell, M., 2006. Clinical findings and risk factors associated with the first report of *Eimeria macusaniensis* in New Zealand alpacas. *Surveillance* 33, 11–15.

1398. Ray, H.N., Sarkar, A., 1967. On a new coccidium, *Tyzzeria chenicusae* n. sp. from cotton teal (*Chenicus coromendelianus*: Aves, Anseriformes). *J. Protozool.* 14, 27.

1399. Rebouças, M.M., Fujii, T.U., Amaral, V., Santos, S.M., Spósito Fa., E., Barci, L.A.G., Fujii, T., 1990. Eimeriídeos parasitas de búfalos (*Bubalus bubalis* L.) da região do vale do Ribeira, Estado de São Paulo, Brasil. *Arq. Inst. Biol.* 57, 1–3.

1400. Rebouças, M.M., Grasso, L.M.P.S., Spósito Filha, E., do Amaral, V., Santos, S.M., Silva, D.M., 1994. Prevalência e distribuição de protozoários do gênero *Eimeria* (Apicomplexa: Eimeriidae) em bovinos nos municípios de Altinópolis, Taquaritinga, São Carlos e Guaíra—estado de São Paulo, Brasil. *Rev. Bras. Parasitol. Vet.* 3, 125–130.

1401. Reeg, K.J., Gauly, M., Bauer, C., Mertens, C., Erhardt, G., Zahner, H., 2005. Coccidial infections in housed lambs: Oocyst excretion, antibody levels and genetic influences on the infection. *Vet. Parasitol.* 127, 209–219.

1402. Regidor-Cerrillo, J., Arranz-Solís, D., Benavides, J., Gómez-Bautista, M., Castro-Hermida, J.A., Mezo, M., Pérez, V., Ortega-Mora, L.M., González-Warleta, M., 2014. *Neospora caninum* infection during early pregnancy in cattle: How the isolate influences infection dynamics, clinical outcome and peripheral and local immune responses. *Vet. Res.* 45, 10.

1403. Reichenow, E., 1940. Ueber das Kokzid der Equiden *Globidium leuckarti*. *Z. Infektionskrankh. Parasitäre Krankh. Hyg. Haustiere* 2, 126–134.

1404. Reid, A.J., Blake, D.P., Ansari, H.R., Billington, K., Browne, H.P., Bryant, J., Dunn, M., et al. 2014. Genomic analysis of the causative agents of coccidiosis in domestic chickens. *Genome Res.* 24, 1676–1685.

1405. Reid, W.M., 1975. Progress in the control of coccidiosis with anticoccidials and planned immunization. *Am. J. Vet. Res.* 36 (4 Pt 2), 593–596.

1406. Reinemeyer, C.R., Lindsay, D.S., Mitchell, S.M., Mundt, H.C., Charles, S.D., Arther, R.G., Settje, T.L., 2007. Development of experimental *Cystoisospora canis* infection models in beagle puppies and efficacy evaluation of 5% ponazuril (toltrazuril sulfone) oral suspension. *Parasitol. Res.* 101, S129–S136.

1407. Ren, C., Yin, G., Qin, M., Suo, J., Lv, Q., Xie, L., Wang, Y., et al. 2014. CDR3 analysis of TCR Vβ repertoire of CD8+ T cells from chickens infected with *Eimeria maxima*. *Exp. Parasitol.* 143, 1–4.

1408. Renaux, S., Drouet-Viard, F., Chanteloup, N.K., Le Vern, Y., Kerboeuf, D., Pakandl, M., Coudert, P., 2001. Tissues and cells involved in the invasion of the rabbit intestinal tract by sporozoites of *Eimeria coecicola*. *Parasitol. Res.* 87, 98–106.

1409. Renaux, S., Quéré, P., Buzoni-Gatel, D., Sewald, B., Le Vern, Y., Coudert, P., Drouet-Viard, F., 2003. Dynamics and responsiveness of T-lymphocytes in secondary lymphoid organs of rabbits developing immunity to *Eimeria intestinalis*. *Vet. Parasitol.* 110, 181–195.

1410. Reppert, J.F., Kemp, R., 1972. Nervous coccidiosis. *Iowa St. Univ. Vet.* 34, 9–12.

1410a. Resende, D.V., Pedrosa, A.L., Correia, D., Cabrine-Santos, M., Lages-Silva, E., Meira, W.S.F., Oliveira-Silva, M.B., 2011. Polymorphisms in the 18S rDNA gene of *Cystoisospora belli* and clinical features of cystoisosporosis in HIV-infected patients. *Parasitol. Res.* 108, 679–685.

1411. Restrepo, C., Macher, A.M., Radany, E.H., 1987. Disseminated extraintestinal isosporiasis in a patient with acquired immune deficiency syndrome. *Am. J. Clin. Pathol.* 87, 536–542.

1412. Revets, H., Dekegel, D., Deleersnijder, W., De Jonckheere, J., Peeters, J., Leysen, E., Hamers, R., 1989. Identification of virus-like particles in *Eimeria stiedae*. *Mol. Biochem. Parasitol.* 36, 209–215.

1413. Reyna, P.S., McDougald, L.R., Mathis, G.F., 1983. Survival of coccidia in poultry litter and reservoirs of infection. *Avian Dis.* 27, 464–473.

1414. Reynaud, M.C., Chauve, C.M., Gastellu, J., Gounel, J.M., 1999. Administration of toltrazuril during experimental coccidiosis in mule ducks: Comparison of the efficacy of a single administration at two different endogenous stages. *Vet. Parasitol.* 81, 265–274.

1415. Ribeiro, M.G., Langoni, H., Jerez, J.A., Leite, D.S., Ferreira, F., Gennari, S.M., 2000. Identification of enteropathogens from buffalo calves with and without diarrhoea in the Ribeira Valley, State of São Paulo, Brazil. *Braz. J. Vet. Res. Anim. Sci.* 37, 159–165.

1416. Rickard, L.G., Bishop, J.K., 1988. Prevalence of *Eimeria* spp. (Apicomplexa: Eimeriidae) in Oregon llamas. *J. Protozool.* 35, 335–336.

1417. Ricketts, A.P., Glazer, E.A., Migaki, T.T., Olson, J.A., 1992. Anticoccidial efficacy of semduramicin in battery studies with laboratory isolates of coccidia. *Poult. Sci.* 71, 98–103.

1418. Riddell, F.G., 2002. Structure, conformation, and mechanism in the membrane transport of alkali metal ions by ionophoric antibiotics. *Chirality* 14, 121–125.

1419. Roberts, L., Walker, E.J., 1981. Coccidiosis in pigs. *Vet. Rec.* 108, 62.

1420. Roberts, L., Walker, E.J., 1982. Field study of coccidial and rotaviral diarrhoea in unweaned piglets. *Vet. Rec.* 110, 11–13.

1421. Roberts, L., Walker, E.J., Snodgrass, D.R., Angus, K.W., 1980. Diarrhoea in unweaned piglets associated with rotavirus and coccidial infections. *Vet. Rec.* 107, 156–157.

1422. Roberts, W.L., Hammond, D.M., 1970. Ultrastructural and cytologic studies of the sporozoites of four *Eimeria* species. *J. Protozool.* 17, 76–86.

1423. Roberts, W.L., Hammond, D.M., Anderson, L.C., Speer, C.A., 1970. Ultrastructural study of schizogony in *Eimeria callospermophili*. *J. Protozool.* 17, 584–592.

1424. Robinson, Y., Morin, M., 1982. Porcine neonatal coccidiosis in Quebec. *Can. Vet. J.* 23, 212–216.

1425. Robinson, Y., Morin, M., Girard, C., Higgins, R., 1983. Experimental transmission of intestinal coccidiosis to piglets: Clinical, parasitological and pathological findings. *Can. J. Comp. Med.* 47, 401–407.

1426. Roditi, I., Wyler, T., Smith, N., Braun, R., 1994. Virus-like particles in *Eimeria nieschulzi* are associated with multiple RNA segments. *Mol. Biochem. Parasitol.* 63, 275–282.

1427. Rodríguez, H.A., Casas, A.E., Luna, E.L., Gavidia Ch., C., Zanabria, H.V., Rosadio, A.R., 2012. Eimeriosis en crías de alpacas: Prevalencia y factores de riesgo. *Rev. Inv. Vet. Perú* 23, 289–298.

1428. Roepstorff, A., Nilsson, O., Oksanen, A., Gjerde, B., Richter, S.H., Örtenberg, E., Christensson, D., et al. 1998. Intestinal parasites in swine in the Nordic countries: Prevalence and geographical distribution. *Vet. Parasitol.* 76, 305–319.

1429. Rohbeck, S., 2006. Parasitosen des Verdauungstrakts und der Atemwege bei Neuweltkameliden: Untersuchungen zu ihrer Epidemiologie und Bekämpfung in einer süd-hessischen Herde sowie zur Biologie von *Eimeria macusaniensis*. Dr. Vet. Med. thesis. Justus-Liebig-University Giessen.

1430. Rojas, M., Manchego, A., Rocha, C.B., Fornells, L.A., Silva, R.C., Mendes, G.S., Dias, H.G., Sandoval, N., Pezo, D., Santos, N., 2016. Outbreak of diarrhea among pre-weaning alpacas (*Vicugna pacos*) in the southern Peruvian highland. *J. Infect. Dev. Ctries.* 10, 269–274.

1431. Rommel, M., 1970. Die Wirkung von Antilymphozytenserum und Kortikosteroiden auf den Übervölkerungseffekt und die Immunität bei der *Eimeria scabra*-Infektion des Schweines. *Zentralbl. Veterinärmed. B* 17, 798–805.

1432. Rommel, M., 1970. Verlauf der *Eimeria scabra*- und *E. polita*-Infektion in vollempfänglichen Ferkeln un Läuferschweinen. *Berl. Münch. tierärztl. Wochenschr* 83, 181–200.

1433. Rommel, M., Ipczynski, V., 1967. Der Lebenszyklus des Schweinekokzids *Eimeria scabra* (Henry, 1931). *Berl. Münch. tierärztl. Woch.* 80, 65–70.

1434. Rommel, M., Zielasko, B., 1981. Untersuchungen über den Lebenszyklus von *Isospora burrowsi* (Trayser und Todd, 1978) aus dem Hund. *Berl. Münch. tierärztl. Wochenschr* 94, 87–90.

1435. Ros Die, A., Nogueira Coito, J.M., 2018. Picture of a microorganism: *Isospora belli*. *Clin. Microbiol. Infect.* 24, 43–44.

1436. Rosadio, R., Londoñe, P., Pérez, D., Castillo, H., Véliz, A., Llanco, L., Yaya, K., Maturrano, L., 2010. *Eimeria macusaniensis* associated lesions in neonate alpacas dying from enterotoxemia. *Vet. Parasitol.* 168, 116–120.

1437. Rosadio, R.H., Ameghino, E.F., 1994. Coccidial infections in neonatal Peruvian alpacas. *Vet. Rec.* 135, 459–460.

1438. Rose, M.E., 1967. Immunity to *Eimeria tenella* and *Eimeria necatrix* infections in the fowl. I. Influence of the site of infection and the stage of the parasite. II. Cross-protection. *Parasitology* 57, 567–583.

1439. Rose, M.E., 1967. The influence of age of host on infection with *Eimeria tenella*. *J. Parasitol.* 53, 924–929.

1440. Rose, M.E., 1972. Immunity to coccidiosis: Maternal transfer in *Eimeria maxima* infections. *Parasitology* 65, 273–282.

1441. Rose, M.E., 1973. Immunity. In Hammond, D.M. and Long, P.L. (Ed.), *The Coccidia: Eimeria, Isospora, Toxoplasma, and Related Genera*. University Park Press. Baltimore, MD, 295–341.

1442. Rose, M.E., 1974. Protective antibodies in infections with *Eimeria maxima*: The reduction of pathogenic effects *in vivo* and a comparison between oral and subcutaneous administration of antiserum. *Parasitology* 68, 285–292.

1443. Rose, M.E., 1982. Host immune responses. In Long, P.L. (Ed.), *The Biology of the Coccidia*. Edward Arnold. London, 329–371.

1444. Rose, M.E., Hesketh, P., 1976. Immunity to coccidiosis: Stages of the life-cycle of *Eimeria maxima* which induce, and are affected by, the response of the host. *Parasitology* 73, 25–37.

1445. Rose, M.E., Hesketh, P., 1979. Immunity to coccidiosis: T-lymphocyte- or B-lymphocyte-deficient animals. *Infect. Immun.* 26, 630–637.

1446. Rose, M.E., Hesketh, P., Ogilvie, B.M., 1979. Peripheral blood leucocyte response to coccidial infection: A comparison of the response in rats and chickens and its correlation with resistance to reinfection. *Immunology* 36, 71–79.

1447. Rose, M.E., Hesketh, P., Wakelin, D., 1992. Immune control of murine coccidiosis: CD4+ and CD8+ T lymphocytes contribute differentially in resistance to primary and secondary infections. *Parasitology* 105 (Pt 3), 349–354.

1448. Rose, M.E., Lawn, A.M., Millard, B.J., 1984. The effect of immunity on the early events in the life-cycle of *Eimeria tenella* in the caecal mucosa of the chicken. *Parasitology* 88 (Pt 2), 199–210.

1449. Rose, M.E., Long, P.L., 1962. Immunity to four species of *Eimeria* in fowls. *Immunology* 5, 79–92.

1450. Rose, M.E., Long, P.L., 1971. Immunity to coccidiosis: Protective effects of transferred serum and cells investigated in chick embryos infected with *Eimeria tenella*. *Parasitology* 63, 299–313.

1451. Rose, M.E., Wakelin, D., Hesketh, P., 1991. Interferon-γ-mediated effects upon immunity to coccidial infections in the mouse. *Parasite Immunol.* 13, 63–74.

1452. Rosenberg, B., Juckett, D.A., Aylsworth, C.F., Dimitrov, N.V., Ho, S.C., Judge, J.W., Kessel, S., et al. 2005. Protein from intestinal *Eimeria* protozoan stimulates IL-12 release from dendritic cells, exhibits antitumor properties *in vivo* and is correlated with low intestinal tumorigenicity. *Int. J. Cancer* 114, 756–765.

1453. Rosenthal, B.M., Dunams-Morel, D., Ostoros, G., Molnár, K., 2016. Coccidian parasites of fish encompass profound phylogenetic diversity and gave rise to each of the major parasitic groups in terrestrial vertebrates. *Infect. Genet. Evol.* 40, 219–227.

1454. Rothwell, L., Gramzinski, R.A., Rose, M.E., Kaiser, P., 1995. Avian coccidiosis: Changes in intestinal lymphocyte populations associated with the development of immunity to *Eimeria maxima*. *Parasite Immunol.* 17, 525–533.

1455. Rothwell, L., Muir, W., Kaiser, P., 2000. Interferon-γ is expressed in both gut and spleen during *Eimeria tenella* infection. *Avian Pathol.* 29, 333–342.

1456. Rothwell, L., Young, J.R., Zoorob, R., Whittaker, C.A., Hesketh, P., Archer, A., Smith, A.L., Kaiser, P., 2004. Cloning and characterization of chicken IL-10 and its role in the immune response to *Eimeria maxima*. *J. Immunol.* 173, 2675–2682.

1457. Ruff, M.D., Doran, D.J., Augustine, P.C., 1980. *Eimeria meleagrimitis* Tyzzer in turkeys: The life cycle and effects of inoculum size and time on severity of infection and intestinal distribution. *J. Protozool.* 27, 186–189.

1458. Ruiz, A., Behrendt, J.H., Zahner, H., Hermosilla, C., Pérez, D., Matos, L., Muñoz, M.C., Molina, J.M., Taubert, A., 2010. Development of *Eimeria ninakohlyakimovae in vitro* in primary and permanent cell lines. *Vet. Parasitol.* 173, 2–10.

1459. Ruiz, A., Gonzalez, J.F., Rodriguez, E., Martin, S., Hernandez, Y.I., Almeida, R., Molina, J.M., 2006. Influence of climatic and management factors on *Eimeria* infections in goats from semi-arid zones. *J. Vet Med. B Infect. Dis. Vet Public Health* 53, 399–402.

1460. Ruiz, A., Guedes, A.C., Muñoz, M.C., Molina, J.M., Hermosilla, C., Martín, S., Hernández, Y.I., et al. 2012. Control strategies using diclazuril against coccidiosis in goat kids. *Parasitol. Res.* 110, 2131–2136.

1461. Ruiz, A., Matos, L., Muñoz, M.C., Hermosilla, C., Molina, J.M., Andrada, M., Rodríguez, F., et al. 2013. Isolation of an *Eimeria ninakohlyakimovae* field strain (Canary Islands) and analysis of its infection characteristics in goat kids. *Res. Vet. Sci.* 94, 277–284.

1462. Ruiz, A., Muñoz, M.C., Molina, J.M., Hermosilla, C., Andrada, M., Lara, P., Bordón, E., et al. 2014. Immunization with *Eimeria ninakohlyakimovae*-live attenuated oocysts protect goat kids from clinical coccidiosis. *Vet. Parasitol.* 199, 8–17.

1463. Ruiz, A., Muñoz, M.C., Molina, J.M., Hermosilla, C., Rodríguez, F., Andrada, M., Martín, S., et al. 2013. Primary infection of goats with *Eimeria ninakohlyakimovae* does not provide protective immunity against high challenge infections. *Small Ruminant Res.* 113, 258–266.

1464. Ruiz, A., Perez, D., Munoz, M.C., Molina, J.M., Taubert, A., Jacobs-Lorena, M., Vega-Rodriguez, J., Lopez, A.M., Hermosilla, C., 2015. Targeting essential *Eimeria ninakohlyakimovae* sporozoite ligands for caprine host endothelial cell invasion with a phage display peptide library. *Parasitol. Res.* 114, 4327–4331.

1465. Ruiz, V.L.A., Bersano, J.G., Carvalho, A.F., Catroxo, M.H.B., Chiebao, D.P., Gregori, F., Miyashiro, S., et al. 2016. Case-control study of pathogens involved in piglet diarrhea. *BMC Res. Notes* 9, 22.

1466. Ruttkowski, B., Joachim, A., Daugschies, A., 2001. PCR-based differentiation of three porcine *Eimeria* species and *Isospora suis*. *Vet. Parasitol.* 95, 17–23.

1467. Ruzicka, C.W., Andrews, J.J., 1983. Porcine neonatal coccidiosis: A clinical review. *Iowa State Univ. Vet.* 45, 90–95.

1468. Ryan, R., Shirley, M., Tomley, F., 2000. Mapping and expression of microneme genes in *Eimeria tenella*. *Int. J. Parasitol.* 30, 1493–1499.

1469. Rychen, G., Aquilina, G., Azimonti, G., Bampidis, V., Bastos, M.L., Bories, G., Chesson, A., et al. 2018. Safety and efficacy of COXAM (amprolium hydrochloride) for chickens for fattening and chickens reared for laying. *EFSA J.* 16 (7), 5338.

1470. Ryff, K.L., Bergstrom, R.C., 1975. Bovine coccidia in American bison. *J. Wildl. Dis.* 11, 412–414.

1471. Ryley, J.F., 1975. Lerbek, a synergistic mixture of methyl benzoquate and clopidol for the prevention of chicken coccidiosis. *Parasitology* 70, 377–384.

1472. Ryley, J.F., Betts, M.J., 1973. Chemotherapy of chicken coccidiosis. *Adv. Pharmacol.* 11, 221–293.

1473. Ryley, J.F., Robinson, T.E., 1976. Life cycle studies with *Eimeria magna* Pérard, 1925. *Z. Parasitenkd.* 50, 257–275.

1474. Ryley, J.F., Wilson, R.G., 1972. The development of *Eimeria brunetti* in tissue culture. *J. Parasitol.* 58, 660–663.

1475. Sagua, H., Soto, J., Delano, B., Fuentes, A., Becker, P., 1978. Brote epidémico de isosporosis por *Isospora belli* en la ciudad de Antofagasta, Chile. Consideraciones sobre 90 casos diagnosticados en 3 meses. *Bol. Chil. Parasitol.* 33, 8–12.

1476. Sahinduran, S., Sezer, K., Buyukoglu, T., Yukari, B.A., Albay, M.K., 2006. Plasma ascorbic acid levels in lambs with coccidiosis. *Turk. J. Vet. Anim. Sci.* 30, 219–221.

1477. Saitoh, Y., Itagaki, H., 1990. Dung beetles, *Onthophagus* spp., as potential transport hosts of feline coccidia. *Jpn. J. Vet. Sci.* 52, 293–297.

1478. Sakr, H.R.M., 1988. *Studies on the Enteric Protozoa of Camel in Egypt*. M.V.Sc thesis. Cairo University. 40 pages.

1479. Salmon, H., Berri, M., Gerdts, V., Meurens, F., 2009. Humoral and cellular factors of maternal immunity in swine. *Dev. Comp. Immunol.* 33, 384–393.

1480. Samarasinghe, B., Johnson, J., Ryan, U., 2008. Phylogenetic analysis of *Cystoisospora* species at the rRNA ITS1 locus and development of a PCR-RFLP assay. *Exp. Parasitol.* 118, 592–595.

1481. Sampson, J.R., Hammond, D.M., 1972. Fine structural aspects of development of *Eimeria alabamensis* schizonts in cell cultures. *J. Parasitol.* 58, 311–322.

1482. Sampson, J.R., Hammond, D.M., Ernst, J.V., 1971. Development of *Eimeria alabamensis* from cattle in mammalian cell cultures. *J. Protozool.* 18, 120–128.

1483. Sanad, M.M., Thagfan, F.A., Al Olayan, E.M., Almogren, A., Al Hammaad, A., Al-Mawash, A., Mohamed, A.A., 2014. Opportunistic coccidian parasites among Saudi cancer patients presenting with diarrhea: Prevalence and immune status. *Res. J. Parasitol.* 9, 55–63.

1484. Sand, J.M., Arendt, M.K., Repasy, A., Deniz, G., Cook, M.E., 2016. Oral antibody to interleukin-10 reduces growth rate depression due to *Eimeria* spp. infection in broiler chickens. *Poult. Sci.* 95, 439–446.

1485. Sanford, S.E., 1983. Porcine neonatal coccidiosis: Clinical, pathological, epidemiological and diagnostic features. *Cal. Vet.* 37, 26–30.

1486. Sanford, S.E., Josephson, G.K.A., 1981. Porcine neonatal coccidiosis. *Can. Vet. J.* 22, 282–285.

1487. Sangster, L.T., Seibold, H.R., Mitchell, F.E., 1976. Coccidial infection in suckling pigs. *Proc. Am. Assoc. Vet. Lab. Diag.* 19, 51–55.

1488. Sangster, L.T., Stuart, B.P., Williams, D.J., Bedell, D.M., 1978. Coccidiosis associated with scours in baby pigs. *Vet. Med. Small Anim. Clin.* 73, 1317–1319.

1489. Sani, R.A., Chandrawathani, P., 1987. Coccidia of buffalo calves. *Trop. Biomed.* 4, 190–191.

1490. Sanyal, P.K., Ruprah, N.S., 1984. Endogenous stages and pathology in *Eimeria zürnii* coccidiosis in buffalo calves. *Sri Lanka Vet. J.* 32, 22–25.

1491. Sanyal, P.K., Ruprah, N.S., Chhabra, M.B., 1985. Attempted transmission of three species of *Eimeria* Schneider, 1875 of buffalo-calves to cow-calves. *Indian J. Anim. Sci.* 55, 301–304.

1492. Sanyal, P.K., Ruprah, N.S., Chhabra, M.B., 1985. Chemotherapeutic efficacy of sulphadimidine, amprolium, halofuginone and chloroquine phosphate in experimental *Eimeria bareillyi* coccidiosis of buffaloes. *Vet. Parasitol.* 17, 117–122.

1493. Sanyal, P.K., Ruprah, N.S., Chhabra, M.B., 1985. Evidence of cell mediated immune response in infection with *Eimeria bareillyi* in buffaloes. *Vet. Parasitol.* 17, 111–115.

1494. Saratsis, A., Joachim, A., Alexandros, S., Sotiraki, S., 2011. Lamb coccidiosis dynamics in different dairy production systems. *Vet. Parasitol.* 181, 131–138.

1495. Saratsis, A., Karagiannis, I., Brozos, C., Kiossis, E., Tzanidakis, N., Joachim, A., Sotiraki, S., 2013. Lamb eimeriosis: Applied treatment protocols in dairy sheep production systems. *Vet. Parasitol.* 196, 56–63.

1496. Saratsis, A., Regos, I., Tzanidakis, N., Voutzourakis, N., Stefanakis, A., Treuter, D., Joachim, A., Sotiraki, S., 2012. *In vivo* and *in vitro* efficacy of sainfoin (*Onobrychis viciifolia*) against *Eimeria* spp. in lambs. *Vet. Parasitol.* 188, 1–9.

1497. Saratsis, A., Voutzourakis, N., Theodosiou, T., Stefanakis, A., Sotiraki, S., 2016. The effect of sainfoin (*Onobrychis viciifolia*) and carob pods (*Ceratonia siliqua*) feeding regimes on the control of lamb coccidiosis. *Parasitol. Res.* 115, 2233–2242.

1498. Sarkar, A.C., Ray, H.N., 1968. On a new coccidium, *Wenyonella gagari* n. sp. from the domestic duck, *Anas boschus.* Proceedings of 55th Indian Scientific Association, pp. 499–500.

1499. Sarvi, S., Daryani, A., Sharif, M., Rahimi, M.T., Kohansal, M.H., Mirshafiee, S., Siyadatpanah, A., Hosseini, S.A., Gholami, S., 2018. Zoonotic intestinal parasites of carnivores: A systematic review in Iran. *Vet. World* 11, 58–65.

1500. Sathyanarayanan, L., Ortega, Y., 2006. Effects of temperature and different food matrices on *Cyclospora cayetanensis* oocyst sporulation. *J. Parasitol.* 92, 218–222.

1501. Sauda, F.C., Zamarioli, L.A., Ebner Filho, W., Mello, L.B., 1993. Prevalence of *Cryptosporidium* sp. and *Isospora belli* among AIDS patients attending Santos Reference Center for AIDS, Sao Paulo, Brazil. *J. Parasitol.* 79, 454–456.

1502. Sayd, S.M.O., Kawazoe, U., 1996. Prevalence of porcine neonatal isosporosis in Brazil. *Vet. Parasitol.* 67, 169–174.

1503. Sayd, S.M.O., Kawazoe, U., 1998. Experimental infection of swine by *Isospora suis* Biester 1934 for species confirmation. *Mem. Inst. Oswaldo Cruz* 93, 851–854.

1504. Sayin, F., 1968. The sporulated oocysts of *E. ankarensis* n. sp. and of other species of *Eimeria* of buffalo in Turkey and transmission of four species of *Eimeria* from buffalo to cow-calves. *Ankara Üniv. Vet. Fak. Derg.* 15, 282–300.

1505. Sayin, F., 1973. The presence of *Eimeria bareillyi* (Gill, Chhabra and Lall, 1963) in buffalo in Turkey. *Ankara Üniv. Vet. Fak. Derg.* 20, 38–42.

1506. Sazmand, A., Hamidinejat, H., Hekmatimoghaddam, S., Asadollahi, Z., Mirabdollahi, S., 2012. *Eimeria* infection in camels (*Camelus dromedarius*) in Yazd province, central Iran. *Trop. Biomed.* 29, 77–80.

1507. Scala, A., Demontis, F., Varcasia, A., Pipia, A.P., Poglayen, G., Ferrari, N., Genchi, M., 2009. Toltrazuril and sulphonamide treatment against naturally *Isospora suis* infected suckling piglets: Is there an actual profit? *Vet. Parasitol.* 163, 362–365.

1508. Schares, G., Pantchev, N., Barutzki, D., Heydorn, A.O., Bauer, C., Conraths, F.J., 2005. Oocysts of *Neospora caninum, Hammondia heydorni, Toxoplasma gondii* and *Hammondia hammondi* in faeces collected from dogs in Germany. *Int. J. Parasitol.* 35, 1525–1537.

1509. Schares, G., Vrhovec, M.G., Pantchev, N., Herrmann, D.C., Conraths, F.J., 2008. Occurrence of *Toxoplasma gondii* and *Hammondia hammondi* oocysts in the faeces of cats from Germany and other European countries. *Vet. Parasitol.* 152, 34–45.

1510. Schneider, K., Klaas, R., Kaspers, B., Staeheli, P., 2001. Chicken interleukin-6 cDNA structure and biological properties. *Eur. J. Biochem.* 268, 4200–4206.

1511. Schneider, K., Puehler, F., Baeuerle, D., Elvers, S., Staeheli, P., Kaspers, B., Weining, K.C., 2000. cDNA cloning of biologically active chicken interleukin-18. *J. Interferon Cytokine Res.* 20, 879–883.

1512. Schnitzler, B.E., Thebo, P.L., Mattsson, J.G., Tomley, F.M., Shirley, M.W., 1998. Development of a diagnostic PCR assay for the detection and discrimination of four pathogenic *Eimeria* species of the chicken. *Avian Pathol.* 27, 490–497.

1513. Schock, A., Bidewell, C.A., Duff, J.P., Scholes, S.F., Higgins, R.J., 2007. Coccidiosis in British alpacas (*Vicugna pacos*). *Vet. Rec.* 160, 805–806.

1514. Scholtyseck, E., 1955. *Eimeria anatis* n. sp., ein neues Coccid aus der Stockente (*Anas platyrhynchos*). *Arch. Protistenkd.* 100, 431–434.

1515. Scholtyseck, E., 1973. Ultrastructure. In Hammond, D.M. and Long, P.L. (Ed.), *The Coccidia. Eimeria, Isospora, Toxoplasma, and Related Genera.* University Park Press. Baltimore, MD, 81–144.

1516. Scholtyseck, E., Entzeroth, R., Pellérdy, L., 1979. Übertragung von *Eimeria stiedai* aus Kaninchen (*Oryctolagus cuniculus*) auf Feldhasen (*Lepus europaeus*). *Acta Vet. Acad. Sci. Hung.* 27, 365–373.

1517. Schrecke, W., Dürr, U., 1970. Excystations- und Infektionsversuche mit Kokzidienoocysten bei neugeborenen Tieren. *Zentralbl. Bakteriol. I. Abt. Orig.* 215, 252–258.

1518. Schrey, C.F., Abbott, T.A., Stewart, V.A., Marquardt, W.C., 1991. Coccidia of the llama, *Lama glama*, in Colorado and Wyoming. *Vet. Parasitol.* 40, 21–28.

1519. Schubnell, F., Von Ah, S., Graage, R., Sydler, T., Sidler, X., Hadorn, D., Basso, W., 2016. Occurrence, clinical involvement and zoonotic potential of endoparasites infecting Swiss pigs. *Parasitol. Int.* 65, 618–624.

1520. Schuhmacher, A., Bafundo, K.W., Islam, K.M.S., Aupperle, H., Glaser, R., Schoon, H.A., Gropp, J.M., 2006. Tiamulin and semduramicin: Effects of simultaneous administration on performance and health of growing broiler chickens. *Poult. Sci.* 85, 441–445.

1521. Schuster, R.K., Sivakumar, S., Nagy, P., Juhasz, J., Ismail, A., Kinne, J., 2017. *Cystoisospora orlovi* (Eimeriorina: Sarcocystidae)—A little known coccidian of the old world camelids. *J. Camel Prac. Res.* 24, 117–122.

1522. Schwarz, L., Joachim, A., Worliczek, H.L., 2013. Transfer of *Cystoisospora suis*-specific colostral antibodies and their correlation with the course of neonatal porcine cystoisosporosis. *Vet. Parasitol.* 197, 487–497.

1523. Schwarz L., Worliczek, H.L., Winkler, M., Joachim, A., 2014. Superinfection of sows with *Cystoisospora suis* ante partum leads to a milder course of cystoisosporosis in suckling piglets. *Vet. Parasitol.* 204, 158–168.

1524. Schwarz, R.S., Fetterer, R.H., Rosenberg, G.H., Miska, K.B., 2010. Coccidian merozoite transcriptome analysis from *Eimeria maxima* in comparison to *Eimeria tenella* and *Eimeria acervulina*. *J. Parasitol.* 96, 49–57.

1525. Schwarz, R.S., Jenkins, M.C., Klopp, S., Miska, K.B., 2009. Genomic analysis of *Eimeria* spp. populations in relation to performance levels of broiler chicken farms in Arkansas and North Carolina. *J. Parasitol.* 95, 871–880.

1526. Scribner, A., Moore, J.A., Ouvry, G., Fisher, M., Wyvratt, M., Leavitt, P., Liberator, P., et al. 2009. Synthesis and biological activity of anticoccidial agents: 2,3-diarylindoles. *Bioorg. Med. Chem. Lett.* 19, 1517–1521.

1527. Sedlak, C., Patzl, M., Saalmüller, A., Gerner, W., 2014. CD2 and CD8α define porcine γδ T cells with distinct cytokine production profiles. *Dev. Comp. Immunol.* 45, 97–106.

1528. Seeger, K.C., 1947. Flock *Eimeria tenella* inoculation followed by sulfaguanidine or sulfamethazine treatment as a method of controlling caecal coccidiosis. *Poult. Sci.* 26, 554–555.

1529. Segev, G., Baneth, G., Levitin, B., Shlosberg, A., Aroch, I., 2004. Accidental poisoning of 17 dogs with lasalocid. *Vet. Rec.* 155, 174–176.

1530. Selan, U., Vittorio, A., 1923. Nuovo coccidio nel cavallo (*Eimeria utinensis*). *Clinica Veterinaria: Rassegna di Polizia Sanitaria e di Igiene (Milano)* 47, 587–592.

1531. Selvaraj, R.K., 2013. Avian CD4⁺CD25⁺ regulatory T cells: Properties and therapeutic applications. *Dev. Comp. Immunol.* 41, 397–402.

1532. Sepp, T., Entzeroth, R., Mertsching, J., Hofschneider, P.H., Kandolf, R., 1991. Novel ribonucleic acid species in *Eimeria nieschulzi* are associated with RNA-dependent RNA polymerase activity. *Parasitol. Res.* 77, 581–584.

1533. Sercy, O., Nie, K., Pascalon, A., Fort, G., Yvoré, P., 1996. Receptivity and susceptibility of the domestic duck (*Anas platyrhynchos*), the Muscovy duck (*Cairina moschata*), and their hybrid, the mule duck, to an experimental infection by *Eimeria mulardi*. *Avian Dis.* 40, 23–27.

1534. Shack, L.A., Buza, J.J., Burgess, S.C., 2008. The neoplastically transformed (CD30ʰⁱ) Marek's disease lymphoma cell phenotype most closely resembles T-regulatory cells. *Cancer Immunol. Immunother.* 57, 1253–1262.

1535. Shah, H.L., 1971. The life cycle of *Isospora felis* Wenyon, 1923, a coccidium of the cat. *J. Protozool.* 18, 3–17.

1536. Shah, H.L., Joshi, S.C., 1963. Coccidia (Protozoa: Eimeriidae) of goats in Madhya Pradesh, with descriptions of the sporulated oocysts of eight species. *J. Vet. Anim. Hus. Res.* 7, 9–20.

1537. Shah, M.A.A., Yan, R., Xu, L., Song, X., Li, X., 2010. A recombinant DNA vaccine encoding *Eimeria acervulina* cSZ-2 induces immunity against experimental *E. tenella* infection. *Vet. Parasitol.* 169, 185–189.

1538. Shahiduzzaman, M., Dyachenko, V., Keidel, J., Schmaschke, R., Daugschies, A., 2010. Combination of cell culture and quantitative PCR (cc-qPCR) to assess disinfectants efficacy on *Cryptosporidium* oocysts under standardized conditions. *Vet. Parasitol.* 167, 43–49.

1539. Shanmugasundaram, R., Selvaraj, R.K., 2011. Regulatory T cell properties of chicken CD4⁺CD25⁺ cells. *J. Immunol.* 186, 1997–2002.

1540. Sharma, D., Singh, N.K., Singh, H., Joachim, A., Rath, S.S., Blake, D.P., 2018. Discrimination, molecular characterisation and phylogenetic comparison of porcine *Eimeria* spp. India. *Vet. Parasitol.* 255, 43–48.

1541. Sharma, N., Bhalla, A., Varma, S., Jain, S., Singh, S., 2005. Toxicity of maduramicin. *Emerg. Med. J.* 22, 880–882.

1542. Sharman, P.A., Smith, N.C., Wallach, M.G., Katrib, M., 2010. Chasing the golden egg: Vaccination against poultry coccidiosis. *Parasite Immunol.* 32, 590–598.

1543. Shastri, U.V., Ghafoor, M.A., 1982. Observations on the developmental stages of *Eimeria bareillyi* Gill, Chhabra and Lall, 1963, in buffalo-calves. *Indian J. Anim. Sci.* 52, 309–313.

1544. Shastri, U.V., Ghafoor, M.A., Krishnamurthy, R., 1976. Some observations on coccidian lesions associated with endogenous phases in buffalo calves. *Indian J. Anim. Sci.* 46, 556–561.

1545. Shastri, U.V., Krishnamurthi, R., 1975. A note on pathological lesions in clinical bubaline coccidiosis due to *Eimeria bareillyi*. *Indian J. Anim. Sci.* 45, 46–47.

1546. Shastri, U.V., Krishnamurthi, R., Ghafoor, M.A., 1973. Some observations on pathogenicity of *Eimeria bareillyi* in buffalo calves. *Indian J. Anim. Res.* 7, 23–25.

1547. Shastri, U.V., Krishnamurthi, R., Ghafoor, M.A., 1974. A note on clinical coccidiosis in buffalo calves due to *Eimeria bariellyi* Gill, Chharbra and Hall, 1963 in Maharashtra. *Indian Vet. J.* 51, 301–302.

1548. Sheahan, B.J., 1976. *Eimeria leuckarti* infection in a thoroughbred foal. *Vet. Rec.* 99, 213–214.

1549. Sheffield, H.G., Hammond, D.M., 1966. Fine structure of first-generation merozoites of *Eimeria bovis*. *J. Parasitol.* 52, 595–606.

1550. Shen, X., Wang, C., Zhu, Q., Li, T., Yu, L., Zheng, W., Fei, C., Qiu, M., Xue, F., 2012. Effect of the diclazuril on Hsp90 in the second-generation merozoites of *Eimeria tenella*. *Vet. Parasitol.* 185, 290–295.

1551. Shen, X.J., Li, T., Fu, J.J., Zhang, K.Y., Wang, X.Y., Liu, Y.C., Zhang, H.J., Fan, C., Fei, C.Z., Xue, F.Q., 2014. Proteomic analysis of the effect of diclazuril on second-generation merozoites of *Eimeria tenella*. *Parasitol. Res.* 113, 903–909.

1552. Sherchan, J.B., Sherpa, K., Tandukar, S., Cross, J.H., Gajadhar, A., Sherchand, J.B., 2010. Infection of *Cyclospora cayetanensis* in diarrhoeal children of Nepal. *J. Nepal Paed. Soc.* 30, 23–30.

1553. Sherchand, J.B., Cross, J.H., 2001. Emerging pathogen *Cyclospora cayetanensis* infection in Nepal. *Southeast Asian J. Trop. Med. Pub. Health* 32 (Suppl 2), 143–150.

1554. Shi, T., Bao, G., Fu, Y., Suo, X., Hao, L., 2014. A low-virulence *Eimeria intestinalis* isolate from rabbit (*Oryctolagus cuniculus*) in China: Molecular identification, pathogenicity, and immunogenicity. *Parasitol. Res.* 113, 1085–1090.

1555. Shi, T., Tao, G., Bao, G., Suo, J., Hao, L., Fu, Y., Suo, X., 2016. Stable transfection of *Eimeria intestinalis* and investigation of its life cycle, reproduction and immunogenicity. *Front. Microbiol.* 7, 807.

1556. Shi, T., Yan, W., Ren, H., Liu, X., Suo, X., 2009. Dynamic development of parasitophorous vacuole of *Eimeria tenella* transfected with the yellow fluorescent protein gene fused to different signal sequences from apicomplexan parasites. *Parasitol. Res.* 104, 315–320.

1557. Shibalova, T.A., 1970. Cultivation of the endogenous stages of chicken coccidia in embryos and in tissue culture. *J. Parasitol.* 56 (4 sec II pt. 1), 315–316.

1558. Shields, J.M., Lee, M.M., Murphy, H.R., 2012. Use of a common laboratory glassware detergent improves recovery of *Cryptosporidium parvum* and *Cyclospora cayetanensis* from lettuce, herbs and raspberries. *Int. J. Food Microbiol.* 153, 123–128.

1559. Shiotani, N., Baba, E., Fukata, T., Arakawa, A., Nakanishi, T., 1992. Distribution of oocysts, sporocysts and sporozoites of *Eimeria tenella* and *Eimeria maxima* in the digestive tract of chicken. *Vet. Parasitol.* 41, 17–22.

1560. Shirley, M.W., 1994. The genome of *Eimeria tenella*: Further studies on its molecular organisation. *Parasitol. Res.* 80, 366–373.

1561. Shirley, M.W., Bellatti, M.A., 1988. Live attenuated coccidiosis vaccine: Selection of a second precocious line of *Eimeria maxima*. *Res. Vet. Sci.* 44, 25–28.

1562. Shirley, M.W., Blake, D., White, S.E., Sheriff, R., Smith, A.L., 2004. Integrating genetics and genomics to identify new leads for the control of *Eimeria* spp. *Parasitology* 128 (Suppl 1), S33–S42.

1563. Shirley, M.W., Harvey, D.A., 1996. *Eimeria tenella*: Genetic recombination of markers for precocious development and arprinocid resistance. *Appl. Parasitol.* 37, 293–299.

1564. Shirley, M.W., Harvey, D.A., 1996. *Eimeria tenella*: Infection with a single sporocyst gives a clonal population. *Parasitology* 112, 523–528.

1565. Shirley, M.W., Lillehoj, H.S., 2012. The long view: A selective review of 40 years of coccidiosis research. *Avian Pathol.* 41, 111–121.

1566. Shirley, M.W., Smith, A.L., Blake, D.P., 2007. Challenges in the successful control of the avian coccidia. *Vaccine* 25, 5540–5547.

1567. Shirley, M.W., Smith, A.L., Tomley, F.M., 2005. The biology of avian *Eimeria* with an emphasis on their control by vaccination. *Adv. Parasitol.* 60, 285–330.

1568. Shlosberg, A., Perl, S., Harmelin, A., Hanji, V., Bellaiche, M., Bogin, E., Cohen, R., et al., 1997. Acute maduramicin toxicity in calves. *Vet. Rec.* 140, 643–646.

1569. Shrestha, A., Abd-Elfattah, A., Freudenschuss, B., Hinney, B., Palmieri, N., Ruttkowski, B., Joachim, A., 2015. *Cystoisospora suis*—A model of mammalian cystoisosporosis. *Front. Vet. Sci.* 2, 68.

1570. Shrestha, A., Freudenschuss, B., Jansen, R., Hinney, B., Ruttkowski, B., Joachim, A., 2017. Experimentally confirmed toltrazuril resistance in a field isolate of *Cystoisospora suis*. *Parasit. Vectors* 10, 317.

1571. Shrestha, A., Freudenschuss, B., Schwarz, L., Joachim, A., 2018. Development and application of a recombinant protein-based indirect ELISA for the detection of serum antibodies against *Cystoisospora suis* in swine. *Vet. Parasitol.* 258, 57–63.

1572. Shrestha, A., Palmieri, N., Abd-Elfattah, A., Ruttkowski, B., Pages, M., Joachim, A., 2017. Cloning, expression and molecular characterization of a *Cystoisospora suis* specific uncharacterized merozoite protein. *Parasit. Vectors* 10, 68.

1573. Shumard, R.F., 1957. Ovine coccidiosis; incidence, possible endotoxin, and treatment. *J. Am. Vet. Med. Assoc.* 131, 559–561.

1574. Sierra-Cifuentes, V., Jiménz-Aguilar, J., Echeverri, A.A., Cardona-Arias, J.A., Ríos-Osorio, L.A., 2015. Prevalencia de parásitos intestinales en perros de dos centros de bienestar animal de Medellín y el oriente antioqueño (Colombia), 2014. *Rev. Med. Vet.* 30, 55–66.

1575. Sifuentes-Osornio, J., Porras-Cortés, G., Bendall, R.P., Morales-Villarreal, F., Reyes-Terán, G., Ruiz-Palacios, G.M., 1995. *Cyclospora cayetanensis* infection in patients with and without AIDS: Biliary disease as another clinical manifestation. *Clin. Infect. Dis.* 21, 1092–1097.

1576. Silva, L.M.R., Caro, T.M., Gerstberger, R., Vila-Viçosa, M.J.M., Cortes, H.C.E., Hermosilla, C., Taubert, A., 2014. The apicomplexan parasite *Eimeria arloingi* induces caprine neutrophil extracellular traps. *Parasitol. Res.* 113, 2797–2807.

1577. Silva, L.M.R., Chávez-Maya, F., Macdonald, S., Pegg, E., Blake, D.P., Taubert, A., Hermosilla, C., 2017. A newly described strain of *Eimeria arloingi* (strain A) belongs to the phylogenetic group of ruminant-infecting pathogenic species, which replicate in host endothelial cells *in vivo*. *Vet. Parasitol.* 248, 28–32.

1578. Silva, L.M.R., Vila-Viçosa, M.J.M., Cortes, H.C.E., Taubert, A., Hermosilla, C., 2015. Suitable in vitro *Eimeria arloingi* macromeront formation in host endothelial cells and modulation of adhesion molecule, cytokine and chemokine gene transcription. *Parasitol. Res.* 114, 113–124.

1579. Siripanth, C., Punpoowong, B., Amarapal, P., Thima, N., 2004. Development of *Isospora belli* in HCT-8, HEP-2, human fibroblast, BEK and VERO culture cells. *Southeast Asian J. Trop. Med. Pub. Health* 35, 796–800.

1580. Sivkova, T.N., Sogrina, A.V., 2015. Parasitoses of domestic carnivores in the Perm city in 2014. *Theory Pract. Struggle Parasit. Dis.* 16, 405–407.

1581. Skampardonis, V., Sotiraki, S., Kostoulas, P., Leontides, L., 2012. Factors associated with the occurrence and level of *Isospora suis* oocyst excretion in nursing piglets of Greek farrow-to-finish herds. *BMC Vet. Res.* 8, 228.

1582. Skírnisson, K., 1997. Mortality associated with renal and intestinal coccidiosis in juvenile eiders in Iceland. *Parassitologia* 39, 325–330.

1583. Skirnisson, K., 2007. *Eimeria* spp. (Coccidia, Protozoa) infections in a flock of sheep in Iceland: Species composition and seasonal abundance. *Icel. Agric. Sci.* 20, 73–80.

1584. Smith, T., 1895. *Investigations Concerning Infectious Diseases among Poultry Bulletin No. 8* (pp. 7–27). U.S. Department of Agriculture, Bureau of Animal Industry, Washington, DC.

1585. Smith, A.L., Hayday, A.C., 2000. Genetic dissection of primary and secondary responses to a widespread natural pathogen of the gut, *Eimeria vermiformis. Infect. Immun.* 68, 6273–6280.

1586. Smith, A.L., Hesketh, P., Archer, A., Shirley, M.W., 2002. Antigenic diversity in *Eimeria maxima* and the influence of host genetics and immunization schedule on cross-protective immunity. *Infect. Immun.* 70, 2472–2479.

1587. Smith, C.K., Galloway, R.B., 1983. Influence of monensin on cation influx and glycolysis of *Eimeria tenella* sporozoites *in vitro. J. Parasitol.* 69, 666–670.

1588. Smith, C.K., Galloway, R.B., White, S.L., 1981. Effect of ionophores on survival, penetration, and development of *Eimeria tenella* sporozoites *in vitro. J. Parasitol.* 67, 511–516.

1589. Smith, C.K., Strout, R.G., 1979. *Eimeria tenella*: Accumulation and retention of anticoccidial ionophores by extracellular sporozoites. *Exp. Parasitol.* 48, 325–330.

1590. Smith, C.K., Strout, R.G., 1980. *Eimeria tenella*: Effect of narasin, a polyether antibiotic on the ultrastructure of intracellular sporozoites. *Exp. Parasitol.* 50, 426–436.

1591. Smith, H.V., Paton, C.A., Mtambo, M.M.A., Girdwood, R.W.A., 1997. Sporulation of *Cyclospora* sp. oocysts. *Appl. Environ. Microbiol.* 63, 1631–1632.

1592. Smith, M.C., Sherman, D.M., 2009. *Goat Medicine, Chapter 10—Digestive System—Protozoan Diseases—Coccidiosis*. Wiley-Blackwell, New York, 2nd ed., 427–437.

1593. Smith, N.C., Wallach, M., Petracca, M., Braun, R., Eckert, J., 1994. Maternal transfer of antibodies induced by infection with *Eimeria maxima* partially protects chickens against challenge with *Eimeria tenella. Parasitology* 109 (Pt 5), 551–557.

1594. Soe, A.K., Pomroy, W.E., 1992. New species of *Eimeria* (Apicomplexa: Eimeriidae) from the domesticated goat *Capra hircus* in New Zealand. *Syst. Parasitol.* 23, 195–202.

1595. Song, H., Dong, R., Qiu, B., Jing, J., Zhu, S., Liu, C., Jiang, Y., Wu, L., Wang, S., Miao, J., Shao, Y., 2017. Potential vaccine targets against rabbit coccidiosis by immunoproteomic analysis. *Korean J. Parasitol.* 55, 15–20.

1596. Song, K.D., Lillehoj, H.S., Choi, K.D., Zarlenga, D., Han, J.Y., 1997. Expression and functional characterization of recombinant chicken interferon-γ. *Vet. Immunol. Immunopathol.* 58, 321–333.

1597. Song, X., Ren, Z., Yan, R., Xu, L., Li, X., 2015. Induction of protective immunity against *Eimeria tenella, Eimeria necatrix, Eimeria maxima* and *Eimeria acervulina* infections using multivalent epitope DNA vaccines. *Vaccine* 33, 2764–2770.

1598. Sorvillo, F.J., Lieb, L.E., Seidel, J., Kerndt, P., Turner, J., Ash, L.R., 1995. Epidemiology of isosporiasis among persons with acquired immunodeficiency syndrome in Los Angeles County. *Am. J. Trop. Med. Hyg.* 53, 656–659.

1599. Sotiraki, S., Roepstorff, A., Nielsen, J.P., Maddox-Hyttel, C., Enøe, C., Boes, J., Murrell, K.D., Thamsborg, S.M., 2008. Population dynamics and intra-litter transmission patterns of *Isospora suis* in suckling piglets under on-farm conditions. *Parasitology* 135, 395–405.

1600. Speer, C.A., 1979. Further studies on the development of gamonts and oocysts of *Eimeria magna* in cultured cells. *J. Parasitol.* 65, 591–598.

1601. Speer, C.A., 1988. Ultrastructure of two types of first-generation merozoites of *Eimeria bovis. J. Protozool.* 35, 379–381.

1602. Speer, C.A., Danforth, H.D., 1976. Fine-structural aspects of microgametogenesis of *Eimeria magna* in rabbits and in kidney cell cultures. *J. Protozool.* 23, 109–115.

1603. Speer, C.A., DeVos, A.J., Hammond, D.M., 1973. Development of *Eimeria zuernii* in cell cultures. *Proc. Helminthol. Soc. Wash.* 40, 160–163.

1604. Speer, C.A., Hammond, D.M., 1971. Development of *Eimeria ellipsoidalis* from cattle in cultured bovine cells. *J. Parasitol.* 57, 675–677.

1605. Speer, C.A., Hammond, D.M., 1971. Development of first- and second-generation schizonts of *Eimeria magna* from rabbits in cell cultures. *Z. Parasitenkd.* 37, 336–353.

1606. Speer, C.A., Hammond, D.M., 1972. Development of gametocytes and oocysts of *Eimeria magna* from rabbits in cell culture. *Proc. Helminthol. Soc. Wash.* 39, 114–118.

1607. Speer, C.A., Hammond, D.M., 1972. Motility of macrogamonts of *Eimeria magna* (Coccidia) in cell culture. *Science* 178, 763–765.

1608. Speer, C.A., Hammond, D.M., 1973. Development of second-generation schizonts, gamonts and oocysts of *Eimeria bovis* in bovine kidney cells. *Z. Parasitenkd.* 42, 105–113.

1609. Speer, C.A., Hammond, D.M., Elsner, Y.Y., 1973. Further asexual development of *Eimeria magna* merozoites in cell cultures. *J. Parasitol.* 59, 613–623.

1610. Speer, C.A., Hammond, D.M., Mahrt, J.L., Roberts, W.L., 1973. Structure of the oocyst and sporocyst walls and excystation of sporozoites of *Isospora canis. J. Parasitol.* 59, 35–40.

1611. Speer, C.A., Reduker, D.W., Burgess, D.E., Whitmire, W.M., Splitter, G.A., 1985. Lymphokine-induced inhibition of growth of *Eimeria bovis* and *Eimeria papillata* (Apicomplexa) in cultured bovine monocytes. *Infect. Immun.* 50, 566–571.

1612. Spitz dos Santos, C., Pereira Berto, B., Teixeira de Jesus, V.L., Gomes Lopes, C.W., 2014. *Eimeria leuckarti* Flesch, 1883 (Apicomplexa: Eimeriidae) from horse foals in Rio de Janeiro. *Coccidia* 2, 40–44.

1613. Stayer, P.A., Pote, L.M., Keirs, R.W., 1995. A comparison of *Eimeria* oocysts isolated from litter and fecal samples from broiler houses at two farms with different management schemes during one growout. *Poult. Sci.* 74, 26–32.

1614. Stepanova, H., Samankova, P., Leva, L., Sinkora, J., Faldyna, M., 2007. Early postnatal development of the immune system in piglets: The redistribution of T lymphocyte subsets. *Cell. Immunol.* 249, 73–79.

1615. Stephan, B., Rommel, M., Daugschies, A., Haberkorn, A., 1997. Studies of resistance to anticoccidials in *Eimeria* field isolates and pure *Eimeria* strains. *Vet. Parasitol.* 69, 19–29.

1616. Stevenson, G.W., Andrews, J.J., 1982. Mucosal impression smears for diagnosis of piglet coccidiosis. *Vet. Med. Small Anim. Clin.* 77, 111–115.

1617. Stockdale, P.H.G., 1977. Proposed life cycle of *Eimeria zuernii*. *Br. Vet. J.* 133, 471–473.

1618. Stockdale, P.H.G., 1977. The pathogenesis of the lesions produced by *Eimeria zuernii* in calves. *Can. J. Comp. Med.* 41, 338–344.

1619. Stockdale, P.H.G., Sheard, A., Tiffin, G.B., 1982. Resistance to *Eimeria bovis* produced after chemotherapy of experimental infections in calves. *Vet. Parasitol.* 9, 171–177.

1620. Straberg, E., 2004. Feldstudie zum Einsatz gezielter Desinfektionsmaßnahmen gegen die Saugferkelkokzidiose. Dr. med. vet. thesis. University of Leipzig.

1621. Straberg, E., Daugschies, A., 2007. Control of piglet coccidiosis by chemical disinfection with a cresol-based product (Neopredisan 135-1). *Parasitol. Res.* 101, 599–604.

1622. Streun, A., Coudert, P., Rossi, G.L., 1979. Characterization of *Eimeria* species. II. Sequential morphologic study of the endogenous cycle of *Eimeria perforans* (Leuckart, 1879; Sluiter and Swellengrebel, 1912) in experimentally infected rabbits. *Z. Parasitenkd.* 60, 37–53.

1623. Stromberg, B.E., Schlotthauer, J.C., Hamann, K.J., Saatara Oz, H., Bemrick, W.J., 1986. Experimental bovine coccidiosis: Control with monensin. *Vet. Parasitol.* 22, 135–140.

1624. Strout, R.G., Ouellette, C.A., 1969. Gametogony of *Eimeria tenella* (coccidia) in cell cultures. *Science* 163, 695–696.

1625. Strout, R.G., Ouellette, C.A., 1970. Schizogony and gametogony of *Eimeria tenella* in cell cultures. *Am. J. Vet. Res.* 31, 911–918.

1626. Strout, R.G., Solis, J., Smith, S.C., Dunlop, W.R., 1965. *In vitro* cultivation of *Eimeria acervulina* (Coccidia). *Exp. Parasitol.* 17, 241–246.

1627. Stuart, B.F., Bedell, D.M., Lindsay, D.S., 1981. Coccidiosis in swine: Effect of disinfectants on in vitro sporulation of *Isospora suis* oocysts. *Vet. Med. Small Anim. Clin.* 76, 1185–1186.

1628. Stuart, B.P., Bedell, D.M., Lindsay, D.S., 1982. Coccidiosis in swine: A search for extraintestinal stages of *Isospora suis*. *Vet. Rec.* 110, 82–83.

1629. Stuart, B.P., Gosser, H.S., Allen, C.B., Bedell, D.M., 1982. Coccidiosis in swine: Dose and age response to *Isospora suis*. *Can. J. Comp. Med.* 46, 317–320.

1630. Stuart, B.P., Lindsay, D.S., 1986. Coccidiosis in swine. *Vet. Clin. North Am. Food Anim. Pract.* 2, 455–468.

1631. Stuart, B.P., Lindsay, D.S., Ernst, J.V., Gosser, H.S., 1980. *Isospora suis* enteritis in piglets. *Vet. Pathol.* 17, 84–93.

1632. Stuart, B.P., Lindsey, D.S., Ernst, J.V., 1978. Coccidiosis as a cause of scours in baby pigs. In: *Proc. 2nd Int. Symp. Neonatal diarrhea in calves and pigs*, Saskatoon, Saskatchewan, Canada, pp. 371–380.

1633. Stuart, B.P., Sisk, D.B., Bedell, D.M., Gosser, H.S., 1982. Demonstration of immunity against *Isospora suis* in swine. *Vet. Parasitol.* 9, 185–191.

1634. Stuart, E.E., Bruins, H.W., Keenum, R.D., 1963. The immunogenicity of a commercial coccidiosis vaccine in conjunction with Trithiadol and Zoalene. *Avian Dis.* 7, 12–18.

1635. Su, H., Liu, X., Yan, W., Shi, T., Zhao, X., Blake, D.P., Tomley, F.M., Suo, X., 2012. PiggyBac transposon-mediated transgenesis in the apicomplexan parasite *Eimeria tenella*. *PLOS ONE* 7, e40075.

1636. Su, S., Hou, Z., Liu, D., Jia, C., Wang, L., Xu, J., Tao, J., 2017. Comparative transcriptome analysis of second- and third-generation merozoites of *Eimeria necatrix*. *Parasit. Vectors* 10, 388.

1637. Su, S., Hou, Z., Liu, D., Jia, C., Wang, L., Xu, J., Tao, J., 2018. Comparative transcriptome analysis of *Eimeria necatrix* third-generation merozoites and gametocytes reveals genes involved in sexual differentiation and gametocyte development. *Vet. Parasitol.* 252, 35–46.

1638. Suárez Fernández, M.L., Engels, K.K., Bender, F., Gassel, M., Marhöfer, R.J., Mottram, J.C., Selzer, P.M., 2012. High-throughput screening with the *Eimeria tenella* CDC2-related kinase2/cyclin complex EtCRK2/EtCYC3a. *Microbiology* 158, 2262–2271.

1639. Suarez, C.E., Bishop, R.P., Alzan, H.F., Poole, W.A., Cooke, B.M., 2017. Advances in the application of genetic manipulation methods to apicomplexan parasites. *Int. J. Parasitol.* 47, 701–710.

1640. Sudhakara Reddy, B., Sivajothi, S., Rayulu, V.C., 2015. Clinical coccidiosis in adult cattle. *J. Parasit. Dis.* 39, 557–559.

1641. Sühwold, A., Hermosilla, C., Seeger, T., Zahner, H., Taubert, A., 2010. T-cell reactions of *Eimeria bovis* primary and challenge-infected calves. *Parasitol. Res.* 106, 595–605.

1642. Sumners, L.H., Miska, K.B., Jenkins, M.C., Fetterer, R.H., Cox, C.M., Kim, S., Dalloul, R.A., 2011. Expression of Toll-like receptors and antimicrobial peptides during *Eimeria praecox* infection in chickens. *Exp. Parasitol.* 127, 714–718.

1643. Sun, H., Wang, L., Wang, T., Zhang, J., Liu, Q., Chen, P., Chen, Z., et al. 2014. Display of *Eimeria tenella* EtMic2 protein on the surface of *Saccharomyces cerevisiae* as a potential oral vaccine against chicken coccidiosis. *Vaccine* 32, 1869–1876.

1644. Sun, H.W., Bernhagen, J., Bucala, R., Lolis, E., 1996. Crystal structure at 2.6-Å resolution of human marophage migration inhibitory factor. *Proc. Natl. Acad. Sci. U.S.A.* 93, 5191–5196.

1645. Sun, L., Dong, H., Zhang, Z., Liu, J., Hu, Y., Ni, Y., Grossmann, R., Zhao, R., 2016. Activation of epithelial proliferation induced by *Eimeria acervulina* infection in the duodenum may be associated with cholesterol metabolism. *Oncotarget* 7, 27627–27640.

1646. Sun, M., Liao, S., Zhang, L., Wu, C., Qi, N., Lv, M., Li, J., et al. 2016. Molecular and biochemical characterization of *Eimeria tenella* hexokinase. *Parasitol. Res.* 115, 3425–3433.

1647. Sun, M., Zhu, G., Qin, Z., Wu, C., Lv, M., Liao, S., Qi, N., Xie, M., Cai, J., 2012. Functional characterizations of malonyl-CoA:acyl carrier protein transacylase (MCAT) in *Eimeria tenella. Mol. Biochem. Parasitol.* 184, 20–28.

1648. Sun, X.M., Pang, W., Jia, T., Yan, W.C., He, G., Hao, L.L., Bentue, M., Suo, X., 2009. Prevalence of *Eimeria* species in broilers with subclinical signs from fifty farms. *Avian Dis.* 53, 301–305.

1649. Suo, X., Li, G., 1998. *Chicken Coccidiosis.* China Agricultural University Press, Beijing, China. 1–438.

1650. Suo, X., Zhang, J.X., Li, Z.G., Yang, C.T., Min, Q.R., Xu, L.T., Liu, Q., Zhu, X.Q., 2006. The efficacy and economic benefits of Supercox, a live anticoccidial vaccine in a commercial trial in broiler chickens in China. *Vet. Parasitol.* 142, 63–70.

1651. Supperer, R., 1961. Die Bedeutung der Sauen und Eber für die Verparasitierung der Schweinebestände. *Wien. tierärztl. Monatsschr.* 48, 201–210.

1652. Suprihati, E., Yunus, M., 2018. Evaluation of the antigenicity and immunogenicity of *Eimeria tenella* by reproductive index and histopathological changes of cecal coccidiosis virulent live vaccine in broiler chickens. *Afr. J. Infect. Dis.* 12, 104–110.

1653. Sutoh, M., Saheki, Y., Ishitani, R., Inui, S., Narita, M., Hamazaki, H., Yokota, T., 1976. *Eimeria leuckarti* infection in foals. *Natl. Inst. Anim. Health Q. (Tokyo)* 16, 59–64.

1654. Svensson, C., 1997. The survival and transmission of oocysts of *Eimeria alabamensis* in hay. *Vet. Parasitol.* 69, 211–218.

1655. Swaggerty, C.L., Genovese, K.J., He, H., Duke, S.E., Pevzner, I.Y., Kogut, M.H., 2011. Broiler breeders with an efficient innate immune response are more resistant to *Eimeria tenella. Poult. Sci.* 90, 1014–1019.

1656. Swanson, E.A., March, J.K., Clayton, F., Couturier, M.R., Arcega, R., Smith, R., Evason, K.J., 2018. Epithelial inclusions in gallbladder specimens mimic parasite infection: Histologic and molecular examination of reported *Cystoisospora belli* infection in gallbladders of immunocompetent patients. *Am. J. Surg. Pathol.* 42, 1346–1352.

1657. Szanto, J., Mohan, R.N., Levine, N.D., 1964. Prevalence of coccidia and gastrointestinal nematodes in beef cattle in Illinois and their relation to shipping fever. *J. Am. Vet. Med. Assoc.* 144, 741–746.

1658. Szkucik, K., Pyz-Lukasik, R., Szczepaniak, K.O., Paszkiewicz, W., 2014. Occurrence of gastrointestinal parasites in slaughter rabbits. *Parasitol. Res.* 113, 59–64.

1659. Tabarés, E., Ferguson, D., Clark, J., Soon, P.E., Wan, K.L., Tomley, F. 2004. *Eimeria tenella* sporozoites and merozoites differentially express glycosylphosphatidylinositol-anchored variant surface proteins. *Mol. Biochem. Parasitol.* 135, 123–132.

1660. Tadayon, S., Razavi, S.M., Nazifi, S., 2016. Dynamic patterns of systemic innate immunity and inflammatory associated factors in experimental caprine coccidiosis. *Korean J. Parasitol.* 54, 719–724.

1661. Talevich, E., Kannan, N., 2013. Structural and evolutionary adaptation of rhoptry kinases and pseudokinases, a family of coccidian virulence factors. *BMC Evol. Biol.* 13, 117.

1662. Talmon, P., Jager, L.P., de Leeuw, W.A., Timmer, W.J., 1989. Coccidiosis in lambs: Observations in the preventive use of an amprolium-containing medicated feed. *Tijdschr. Diergeneeskd.* 114, 611–617.

1663. Tan, C.Y., Chen, J.M., Ji, L.Q., 2014. Diagnosis and treatment of coccidiosis in Taiwanese hybrid white duck. *Poultry Husb. Dis. Control* 4, 5 (in Chinese).

1664. Tan, L., Li, Y., Yang, X., Ke, Q., Lei, W., Mughal, M.N., Fang, R., Zhou, Y., Shen, B., Zhao, J., 2017. Genetic diversity and drug sensitivity studies on *Eimeria tenella* field isolates from Hubei Province of China. *Parasit. Vectors* 10, 137.

1665. Tandukar, S., Ansari, S., Adhikari, N., Shrestha, A., Gautam, J., Sharma, B., Rajbhandari, D., Gautam, S., Nepal, H.P., Sherchand, J.B., 2013. Intestinal parasitosis in school children of Lalitpur district of Nepal. *BMC Res. Notes* 6, 449.

1666. Tang, K., Guo, Y., Zhang, L., Rowe, L.A., Roellig, D.M., Frace, M.A., Li, N., Liu, S., Feng, Y., Xiao, L., 2015. Genetic similarities between *Cyclospora cayetanensis* and cecum-infecting avian *Eimeria* spp. in apicoplast and mitochondrial genomes. *Parasit. Vectors* 8, 358.

1667. Tang, K.L., Caffrey, N.P., Nóbrega, D.B., Cork, S.C., Ronksley, P.E., Barkema, H.W., Polachek, A.J., et al. 2017. Restricting the use of antibiotics in food-producing animals and its associations with antibiotic resistance in food-producing animals and human beings: A systematic review and meta-analysis. *Lancet Planet Health* 1, e316–e327.

1668. Tang, X., Huang, G., Liu, X., El-Ashram, S., Tao, G., Lu, C., Suo, J., Suo, X., 2018. An optimized DNA extraction method for molecular identification of coccidian species. *Parasitol. Res.* 117, 655–664.

1669. Tang, X., Li, C., Hu, D., Zhang, S., Duan, C., Bi, F., Liu, J., Liu, X., Suo, X., 2019. The past, present and future of chicken coccidiosis research in China. *Acta Parasitol. Med. Entomol. Sinica*, xx (in Chinese). 26, 206–211.

1670. Tang, X., Liu, X., Tao, G., Qin, M., Yin, G., Suo, J., Suo, X., 2016. "Self-cleaving" 2A peptide from porcine teschovirus-1 mediates cleavage of dual fluorescent proteins in transgenic *Eimeria tenella. Vet. Res.* 47, 68.

1671. Tang, X., Liu, X., Yin, G., Suo, J., Tao, G., Zhang, S., Suo, X., 2018. A novel vaccine delivery model of the apicomplexan *Eimeria tenella* expressing *Eimeria maxima* antigen protects chickens against infection of the two parasites. *Front Immunol.* 8, 1982.

1672. Tang, X., Suo, J., Li, C., Du, M., Wang, C., Hu, D., Duan, C., Lyu, Y., Liu, X., Suo, X., 2018. Transgenic *Eimeria tenella* expressing profilin of *Eimeria maxima* elicits enhanced protective immunity and alters gut microbiome of chickens. *Infect. Immun.* 86, e00888–17.

1673. Tang, X., Suo, X., Liu, X., 2018. Control of chicken coccidiosis in the modern poultry industry in China. *Acta Parasitol. Med. Entomol. Sinica* 25, 279–286 (in Chinese).

1674. Tang, X., Yin, G., Qin, M., Tao, G., Suo, J., Liu, X., Suo, X., 2016. Transgenic *Eimeria tenella* as a vaccine vehicle: Expressing TgSAG1 elicits protective immunity against *Toxoplasma gondii* infections in chickens and mice. *Sci. Rep.* 6, 29379.

1675. Taniuchi, M., Verweij, J.J., Sethabutr, O., Bodhidatta, L., Garcia, L., Maro, A., Kumburu, H., Gratz, J., Kibiki, G., Houpt, E.R., 2011. Multiplex polymerase chain reaction method to detect *Cyclospora*, *Cystoisospora*, and Microsporidia in stool samples. *Diagn. Microbiol. Infect. Dis.* 71, 386–390.

1676. Tao, G., Shi, T., Tang, X., Duszynski, D.W., Wang, Y., Li, C., Suo, J., Tian, X., Liu, X., Suo, X., 2017. Transgenic *Eimeria magna* Pérard, 1925 displays similar parasitological properties to the wild-type strain and induces an exogenous protein-specific immune response in rabbits (*Oryctolagus cuniculus* L.). *Front. Immunol.* 8, 2.

1677. Tarlatzis, C., Panetsos, A., Dragonas, P., 1957. Further experiences with furacin in treatment of ovine and caprine coccidiosis. *J. Am. Vet. Med. Assoc.* 131, 474.

1678. Taubert, A., Behrendt, J.H., Sühwold, A., Zahner, H., Hermosilla, C., 2009. Monocyte- and macrophage-mediated immune reactions against *Eimeria bovis*. *Vet. Parasitol.* 164, 141–153.

1679. Taubert, A., Zahner, H., Hermosilla, C., 2006. Dynamics of transcription of immunomodulatory genes in endothelial cells infected with different coccidian parasites. *Vet. Parasitol.* 142, 214–222.

1680. Tavassoli, M., Dalir-Naghadeh, B., Valipour, S., Maghsoudlo, M., 2018. Prevalence of gastrointestinal parasites in water buffalo (*Bubalus bubalis*) calves raised with cattle in smallholder farming system in the northwest of Iran. *Acta Vet. Eurasia* 44, 6–11.

1681. Tawfik, M.A., 1976. Parasitic infestation as a cause of diarrhoea in buffalo-calves. *Assiut Vet. Med. J.* 4, 162–168.

1682. Taylor, J.R., 1984. Immune response of pigs to *Isospora suis* (Apicomplexia, Eimeriidae). Doctoral thesis. Auburn University. Auburn, AL.

1683. Taylor, M., 1995. Diagnosis and control of coccidiosis in sheep. *In Practice* 172–177.

1684. Taylor, M.A., 2016. Antiparasitics. In Taylor, M.A., Coop, R.L., and Wall, R.L. (Ed.), *Veterinary Parasitology*. John Wiley and Sons. West Sussex, United Kingdom. 4th ed., 318–323.

1685. Taylor, M.A., Bartram, D.J., 2012. The history of decoquinate in the control of coccidial infections in ruminants. *J. Vet. Pharmacol. Therap.* 35, 417–427.

1686. Taylor, M.A., Catchpole, J., 1994. Review article: Coccidiosis of domestic ruminants. *Appl. Parasitol.* 35, 73–86.

1687. Taylor, M.A., Catchpole, J., Marshall, J., Marshall, R.N., Hoeben, D., 2003. Histopathological observations on the activity of diclazuril (Vecoxan) against the endogenous stages of *Eimeria crandallis* in sheep. *Vet. Parasitol.* 116, 305–314.

1688. Taylor, M.A., Coop, R.L., Wall, R.L., 2007. Parasites of sheep and goats. In Taylor, M.A., Coop, R.L., and Wall, R.L. (Ed.), *Veterinary Parasitology*. Blackwell Publishing. Oxford, UK, 3rd ed., 152–258.

1689. Taylor, M.A., Marshall, R.N., Marshall, J.A., Catchpole, J., Bartram, D., 2011. Dose-response effects of diclazuril against pathogenic species of ovine coccidia and the development of protective immunity. *Vet. Parasitol.* 178, 48–57.

1690. Tehrani, A.A., Yakhchali, M., Beikzadeh, B., Morvaridi, A., 2013. Prevalence of rabbit hepatic coccidiosis in north west of Iran. *Arch. Razi Institute* 68, 65–69.

1691. Teixeira Filho, W.L., Gonçalves, L.R., Lopes, C.W.G., 2016. Natural coccidiosis in water buffaloes (*Bubalus bubalis* L. 1875) in Southeastern Brazil. *Rev. Bras. Med. Vet.* 38 (Suppl 3), 1–8.

1692. Temperley, N.D., Berlin, S., Paton, I.R., Griffin, D.K., Burt, D.W., 2008. Evolution of the chicken Toll-like receptor gene family: A story of gene gain and gene loss. *BMC Genomics* 9, 62.

1693. ten Hove, R.J., van Lieshout, L., Brienen, E.A.T., Perez, M.A., Verweij, J.J., 2008. Real-time polymerase chain reaction for detection of *Isospora belli* in stool samples. *Diagn. Microbiol. Infect. Dis.* 61, 280–283.

1694. Tensa, L.R., Jordan, B.J., 2019. Comparison of the application parameters of coccidia vaccines by gel and spray. *Poult. Sci.* 98, 634–641.

1695. Tewari, A.K., Maharana, B.R., 2011. Control of poultry coccidiosis: Changing trends. *J. Parasit. Dis.* 35, 10–17.

1696. Thomas, M.K., Murray, R., Flockhart, L., Pintar, K., Pollari, F., Fazil, A., Nesbitt, A., Marshall, B., 2013. Estimates of the burden of foodborne illness in Canada for 30 specified pathogens and unspecified agents, circa 2006. *Foodborne Pathog. Dis.* 10, 639–648.

1697. Tian, S.Q., Cui, P., Fang, S.F., Liu, G.H., Wang, C.R., Zhu, X.Q., 2015. The complete mitochondrial genome sequence of *Eimeria magna* (Apicomplexa: Coccidia). *Mitochondrial DNA* 26, 714–715.

1698. Tohno, M., Ueda, W., Azuma, Y., Shimazu, T., Katoh, S., Wang, J.M., Aso, H., et al. 2008. Molecular cloning and functional characterization of porcine nucleotide-binding oligomerization domain-2 (NOD2). *Mol. Immunol.* 45, 194–203.

1699. Tomczuk, K., Grzybek, M., Szczepaniak, K., Studzinska, M., Demkowska-Kutrzepa, M., Roczen-Karczmarz, M., Klockiewicz, M., 2015. Analysis of intrinsic and extrinsic factors influencing the dynamics of bovine *Eimeria* spp. from central-eastern Poland. *Vet. Parasitol.* 214, 22–28.

1700. Torres, A., 2004. Prevalence survey of *Isospora suis* in twelve Europea countries. In: *Proc. 18th IPVS Congr.*, Hamburg, p. 243.

1701. Tram, N.T., Hoang, L.M.N., Cam, P.D., Chung, P.T., Fyfe, M.W., Isaac-Renton, J.L., Ong, C.S.L., 2008. *Cyclospora* spp. in herbs and water samples collected from markets and farms in Hanoi, Vietnam. *Trop. Med. Int. Health* 13, 1415–1420.

1702. Trasviña-Muñoz, E., López-Valencia, G., Álvarez Centeno, P., Cueto-González, S.A., Monge-Navarro, F.J., Tinoco-Gracia, L., Núñez-Castro, K., et al. 2017. Prevalence and distribution of intestinal parasites in stray dogs in ther northwest area of Mexico. *Austral J. Vet. Sci.* 49, 105–111.

1703. Trayser, C.V., Todd, K.S., 1978. Life cycle of *Isospora burrowsi* n sp (Protozoa: Eimeriidae) from the dog *Canis familiaris*. *Am. J. Vet. Res.* 39, 95–98.

1704. Trentini, A., Stancampiano, L., Usai, F., Micagni, G., Poglayen, G., 2010. Donkey endoparasites in an organic farm. *Proc. 26th Congr. Naz. Soc. Italia Parassitologia 2010. Parassitologia* 52, p. 336.

1705. Trier, J S., Moxey, P.C., Schimmel, E.M., Robles, E., 1974. Chronic intestinal coccidiosis in man: Intestinal morphology and response to treatment. *Gastroenterology* 66, 923–935.

1706. Trout, J.M., Lillehoj, H.S., 1995. *Eimeria acervulina* infection: Evidence for the involvement of CD8+ T lymphocytes in sporozoite transport and host protection. *Poult. Sci.* 74, 1117–1125.

1707. Trout, J.M., Lillehoj, H.S., 1996. T lymphocyte roles during *Eimeria acervulina* and *Eimeria tenella* infections. *Vet. Imriunol. Immunopathol.* 53, 163–172.

1708. Trout, J.M., Santín, M., Fayer, R., 2008. Detection of assemblage A, *Giardia duodenalis* and *Eimeria* spp. in alpacas on two Maryland farms. *Vet. Parasitol.* 153, 203–208.

1709. Tscherner, W., 1978. Koprologische Untersuchungen bei Huftieren des Tierparks Berlin. *Verhandlungsber. Int. Symp. Erkr. Zoo- und Wildtiere* 20, 137–143.

1710. Tsiouris, V., 2016. Poultry management: A useful tool for the control of necrotic enteritis in poultry. *Avian Pathol.* 45, 323–325.

1711. Tsygankov, A.A., 1950. To revision of species composition of camel coccidia. *Investiya of the Acad. Sci. Kazakh SSP* 8, 174–185.

1712. Tu, Y., 2011. The discovery of artemisinin (qinghaosu) and gifts from Chinese medicine. *Nature Med.* 17, 1217.

1713. Tubbs, R.C., 1987. Controlling coccidiosis in neonatal pigs. *Vet. Med.* 82, 646–650.

1714. Twomey, D.F., Allen, K., Bell, S., Evans, C., Thomas, S., 2010. *Eimeria ivitaensis* in British alpacas. *Vet. Rec.* 167, 797–798.

1715. Tynan, E J., Nelson, T.H., Davies, R.A., Wernau, W.C., 1992. The production of semduramicin by direct fermentation. *J. Antibiot.* 45, 813–815.

1716. Tyzzer, E.E., 1927. Species and strains of coccidia in poultry. *J. Parasitol.* 13, 215.

1717. Tyzzer, E.E., 1929. Coccidiosis in gallinaceous birds. *Am. J. Hyg.* 10, 269–383.

1718. Tyzzer, E.E., Theiler, H., Jones, E.E., 1932. Coccidiosis in gallinaceous: II. A comparative study of species of *Eimeria* of the chicken. *Am. J. Hyg.* 15, 319–393.

1719. Uebe, F., 2011. Studien zur Behandlung der *Eimeria bovis*—Kokzidiose des Kalbes mit Toltrazuril. Dr. med. vet. thesis. Universität Leipzig.

1720. Umemura, T., Nakamura, H., Goryo, M., Itakura, C., 1984. Histopathology of monensin-tiamulin myopathy in broiler chicks. *Avian Pathol.* 13, 459–468.

1721. Umemura, T., Nakamura, H., Goryo, M., Itakura, C., 1984. Ultrastructural changes of monensin-oleandomycin myopathy in broiler chicks. *Avian Pathol.* 13, 743–751.

1722. U.S. Food and Drug Administration, 2016. Bluebird Label: Sulfadimethoxine and ormetoprim Type C medicated feed https://www.fda.gov/food/laboratory-methods-food/bam-19b-molecular-detection-cyclospora-cayetanensis-fresh-produce-using-real-time-pcr

1723. Upton, S., 2001. Suborder Eimeriorina Leger, 1911. In Anonymous (Ed.), *The Illustrated Guide to the Protozoa.* Allen Press. Lawrence, KS, 2nd ed., 318–339.

1724. Upton, S.J., McAllister, C.T., Brillhart, D.B., Duszynski, D.W., Wash, C.D., 1992. Cross-transmission studies with *Eimeria arizonensis*-like oocysts (Apicomplexa) in New World rodents of the genera *Baiomys*, *Neotoma*, *Onychomys*, *Peromyscus*, and *Reithrodontomys* (Muridae). *J. Parasitol.* 78, 406–413.

1725. Vadlejch, J., Petrtýl, M., Lukešová, D., Cadková, Z., Kudrnácová, M., Jankovská, I., Langrová, I., 2013. The concentration McMaster technique is suitable for quantification of coccidia oocysts in bird droppings. *Pakistan Vet. J.* 33, 291–295.

1726. Vadlejch, J., Petrtýl, M., Zaichenko, I., Cadková, Z., Jankovská, I., Langrová, I., Moravec, M., 2011. Which McMaster egg counting technique is the most reliable? *Parasitol. Res.* 109, 1387–1394.

1727. Valdivieso, M.C.R., 2015. Prevalencia de parásitos gastrointestinales en alpacas (*Lama pacos*) del sector Pedregal-Mejía en la Provincia de Cotopaxi. *Bacheolar thesis in Veterinary Medicine.* Universidad San Francisco de Quito Ecudor.

1728. van Doorninck, W.M., Becker, E.R., 1957. Transport of sporozoites of *Eimeria necatrix* in macrophages. *J. Parasitol.* 43, 40–44.

1729. Vanparijs, O., Desplenter, L., Marsboom, R., 1989. Efficacy of diclazuril in the control of intestinal coccidiosis in rabbits. *Vet. Parasitol.* 34, 185–190.

1730. Varea, M., Clavel, A., Doiz, O., Castillo, F.J., Rubio, M.C., Gómez-Lus, R., 1998. Fuchsin fluorescence and autofluorescence in *Cryptosporidum*, *Isospora* and *Cyclospora* oocysts. *Int. J. Parasitol.* 28, 1881–1883.

1731. Varga, I., 1976. Experimental transmission of *Eimeria stiedai* to the hare. *Acta Vet. Acad. Sci. Hung.* 26, 105–112.

1732. Varghese, T., 1986. Porcine coccidia in Papua New Guinea. *Vet. Parasitol.* 21, 11–20.

1733. Varma, M., Hester, J.D., Schaefer, F.W., III, Ware, M.W., Lindquist, H.D.A., 2003. Detection of *Cyclospora cayetanensis* using a quantitative real-time PCR assay. *J. Microbiol. Methods* 53, 27–36.

1734. Velkers, F.C., Bouma, A., Stegeman, J.A., de Jong, M.C., 2012. Transmission of a live *Eimeria acervulina* vaccine strain and response to infection in vaccinated and contact-vaccinated broilers. *Vaccine* 30, 322–328.

1735. Verdier, R.I., Fitzgerald, D.W., Johnson, W.D., Jr., Pape, J.W., 2000. Trimethoprim-sulfamethoxazole compared with ciprofloxacin for treatment and prophylaxis of *Isospora belli* and *Cyclospora cayetanensis* infection in HIV-infected patients: A randomized, controlled trial. *Ann. Intern. Med.* 132, 885–888.

1736. Verhelst, D., de Craeye, S., Jennes, M., Dorny, P., Goddeeris, B., Cox, E., 2015. Interferon-γ expression and infectivity of *Toxoplasma* infected tissues in experimentally infected sheep in comparison with pigs. *Vet. Parasitol.* 207, 7–16.

1737. Verheyen, A., Maes, L., Coussement, W., Vanparijs, O., Lauwers, F., Vlaminckx, E., Borgers, M., Marsboom, R., 1988. *In vivo* action of the anticoccidial diclazuril (Clinacox) on the developmental stages of *Eimeria tenella*: An ultrastructural evaluation. *J. Parasitol.* 74, 939–949.

1738. Verheyen, A., Maes, L., Coussement, W., Vanparijs, O., Lauwers, F., Vlaminckx, E., Marsboom, R., 1989. Ultrastructural evaluation of the effects of diclazuril on the endogenous stages of *Eimeria maxima* and *E. brunetti* in experimentally inoculated chickens. *Parasitol. Res.* 75, 604–610.

1739. Verma, S.K., Cerqueira-Cézar, C.K., Murata, F.H.A., Lovallo, M.J., Rosenthal, B.M., Dubey, J.P., 2017. Bobcats (*Lynx rufus*) are natural definitive host of *Besnoitia darlingi*. *Vet. Parasitol.* 248, 84–89.

1740. Vermeire, J.J., Cho, Y., Lolis, E., Bucala, R., Cappello, M., 2008. Orthologs of macrophage imgration inhibitory factor from parasitic nematodes. *Trends Parasitol.* 24, 355–363.

1741. Versényi, L., 1967. Studies on the endogenous cycle of *Tyzzeria perniciosa* (Allen, 1935). *Acta Vet. Acad. Sci. Hung.* 17, 449–456.

1742. Vervelde, L., Vermeulen, A.N., Jeurissen, S.H.M., 1996. *In situ* characterization of leucocyte subpopulations after infection with *Eimeria tenella* in chickens. *Parasite Immunol.* 18, 247–256.

1743. Verweij, J.J., Laeijendecker, D., Brienen, E.A.T., van Lieshout, L., Polderman, A.M., 2003. Detection of *Cyclospora cayetanensis* in travellers returning from the tropics and subtropics using microscopy and real-time PCR. *Int. J. Med. Microbiol.* 293, 199–202.

1744. Veterinary Medicines Directorate, 2012. Sales of Antimicrobial Products Authorised for Use as Veterinary Medicines. Antiprotozoals, Antifungals, Growth Promoters and Coccidiostats in the UK in 2001. Veterinary Medicines Directorate (https://www.fda.gov/regulatory-information/search-fda-guidance-documents/cvm-gfi-181-blue-bird-medicated-feed-labels),.

1745. Vetterling, J.M., 1965. Coccidia (Protozoa: Eimeriidae) of swine. *J. Parasitol.* 51, 897–912.

1746. Vetterling, J.M., Doran, D.J., 1966. Schizogony and gametogony in the life cycle of the poultry coccidium, *Eimeria acervulina* Tyzzer, 1929. *J. Parasitol.* 52, 1150–1157.

1747. Vieira, L.S., Lima, J.D., Ribeiro, M.F.B., Bozzi, I.A., Camargos, E.R.S., 1997. Ultrastructure of endogenous stages of *Eimeria ninakohlyakimovae* Yakimoff and Rastegaieff, 1930 Emend. Levine, 1961 in experimentally infected goat. *Mem. Inst. Oswaldo Cruz* 92, 533–538.

1748. Vieira, L.S., Lima, J.D., Rosa, J.S., 1997. Development of *Eimeria ninakohlyakimovae* Yakimoff and Rastegaieff, 1930 emend. Levine, 1961 in experimentally infected goats (*Capra hircus*). *J. Parasitol.* 83, 1015–1018.

1749. Visvesvara, G.S., Moura, H., Kovacs-Nace, E., Wallace, S., Eberhard, M.L., 1997. Uniform staining of *Cyclospora* oocysts in fecal smears by a modified safranin technique with microwave heating. *J. Clin. Microbiol.* 35, 730–733.

1750. Vítovec, J., Koudela, B., 1987. Pathology of natural isosporosis in nursing piglets. *Folia Parasitol. (Praha)* 34, 199–204.

1751. Vítovec, J., Koudela, B., 1990. Double alteration of the small intestine in conventional and gnotobiotic piglets experimentally infected with the coccidium *Isospora suis* (Apicomplexa, Eimeriidae). *Folia Parasitol. (Praha)* 37, 21–33.

1752. Vítovec, J., Koudela, B., 1990. Pathogenicity and ultrastructural pathology of *Eimeria debliecki* (Douwes, 1921) in experimentally infected pigs. *Folia Parasitol. (Praha)* 37, 193–199.

1753. Vítovec, J., Koudela, B., Kudweis, M., Stepanek, J., Smid, B., Dvorak, R., 1991. Pathogenesis of experimental combined infections with *Isospora suis* and rotavirus in conventional and gnotobiotic piglets. *J. Vet. Med. B* 38, 215–226.

1754. Vítovec, J., Koudela, B., Sterba, J., 1987. Pathology and pathogenicity of *Eimeria scabra* (Henry, 1931) in experimentally infected pigs. *Folia Parasitol. (Praha)* 34, 299–304.

1755. Vrba, V., Blake, D.P., Poplstein, M., 2010. Quantitative real-time PCR assays for detection and quantification of all seven *Eimeria* species that infect the chicken. *Vet. Parasitol.* 174, 183–190.

1756. Vrba, V., Pakandl, M., 2014. Coccidia of turkey: From isolation, characterization and comparison to molecular phylogeny and molecular diagnostics. *Int. J. Parasitol.* 44, 985–1000.

1757. Vrba, V., Pakandl, M., 2015. Host specificity of turkey and chicken *Eimeria*: Controlled cross-transmission studies and a phylogenetic view. *Vet. Parasitol.* 208, 118–124.

1758. Vrba, V., Poplstein, M., Pakandl, M., 2011. The discovery of the two types of small subunit ribosomal RNA gene in *Eimeria mitis* contests the existence of *E. mivati* as an independent species. *Vet. Parasitol.* 183, 47–53.

1759. Waap, H., Gomes, J., Nunes, T., 2014. Parasite communities in stray cat populations from Lisbon, Portugal. *J. Helminthol.* 88, 389–395.

1760. Wahba, A.A., Radwan, I.G.H., 2009. Some studies on protozoal parasites of camels in Egypt. *Egypt. J. Comp. Pathol. Clin. Pathol.* 22, 41–53.

1761. Wakelin, D., Rose, M.E., Hesketh, P., Else, K.J., Grencis, R.K., 1993. Immunity to coccidiosis: Genetic influences on lymphocyte and cytokine responses to infection with *Eimeria vermiformis* in inbred mice. *Parasite Immunol.* 15, 11–19.

1762. Waldén, H.W., 1961. Observations on renal coccidia in Swedish anseriform birds, with notes concerning two new species, *Eimeria boschadis*, and *Eimeria christianseni* (Sporozoa, Telosporidia). *Arkiv för Zoologi* 15, 97–104.

1763. Waldenstedt, L., Elwinger, K., Lundén, A., Thebo, P., Uggla, A., 2001. Sporulation of *Eimeria maxima* oocysts in litter with different moisture contents. *Poult. Sci.* 80, 1412–1415.

1764. Walker, R.A., Ferguson, D.J.P., Miller, C.M.D., Smith, N.C., 2013. Sex and *Eimeria*: A molecular perspective. *Parasitology* 140, 1701–1717.

1765. Walker, R.A., Sharman, P.A., Miller, C.M., Lippuner, C., Okoniewski, M., Eichenberger, R.M., Ramakrishnan, C., Brossier, F., Deplazes, P., Hehl, A.B., Smith, N.C., 2015. RNA Seq analysis of the *Eimeria tenella* gametocyte transcriptome reveals clues about the molecular basis for sexual reproduction and oocyst biogenesis. *BMC Genomics* 16, 94.

1766. Wallach, M., 2010. Role of antibody in immunity and control of chicken coccidiosis. *Trends Parasitol.* 26, 382–387.

1767. Wallach, M., Smith, N.C., Miller, C.M.D., Eckert, J., Rose, M.E., 1994. *Eimeria maxima*: ELISA and Western blot analyses of protective sera. *Parasite Immunol.* 16, 377–383.

1768. Wallach, M.G., Mencher, D., Yarus, S., Pillemer, G., Halabi, A., Pugatsch, T., 1989. *Eimeria maxima*: Identification of gametocyte protein antigens. *Exp. Parasitol.* 68, 49–56.

1769. Walther, Z., Topazian, M.D., 2009. *Isospora* cholangiopathy: Case study with histologic characterization and molecular confirmation. *Hum. Pathol.* 40, 1342–1346.

1770. Wan, K.L., Chong, S.P., Ng, S.T., Shirley, M.W., Tomley, F.M., Jangi, M.S., 1999. A survey of genes in *Eimeria tenella* merozoites by EST sequencing. *Int. J. Parasitol.* 29, 1885–1892.

1771. Wang, C., Han, C., Li, T., Yang, D., Shen, X., Fan, Y., Xu, Y., et al. 2013. Nuclear translocation and accumulation of glyceraldehyde-3-phosphate dehydrogenase involved in diclazuril-induced apoptosis in *Eimeria tenella* (*E. tenella*). *Vet. Res.* 44, 29.

1772. Wang, C.C., 1975. Studies of the mitochondria from *Eimeria tenella* and inhibition of the electron transport by quinolone coccidiostats. *Biochim. Biophys. Acta* 396, 210–219.

1773. Wang, C.C., 1976. Inhibition of the respiration of *Eimeria tenella* by quinolone coccidiostats. *Biochem. Pharmacol.* 25, 343–349.

1774. Wang, C.C., 1978. Biochemical and nutritional aspects of coccidia. In Long, P.L., Boorman, K.N., and Freeman, B.M. (Ed.), *Avian coccidiosis: Proceedings of the Thirteenth Poultry Science Symposium*, September 14–16, 1977. British Poultry Science Ltd. Edinburgh, pp. 135–184.

1775. Wang, C.C., 1982. Biochemistry and physiology of coccidia. In Long, P.L. (Ed.), *The Biology of the Coccidia*. University Park Press. Baltimore, MD, 167–228.

1776. Wang, C.R., Xiao, J.Y., Chen, A.H., Chen, J., Wang, Y., Gao, J.F., Zhu, X.Q., 2010. Prevalence of coccidial infection in sheep and goats in northeastern China. *Vet. Parasitol.* 174, 213–217.

1777. Wang, K.X., Li, C.P., Wang, J., Tian, Y., 2002. *Cyclospora cayetanensis* in Anhui, China. *World J. Gastroenterol.* 8, 1144–1148.

1778. Wang, Q., Li, J., Zhang, X., Liu, Q., Liu, C., Ma, G., Cao, L., Gong, P., Cai, Y., Zhang, G., 2009. Protective immunity of recombinant *Mycobacterium bovis* BCG expressing rhomboid gene against *Eimeria tenella* challenge. *Vet. Parasitol.* 160, 198–203.

1779. Wang, T., Sun, H., Zhang, J., Liu, Q., Wang, L., Chen, P., Wang, F., Li, H., Xiao, Y., Zhao, X., 2014. The establishment of *Saccharomyces boulardii* surface display system using a single expression vector. *Fungal Genet. Biol.* 64, 1–10.

1780. Wang, X., Gong, P.T., Li, J.H., Yang, J., Zhang, X.C., 2018. Identificaiton of interaction between *Eimeria tenella* apical membrane antigen-1 and microneme protein-2. *J. Pathog. Biol.* 13, 267–273.

1781. Wang, Y., Tao, G., Cui, Y., Lv, Q., Xie, L., Li, Y., Suo, X., Qin, Y., Xiao, L., Liu, X., 2014. Molecular analysis of single oocyst of *Eimeria* by whole genome amplification (WGA) based nested PCR. *Exp. Parasitol.* 144, 96–99.

1782. Wang, Z., Huang, B., Dong, H., Zhao, Q., Zhu, S., Xia, W., Xu, S., et al. 2016. Molecular characterization and functional analysis of a novel calcium-dependent protein kinase 4 from *Eimeria tenella*. *PLOS ONE* 11, e0168132.

1783. Wang, Z., Shen, J., Suo, X., Zhao, S., Cao, X., 2006. Experimentally induced monensin-resistant *Eimeria tenella* and membrane fluidity of sporozoites. *Vet. Parasitol.* 138, 186–193.

1784. Wang, Z., Suo, X., Xia, X., Shen, J., 2006. Influence of monensin on cation influx and Na+ -K+ -ATPase activity of *Eimeria tenella* sporozoites *in vitro*. *J. Parasitol.* 92, 1092–1096.

1785. Warren, E.W., Ball, S.J., Fagg, J.R., 1963. Age resistance by turkeys to *Eimeria meleagrimitis* Tyzzer, 1929. *Nature* 200, 238–240.

1786. Weber, F.H., Evans, N.A., 2003. Immunization of broiler chicks by *in ovo* injection of *Eimeria tenella* sporozoites, sporocysts, or oocysts. *Poult. Sci.* 82, 1701–1707.

1787. Weber, F.H., Farrand, M., LeMay, M.A., Lewis, D.O., Genteman, K.C., Evans, N.A., 2001. Movement of oocysts within chicken embryos after *in ovo* vaccination with *Eimeria maxima*. *Proceedings of the VIIIth International Coccidiosis Conference*, Sydney, Australia, p. 184.

1788. Weber, F.H., Genteman, K.C., LeMay, M.A., Lewis, D.O., Sr., Evans, N.A., 2004. Immunization of broiler chicks by *in ovo* injection of infective stages of *Eimeria*. *Poult. Sci.* 83, 392–399.

1789. Wei, J., Wang, Z., 1990. Survey of *Eimeria* sp. in Bactrian camels in Inner Mongolia. *Chin. Vet. J.* 16, 23–24 (in Chinese).

1790. Welter, M.W., Quick, D.P., Steger, A.M., Welter, L.M., 1996. Vaccine potential of a plasmid encoding for the sporozoite attachment protein of *Isospora suis*. In: *Proc. 14th IPVS Congr.*, Bologna, Italy, p. 349.

1791. Wenyon, C.M., 1923. Coccidiosis of cats and dogs and the status of the *Isospora* of man. *Ann. Trop. Med. Parasitol.* 17, 231–288.

1792. Wheat, B.E., 1979. Pathogenesis of the swine coccidia in natural and experimental infections and the life cycles of two *Eimeria* species. Doctoral thesis. University of Illinois at Urbana-Champaign.

1793. Wheeldon, E.B., Greig, W.A., 1977. *Globidium leuckarti* infection in a horse with diarrhoea. *Vet. Rec.* 100, 102–104.

1794. Whitehead, C.E., Anderson, D.E., 2006. Neonatal diarrhea in llamas and alpacas. *Small Ruminant Res.* 61, 207–215.

1795. WHO, 2017. WHO guidelines on use of medically important antimicrobials in food-producing animals. http://www.who.int/foodsafety/publications/cia_guidelines/en/.

1796. Wiedmer, S., Erdbeer, A., Volke, B., Randel, S., Kapplusch, F., Hanig, S., Kurth, M., 2017. Identification and analysis of *Eimeria nieschulzi* gametocyte genes reveal splicing events of *gam* genes and conserved motifs in the wall-forming proteins within the genus *Eimeria* (Coccidia, Apicomplexa). *Parasite* 24, 50.

1797. Wiedmer, S., Stange, J., Kurth, T., Bleiss, W., Entzeroth, R., Kurth, M., 2011. New insights into the excystation process and oocyst morphology of rodent *Eimeria* species. *Protist* 162, 668–678.

1798. Wiesenhütter, E., 1962. Ein Beitrag zur Kenntnis der endogenen Entwicklung von *Eimeria spinosa* des Schweines. *Berl. Münch. tierärztl. Wochenschr.* 75, 172–173.

1799. Williams, R.B., 1995. Epidemiological studies of coccidiosis in the domesticated fowl (*Gallus gallus*): I. The fate of ingested oocysts of *Eimeria tenella* during the prepatent period in susceptible chicks. *Appl. Parasitol.* 36, 83–89.

1800. Williams, R.B., 1997. The mode of action of anticoccidial quinolones (6-decyloxy-4-hydroxyquinoline-3-carboxylates) in chickens. *Int. J. Parasitol.* 27, 101–111.

1801. Williams, R.B., 1998. Epidemiological aspects of the use of live anticoccidial vaccines for chickens. *Int. J. Parasitol.* 28, 1089–1098.

1802. Williams, R.B., 1999. A compartmentalised model for the estimation of the cost of coccidiosis to the world's chicken production industry. *Int. J. Parasitol.* 29, 1209–1229.

1803. Williams, R.B., 2001. Quantification of the crowding effect during infections with the seven *Eimeria* species of the domesticated fowl: Its importance for experimental designs and the production of oocyst stocks. *Int. J. Parasitol.* 31, 1056–1069.

1804. Williams, R.B., 2002. Anticoccidial vaccines for broiler chickens: Pathways to success. *Avian Pathol.* 31, 317–353.

1805. Williams, R.B., 2002. Fifty years of anticoccidial vaccines for poultry (1952–2002). *Avian Dis.* 46, 775–802.

1806. Williams, R.B., 2003. Anticoccidial vaccination: The absence or reduction of numbers of endogenous parasites from gross lesions in immune chickens after virulent coccidial challenge. *Avian Pathol.* 32, 535–543.

1807. Williams, R.B., 2006. Tracing the emergence of drug-resistance in coccidia (*Eimeria* spp.) of commercial broiler flocks medicated with decoquinate for the first time in the United Kingdom. *Vet. Parasitol.* 135, 1–14.

1808. Williams, R.B., Catchpole, J., 2000. A new protocol for a challenge test to assess the efficacy of live anticoccidial vaccines for chickens. *Vaccine* 18, 1178–1185.

1809. Williams, R.B., Johnson, J.D., Andrews, S.J., 2000. Anticoccidial vaccination of broiler chickens in various management programmes: Relationship between oocyst accumulation in litter and the development of protective immunity. *Vet. Res. Commun.* 24, 309–325.

1810. Windingstad, R.M., McDonald, M.E., Locke, L.N., Kerr, S.M., Sinn, J.A., 1980. Epizootic of coccidiosis in freeflying lesser scaup. *Avian Dis.* 24, 1044–1049.

1811. Witcombe, D.M., Smith, N.C., 2014. Strategies for anticoccidial prophylaxis. *Parasitology* 141, 1379–1389.

1812. Wobeser, G., 1974. Renal coccidiosis in mallard and pintail ducks. *J. Wildl. Dis.* 10, 249–255.

1813. Wolters, E., Heydorn, A.O., Laudahn, C., 1980. Das Rind als Zwischenwirt von *Cystoisospora felis. Berl. Münch. tierärztl. Wochenschr.* 93, 207–210.

1814. Wong, D.T., Horng, J.S., Wilkinson, J.R., 1972. Robenzidene, an inhibitor of oxidative phosphorylation. *Biochem. Biophys. Res. Commun.* 46, 621–627.

1815. Woon, S.A., Yang, R., Ryan, U., Boan, P., Prentice, D., 2016. Chronic *Cystoisospora belli* infection in an immunocompetent Myanmar refugee—Microscopy is not sensitive enough. *BMC Infect. Dis.* 16, 221.

1816. Worliczek, H.L., Buggelsheim, M., Alexandrowicz, R., Witter, K., Schmidt, P., Gerner, W., Saalmüller, A., Joachim, A., 2010. Changes in lymphocyte populations in suckling piglets during primary infections with *Isospora suis. Parasite Immunol.* 32, 232–244.

1817. Worliczek, H.L., Buggelsheim, M., Saalmüller, A., Joachim, A., 2007. Porcine isosporosis: Infection dynamics, pathophysiology and immunology of experimental infections. *Wien. klin. Wochenschr.* 119 (19–20 Suppl 3), 33–39.

1818. Worliczek, H.L., Gerner, W., Joachim, A., Mundt, H.C., Saalmüller, A., 2009. Porcine coccidiosis—Investigations on the cellular immune response against *Isospora suis. Parasitol. Res.* 105 (Suppl 1), S151–S155.

1819. Worliczek, H.L., Mundt, H.C., Ruttkowski, B., Joachim, A., 2009. Age, not infection dose, determines the outcome of *Isospora suis* infections in suckling piglets. *Parasitol. Res.* 105 (Suppl 1), S157–S162.

1820. Worliczek, H.L., Ruttkowski, B., Joachim, A., Saalmüller, A., Gerner, W., 2010. Faeces, FACS, and functional assays—Preparation of *Isospora suis* oocyst antigen and representative controls for immunoassays. *Parasitology* 137, 1637–1643.

1821. Worliczek, H.L., Ruttkowski, B., Schwarz, L., Witter, K., Tschulenk, W., Joachim, A., 2013. *Isospora suis* in an epithelical cell culture system—An *in vitro* model for sexual development in coccidia. *PLOS ONE* 8, e69797.

1822. Wright, S.E., Coop, R.L., 2007. Cryptosporidiosis and coccidiosis. In Aitken, I.D. (Ed.), *Diseases of Sheep.* 4th ed., Blackwell Publishing, Oxford, U.K., 179–184.

1823. Wu, B., Zhang, X., Gong, P., Li, M., Ding, H., Xin, C., Zhao, N., Li, J., 2016. *Eimeria tenella*: A novel dsRNA virus in *E. tenella* and its complete genome sequence analysis. *Virus Genes* 52, 244–252.

1824. Wu, C., Sun, M., Qi, N., Liao, S., Li, J., Lv, M., Xie, M., 2014. Antigenicity analysis of three strains of *Eimeria maxima. Anim. Husb. Vet. Med.* 46, 67–69 (in Chinese).

1825. Wu, H.L., 2016. Prevalence of *Wenyonella philiplevinei* infection in Linwu ducks in Linwu county, subtropical China. *Trop. Anim. Health Prod.* 48, 659–662.

1826. Wu, S.H., Jiang, B., Lin, L., Wu, N.Y., Zhang, S.Z., 2005. Diagnosis and treatment of a Muscovy duck coccidiosis. *Fujian Anim. Sci. Vet. Med.* 27, 71 (in Chinese).

1827. Wu, S.H., Jiang, B., Lin, L., Zhang, S.Z., 2011. A preliminary survey of duck coccidiosis in Fuzhou. *Fujian Anim. Sci. Vet. Med.* 33, 17–20 (in Chinese).

1828. Wu, S.H., Jiang, B., Lin, L., Zhang, S.Z., 2012. The species and prevalence research of 106 duck coccidiosis. *Fujian Anim. Sci. Vet. Med.* 34, 8–10 (in Chinese).

1829. Xavier, R., Santos, J.L., Veríssimo, A., 2018. Phylogenetic evidence for an ancestral coevolution between a major clade of coccidian parasites and elasmobranch hosts. *Syst. Parasitol.* 95, 367–371.

1830. Xie, M.Q., Gilbert, J.M., Fuller, A.L., McDougald, L.R., 1990. A new method for purification of *Eimeria tenella* merozoites. *Parasitol. Res.* 76, 566–569.

1831. Xie, Y.H., 2007. Diagnosis and treatment of coccidiosis in Yingtao Valley. *Fujian Anim. Sci. Vet. Med.* 29, 58 (in Chinese).

1832. Xin, C., Wu, B., Li, J., Gong, P., Yang, J., Li, H., Cai, X., Zhang, X., 2016. Complete genome sequence and evolution analysis of *Eimeria stiedai* RNA virus 1, a novel member of the family *Totiviridae*. *Arch. Virol.* 161, 3571–3576.

1833. Xu, B., Fu, Y., Pei, M.M., 2005. Diagnosis and treatment of duck coccidiosis. *Tech. Advis. Anim. Husb.* 24, 25 (in Chinese).

1834. Xu, B.G., Yu, S.J., Chu, Z.P., 2014. A clinical report on diagnosis and treatment of duck coccidiosis. *Modern Anim. Husb.* 2, 36–37 (in Chinese).

1835. Xu, J.H., Qin, Z.H., Liao, Y.S., Xie, M.Q., Li, A.X., Cai, J.P., 2008. Characterization and expression of an actin-depolymerizing factor from *Eimeria tenella*. *Parasitol. Res.* 102, 263–270.

1836. Xun, S., Fang, W., Liu, X.Y., Song, Y.H., Wang, Y.Z., Xue, J.B., Tao, G.R., et al. 2016. Control of rabbit coccidiosis and rabbit haemorrhagic disease: Impact of recombinant DNA technology. *Proceedings of the 11th World Rabbit Congress*, June 15–18, 2016, Qingdao, China, pp. 477–489.

1837. Yagoub, I.A., 1989. Coccidiosis in Sudanese camels (*Camelus dromedarius*): 1—First record and description of *Eimeria* spp. harboured by camels in the eastern region of Sudan. *J. Protozool.* 36, 422–423.

1838. Yakhchali, M., Athari, S., 2010. A study on prevalence of *Eimeria* spp. infection in camels of Tabriz region. *Arch. Razi Inst.* 65, 111–115.

1839. Yakhchali, M., Cheraghi, E., 2007. Eimeriosis in Bactrian and Dromedary camels in the Miandoab Region, Iran. *Acta Vet. (Beograd)* 57, 545–552.

1840. Yakhchali, M., Golami, E., 2008. *Eimeria* infection (Coccidia: Eimeriidae) in sheep of different age groups in Sanandaj city, Iran. *Veterinarski Arhiv.* 78, 57–64.

1841. Yakhchali, M., Zareei, M., 2008. A survey of frequency and diversity of *Eimeria* species in cattle and buffalo in Tabriz Region. *Sci. Res. Iranian Vet. J.* 4, 94–102.

1842. Yan, W., Liu, X., Shi, T., Hao, L., Tomley, F.M., Suo, X., 2009. Stable transfection of *Eimeria tenella*: Constitutive expression of the YFP-YFP molecule throughout the life cycle. *Int. J. Parasitol.* 39, 109–117.

1843. Yan, W., Wang, W., Wang, T., Suo, X., Qian, W., Wang, S., Fan, D., 2013. Simultaneous identification of three highly pathogenic *Eimeria* species in rabbits using a multiplex PCR diagnostic assay based on ITS1-5.8S rRNA-ITS2 fragments. *Vet. Parasitol.* 193, 284–288.

1844. Yan, X., Liu, X., Ji, Y., Tao, G., Suo, X., 2015. Ethanol and isopropanol trigger rapid egress of intracellular *Eimeria tenella* sporozoites. *Parasitol. Res.* 114, 625–630.

1845. Yan, X., Tao, G., Liu, X., Ji, Y., Suo, X., 2016. Calcium-dependent microneme protein discharge and in vitro egress of *Eimeria tenella* sporozoites. *Exp. Parasitol.* 170, 193–197.

1846. Yang, G., Li, J., Zhang, X., Zhao, Q., Gong, P., Ren, B., Zhang, G., 2010. *Eimeria tenella*: Cloning and characterization of telomerase reverse transcriptase gene. *Exp. Parasitol.* 124, 380–385.

1847. Yang, G., Wang, C., Hao, F., Zhao, D., Zhang, Y., Li, Y., 2010. Studies on construction of a recombinant *Eimeria tenella* SO7 gene expressing *Escherichia coli* and its protective efficacy against homologous infection. *Parasitol. Int.* 59, 517–523.

1848. Yang, G., Yao, J., Yang, W., Jiang, Y., Du, J., Huang, H., Gu, W., et al. 2017. Construction and immunological evaluation of recombinant *Lactobacillus plantarum* expressing SO7 of *Eimeria tenella* fusion DC-targeting peptide. *Vet. Parasitol.* 236, 7–13.

1849. Yang, N., Ning, C., Qi, M., Zhang, L., 2011. Single oocyst separation of *Eimeria* and oocyst amplification on chicken. *Chin. J. Anim. Husb. Vet. Med.* 38, 172–174 (in Chinese).

1850. Yang, R., Jacobson, C., Gardner, G., Carmichael, I., Campbell, A.J.D., Ryan, U., 2014. Longitudinal prevalence, oocyst shedding and molecular characterisation of *Eimeria* species in sheep across four states in Australia. *Exp. Parasitol.* 145, 14–21.

1851. Yang, X., Guo, Y., Wang, Z., Nie, W., 2006. Fatty acids and coccidiosis: Effects of dietary supplementation with different oils on coccidiosis in chickens. *Avian Pathol.* 35, 373–378.

1852. Yang, Z., Peng, H., Lu, X., Liu, Q., Huang, R., Hu, B., Kachanoski, G., Zuidhof, M.J., Le, X.C., 2016. Arsenic metabolites, including n-acetyl-4-hydroxy-m-arsanilic acid, in chicken litter from a roxarsone-feeding study involving 1600 chickens. *Environ. Sci. Technol.* 50, 6737–6743.

1853. Yao, Q., Han, H.Y., Huang, B., Dong, H., Zhao, Q.P., Jiang, L.L., Guo, T., Li, Y., Li, Y.J., Fan, Y.J., 2009. A preliminary survey of duck coccidiosis in Shanghai. Prevalence of coccidian among domestic ducks in suburban district of Shanghai. *China Poultry* 31, 23–26 (in Chinese).

1854. Yap, G.S., Sher, A., 1999. Cell-mediated immunity to *Toxoplasma gondii*: Initiation, regulation and effector function. *Immunobiology* 201, 240–247.

1855. Yarovinsky, F., Zhang, D., Andersen, J.F., Bannenberg, G.L., Serhan, C.N., Hayden, M.S., Hieny, S., Sutterwala, F.S., Flavell, R.A., Ghosh, S., Sher, A., 2005. TLR11 activation of dendritic cells by a protozoan profilin-like protein. *Science* 308, 1626–1629.

1856. Yastreb, V.B., Shaytanov, V.M., 2017. Intestinal parasitoses in adult dogs and cats kept in shelters for stray animals. *Russian J. Parasitol.* 39, (1).

1857. Yin, G., Goraya, M.U., Huang, J., Suo, X., Huang, Z., Liu, X., 2016. Survey of coccidial infection of rabbits in Sichuan Province, Southwest China. *SpringerPlus* 5, 870.

1858. Yin, G., Lin, Q., Wei, W., Qin, M., Liu, X., Suo, X., Huang, Z., 2014. Protective immunity against *Eimeria tenella* infection in chickens induced by immunization with a recombinant C-terminal derivative of EtIMP1. *Vet. Immunol. Immunopathol.* 162, 117–121.

1859. Yin, G., Qin, M., Liu, X., Suo, J., Suo, X., 2013. Interferon-γ enzyme-linked immunosorbent spot assay as a tool to study T cell responses to *Eimeria tenella* infection in chickens. *Poult. Sci.* 92, 1758–1763.

1860. Yin, G., Qin, M., Liu, X., Suo, J., Tang, X., Tao, G., Han, Q., Suo, X., Wu, W., 2013. An *Eimeria* vaccine candidate based on *Eimeria tenella* immune mapped protein 1 and the TLR-5 agonist *Salmonella typhimurium* FliC flagellin. *Biochem. Biophys. Res. Commun.* 440, 437–442.

1861. Yin, P.Y., Jiang, J.S., Kong, F.Y., Lin, K.H., Fan, G.X., Liu, G.Y., Wu, J., Yang, H.X., 1983. Endogenous development of *Tyzzeria perniciosa* in Pekin duck. *Acta Vet. Zootech. Sinica* 14, 257–262 (in Chinese).

1862. Yin, P.Y., Jiang, J.S., Kong, F.Y., Lin, K.H., Fan, G.X., Liu, G.Y., Wu, J., Yang, H.X., 1984. Endogenous development of *Wenyonella philiplevinei* in Pekin duck. *Acta Vet. Zootech. Sinica* 15, 115–120 (in Chinese).

1863. Yin, P.Y., Jiang, J.S., Kong, F.Y., Lin, K.H., Liu, G.Y., 1983. A study of the pathogenicity of *Tyzzeria perniciosa* and *Wenyonella philiplevinei*, and a comparative test on the preventive effects of eight kinds of anticoccidial drugs against duck coccidiosis. *Acta Vet. Zootech. Sinica* 14, 263–270 (in Chinese).

1864. Yin, P.Y., Jiang, J.S., Lin, K.H., Liu, G.Y., Qiu, L.Y., 1982. A preliminary research of duck coccidia in Pekin duck. *Acta Vet. Zootech. Sinica* 13, 119–124 (in Chinese).

1865. Ying, S., 1985. Symposium on poultry coccidiosis control held at Laohekou. *Chin. J. Vet. Med.* 12, 46–47 (in Chinese).

1866. Yoder, C.A., Graham, J.K., Miller, L.A., 2006. Molecular effects of nicarbazin on avian reproduction. *Poult. Sci.* 85, 1285–1293.

1867. Yoo, J., Jang, S.I., Kim, S., Cho, J.H., Lee, H.J., Rhee, M.H., Lillehoj, H.S., Min, W., 2009. Molecular characterization of duck interleukin-17. *Vet. Immunol. Immunopathol.* 132, 318–322.

1868. Younan, M., McDonough, S.P., Herbert, D., Saez, J., Kibor, A., 2002. *Isospora* excretion in scouring camel calves (*Camelus dromedarius*). *Vet. Rec.* 151, 548–549.

1869. Yun, C.H., Lillehoj, H.S., Choi, K.D., 2000. Chicken IFN-γ monoclonal antibodies and their application in enzyme-linked immunosorbent assay. *Vet. Immunol. Immunopathol.* 73, 297–308.

1870. Yun, C.H., Lillehoj, H.S., Lillehoj, E.P., 2000. Intestinal immune responses to coccidiosis. *Dev. Comp. Immunol.* 24, 303–324.

1870a. Yvoré, P., Peloille, M., Bernard, F., Cothenet, C., 1976. Coccidiosis in swine: Species present in France. Experimental infection. *Rec. Méd. Vét.* 152, 25–32.

1871. Zaionts, V.I., Krylov, M.V., Loskot, V.I., Kirillov, A.I., 1978. Biosynthesis of folic acid in *Eimeria tenella* (Coccidia). *Parazitologiia* 12, 3–8.

1872. Zanetti Lopes, W.D., Borges, F.A., Faiolla, T.P., Antunes, L.T., Borges, D.G.L., de Souza Rodrigues, F., Ferraro, G., et al. 2013. *Eimeria* species in young and adult sheep raised under intensive and/or semi-intensive systems of a herd from Umuarama city, Parana State, Brazil. *Ciência Rural* 43, 2031–2036.

1873. Zar, F.A., El-Bayoumi, E., Yungbluth, M.M., 2001. Histologic proof of acalculous cholecystitis due to *Cyclospora cayetanensis*. *Clin. Infect. Dis.* 33, E140–E141.

1874. Zayed, A.A., El-Ghaysh, A., 1998. Pig, donkey and buffalo meat as a source of some coccidian parasites infecting dogs. *Vet. Parasitol.* 78, 161–168.

1875. Zhang, D.F., Sun, B.B., Yue, Y.Y., Yu, H.J., Zhang, H.L., Zhou, Q.J., Du, A.F., 2012. Anticoccidial effect of halofuginone hydrobromide against *Eimeria tenella* with associated histology. *Parasitol. Res.* 111, 695–701.

1876. Zhang, D.F., Sun, B.B., Yue, Y.Y., Zhou, Q.J., Du, A.F., 2012. Anticoccidial activity of traditional Chinese herbal *Dichroa febrifuga* Lour. extract against *Eimeria tenella* infection in chickens. *Parasitol. Res.* 111, 2229–2233.

1877. Zhang, F.Y., Liu, Y.M., Chen, J.H., Huang, S., 2007. Diagnosis and treatment of coccidiosis in Yingtao Valley. *Poultry Poultry Dis. Prev.* 12, 18–19 (in Chinese).

1878. Zhang, J., Chen, P., Sun, H., Liu, Q., Wang, L., Wang, T., Shi, W., et al. 2014. *Pichia pastoris* expressed EtMic2 protein as a potential vaccine against chicken coccidiosis. *Vet. Parasitol.* 205, 62–69.

1879. Zhang, J.J., Wang, L.X., Ruan, W.K., An, J., 2013. Investigation into the prevalence of coccidiosis and maduramycin drug resistance in chickens in China. *Vet. Parasitol.* 191, 29–34.

1880. Zhang, L., Liu, M., Lu, C., Ren, D., Fan, G., Liu, C., Liu, M., et al. 2018. The hydroxypropyl-β-cyclodextrin complexation of toltrazuril for enhancing bioavailability. *Drug Des. Dev. Ther.* 12, 583–589.

1881. Zhang, L., Liu, R., Ma, L., Wang, Y., Pan, B., Cai, J., Wang, M., 2012. *Eimeria tenella*: Expression profiling of toll-like receptors and associated cytokines in the cecum of infected day-old and three-week old SPF chickens. *Exp. Parasitol.* 130, 442–448.

1882. Zhang, L., Liu, R., Song, M., Hu, Y., Pan, B., Cai, J., Wang, M., 2013. *Eimeria tenella*: Interleukin 17 contributes to host immunopathology in the gut during experimental infection. *Exp. Parasitol.* 133, 121–130.

1883. Zhang, L., Ma, L., Liu, R., Zhang, Y., Zhang, S., Hu, C., Song, M., Cai, J., Wang, M., 2012. *Eimeria tenella* heat shock protein 70 enhances protection of recombinant microneme protein MIC2 subunit antigen vaccination against *E. tenella* challenge. *Vet. Parasitol.* 188, 239–246.

1884. Zhang, L.X., Ning, C.S., Li, J.Z., 1999. A preliminary survey of duck coccidiosis in Henan province. *J. Anim. Sci Vet. Med.* 18, 8–10 (in Chinese).

1885. Zhang, N.G., 2017. A case report of diagnosis and treatment of Muscovy duck coccidiosis. *Chin. J. Vet. Med.* 53, 104 (in Chinese).

1886. Zhang, N.G., 2017. Diagnosis and treatment of a Muscovy duck coccidiosis. *Basic Agric. Technol. Extension* 5, 103–106 (in Chinese).

1887. Zhang, S., Lillehoj, H.S., Ruff, M.D., 1995. Chicken tumor necrosis-like factor. I. *In vitro* production by macrophages stimulated with *Eimeria tenella* or bacterial lipopolysaccharide. *Poult. Sci.* 74, 1304–1310.

1888. Zhang, S., Tang, X., Li, C., Liu, X., Lv, Y., Suo, X., 2018. Progress in coccidiosis vaccine development for chickens in China. *Acta Parasitol. Med. Entomol. Sinica* 25, 254–261 (in Chinese).

1889. Zhang, W., Wang, Y., Wang, M., Li, Y., Xue, F., 2018. The degradation properties and biological effects of ethanamizuril in soils. *J. Agro-Environ. Sci.* 37, 478–484 (in Chinese).

1890. Zhang, W.J., Xu, L.H., Liu, Y.Y., Xiong, B.Q., Zhang, Q.L., Li, F.C., Song, Q.Q., et al. 2012. Prevalence of coccidian infection in suckling piglets in China. *Vet. Parasitol.* 190, 51–55.

1891. Zhang, W.X., Zhang, X.C., Li, J.H., Zhao, Q., Qin, J.H., Yin, J.G., Yang, J., 2004. Development of hybrid strains from geographic isolates of *Eimeria tenella* and their immunoprotection. *Chin. J. Parasitol. Parasit. Dis.* 22, 37–41.

1892. Zhang, Y., Wang, L., Ruan, W., Zhang, J., Yao, P., Zhou, S., An, J., 2014. Immunization with recombinant 3-1E protein in AbISCO-300 adjuvant induced protective immunity against *Eimeria acervulina* infection in chickens. *Exp. Parasitol.* 141, 75–81.

1893. Zhang, Z., Huang, J., Li, M., Sui, Y., Wang, S., Liu, L., Xu, L., Yan, R., Song, X., Li, X., 2014. Identification and molecular characterization of microneme 5 of *Eimeria acervulina*. *PLOS ONE* 9, e115411.

1894. Zhang, Z., Liu, L., Huang, J., Wang, S., Lu, M., Song, X., Xu, L., Yan, R., Li, X., 2016. The molecular characterization and immune protection of microneme 2 of *Eimeria acervulina*. *Vet. Parasitol.* 215, 96–105.

1895. Zhang, Z., Liu, X., Yang, X., Liu, L., Wang, S., Lu, M., Ehsan, M., et al. 2016. The molecular characterization and immunity identification of microneme 3 of *Eimeria acervulina*. *J. Eukaryot. Microbiol.* 63, 709–721.

1896. Zhang, Z., Wang, S., Huang, J., Liu, L., Lu, M., Li, M., Sui, Y., et al. 2015. Proteomic analysis of *Eimeria acervulina* sporozoite proteins interaction with duodenal epithelial cells by shotgun LC-MS/MS. *Mol. Biochem. Parasitol.* 202, 29–33.

1897. Zhang, Z., Wang, S., Li, C., Liu, L., 2017. Immunoproteomic analysis of the protein repertoire of unsporulated *Eimeria tenella* oocysts. *Parasite* 24, 48.

1898. Zhang, Z.H., Hou, Z.F., Zang, C.J., Zhu, S.M., Tao, J.P., 2015. Oocyst shedding pattern in cats infected with *Isospora rivolta*. *Chin. J. Anim. Infect. Dis.* 23, 51–53.

1899. Zhao, A.Y., Jing, B., Jia, G.Z., 2008. A preliminary survey of duck coccidiosis in Keshi. *J. Tarim Univ.* 20, 30–31 (in Chinese).

1900. Zhao, G.H., Lei, L.H., Shang, C.C., Gao, M., Zhao, Y.Q., Chen, C.X., Chen, D.K., 2012. High prevalence of *Eimeria* infection in dairy goats in Shaanxi province, northwestern China. *Trop. Anim. Health Prod.* 44, 943–946.

1901. Zhao, J., Guo, Y., Suo, X., Yuan, J., 2006. Effect of dietary zinc level on serum carotenoid levels, body and shank pigmentation of chickens after experimental infection with coccidia. *Arch. Anim. Nutr.* 60, 218–228.

1902. Zhao, N., Gong, P., Li, Z., Cheng, B., Li, J., Yang, Z., Li, H., Yang, J., Zhang, G., Zhang, X., 2014. Identification of a telomeric DNA-binding protein in *Eimeria tenella*. *Biochem. Biophys. Res. Commun.* 451, 599–602.

1903. Zhao, X., Xu, Y., Zhang, L., Wang, C., Guo, C., Fei, C., Zhang, K., et al. 2017. Development and validation of an UPLC-UV method for determination of a novel triazine coccidiostat ethanmizuril and its metabolite M3 in chicken tissues. *J. Chromatogr. B Analyt. Technol. Biomed. Life Sci.* 1059, 1–6.

1904. Zhao, Y., Amer, S., Wang, J., Wang, C., Gao, Y., Kang, G., Bao, Y., He, H., Qin, J., 2010. Construction, screening and identification of a phage display antibody library against the *Eimeria acervulina* merozoite. *Biochem. Biophys. Res. Commun.* 393, 703–707.

1905. Zhao, Y., Xu, R., Zhang, Y., Ji, X., Zhang, J., Liu, Y., Bao, Y., Qin, J., 2014. Protective efficacy in chickens of recombinant plasmid pET32a(+)-ADF-3-1E of *Eimeria acervulina*. *Parasitol. Res.* 113, 3007–3014.

1906. Zhou, B., Wang, H., Xue, F., Wang, X., Fei, C., Wang, M., Zhang, T., Yao, X., He, P., 2010. Effects of diclazuril on apoptosis and mitochondrial transmembrane potential in second-generation merozoites of *Eimeria tenella*. *Vet. Parasitol.* 168, 217–222.

1907. Zhou, B.H., Shen, X.J., Wang, H.W., Li, T., Xue, F.Q., 2012. Receptor for activated C kinase ortholog of second-generation merozoite in *Eimeria tenella*: Clone, characterization, and diclazuril-induced mRNA expression. *Parasitol. Res.* 111, 1447–1455.

1908. Zhou, B.H., Wang, H.W., Wang, X.Y., Zhang, L.F., Zhang, K.Y., Xue, F.Q., 2010. *Eimeria tenella*: Effects of diclazuril treatment on microneme genes expression in second-generation merozoites and pathological changes of caeca in parasitized chickens. *Exp. Parasitol.* 125, 264–270.

1909. Zhou, B.H., Wang, H.W., Xue, F.Q., Wang, X.Y., Yang, F.K., Ban, M.M., Xin, R.X., Wang, C.C., 2010. Actin-depolymerizing factor of second-generation merozoite in *Eimeria tenella*: Clone, prokaryotic expression, and diclazuril-induced mRNA expression. *Parasitol. Res.* 106, 571–576.

1910. Zhou, B.H., Wang, H.W., Zhao, Z.S., Liu, M., Yan, W.C., Zhao, J., Zhang, Z., Xue, F.Q., 2013. A novel serine/threonine protein phosphatase type 5 from second-generation merozoite of *Eimeria tenella* is associated with diclazuril-induced apoptosis. *Parasitol. Res.* 112, 1771–1780.

1911. Zhou, K., Wang, Y., Chen, M., Wang, L., Huang, S., Zhang, J., Liu, R., Xu, H., 2006. *Eimeria tenella*: Further studies on the development of the oocyst. *Exp. Parasitol.* 113, 174–178.

1912. Zhou, Q., Chen, F., Fan, J., 1981. The gas chromatographic determination of D.O.T., 3,5-dinitro-o-toluic acid and o-toluic acid. *Acta Agr. Univ. Pekin.* 7(3), 31–34 (in Chinese).

1913. Zhou, S., Wang, L., Zhang, Y., Liu, X., Zhang, C., Zhang, J., An, J., 2013. On the protective efficiency of *Eimeria tenella* recombinant protein EtMic4-N AbISCO-100 vaccine. *J. Beijing Univ. Agr.* 28, 29–32 (in Chinese).

1914. Zhou, Y., Lv, B., Wang, Q., Wang, R., Jian, F., Zhang, L., Ning, C., et al. 2011. Prevalence and molecular characterization of *Cyclospora cayetanensis*, Henan, China. *Emerg. Infect. Dis.* 17, 1887–1890.

1915. Zhou, Z., Nie, K., Huang, Q., Li, K., Sun, Y., Zhou, R., Wang, Z., Hu, S., 2017. Changes of cecal microflora in chickens following *Eimeria tenella* challenge and regulating effect of coated sodium butyrate. *Exp. Parasitol.* 177, 73–81.

1916. Zhou, Z., Wang, Z., Cao, L., Hu, S., Zhang, Z., Qin, B., Guo, Z., Nie, K., 2013. Upregulation of chicken TLR4, TLR15 and MyD88 in heterophils and monocyte-derived macrophages stimulated with *Eimeria tenella in vitro*. *Exp. Parasitol.* 133, 427–433.

1917. Zhu, G., Wu, B., 1986. Preliminary survey on chicken coccidia species in Hangzhou. *J. Hangzhou Univ. (Nat. Sci. Ed.)*, 13, 224–230 (in Chinese).

1918. Zhu, H., Xu, L., Yan, R., Song, X., Tang, F., Wang, S., Li, X., 2012. Identification and characterization of a cDNA clone-encoding antigen of *Eimeria acervulina*. *Parasitology* 139, 1711–1719.

1919. Zhu, H., Yan, R., Wang, S., Song, X., Xu, L., Li, X., 2012. Identification and molecular characterization of a novel antigen of *Eimeria acervulina*. *Mol. Biochem. Parasitol.* 186, 21–28.

1920. Zhu, Y., Wang, R., Liu, Zh., 1981. Efficacy of *Artemisia* ethanol-extract and robenidine against *Eimeria tenella* in chicks. *Chin. J. Trad. Vet. Sci.* 1, 5–7 (in Chinese).

1921. Zimmerman, J.J., Karriker, L.A., Ramirez, A., Schwartz, K.J., Stevenson, G.W., 2012. *Diseases of Swine*. Wiley-Blackwell. Hoboken, NJ, 10th ed., 709–794.

1922. Zuo, Y., Ma, X., Dong, Z., Yin, H., Liu, B., Han, Z., Cai, J., 2016. Cloning and expression profiling of sirtuin-like histone deacetylase 2A during *Eimeria tenella* developmental cycle. *Anim. Husb. Vet. Med.* 48, 7–12 (in Chinese).

1923. Zuo, Y.X., Song, X.L., Lin, Y.Y., Tu, Y., 1990. The prevalence of duck coccidia in Yunnan Province. *Vet. Sci. China* 20, 13–16 (in Chinese).

1924. Zvinorova, P.I., Halimani, T.E., Muchadeyi, F.C., Matika, O., Riggio, V., Dzama, K., 2016. Prevalence and risk factor of gastrointestinal parasitic infections in goats in low-input low-output farming systems in Zimbabwe. *Small Ruminant Res.* 143, 75–83.

Index

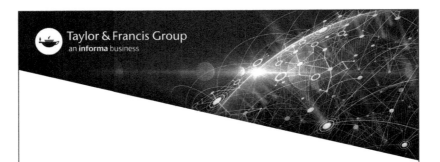